Principles and Practice of Pharmacovigilance and Drug Safety

Jimmy Jose • Anthony R. Cox
Vibhu Paudyal
Editors

Principles and Practice of Pharmacovigilance and Drug Safety

Springer

Editors
Jimmy Jose
Pharmacy Practice
School of Pharmacy
College of Health Sciences
University of Nizwa
Nizwa, Oman

Anthony R. Cox
Clinical Pharmacy and Drug Safety
School of Pharmacy
College of Medical and Dental Sciences
University of Birmingham
Birmingham, UK

Vibhu Paudyal
Clinical Pharmacy
School of Pharmacy
College of Medical and Dental Sciences
University of Birmingham
Birmingham, UK

Health Services Research and
Inequalities
Florence Nightingale Faculty of
Nursing, Midwifery and Palliative Care
King's College London
London, UK

ISBN 978-3-031-51088-5 ISBN 978-3-031-51089-2 (eBook)
https://doi.org/10.1007/978-3-031-51089-2

This Springer imprint is published by the registered company Springer Nature Switzerland AG
The registered company address is: Gewerbestrasse 11, 6330 Cham, Switzerland

This book is dedicated to our spouses Beena, Dianne, and Pawana, and also to our children Marita, Norah, Leana, Lauren, James, Tanisi, and Avyan who greatly supported and sacrificed much to complete this project.

Thanks to our parents, brothers and sisters, and other family members who always inspired us to do our best.

We are thankful to our friends who supported us always, teachers who inculcated the passion for promoting safer drug use, students who helped us to be better teachers, and patients who motivated us to be better practitioners. Finally, we would like to gratefully remember the support of one of the pioneers in the field of pharmacovigilance, Sten Olson (1950–2023). He was a dear friend to the pharmacovigilance community.

Foreword

Drug safety is like automobile safety—perfection is unachievable. The pharmacological actions of drugs inevitably can cause harm, just as the social and economic benefits of cars to individuals can only be realised if their risks are accepted. We should, nonetheless, try to use medicines as safely as possible. The authors are to be congratulated, therefore, on providing a guide to detecting and avoiding harm from medicines suitable for a wide audience.

The reader is introduced to the main terms and concepts in drug safety. This is a difficult task both for adverse drug reactions and for medication errors, which have been variously defined by different groups. The old binary classification into Type A, 'augmented', adverse drug reactions that can be explained by the known pharmacology of a drug and Type B, 'bizarre', reactions that cannot is of limited use. The authors overcome this difficulty by describing fully the Type A/B dichotomy, the expansion to Types A–F, and the DoTS classification.

There is also discussion of those factors that predispose to adverse reactions. These predisposing factors depend partly on the properties of the drug and its formulation, and partly on the susceptibilities of the person to whom it is prescribed, including the other drugs that they may be taking. This leads to important considerations of drug–drug interactions. Increasing the number of prescribed drugs increases the risk of interactions, so it is timely that the authors consider polypharmacy and how the burden of drug treatments may be reduced while benefiting patients—deprescribing.

Detection of adverse drug reactions, initially reliant on clinical observation and then on spontaneous reporting systems, has advanced with the more widespread introduction of patient reporting, and the use of large databases to confirm pharmacovigilance signals—indications of effects, causally related to medicines, that require verification—and the introduction of increasingly sophisticated statistical methods and artificial intelligence. This text rightly stresses the need for cooperation between different professionals, patients, and agencies in the detection and verification of signals of harm, and in the evaluation of their harmful impact. The chapter on patient and public involvement in pharmacovigilance is an important contribution.

Detecting errors in medical treatment can be much harder than detecting adverse drug reactions, and there remain real uncertainties about the frequency, consequences, and remedies for medication errors. That makes it hard to know how far the measures adopted since the influential report *To Err Is Human* was published by the Institute of Medicine in 2000 have led to systemic improvements. There is also uncertainty about the extent to which electronic prescribing systems have reduced the risk of error. What is clear, though, is that awareness of the possibility of error, and repeated checking to reduce errors in the medication process, from prescribing, through dispensing, to administration, can make the process safer.

Unusually, the authors consider the communication of risk from medicines, the ethics of pharmacovigilance, and the need to balance the needs of individual patients against the wider public good. Students, practitioners, and educators should find this book very useful.

Department of Clinical Pharmacology
University of Birmingham
Birmingham, UK

Robin Ferner

Preface

It is our great pleasure to finally introduce this book, *Pharmacovigilance and Drug Safety in Practice*, to our readers. This book was inspired by our own quest for a single reference text that captures the needs of educators, clinical practitioners, researchers, policymakers, patient/public societies, and wider stakeholders. The concept of pharmacovigilance and drug safety has evolved over the years in the light of emerging research, policy, practice, and technological changes. However, the development and challenges vary across different countries and continents. An increasing number of drug therapies have been developed to manage a wide range of complex health states, including treatments, diagnostic drugs, and disease prevention. Emergent health technologies including pharmacogenomics, precision medicine, biological therapies, and novel formulations provide both solutions and challenges to safety. The need for ethical, responsible, and accountable safety practices in the use and monitoring of drugs has never been higher.

We have excellent textbooks written by experienced professionals in the field of pharmacovigilance. As educators, we have faced difficulties finding a reference which discusses pharmacovigilance and drug safety from different perspectives, as others may have. We observed that most of the books on pharmacovigilance are written from an industry or regulatory perspective or presented as a detailed description of adverse drug reactions (ADRs) for individual drugs or affecting individual body systems. Books which discuss the various aspects of safe use of medications in clinical practice in one volume are lacking though they are discussed as part of the references of clinical pharmacy, clinical pharmacology, and pharmacotherapy.

It would be wise to clarify what we mean by the terms 'pharmacovigilance' and 'drug safety'. At times, these are often treated as synonyms, and many would consider them mutually inclusive. For the purpose of discussion in this book, drug safety is a broad concept that refers to the overall safety of a drug product throughout its life cycle right from its development phase to post-market surveillance and ongoing monitoring during clinical use by healthcare professionals. This includes clinical practice of drug safety principles encompassing the prevention, monitoring, identification, and management of adverse effects, medication errors, and other drug-related problems. It includes the individual clinical decision-making in patients to ensure safe use of drugs. We have tended to restrict pharmacovigilance to a focus on theories, research, and practices related to monitoring and managing the safety of drugs (adverse effects and other drug-related issues) mainly in the post-marketing phase. It gives greater focus on the industrial or regulatory side of pharmacovigilance. However, the overlap at times can be hard to assess, and some cross-over may have crept in despite our best efforts.

We hope that this book will serve teachers and students who would like to enhance or deliver knowledge on pharmacovigilance and drug safety. At the same time, it is expected to function as a 'reference source' for clinical practitioners, researchers, industry professionals, and policymakers. The book will address an important gap between clinical practice and pharmacovigilance, by integrating pharmacovigilance, drug safety, pharmacoepidemiology, medication errors, and prescribing skills into clinical practice, providing a more holistic view of the broad topic of drug safety. It will also be useful for those professionals moving from a clinical practice role to a pharmacovigilance role. Taking the reader through the key material in ADRs, medication errors, prescribing safety, as well as data sources used in drug safety and pharmacovigilance, the key benefit of our text will be in bridging the divide between the pharmacovigilance, pharmacoepidemiology, and wider drug safety matters and clinical practice.

The book is designed to be a multidisciplinary resource, both for undergraduate healthcare professionals (in fields such as medical, pharmacy, nursing, and dental science) and for those in postgraduate studies. Particularly for those with prescribing responsibilities, the book aims to improve the safety of medicines. The book is aimed to be international in scope and context. Each of the chapters is structured as a self-contained learning resource, with learning objectives, key points, worked cases, and additional reading materials alongside the main text.

We would like to share in brief the steps involved in publishing this book. All the authors are very passionate about the topic of pharmacovigilance and drug safety and have significant years of experience in teaching pharmacovigilance, clinical practice, and conducting research in this specific field. Interestingly, we feel that this book is a positive outcome of the COVID pandemic as the initiation of the idea and discussions in preparing the book happened during that period. Communications through online meetings became so common and easy during the period that it gave us confidence in contacting, interacting, and planning the work related to the book with people whom we had not interacted with before. To ensure that the potential authors selected were experts in various fields, academia, clinical practice, research, industry, and regulatory, from multidisciplinary backgrounds and from around the globe, we took initiative in identifying the authors based on their research output and helped in forming teams to write the chapter. We believe this has created a diverse and informed perspective. From the time the idea of the book was initiated until its publication, there were lots of ups and downs with the project over these years before the book could take its present shape. It was not an easy task to take along this project with our other commitments, but we are glad that we stayed together as a team and exhibited perseverance in tackling these challenges and reached the present stage.

The first two-thirds of the book focus on the principles and practice in pharmacovigilance, covering core conceptual areas and the pharmacovigilance system at a population level, with the last third examining the use of medicines at the level of the individual patient.

Chapter 1 introduces key concepts related to pharmacovigilance and drug safety including epidemiology, definitions, classification, and predisposing factors of ADRs, including a holistic view of drug safety in relation to medication errors, prescribing issues, and regulatory approaches. Chapter 2 focuses on the important area of drug allergy and hypersensitivity reactions. Chapter 3 describes the predisposing factors for ADRs.

The ageing global population and associated comorbidities is linked to an increase in polypharmacy. Preventing drug interactions, particularly those that are clinically significant, has become ever more important. Chapter 4 defines and describes various types of drug interactions, their mechanisms, and the factors that increase the risk of their occurrence. It provides specific details of important interactions and ways in which healthcare professionals can prevent and manage drug interactions. An under-examined area of drug safety has been the economic aspects. Chapter 5 explains how the economic burden may be defined and measured, and lists associated challenges and methods used to assess cost-effectiveness in relation to strategies used to improve medication safety. The principles of pharmacovigilance and medicines regulation are discussed in Chap. 6, providing a comprehensive history of the development of pharmacovigilance regulations over the years and international effects on harmonisation. Laws governing pharmacovigilance throughout the drug development life cycle, including post-authorisation studies, are discussed. Safety monitoring is a critical component in the clinical development process. It is important to understand the process, guidelines, and outcome pertaining to this important component of clinical trials, and these are discussed in Chap. 7. Chapter 8 discusses causality assessment, which is an essential component and routine procedure in the pharmacovigilance system.

Pharmacoepidemiology and pharmacovigilance are very closely related, and Chap. 9 outlines the most common epidemiological study designs using real-world data sources. Even with the advancement of various methods to monitor and capture adverse reactions to a drug during its life cycle, spontaneous reports still represent an irreplaceable source of information for pharmacovigilance. The role of spontaneous reporting in pharmacovigilance, the contribution of various stakeholders, and the strengths and limitations of pharmacovigilance are discussed in Chap. 10. Chapter 11 is about communicating drug safety and it focuses on risk communications. Patients have played an increasing role in drug safety, and there should be an active and collaborative interaction between patients and other stakeholders. Chapter 12 discusses the evolving role of patients in different areas of pharmacovigilance. An increasingly complex healthcare system requires collaborative approaches to establishing and implementing pharmacovigilance systems. Chapter 13 discusses the importance of collaboration and cooperation across diverse disciplines, stakeholders, academia, patients, and carers as well as capacity building in pharmacovigilance. The ethics of pharmacovigilance is covered in depth in Chap. 14, outlining key ethical principles including the fiduciary duty, the duty to protect the public from harm, privacy, consent, scientific integrity, and conflicts of interest.

The last third of the book moves to safe prescribing and practice, opening with the errors associated with the medication use process in Chap. 15. The various types of medication errors, methods of detection, factors that contribute to error, and strategies for risk mitigation are discussed—including educational interventions, error reporting systems, and the role of medication safety officers. Chapter 16 outlines the various study designs of Post-Authorisation Safety Studies (PASS) used to identify ADRs, and the various challenges in diagnosing and managing ADRs. This chapter also summarises various strategies to predict and thereby prevent ADRs such as pharmacogenetics, use of omics, and in silico approaches including artificial intelligence.

To facilitate the decision-making process in drug safety and subsequent communication of drug safety issues to patients and their families, identifying and utilising appropriate health and medicines information sources is critical. Chapter 17 discusses various information sources for drug safety and communicating risks in practice. Chapter 18 describes and distinguishes appropriate and inappropriate polypharmacy, and outlines the tools to identify inappropriate prescribing, and the approaches to involving patients in discussions about their medicines. The concept of deprescribing, and the purpose and process involved is discussed in this chapter. The complexities of special patient groups are covered in Chaps. 19 to 22, including the paediatric population (Chap. 19), older people (Chap. 20), pregnancy and breast feeding (Chap. 21), and renal and hepatic diseases (Chap. 22). These chapters outline the main factors that increase the risk of medication safety incidents in these special patient populations. Key safety considerations for prescribing medications in these populations are discussed. The benefits of pharmacogenomics have been forecast for many years, with a tipping point into wider utility occurring in recent years. Chapter 23 covers the key developments in the application of pharmacogenetics in improving drug safety and the exciting possibilities to reduce the harm of medicines they promise.

As with any human task, our achievements may not meet our original vision, but we hope that we have covered most of the key aspects of pharmacovigilance and drug safety. However, we are aware that some areas covered as elements of a chapter might be thought to deserve a chapter in their own right by some readers. The field of industry and regulatory pharmacovigilance is very wide, as are the issues in clinical practice, and we welcome feedback on the content of the book. Although we took utmost care in avoiding errors through a two-tier review; editors and expert reviewers, any suggestions, feedback, errors noticed, and ideas for additional elements would be welcomed.

We hope you enjoy the book and find it useful.

Nizwa, Oman — Jimmy Jose
Birmingham, UK — Anthony R. Cox
London, UK — Vibhu Paudyal

Acknowledgements

We are immensely grateful for the contributions made by all authors involved from across the globe who gave their valuable time to complete this book. The authors represent a wealth of expertise and interest in pharmacovigilance in the pharmaceutical industry, healthcare practice, drug safety research, health economics, policy, and patient and public involvement, and we are humbled by their dedication to this project. Additionally, these independent experts and researchers selflessly invested time as peer reviewers during the production of this book, providing thorough and constructive insights. We would particularly like to thank Brian Edwards, Olav Spigset, and Francisco J. de Abajo for their outsized contributions.

In addition to the chapter authors who performed this role, we would like to thank Andrew McLachlan, Ann Daly, Christine Erikstrup Hallgreen, Deb Pasko, Derek Stewart, Gianluca Trifiro, James Stevenson, Kavitha Saravu, Kumi Om, Marleen van Gelder, Patrick Edwards, Pramod Kumar, Saval Khanal, Shusen Sun, and Tanja Fens for their time and efforts in reviewing the manuscripts.

We are thankful to our parent institutions for the support provided in our endeavours. We are also indebted to the support offered by Springer staff, especially Susanne Dathe, the project editor, and the production editors. Susanne supported us relentlessly from the initial proposal during the pandemic to completion, and her sincere regular follow-ups and responses to queries were a welcome boost during difficult times.

Vibhu and Anthony would also like to personally thank Jimmy for his leadership as lead editor throughout this process.

Contents

Part I

Principles and Practice of Pharmacovigilance and Drug Safety

Introduction to Drug Safety and Pharmacovigilance

1

Jimmy Jose, Anthony R. Cox, and Andrew Bate

Abstract

This chapter will introduce the main terms and concepts related to drug safety. This includes definitions, epidemiology, diagnosis, and classification of adverse drug reactions (ADRs) as well as the shift to a more holistic view of drug safety in relation to medication errors, issues in clinical practice, and regulatory approaches. The development of modern pharmacovigilance and drug safety practices can be attributed to a series of drug safety events that took place throughout the twentieth century. Even with high-quality randomized controlled trials, the safety of new medicines is not guaranteed due to limitations of the clinical trials, such as trial size, exclusion of subjects at risk of developing ADRs, short trial durations, and the nature of potential ADRs. Clinical trials are unlikely to detect infrequent ADRs or those that are delayed. Once marketed, large numbers of individuals can be exposed to the drug and detection of new ADRs is possible.

Spontaneous reporting of ADRs by healthcare professionals and patients is one of the primary methods of detecting new safety signals, and post-marketing observational studies using real-world data are used to investigate potential signals. For methodological reasons, several terms related to ADRs, as well as dictionaries of ADRs, have been developed, which are essential for the quantitative examination of drug safety issues. Pharmacovigilance is a collaborative venture including healthcare professionals, patients, regulators, and pharmaceutical companies to ensure that the chances of finding new safety issues are maximized.

Even following successful detection of an ADR, the complex communication and ethical issues present challenges. In clinical practice, the burden of harms generally comes from the most frequently used drugs, and good patient management is enhanced by understanding of the principles and methods in pharmacovigilance and the safe use of medicines. At the local level, managing polypharmacy in an aging population will become increasingly challenging. The future of pharmacovigilance

J. Jose (✉)
Pharmacy Practice, School of Pharmacy, College of Health Sciences, University of Nizwa, Nizwa, Oman
e-mail: jimmy.jose@unizwa.edu.om

A. R. Cox
Clinical Pharmacy and Drug Safety School of Pharmacy, College of Medical and Dental Sciences University of Birmingham, Birmingham, UK

A. Bate
GSK, Brentford, UK

London School of Hygiene and Tropical Medicine, London, UK

J. Jose et al. (eds.), *Principles and Practice of Pharmacovigilance and Drug Safety*,
https://doi.org/10.1007/978-3-031-51089-2_1

will see major developments in pharmacoinformatics, artificial intelligence, and pharmacogenomics. Continued educational efforts at both the undergraduate and postgraduate levels are required to enhance the effective practice of drug safety and pharmacovigilance.

Keywords

Adverse drug reactions · Adverse events · Pharmacovigilance · Drug safety · Patient safety

Learning Objectives

After reading this chapter, the reader should be able to:

- Understand the origins of drug safety and pharmacovigilance.
- Understand the importance of drug safety at population and individual patient levels.
- Describe the various definitions of the key terms in drug safety and pharmacovigilance.
- Understand the basic principles that govern the practice of drug safety.
- Describe the key aspects of pharmacovigilance systems and regulation.

Key Points

- Pharmacovigilance is an evolving science consisting of multiple methodologies, with complex communication issues with health-care professionals, patients, and broader society.
- Understanding the key terminology is useful for applying pharmacovigilance in clinical practice.
- Among other skills, quantitative and clinical skills are important for pharmacovigilance science, which underscores the importance of multidisciplinary pharmacovigilance teams.
- Pharmacovigilance has the safety of individual patients and the assessment of the harm of medicines at the population level as its central tenets.

1 Introduction

Drug safety and pharmacovigilance encompass a wide field of knowledge, from individual risk factors and management of adverse effects in patients to population-level science to detect the novel risks of medicines. This includes complex and evolving methodologies as well as difficult communication issues regarding the risks. This opening chapter puts the knowledge in context, provides a brief overview of the field, and outlines the key concepts and definitions that are needed to negotiate the remaining chapters in this book.

The science of optimizing the safety of medicines is called pharmacovigilance, which comes from the Greek word *pharmakon* (medicinal substance) and the Latin word *vigilia* (to keep watch). A relatively new science, it has largely developed since the middle of the twentieth century. Pharmacovigilance has been defined by Rawlins as 'the process of identifying, and then responding to, safety issues about marketed drugs' [1] and by Mann and Andrews as 'the study of the safety of marketed drugs under the practical conditions of clinical use in large communities' [2]. These definitions help capture the core element of pharmacovigilance, which is focused on detecting the harms of a medicine following its marketing among the general population. However, as noted by Rawlins, pharmacovigilance is more than the detection of safety issues. Knowledge of a problem is nothing without an effective process of choosing the right action to take once it is found and being able to communicate that action well. The concise definition of pharmacovigilance by the World Health Organization (WHO) captures these elements: 'Pharmacovigilance is the science and activities relating to the detection, assessment, understanding and prevention of adverse effects or any other medicine/vaccine related problem' [3]. Considering the activities specifically related to vaccines, the Council for International Organizations of Medical Sciences (CIOMS)/WHO Working group on vaccine pharmacovigilance defined vaccine pharmacovigilance 'as the science and activities relating to the detection, assessment, understanding and communication of adverse events following immunization and other vaccine- or immunization-related issues, and to the prevention of untoward effects of the vaccine or immunization' [4].

Being able to detect a signal of potential harm is the first step, but, without further case assessments and signal testing with pharmacoepidemiological methodologies, only a limited understanding can be obtained. Understanding the potential mechanisms of an adverse drug reaction (ADR) may provide a clue to the risk factors or mechanisms to prevent such harm. For the purpose of simplicity and following the usual method of representation, the term 'drug' used in the remainder of this chapter and the entire book also encompasses the term 'vaccines', unless otherwise specified. While harm can be prevented by the withdrawal of a drug from the market, its restricted use, or labelling changes facilitating its safer use, much of pharmacovigilance deals with the communication of the complex balances between benefits and harms to professionals and the public. Even so, a drug's withdrawal requires a well-justified and clear communication plan to avoid raising disproportionate public concern. Pharmacovigilance is therefore an activity that surrounds the entire life of a medicine and is related to all aspects of a drug's continued safety.

2 History

Medicines are intended to exert a beneficial pharmacological effect on patients. Sometimes such effects work as intended, whereas, at other times, unintended harmful effects may occur. At both the population and individual levels, a mix of both benefits and harms will coexist, with complex decisions and personal preferences influencing drug therapy. The complexity of modern medicine, an aging world population, and the increase in polypharmacy all mean that the challenges in pharmacovigilance are increasing, despite the improvements in the field over the past century.

The history of harmful effects of medicines has been punctuated with tragedies, some of which may have been preventable with knowledge at that time. It is beyond the scope of this chapter to comprehensively review the history of pharmacovigilance, which is covered in several other texts [5–8], but a brief overview of some historical cases can help understand the context of modern pharmacovigilance—which has often proceeded in a paroxysmal manner following tragic events. Further details can be found in Chap. 6.

Although the adverse effects of medicines have been noted since ancient times, one of the first systematic attempts to do so was made in the nineteenth century following several deaths related to early general anesthetic use. A collaborative commission was set up by *The Lancet* and *The British Medical Journal* to examine the safety of chloroform. Published in 1893, it is notable that this commission set up a reporting system for physicians to report anesthesia-related deaths [6]. In 1937, an early antibiotic, sulfanilamide, was reformulated into a liquid preparation by the Massengill Company, leading to the deaths of 107 people, most of whom were children. Diethylene glycol had been used in the formulation, with the company scientists being unaware of its already known toxicity. This led to an amendment of the United States 1906 Food and Drug Administration Act in 1938 to avoid such incidences in the future [9]. Tragically, outbreaks of diethylene glycol contamination of medicines have still been leading to poisoning and deaths periodically ever since, with more than 300 deaths occurring in 2022, mostly of children under 5 years of age, in Uzbekistan, Ghana, and The Gambia [10].

The development of modern pharmacovigilance as an international collaborative science arose because of the thalidomide tragedy in the 1960s. Thalidomide was first marketed in 1957 and had been declared suitable for use in pregnancy and nursing mothers by the company Chemie Grünenthal without supporting evidence of safety [11]. In 1961, an Australian doctor,

William McBride, who had prescribed the drug to several female patients, drew attention to a potential causal link to deformities in the babies of the women he had treated [12]. Despite increasing concerns, the company continued to market the drug as safe, until eventual withdrawal. At this point, thousands of babies had been born with congenital malformations because of maternal exposure to thalidomide, with no awareness that a teratogenic effect existed [13].

A widespread effect had been missed, with no central overview of the incidence of the congenital defects. This direct articulation of the need to effectively compare experiences of suspected adverse effects of medicines was the spur that led to the widespread setting up of organized national surveillance systems in the early 1960s as well as the WHO Program to collect such data internationally in 1968 [14]. Major advances in monitoring capability, or legislative responsibilities regarding pharmacovigilance, have arisen because of further drug or vaccine safety events. Examples include the late detection of sclerosing peritonitis caused by practolol in 1975 [15], the withdrawal of benoxaprofen in 1982 following reports of hepatotoxicity and deaths [16], and the withdrawal of the cyclooxygenase (COX)-2-selective nonsteroidal anti-inflammatory drug (NSAID) rofecoxib in 2004 following the finding of a significantly increased risk of cardiovascular events in clinical trials [17]. In the latter case, as one example, this led to the Food and Drug Administration (FDA) Amendments Act of 2007, which, in turn, led to the creation of the FDA Sentinel Initiative, a national resource for monitoring safety across more than 100 million patient lives with data captured during routine care delivery [18].

3 The Importance of Pharmacovigilance

The modern drug development process has the ability to expediently test and identify safety issues in the developmental stages of a drug, even before it is used in human trials. Safety has an increased focus in the clinical development life cycle, and data regarding safety issues not only form part of the safety assessment of new drugs entering the market but also inform pharmacovigilance plans to monitor the product once it is released to the wider population. However, the inherent weakness of premarketing studies, such as the highly selective patient group, the relatively small size of clinical trials compared to real-world exposure to new drugs, and the limited duration of therapy and follow-up, make continued post-marketing surveillance essential. In addition, routine health care is unavoidably significantly different to controlled trials. It is therefore essential to continue to monitor for emerging safety issues, or for new information on known safety issues, once medicinal products are used as part of routine real-world health-care delivery—where practice often differs from clinical trials.

Pharmacovigilance is critically important not only for individual patients but also at the public health level, both in identifying new issues and in managing known safety issues. In addition to individual patient suffering, the impact and scale of drug safety failure on a population can be high. This varies by setting and the nature of exposure and outcome, and there is a wide variation in estimates, but one such analysis conducted across multiple US hospital databases estimated that adverse drug events occurred in 2.1% of all inpatient stays and were present on admission in 5.1% of stays, with the management of such adverse drug events estimated to cost US $28 billion annually [19]. More details on the economic burden of drug safety can be found in Chap. 5. In the case of new medicines, the importance of the rapid detection of safety signals is highlighted by the fact that nearly 20 million people were exposed to 5 drugs in the US market that were later withdrawn for safety issues [20]. Although media reporting may fixate on the failures of drug regulation, modern pharmacovigilance science, which started during the latter part of the twentieth century, has undoubtedly saved lives and averted widespread misery.

4 The Principles of Pharmacovigilance and Drug Regulation

Pharmacovigilance is essential to ensure safety whenever people take medicines, whether the medicine is under development or as part of routine health care. Thus, pharmacovigilance should be in place across all clinical trial phases and for post-marketing usage. Its objective is to ultimately identify and understand safety issues as precisely and promptly as possible so that the benefit–harm of marketed medicines is favourable in a specific defined population, the risk is communicated, and, when there is differential risk across individuals, it is managed appropriately to minimize it. Usage is monitored for as long as medicines are marketed, and, if, for example, in subpopulations the benefit–harm is unfavourable, then this will be identified and steps taken to mitigate it, such as by the inclusion of new contraindications. Medicines regulation around the world defines how this is done and ensures that the pharmaceutical industry complies with the regulation all with the ultimate goal of ensuring patient safety and trust in the system. Accordingly, pharmacovigilance legalization covers all phases of the evaluation and usage of medicines. For more details on how medicines regulation is coordinated, please refer to Chap. 6. Additionally, please refer to the following articles as examples: Santoro et al. [21] and Park [22]. Although there is much international variability, there are efforts to harmonize approaches through international organizations like the International Council for Harmonisation of Technical Requirements for Pharmaceuticals for Human Use (ICH), which is particularly valuable to international organizations and companies that market medicines across different geographies [23].

5 Terminology

Consistent drug safety terminology, with clear and unambiguous definitions is critical to enable prescribers, patients, manufacturers, and regulators to understand each other. The confusion that exists due to different terms and definitions used in the field of drug safety by researchers, practitioners, and regulatory agencies is a concern [24]. This can influence various activities related to drug safety such as in routine clinical practice, safety reporting, and communications. A complete description of all the terms used in pharmacovigilance in the pharmaceutical industry and the regulatory field can be obtained from the specialist chapters in this book, but the fundamental terms frequently used in clinical practice are discussed below.

Two commonly used terms in drug safety, namely 'adverse drug reactions (adverse reactions)' and 'adverse drug effects (adverse effects),' refer to the same phenomenon, though they are different in perspective. While an adverse effect is seen from the point of view of the drug, an adverse reaction is seen from the point of view of the patient [24]. Drug X caused an 'adverse effect' in patient Y, whereas patient Y developed an 'adverse reaction' from drug X. Terms that are commonly used to denote all the harmful effects of drugs in the general sense are 'toxic effect' and 'side effect'. Technically, an 'adverse reaction' or an 'adverse effect' seems to be a better term to use than the above two [24]. It is worth noting that a side effect can be beneficial and is often used as a lay term for an ADR and that a toxic effect is not common at normal doses.

The WHO's definition of an ADR is 'a response to a drug that is noxious and unintended and occurs at doses normally used in man for the prophylaxis, diagnosis or therapy of disease, or for modification of physiological function' [25]. Although this definition, which was first published in 1972, is still widely used, it has certain drawbacks. Adverse effects can occur at doses other than those that are used in the way that the definition describes, for example, after a test dose. All adverse effects need not be noxious or harmful as the definition indicates and can include those effects that are inconvenient and not harmful per se [24]. Although there are many other definitions available in the literature, as additional information, few other definitions for ADRs are included in Table 1.1. The common

Table 1.1 Definitions (commonly used) for adverse drug reactions in the literature

Definition	References
An ADR[a] is defined as a response to a drug that is noxious and unintended and occurs at doses normally used in man for the prophylaxis, diagnosis or therapy of disease, or for modification of physiological function.	World Health Organization [25]
An ADR is 'a response to a medicinal product which is noxious and unintended. Response in this context means that a causal relationship between a medicinal product and an adverse event is at least a reasonable possibility. Adverse reactions may arise from use of the product within or outside the terms of the marketing authorisation or from occupational exposure. Conditions of use outside the marketing authorisation include off-label use, overdose, misuse, abuse and medication errors.' This definition is adopted from Definition EU Guideline on good pharmacovigilance practices (GVP)—Annex-I—Definitions (8 January 2014) (Rev 2). https://www.ema.europa.eu/en/documents/scientific-guideline/guideline-good-pharmacovigilance-practices-annex-i-definitions-rev-2-superseded_en.pdf	Council for International Organizations of Medical Sciences[b] [26]
As described in the ICH[c] Topic E 2 A Clinical Safety Data Management: Definitions and Standards for Expedited Reporting: 'in the pre-approval *clinical experience* with a new medicinal product or its new usages, particularly as the therapeutic dose(s) may not be established: *all noxious and unintended responses to a medicinal product related to any dose should be considered adverse drug reactions'*.	ICH [27]
An ADR is defined as 'a response to a medicinal product which is noxious and unintended' (Article 1 of Directive 2001/83/EC).	European Medicine Agency [28]
'For purposes of prescription drug labeling, an adverse reaction is an undesirable effect, reasonably associated with use of a drug, that may occur as part of the pharmacological action of the drug or may be unpredictable in its occurrence. This definition does not include all adverse events observed during use of a drug, only those adverse events for which there is some basis to believe there is a causal relationship between the drug and the occurrence of the adverse event.'	US Food and Drug Administration [29]
According to Food and Drug Regulations of Canada, an ADR is 'a noxious and unintended response to a drug which occurs at doses normally used or tested for the diagnosis, treatment or prevention of a disease or the modification of an organic function.'	Health Canada— Canada Vigilance Program [30]
The American Society of Health-System Pharmacists defines a significant ADR as 'any unexpected, unintended, undesired, or excessive response to a drug that requires discontinuing the drug (therapeutic or diagnostic), requires changing the drug therapy, requires modifying the dose (except for minor dosage adjustments), necessitates admission to a hospital, prolongs stay in a health care facility, necessitates supportive treatment, significantly complicates diagnosis, negatively affects prognosis, or results in temporary or permanent harm, disability, or death.'	American Society of Health-System Pharmacists [31]
An ADR is an 'An appreciably harmful or unpleasant reaction, resulting from an intervention related to the use of a medicinal product; adverse effects usually predict hazard from future administration and warrant prevention, or specific treatment, or alteration of the dosage regimen, or withdrawal of the product.'	Aronson and Ferner [24]

[a] *ADR* adverse drug reaction
[b] *CIOMS* Council for International Organizations of Medical Sciences
[c] *ICH* International Council for Harmonisation of Technical Requirements for Pharmaceuticals for Human Use

theme in all definitions is that the reaction is undesired and unintended [32].

The use of the term 'at doses normally used in man' in the WHO definition tries to differentiate an ADR from 'toxicity', which is a harmful effect that occurs due to overexposure either due to acute (acute drug toxicity) or chronic (chronic drug toxicity) use. Drug toxicity is always considered to be dose-related, whereas the manifestations of drug toxicity may be related to therapeutic effects or otherwise. Liver toxicity because of acute exposure to higher doses of paracetamol (paracetamol overdose) could be considered as acute drug toxicity, which is unrelated to the therapeutic effect of the drug. On the other hand, excessive bleeding caused by acute exposure to higher doses of warfarin (warfarin overdose) could also be considered as acute toxicity but is related to the therapeutic effect of the drug.

Even though the terms 'side effect' and 'ADR' are used interchangeably, they are distinct by nature. By the definition of the WHO, a side effect is 'any unintended effect of a pharmaceutical product occurring at doses normally used in man, which is related to the pharmacological properties of the drug'. The essential elements of this definition are the pharmacological nature of the effect, that the phenomenon is unintended, and that it is in its normal dose [24, 33]. The term mainly aims to indicate those unintended effects of the drug that may occur side by side with its main therapeutic effect and may include its beneficial or harmful effects. In practice, it refers more commonly to the harmful effects caused by the drug. To elucidate the concept of the beneficial part of the term 'side effect', let us consider the anticholinergic effect of a tricyclic antidepressant (TCA). Since the anticholinergic effect with a TCA is not associated with the main therapeutic effect (antidepressant effect), it could be considered as a side effect. This side effect may be troublesome for some individuals, whereas it may be beneficial for some others. A depressed patient with irritable bowel syndrome may incidentally benefit from the anticholinergic side effect of a TCA when it is administered to the patient as an antidepressant. The term 'side effect' is more of a layman's term to indicate the negative effects of drugs and, ideally, should be avoided professionally to avoid ambiguity and risk of misclassification [34, 35]. The term 'adverse effect' encompasses all unwanted effects; it makes no assumptions about the mechanism, evokes no ambiguity, and avoids the risk of misclassification [24].

A term commonly used in the field of drug safety and used interchangeably with an ADR is 'adverse event'. An adverse event (AE) or an adverse experience in drug safety is defined by the WHO as 'any untoward medical occurrence that may present during treatment with a medicine, but which does not necessarily have a causal relationship with this treatment'. To label an untoward medical event as AE, there need not be suspicion of a causal relationship. The basic point is the coincidence of the time of the event with the use of the drug [36]. The CIOMS has presented the definition with a slight modification to include the events observed during clinical trials: 'any untoward medical occurrence in a patient or clinical trial subject administered a medicinal product and which does not necessarily have a causal relationship with this treatment' [26]. For vaccines, a specific term of art is often used: adverse event following immunization (AEFI). An AEFI is defined as 'any untoward medical occurrence following immunization, which does not necessarily have a causal relationship with the vaccine'. This AE may be any unfavourable or unintended sign, an abnormal laboratory finding, a symptom, or a disease [37].

Looking at the difference between an ADR and an AE, an ADR is an adverse outcome that can be attributed, with some degree of probability, to the use of the drug. An AE can be any unfavourable or unintended sign, a symptom, or a disease temporally associated with the use of a medicinal product, whether or not considered related to the medicinal product [35]. The term 'AE' can be used when a causal link between the drug and the untoward medical occurrence has not been proven, whereas suspicion of a causal relationship between the drug and the AE is essential to use the term 'ADR' [33]. In effect, all ADRs are AEs, but not all AEs are ADRs. The use of this term is particularly important in clinical trials in which not all events are necessarily drug-induced [24]. It is important to document all the events occurring in the clinical trial subjects, as data regarding the possible adverse effects of the investigational drug are not much known during the clinical trial. After identifying any possible relationship of the AEs with the drug, the ADRs of the investigational drug could be better identified and documented at the time of marketing.

A few of the other commonly used terms and definitions in drug safety are presented in Table 1.2, and they will be appropriately discussed in the respective sections of this book.

It is important to differentiate between the terms 'serious' and 'severe' adverse reaction and use them appropriately. The 'seriousness' of an ADR is a measure of the extent to which the reaction developed can or does cause harm. On the other hand, the 'severity' of an ADR is a measure of the extent to which the adverse effect develops in an individual. For example, nitrates may cause severe headache in a patient, which may not be serious, whereas drug-induced ventricular tachycardia of any severity is serious [24]. The approach is somewhat different when severity is assessed using standard scales, and the same is discussed in Chap. 16.

Table 1.2 Definitions of a few other commonly used terms in drug safety

Term	Definition
Unexpected adverse reaction	'An adverse reaction, the nature or severity of which is not consistent with domestic labelling or market authorisation, or expected from characteristics of the drug' [36]
Signal	'A reported information on a possible causal relationship between an adverse event and a drug, the relationship being unknown or incompletely documented previously' [36]
Serious adverse event (experience) or reaction	'Any untoward medical occurrence that at any dose: results in death; is life-threatening; requires inpatient hospitalization or prolongation of hospitalization; results in persistent or significant disability/incapacity; is a congenital anomaly/birth defect' [26]

Medication errors may be a cause of AEs, but it is not always so. Consequently, the term 'medication error' cannot be used interchangeably with ADRs or AEs. The National Coordinating Council for Medication Error Reporting and Prevention defines it as 'A medication error is any preventable event that may cause or lead to inappropriate medication use or patient harm while the medication is in the control of the health care professional, patient, or consumer. Such events may be related to professional practice, health care products, procedures, and systems, including prescribing, order communication, product labelling, packaging and nomenclature, compounding, dispensing, distribution, administration, education, monitoring, and use' [38]. The approach is somewhat different when severity is assessed using standard scales and the same is discussed in Chap. 16. Since medication errors are preventable, AEs or ADRs caused by medication errors are preventable as well. The relationship between medication errors, AEs, and ADRs is depicted in Fig. 1.1. In everyday drug use, the

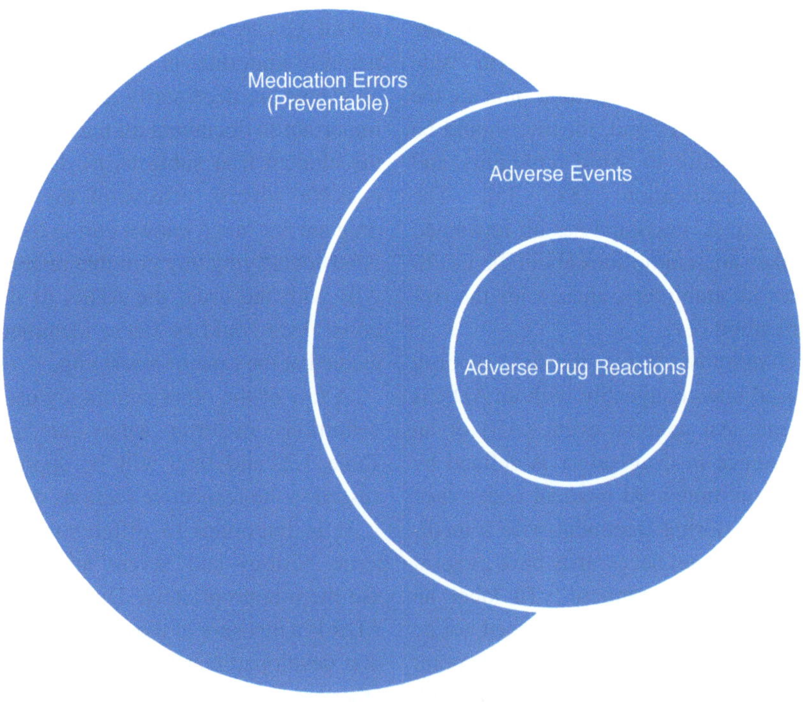

Fig. 1.1 Relationship between medication errors, adverse events, and adverse drug reactions

focus should always be on avoiding these preventable ADRs. Further details on medication errors, including their types and severity, are provided in Chap. 15.

6 Classification of Adverse Drug Reactions

The classification of ADRs is essential to the practice of pharmacovigilance and its clinical understanding. Classification can help reveal the mechanism behind the ADR and inform practical considerations to prevent and manage the same. It is useful for educational and practical purposes for those working in regulatory and clinical settings [33]. It is also important in regulatory and health-care settings where ADRs are evaluated. Multiple methods of classifying ADRs have been developed over the years. The most commonly used is the Rawlins and Thompson's classification of ADRs [39].

6.1 Rawlins and Thompson's Classification of Adverse Drug Reactions

Rawlins and Thompson suggested that adverse reactions and interactions can usually be logically, and clinically, divided into those that form part of a drug's normal pharmacological actions (type A: augmented) and those that represent a novel response (type B: bizarre) [39]. The major differences between these two types of ADRs are summarized in Table 1.3.

6.1.1 Type A Reactions

Type A reactions are the results of quantitatively abnormal, pharmacological effects of drugs. They are the most common type of ADRs, responsible for 80% of the reactions [33]. Type A reactions can be due to the primary (or intended) pharmacological property of a compound, such as hypotension with antihypertensive agents and hypoglycemia with antidiabetic agents. Other than the primary pharmacological effects, type A reactions could be due to the drug's secondary pharmacological effects. An example is the anticholinergic effects of tricyclic antidepressants and many antipsychotics causing tachycardia, constipation, dryness of the mouth, and blurring of vision [33].

Table 1.3 The major differences between type A and type B reactions [33, 39, 40]

Features	Type A	Type B
Pharmacologically predictable	Yes	No
Dose-dependent	Yes	No
Incidence	Common	Uncommon
Morbidity	High	Low
Mortality	Low	High
Preventability	More likely by appropriate drug and dose selection	Less likely
Management	Dose adjustment might be sufficient usually or withhold temporarily	Usually require complete withdrawal of drug. Avoid use in future

Type A reactions are usually considered to be predictable, dose-dependent, common, are rarely life-threatening, and occur in individuals lying at the top of dose–response curves for pharmacological effects. Three potential causes for this type of response include pharmaceutical, pharmacokinetic, and pharmacodynamic. Pharmaceutical factors such as differences in pharmaceutical formulation can give rise to substantial alterations in the quantity of the drug that is 'available' to reach its site of action. Individual differences in the pharmacokinetic variables of absorption, distribution, and elimination result in differences in drug concentrations at the site of action. Pharmacodynamic factors are due to the altered target organ sensitivity, which results in differing individual susceptibilities to drugs [39].

6.1.2 Type B Reactions

Type B reactions are bizarre, qualitatively abnormal effects, which are seemingly unrelated to a drug's desired pharmacological effect. Examples include the severe skin reactions to some antiseizure drugs or antibiotics or hepatoxicity associated with statins [39]. They are infrequent, are usually unknown before the drug is marketed, and are first identified after use in the wider population [33]. Different mechanisms may play a role in the development of type B reactions. By-products of chemical synthesis can be involved, for instance, aspirin anhydride, a contaminant found in the commercial samples of aspirin, or in vitro degradation products, such as those arising from tetracyclines, may give rise to toxic effects, which cannot be explained by the pharmacological properties of the drugs. The components of a pharmaceutical product such as additives, excipients, colorizers, and binders may themselves cause toxicity, or may react with the drug, thus resulting in toxic derivatives leading to type B reactions. Development of unusual, or novel, drug metabolites in the body can also lead to these bizarre reactions. Genetic factors resulting in altered target organ responses can explain some type B reactions. Examples are development of hemolysis with oxidant drugs in patients with red cell glucose-6-phosphate dehydrogenase deficiency or certain hemoglobinopathies and the precipitation of acute porphyria with enzyme-inducing agents. Many of the type B reactions have an immunological basis [39]. The immunological basis of ADRs is discussed in detail in Chap. 2.

6.1.3 Clinical Implications

In clinical practice, the focus of health-care professionals should be on preventing and reducing the occurrence of both type A and type B ADRs. Reductions in type A reactions can be achieved by ensuring appropriate drug and dose selection for individual patients based on their unique characteristics and disease details, including comorbid conditions. Ensuring patient compliance and appropriate monitoring of therapeutic and toxic parameters in the patient can contribute toward reducing these predictable and dose-dependent effects. On the other hand, obtaining an appropriate medication history, use of ADR-alert mechanisms, close monitoring of predisposing factors before and during medication use, using pharmacogenomic screening wherever applicable, and patient education may be beneficial in reducing type B reactions.

6.1.4 Extended Classification

A number of ADRs vary from type A and type B reactions, and the classification system of Rawlins and Thompson's underwent expansion to accommodate those reactions which do not appropriately fit into this basic classification. The classes, as per the expanded version of the basic classification, are listed in Table 1.4.

6.2 DoTS (Dose Relatedness, Timing, and Patient Susceptibility) Classification

Several criticisms of the Rawlins and Thompson's classification have been made over the years, especially as it has expanded in complexity. For example, the concept that some ADRs are not dose-related

Table 1.4 Extended classification of Rawlins and Thompson's classification [33, 40]

Classes	Features	Examples
Type C (chronic): dose- and time-related	Uncommon Related to cumulative dose	Hypothalamus–pituitary–adrenal axis suppression by corticosteroids Retinal toxicity with hydroxychloroquine
Type D (delayed): time-related	Uncommon Usually dose-related Occurs or becomes apparent sometime after use of the drug	Carcinogenesis
Type E (exit): withdrawal	Uncommon Occurs soon after withdrawal of the drug	Opiate withdrawal syndrome Benzodiazepine withdrawal syndrome Beta-blocker rebound effects after abrupt discontinuation
Type F (failure): unexpected failure of therapy	Common Dose-related Often caused by drug interactions	Inadequate dose/level of contraceptives in the presence of enzyme inducers resulting in contraceptive failure

has been criticized [41]. A new three-dimensional classification system for ADRs based on dose relatedness, timing, and patient susceptibility (DoTS) was proposed by Aronson & Ferner [42] and can theoretically classify any ADR without further expansions, and thus removes the concept of a non-dose-related ADR. This comprehensive classification includes properties of both the reaction (the time course of its appearance and its severity) and the individual (the genetic, pathological, and other biological differences that confer susceptibility). An advantage of the DoTS system is its ability to focus on examining the key risk factors and nature of the ADR, which can inform future prevention and management of the ADR.

6.2.1 Dose Relatedness

According to this classification, all adverse effects by drugs, including type B reactions, have a relation with the dose. ADRs can be classified as toxic, collateral, or hypersusceptible. Toxic reactions are those that occur at supratherapeutic doses; collateral reactions are those that occur at standard therapeutic doses; and hypersusceptible reactions are those that occur at subtherapeutic doses in susceptible patients. Collateral reactions can include those that occur due to a different pharmacological effect from the therapeutic action and also those that occur through the therapeutic pharmacological effect but at another site of action.

6.2.2 Time Relatedness

Many pharmacological effects depend on the time course of its appearance. The time course of ADRs is considered to be either time-dependent or time-independent. Time-independent reactions may occur at any time during treatment, independent of the duration of the course, either when the concentration of the drug at the site of action changes (for example, digoxin toxicity in patients with renal dysfunction) or when the pharmacological response is altered without a change in concentration (for example, digoxin toxicity in patients with hypokalemia).

On the other hand, time-dependent reactions arise in relation to the duration of treatment. Six subtypes of time-dependent reactions are described—rapid, first-dose, early, intermediate, late, and delayed. Rapid reactions occur only when a drug is administered too rapidly as in the case of development of red man syndrome after rapid administration of vancomycin. First-dose reactions occur after the first dose of a course of treatment and not necessarily thereafter. An example of this is the development of hypotension after the first dose of an angiotensin-converting enzyme inhibitor. Early reactions occur early in treatment and then subside with continuing treatment. Examples include the early symptoms of gastrointestinal adverse effects with orlistat or the headache following the first use of nitrates [43]. Intermediate reactions occur after some delay, but if the reaction has not occurred after a certain time, then it is unlikely to develop at a later stage. Examples are hypersensitivity reactions of type II (thrombocytopenia due to quinine). In late reactions, the risk of developing the reaction at the beginning of treatment is rare or nil, but the risk increases with continued or repeated use; examples include many of the adverse effects of corticosteroids and the ophthalmic adverse effects of hydroxychloroquine. Delayed reactions are observed sometime after exposure and can occur even after the drug is withdrawn; examples include carcinogenesis (such as the vaginal adenocarcinoma in female children whose mothers used diethylstilbesterol during pregnancy) and teratogenesis.

6.2.3 Susceptibility

The risk of an ADR differs among members of an exposed population depending on the presence of a single or multiple factors such as genetic variation, age, sex, physiological variation, exogenous factors, and disease.

Table 1.5 presents examples of different ADRs of the same drug enalapril classified under the DoTS system.

One potential limitation of the DoTS classification system is that it may not be always easy to fit an individual ADR into a specific type based on dose, time relatedness, and susceptibility. In regular clinical practice, the application of the DoTS system may enable practitioners to have a better understanding of the pattern and contributing factors to a particular ADR, focusing the mind of the prescribers on prevention and monitoring of adverse effects. An increased under-

Table 1.5 Examples of DoTS classification applied to differing adverse effects of enalapril

Dry cough with enalapril	*Angioedema with enalapril*	*Hypotension after the first dose of enalapril*
Do—collateral effect; T—intermediate[a]; S—sex (female)	Do—hypersusceptible; T—[b]early; S—race (Black patients)	Do—collateral; T—first dose; S—volume-depleted individuals, patients additionally on diuretics

[a] At times dry cough develops with the first dose or could develop extremely late as well

[b] Angioedema may develop later during treatment as well. Furthermore, it does not go away with continuing treatment

standing of the susceptibility factors helps in safer prescribing considering the patient and drug-specific factors, such as the need for dose reductions in renal failure.

6.3 Classification of Adverse Effects Induced by Biological Agents

ADRs induced by biological agents are often target-related and linked to the biological outcomes of their action [44]. Based on the peculiar features of biological agents, a new classification of the adverse effects of biological agents has been proposed [45].

This classification system differentiates adverse effects into five distinct types, namely, clinical reactions because of high cytokine levels (type α), hypersensitivity because of an immune reaction against the biological agent (type β), immune or cytokine imbalance syndromes (type γ), symptoms because of cross-reactivity (type δ), and symptoms not directly affecting the immune system (type ε). This unique classification could help better deal with the clinical features of side effects with this specific class of drugs, to identify possible individual and general risk factors.

6.4 Classification Based on Predictability, Frequency of Occurrence, and Preventability

ADRs can also be categorized as either predictable or unpredictable. Predictable ADRs include (1) toxicity from medication, (2) unavoidable side effects, (3) pharmacological actions, and (4) drug–drug interactions. Unpredictable adverse reactions include (1) intolerance, in which the patient experiences expected reactions at much lower doses or blood concentrations than usual; (2) idiosyncratic reactions, which are often attributable to genetic or pharmacokinetic responses that cause reactions not occurring in other subjects; and (3) allergic (immunoglobulin [IgE-mediated]) or pseudo-allergic (non-IgE-mediated) reactions [46, 47]. Knowledge of the predictability of individual ADRs is of benefit in clinical practice to prevent, identify, manage, and communicate information about ADRs.

Based on the frequency of occurrence of ADRs, they are often classified as very common (≥1/10), common (≥1/100 to <1/10), uncommon (≥1/1000 to <1/100), rare (≥1/10,000 to <1/1000), and very rare <1/10,000). This categorization is especially important for prescribing decisions, reporting and managing ADRs, patient communication, and regulatory actions. This classification is beneficial for categorizing ADRs as either predictable or unpredictable and is further discussed in Chap. 16 [48].

ADRs could be classified as preventable and nonpreventable reactions based on assessment of preventability of reactions based on specific scales, as discussed in Chap. 16.

7 Taxonomies

The adverse effects themselves require specific definitions for uniform use in various situations such as collating ADR reports to enable the quantitative evaluation of drug safety signals. Various dictionaries have been developed [24]. The Medical Dictionary for Regulatory Activities (MedDRA) Terminology is the international medical terminology developed under the auspices of the ICH. It was developed in the 1990s with version 1 adopted by the ICH in 1994 with the latest edition being version 26, March 2023 [49].

Another classification system is the WHO Adverse Reaction Terminology (WHO-ART), which was developed and maintained by the Uppsala Monitoring Centre (UMC) to serve as a terminology for coding adverse reaction terms, covering most medical terms needed in adverse reaction reporting. Although its use has been replaced by MedDRA, any user who requires it for a specific purpose can contact the UMC [50].

Similar coding systems exist in other data collection systems. One example is the International Classification of Diseases (ICD) now in its 11th edition (ICD-11). Published by the WHO, it serves a broad range of uses globally. For example, the clinical terms coded with the ICD are the main basis for health recording and statistics on diseases in primary, secondary, and tertiary care as well as on cause of death certificates [51]. Although not specifically created for the purpose of ADR reporting, data coded by the ICD can be used for specific and general purposes in post-authorization safety studies for identification, reporting, and data analysis. The Systemized Nomenclature of Medicine—Clinical Terminology (SNOMED-CT) is another similar standardized, international, multilingual core set of clinical health-care terminologies that can be used in electronic health records [52].

A series of international working groups was convened by the CIOMS, in which representatives of regulatory bodies and pharmaceutical companies, together with clinical experts and staff members of the WHO and CIOMS, agreed on standard definitions of selected terms for ADRs and on the minimum requirements for the use of the terms in international reporting, in the framework of post-marketing surveillance [53]. The resulting publication *Definitions and Basic Requirements for the Use of Terms for Reporting Adverse Drug Reactions* aims to facilitate efficient communication between people of diverse cultural and linguistic backgrounds, and from different medical care and education systems. It was primarily designed to meet the needs of drug regulatory authorities and drug safety departments of pharmaceutical companies as well as for medical or other reporters of ADRs, to help them document their case reports and communicate them to regulatory authorities or drug manufacturers.

WHODrug Global is the international reference for medicinal product information and is maintained by the UMC. The dictionary is used to identify drug names and evaluate medicinal product information, including active ingredients and products' anatomical and therapeutic classifications, from nearly 150 countries. It consists of medications with individual trade names linked to the active ingredients, pharmaceutical form, strength, marketing authorization holder, and country of sales as well as a classification according to the WHO Anatomical Therapeutic Chemical (ATC) classification [54]. WHODrug Global's standardized data help identify drug-related problems in clinical trials and pharmacovigilance [55]. The eXtended EudraVigilance Medicinal Product Dictionary (XEVMPD) is a database designed to support the collection, reporting, coding, and evaluation of medicinal product data in a standardized and structured way [56]. The main objective of the XEVMPD is to assist the pharmacovigilance activities in the European Economic Area (EEA).

8 Predisposing Factors

As noted earlier, the risk of an adverse reaction differs among different members of an exposed population [24]. Many factors can predispose individuals to an ADR, including polypharmacy, age (the elderly and children are more prone), genetic variation (porphyria, CYP isoenzyme polymorphisms), sex (with females being more susceptible in general and some sex-specific ADRs in both sexes), physiological variation (for example, pregnancy can influence the development of specific ADRs), exogenous factors (drug–drug or drug–food interactions), disease (renal and hepatic insufficiency), and variations in drug formulations [42, 57]. It is important as far as possible to identify and have an appropriate understanding of the predisposing factors for specific ADRs with specific drugs.

Although basic information on the predisposing factors may be available at the time of marketing of the drug, much of this is obtained after the drug is in general use. This highlights the importance of spontaneous reporting, post-marketing studies, and timely evaluation of post-marketing safety data. Appropriate knowledge of health-care professionals on predisposing factors is essential for safe prescribing, dispensing, and monitoring of medications. Patient education is equally important based on the predisposing factors present for individual drugs. A further in-depth discussion of these issues can be found in Chap. 3.

Genetics plays a major role in interindividual variability in the response to drug therapy in terms of both efficacy and safety. The pathogenesis of an ADR could be influenced by genomics, and the identification of subpopulations with altered sensitivity to medicines due to genomic factors could provide important information that could be used to mitigate the risk of ADRs [58]. Personalized medicine aims to provide individualized treatment and to predict the clinical outcome of different treatments in diverse patients [59]. Pharmacogenetics, the study of genetic causes of individual variations in drug response, is one of the core elements of personalized medicine [59, 60]. Translational medicine, which is an interdisciplinary science that links laboratory research to clinical research, has been instrumental in bringing about drug safety-related applications of pharmacogenetics in clinical practice [60]. The influence of pharmacogenetics on drug safety is further discussed in Chap. 23.

9 An Overview of Pharmacovigilance Systems

As already noted, the drug safety information collected during the premarketing phase of drug development is incomplete and post-marketing surveillance after a drug launch is crucial. Much of the world now has an established pharmacovigilance system, with the WHO Program for International Drug Monitoring having more than 170 members and associates who cover 99% of the world's population. These pharmacovigilance systems depend on spontaneous reporting of suspected ADRs by health-care professionals and patients [36].

The primary AE reporting system in the United States is MedWatch, the FDA Safety Information and Adverse Event Reporting Program where health-care professionals and consumers voluntarily report ADRs, AEs, and medication errors for entry into the FDA Adverse Event Reporting System (FAERS) database, with vaccine reports in a separate system called the Vaccine Adverse Event Reporting System (VAERS). Other examples of established pharmacovigilance systems include The Canada Vigilance Program and the Yellow Card Scheme operated by the Medicines, and Health-care Products Regulatory Agency (MHRA) and the Commission on Human Medicines in the United Kingdom (UK). National regulators and the industry in Europe contribute to EudraVigilance, a system for managing and analysing information on suspected adverse reactions to medicines, which have been authorized or are under study in clinical trials in the EEA. Such pooling of spontaneous ADR reports, both nationally and internationally, can expedite ADR identification. The WHO, using the UMC in Sweden, aims to assist in global ADR signal detection through a database called VigiBase. Individual countries throughout the world submit ADR reports to VigiBase, and the trends are tracked to identify signals [32]. There are deeper discussions on pharmacovigilance systems throughout this book, mainly in Chaps. 6, 7, 9, and 13.

10 Methods in Pharmacovigilance

Although early clinical studies, toxicology reports, and clinical trials may provide evidence for some of the frequent adverse effects expected from the pharmacology of a drug (the known knowns) and potentially future possible ADRs (the known unknowns), pharmacovigilance must often deal with the unexpected ADRs that cannot be predicted (the unknown unknowns). As already noted, although randomized controlled trials (RCTs) are considered the gold standard for discovering efficacy and are high in some hierarchies of evidence, evidence for harms comes from a more varied evidence base.

The idea of a reliable hierarchy of evidence that fits any clinical topic has been described as illusory by Rawlins [61], and there are various arguments against the rigid use of categorical hierarchies [62–64]. It has been argued that a 'network of evidence' may be a better term [65], and there are instances in which forms of evidence considered lower in the usual hierarchical structures of medicine are more important. Harms is one of these areas.

As discussed previously, RCTs are poor at identifying all relevant harms since they were primarily designed to detect efficacy in a single outcome. Although randomization is important for studying efficacy, it can also be beneficial for identifying or studying safety issues, e.g. APPROVe (Adenomatous Polyp Prevention on Vioxx) Trial for rofecoxib [66]. Randomization helps look for an imbalance in the rate of recording of outcomes across exposed and nonexposed events, which can be indicative of safety issues. However, many clinical trials fail to report ADRs adequately when published. An examination of clinical trials in six major medical journals found that descriptions of AEs were missing in 18% of the reports. A presentation of the severity of the AEs was missing in 27.1% of studies, and reporting of withdrawals from the trial because of AEs was absent in 47.4% of the studies [67]. Even when AEs are adequately reported, RCTs cannot detect relatively rare but important harms of treatments, which can be varied and multiple. Harms found during the post-marketing phase of a medicine most commonly arise from spontaneous case reports and can be hypothesis-generating. The next common source is observational studies. In a review of 462 medications withdrawn from the market between 1953 and 2013, 72% were withdrawn based on 'anecdotal reports', i.e. spontaneous reports alone [68]. Some anecdotes may provide strong certainty of a drug cause. Aronson and Hauben described four types of spontaneously reported ADRs to which a high level of confidence of causality could be attributed [69]:

- Extracellular or intracellular tissue deposition of the drug or metabolite.
- Specific anatomical location or pattern of injury.
- Physiological dysfunction or direct tissue damage that can be proved by physicochemical testing.
- Infection because of administration of a potentially infective agent or because of demonstrable contamination.

Spontaneous reports are also important for discovering drug–drug and drug–food interactions. The incidence of drug interactions may be low in the general population since they may require specific comorbidities and other risk factors in the patients to manifest. This means that the design of an RCT to assess the risk or reality of a drug interaction may be prohibitively expensive or large. The best evidence may initially come from case reports, an inversion of the usual hierarchy of evidence, although they require a thorough causality evaluation [70].

Following the detection of a drug signal, post-marketing studies can be undertaken for signal testing. They can take the form of observational studies, such as cohort studies or case–control studies depending on the nature of the event being examined. Such studies may be able to prove associations, although causality may still be difficult to ascertain. Increasingly, there is use of big data for data mining in novel real-world datasets from health-care systems [71]. Chapter 6 elaborates on pharmacoepidemiology and the use of real-world data. Further on, Chap. 16 outlines the various study designs of post-authorization safety studies (PASSs) used to identify ADRs and summarizes the various strategies to predict and thereby prevent ADRs such as pharmacogenetics, use of omics, and in silico approaches, including artificial intelligence. Increasingly, the electronic health-care database studies that are used for hypothesis testing are also being explored for near real-time monitoring and rapid response analyses [72, 73]. Such databases can be used for hypothesis generation, i.e. signal detection, although for the latter there is little compelling evidence to date that signals can be consistently identified earlier through spontaneous reporting [74].

11 Pharmacovigilance in the Industry

The pharmaceutical industry has ensured that it has processes in place to monitor the benefit–harm ratio of its products under development and also after it has been marketed. As safety issues arise, action is taken as needed. In addition to conducting pharmacovigilance activities across the life cycle of a drug, companies must also ensure that they have set up approaches, including safety governance. To achieve these objectives, quality processes need to be clear and fit for purpose. These processes should be open to and be frequently inspected by regulatory authorities to assess how well companies are meeting pharmacovigilance requirements.

Pharmacovigilance has become increasingly intricate and multifaceted, looking at all the safety elements of a drug from the inherent properties of a molecule to the licensed and unlicensed uses of the drug in clinical practice. This requires multiple types of expertise, including experts in risk management and risk minimization, epidemiologists, statisticians, and clinical experts with disease and therapeutic knowledge. Scanning for safety outcomes from unlicensed usage and medical errors as well as manufacturing issues are also part of modern pharmacovigilance, as is implementing and measuring the effectiveness of risk mitigation strategies. The principles and practice of pharmacovigilance in the industry are discussed in the first part of this book from Chaps. 6 to 14. For more details on pharmacovigilance in the industry, see Gatto et al. [75], Talbot and Nilsson [76], and Hartford et al. [77].

12 Communications in Pharmacovigilance

Detecting new ADRs and the subsequent regulatory decisions, short of withdrawing a drug from the market, may have limited impact without good communication. There are two main areas where particular complexity exists. First, the communication of benefits and harms to stakeholders, including patients and the public and, second, influencing the prescribing and monitoring of medicines by health-care professionals.

Communicating the risk of harms to patients and the public is hard, even when the facts are clear. However, pharmacovigilance is a complex science, using multiple sources of data. There is a large amount of uncertainty inherent in the field. This makes communication critical and challenging when communicating risks of harms and benefits clearly to health-care professionals and patients. Much effort in recent years has considered approaches for effective communication to stakeholders and enabling informed decision-making [78]. Openness and clarity on uncertainties is important in communication. Yet, the open availability of pharmacovigilance data carries dangers, since it can be taken out of context and misused either unknowingly by those who misunderstand the nature of the data sources or by bad actors. This has been demonstrated by often deliberate attempts by bad actors to use data from the US VAERS system to create narratives around the coronavirus disease of 2019 (COVID-19) vaccines, and such data have been misused in the past around previous vaccine scares. Chapter 11 provides a broad overview of this component from various perspectives. It is important for practitioners, regulators, and other stakeholders to be aware of information sources for drug safety and communicating risks in clinical practice, which is discussed in Chap. 17.

The use of a clear risk management plan based on best practice and influencing prescribers to change practice can be difficult [79], and there are many examples of the failure of warnings to change prescribing practice [80]. However, there are examples of how sustained efforts can lead to significant improvements in prescribing. Following the voluntary withdrawal of rofecoxib in 2004, the UK's MHRA issued guidance in 2005 on the increased thrombotic risk associated with other NSAIDs and the relative safety of some NSAIDs (naproxen, ibuprofen) compared to others (diclofenac). The UK's National Prescribing Centre carried out a series of interventions, including therapeutic bulletins, e-learning materials, and therapeutic workshops, which was associated with a significant fall in diclofenac prescribing and a proportionate increase in the use of naproxen and ibuprofen [81]. Changing ingrained practices and clinical decision-making requires long-term multidisciplinary efforts.

13 A Multidisciplinary Approach to Pharmacovigilance

A multidisciplinary approach is essential to address drug safety challenges. Pharmacovigilance is a challenge that is increasingly taken up by multilateral organizations and institutions, including hospitals, academia, community pharmacies, pharmaceutical companies, medicine regulatory authorities, and other independent institutions [27]. Along with health-care professionals, patients increasingly play a noteworthy role in pharmacovigilance. At the same time, patient organizations progressively position themselves as stakeholders in pharmacovigilance, carrying out many activities that stimulate awareness and participation of the public in drug safety [82]. Pharmacovigilance systems face a common set of ongoing challenges in drug safety surveillance in five principal interrelated areas: engaging the public, collaboration and partnerships, incorporating informatics, adopting a global approach, and assessing the impact of efforts. Accordingly, to tackle the multifaceted challenges of pharmacovigilance, a science-based, public health-focused, collaborative, and global approach is needed. Active engagement of patients and practitioners in pharmacovigilance, collaboration of pharmacovigilance centres with other public health agencies, appropriate utilization of informatic systems, and assessment of the impact of various strategies on improving health outcomes are all crucial [83]. The importance of multidisciplinary approach in pharmacovigilance and contribution of various stakeholders is discussed in Chap. 13. The involvement of patients, specifically in the entire process of pharmacovigilance and drug safety, is discussed in Chap. 12.

13.1 Pharmacovigilance Education

The burden of known AEs from medicines and the importance of detecting new signals of potential harms mean that education on the importance of pharmacovigilance is essential for health-care practitioners to play their part. The underreporting of suspected ADRs to regulators has led to various attempts to improve the reporting of adverse reactions. Limited pharmacovigilance knowledge demonstrated by health-care professionals is one among the main reasons for the underreporting of ADRs [84]. In practice settings with multiple medications, complex regimens, and better health-literate patients, there is an additional demand for health-care professionals to have up-to-date knowledge on drug safety [85].

Concern about the state of pharmacovigilance knowledge within professions [86] has led to the development of model curricula to inform educators [87] as well as to the incorporation of pharmacovigilance into the educational standards of professional regulatory bodies. More recently, it appears that there has been a greater uptake of pharmacovigilance in undergraduate programs worldwide [88]. There have also been interesting experiments such as including undergraduates directly in pharmacovigilance by evaluating spontaneous ADR reports and writing feedback letters with regulatory oversight and imparting medication safety education through games [89, 90].

At the postgraduate level, various attempts to insert the key concepts of pharmacovigilance into education have been made, including by continuing professional development, by providing online education about pharmacovigilance (as done by many drug regulatory agencies), and by engaging with professional regulatory bodies to ensure that the commitment to improve medicine safety is highlighted. Additionally, the WHO UMC provides news updates on the current issues in pharmacovigilance via publications, podcasts, and training. The International Society of Pharmacovigilance (ISoP) holds various meetings centred on training and education, including a major conference with pre-conference educational sessions.

For those whose primary role is pharmacovigilance, either working in regulation or in the pharmaceutical industry, there are specialist qualifications in pharmacovigilance. There is a growing need for pharmacovigilance capacity building among various stakeholders, including health-care professionals, industry, local health workers, regulators, policy makers, health care-related nongovernmental organizations, researchers in health-care disciplines, and teachers at universities and hospitals. The WHO-International Society of Pharmacovigilance (ISoP) Core Elements of a Comprehensive Modular Curriculum is a broad pharmacovigilance curriculum, which lists the essential elements of pharmacovigilance education and training [85].

In general, education of health-care professionals should also focus on awareness, on considering ADRs as part of the differential diagnosis, and knowledge on having a sound understanding of the most frequently used drugs and their ADRs, on the predisposing factors for ADRs, on the causes of medication errors, and on the reporting of ADRs and medication errors. Clinical appraisal skills and pharmacovigilance competencies in clinical practice should be inculcated as part of training, which must include prevention, identification, analysis, management, and patient communication related to drug safety issues. Both current and future health-care professionals should be aware of the need for and the outcome of pharmacovigilance and reporting of ADRs and the process of ADR reporting [87, 91–93].

Patients should also be encouraged to take an active step in promoting drug safety by educating them on the safe use of medications, monitoring, and reporting drug safety issues. Many countries allow and encourage patients to report ADRs, and such reports can be complementary to those reported by health-care professionals. To achieve patient reporting, it is of importance to create awareness among the public on the need to report

ADRs and how to report them. The reporting system should be patient- and carer-friendly [94].

14 Drug Safety in Clinical Practice

In clinical practice, the concern shifts to the individual care of patients and the associated clinical decision-making, rather than the population-level concerns about drug safety. Although there is variation in the prevalence of preventable ADRs, it is clear that there are ways in which the exposure to potential harms from medicines can be reduced. These can be summarized as follows:

1. Careful initiation of medicines
2. Timely and regular review of medicine use
3. The use of additional technologies such as pharmacogenetics and decision support tools in 1 and 2

At least 1 in 20 admissions to a hospital are associated with the harmful effects of medicines [95]. The increasing issue of harmful polypharmacy, linked to increasing comorbidities, is a call to action. There is now a global movement, termed 'deprescribing', to remove inappropriate medicines. Deprescribing has been defined as 'the process of withdrawal of an inappropriate medication, supervised by a health-care professional with the goal of managing polypharmacy and improving outcomes' [96].

The causes of polypharmacy are many and pharmaceutical marketing, multiple disease state, evidence-based medicine guidelines, government targets, and sociocultural expectations of treatment are just some of them. However, there is some optimism that despite the demographic changes that will lead to an increasing potential of inappropriate prescribing, changes in health-care systems, such as the extension of clinical pharmacists into primary care, increasing prescribing rights, and the development of pharmacogenetics, may attenuate the risks. There are also several screening tools (such as the Screening Tool of Older People's Prescriptions [STOPP]/Screening Tool to Alert to Right Treatment [START] criteria), which may help. Chapter 18 describes several screening tools and provides an extended discussion of polypharmacy and deprescribing. With the increasing prevalence of polypharmacy, the significance of considering drug interactions in clinical practice has increased. Chapter 4 discusses the mechanisms by which drug interactions occur and outlines how drug interactions can be managed and prevented in practice.

Elements of pharmacovigilance training are directly useful at the individual patient level, as much as they are in the regulatory environment, or for encouraging the reporting of ADRs. For example, an understanding of the principles of causality assessment is useful for clinical decision-making when an ADR is suspected in a patient (Chap. 8), as are the issues around patient susceptibilities and prescribing in selected groups: children, elderly, pregnant and breastfeeding mothers, and patients with renal and hepatic dysfunction (see Chaps. 19 to 22).

An increasing number of drugs now have pharmacogenetic guidance. A recent cluster randomized, cross-over implementation of a 12-gene panel, covering 6944 patients in 7 European countries, has found that the incidence of clinically relevant ADRs was significantly reduced (21.0% with screening versus 27.7% without) [97]. The implementation of screening more widely could thus have beneficial effects in clinical practice. Pharmacogenetics is further discussed in Chap. 23.

Reducing medication errors has been a point of focus in recent years, with the WHO's third Global Patient Safety Challenge attempting to reduce the global burden of iatrogenic medication-related harm by 50% [98]. In the case of prescribing errors, the UK's EQUIP study found a rate of 8.9 errors per 100 medication orders (11,077 errors were detected in 124,260 medication orders). Other studies have shown that as many as a quarter of all prescribing errors could have been prevented using electronic prescribing systems [99]. Such reductions can be achieved through the removal of legibility issues and computer-aided prescribing decisions. There is strong evidence that the use of electronic prescribing reduces the number of prescribing errors [100], although they have also led to novel forms of errors and, in some cases, more severe errors [101]. Poorly designed electronic prescribing systems can also be associated with new forms of errors, such as drop-down menus leading to picking errors, causing incorrect dosing. Overall, the effect of electronic prescribing will lead to improved patient safety, but it is important that users are actively engaged and trained. A detailed discussion of medication errors, including the components of medication errors, its detection, and mitigation strategies, can be found in Chap. 15.

15 Pharmacoinformatics and Artificial Intelligence in Pharmacovigilance

15.1 Pharmacoinformatics and Pharmacovigilance

The influences of information technology in drug-related areas have resulted in the application of a specific branch of medical informatics known as pharmacoinformatics [102]. The specialty of 'pharmacoinformatics' combines bio- and chemoinformatic approaches as well as artificial intelligence (AI) to support drug design and development at various stages, starting from preclinical research support to clinical trial design and execution support, as well as pharmacovigilance, pharmacoeconomics, and personalized medicine [103]. Pharmacoinformatics has an important role to play in the success of pharmacovigilance at the hospital, industry, and regulatory levels. It will facilitate reporting of ADRs, and, in addition, it will revolutionize signal detection using data mining techniques. At the clinical level, as more health-care settings implement computerized physician order entry along with advanced decision support systems, this can greatly influence the prevention of medication errors [102].

15.2 Artificial Intelligence and Pharmacovigilance

There are significant opportunities and challenges in utilizing advanced information technology within pharmacovigilance systems and across the pharmaceutical industry [104]. There is great interest in the application of AI to pharmacovigilance [105]. AI is a broad field, including replicating human cognition by machines and computers [106]. Machine learning (ML) is a subset of AI that automatically enables a machine or system to learn and improve from experience [107]. Pharmacovigilance's broad scope, with the need for processing extensive data to achieve regulatory, scientific, and clinical objectives, plus a growing treasure of data and technology, makes it a high-grade ore for mining by AI [106]. Pharmacovigilance requires ongoing surveillance of the known side effects of medicines as well as sifting through large volumes of data to identify and act on emerging, previously unknown side effects [108]. AI could tackle large, complex, high-dimensional data containing complex nonlinear relationships [106].

Various aspects of pharmacovigilance will benefit from automation, subject to good pharmacovigilance standards of practice. These include individual case safety report (ICSR) processing, signal management, pharmacovigilance quality management systems, and risk management systems [104]. ICSRs will very likely remain an important part of pharmacovigilance for the foreseeable future. The continually growing number of ICSRs from an increasing number and variety of data sources that are processed, submitted, and assessed for safety signals leads to increased costs and workloads for a limited supply of human safety experts [105]. The overall goal of automation is to provide high-quality safety data in the correct format, in context, more quickly, and with less manual effort, and AI potentially plays an important role in improving the efficiency and scientific value of ICSRs [104, 105].

In a recent paper that has analysed the studies related to use of AI in the pharmacovigilance industry, the major trends and opportunities included data ingestion, disease-specific studies, literature reviews (i.e. for signal detection), leveraging real-world data, signal detection in spontaneous safety reports, and the use of social media data [109]. The current areas of AI activities in assessment, proof of concept, or development for production include digital media screening, extracting data from source documents, checking for duplicate reports, case validation, triage, and initial assessment of cases and data entry, medical assessment, including causality, narrative writing, and coding AE concepts [110, 111]. Furthermore, AI has been used to search for leads in vast amounts of social media data for real-time signal detection but with several associated limitations [106]. To date, such approaches have had a limited practical impact.

According to a recent systematic review assessing the role of AI in pharmacovigilance and drug safety, it has been reported that the most identified uses include identification and prediction of ADRs, followed by the processing of safety reports or clinical narratives and extraction or prediction of the effects of drug–drug interactions [112]. Application of AI technology in clinical practice could assist in safer use of medications in practice by its potential to improve disease diagnosis, treatment selection, clinical laboratory testing, and minimize human errors [113]. AI could be used to identify populations at high risk of experiencing ADRs, to predict ADRs, to identify potential drug interactions, to optimize medication dosages, to guide personalized medicine, and to improve patient education using innovative and effective ways [112, 113]. AI could also be utilized in drug information and consultation, thereby promoting drug safety by designing a new support system to assist practical decision-making tools for health-care providers [113].

Table 1.6 Potential applications of artificial intelligence in promoting drug safety and facilitating pharmacovigilance activities

Industry and regulatory agencies
Monitoring large volumes of complex, high-dimensional data to identify and act on emerging, previously unknown side effects
Individual case safety report (ICSR) processing, including data ingestion, case validation, triage, and initial assessment of cases, medical assessment, including causality, narrative writing, and coding AE concepts
Signal detection and management from spontaneous reports, literature reviews, digital media screening
Pharmacovigilance quality management systems
Risk management systems
Leveraging real-world data
Identifying clusters and patterns in data that might not be possible with rules-based systems.
Clinical/health-care settings
Improving disease diagnosis and clinical laboratory testing
Assisting in treatment selection and medication use using practical decision-making tools for health-care providers
Optimizing medication dosages and guiding personalized medicine
Improving patient education
Identifying populations at high risk of experiencing ADRs and potential drug interactions
Minimizing human errors related to medications

[104–106, 108–112].

The potential applications of AI in promoting drug safety and facilitating pharmacovigilance activities from the perspective of the industry, regulatory agencies, and health-care settings are summarized in Table 1.6.

15.2.1 Challenges in Using Artificial Intelligence in Pharmacovigilance

There are multiple challenges or limitations associated with the use of AI in real practice. AI should be implemented in pharmacovigilance only when it can help provide solutions that reduce the workload, complexity, or budget associated with pharmacovigilance or, otherwise, it could potentially make the pharmacovigilance system inconsistent and decrease public trust and patient safety [108]. It is not always possible for machines to match the accuracy/compliance of pharmacovigilance professionals, especially in a highly regulated area, thus underscoring the need to precisely define operational objectives of using AI in pharmacovigilance [106]. The performance of the current AI algorithms for ICSR processing and evaluation requires a 'human in the loop' to ensure good quality [104]. As there are concerns about the clarity and ease of interpretation of outputs, we must ensure that humans are in the loop so that they are able to make appropriate decisions based on the AI output, given that AI outputs are not perfect. The need for human expertise must be addressed for the ethical and effective implementation of AI in health care [113]. Considering that the data obtained through pharmacovigilance activities are likely to be heterogeneous, data are captured and shared imperfectly, analytics through AI could be challenging, especially to determine the validity of the data [108]. Challenges related to data privacy, misuse of data, bias, and dangers of sharing data might deter from free sharing of data for analysis by AI tools, which can decrease the performance of such analysis and hinder the real implications [108, 113]. The quality of AI and ML studies will improve over time, providing more robust studies with better generalizability. The challenge of converting ML research studies into production AI for effective trusted routine use has not yet been resolved, except for highly limited specific pieces of the pharmacovigilance life cycle (such as surveillance of the published literature for identification of reportable safety events). Although we expect progress in this area, it is unclear how rapidly advances will occur.

15.2.2 Future of Using Artificial Intelligence in Pharmacovigilance

Technology does hold increasing potential for automating pharmacovigilance functions. Although progress has been uneven, there have been successes so that barriers to development and implementation can be reduced or resolved, making the routine use of AI to perform pharmacovigilance functions more likely [109]. Several measures must be taken to ensure responsible and effective implementation of AI in health care, including developing and implementing comprehensive cybersecurity strategies to protect patient data and critical health-care operations [113]. Collaboration between industry personnel, health-care organizations, AI researchers, and regulatory bodies is crucial to establish guidelines and standards for the development and trusted deployment of AI algorithms as part of routine pharmacovigilance [108, 113].

16 Ethics in Pharmacovigilance

Ensuring that patient data are securely managed and that understanding of the benefits and harms of medicines is communicated to them appropriately and in a timely manner for informed decision-making is central to pharmacovigilance. As discussed, pharmacovigilance deals with considerable uncertainty.

Ethics in pharmacovigilance can be complex. The risks of harms should be identified and fully understood as quickly as possible and constantly evaluated against expected and actual benefits. The decision to remove a medicine from the market is not a neutral act since it removes the benefits of a drug from patients.

It has been argued that the precautionary principle should be applied within the context of drug safety, particularly when it comes to vulnerable patient groups such as the elderly and the children [114]. It has also been suggested that if there is any risk of a safety issue, then therapeutic intervention should be avoided and, in some cases, even to the extreme of product withdrawal from the market worldwide.

However, since potential safety signals arise quite often, and many may ultimately be refuted, the precautionary principle may be an ill fit when the benefits are high. Misapplication of the precautionary principle could lead to erratic decision-making, leading to a net increase in harm caused by market withdrawal of a drug providing a net benefit. An example might be the European pause in the use of the AstraZeneca COVID-19 vaccine in older patients following the discovery of a rare clotting disorder, when there were limited alternate vaccines, and a high prevalence of COVID-19 infections. Clearly, caution should be exercised when applying the precautionary principle in pharmacovigilance.

However, what is clear is that there should be open and continued discussion on the expected benefits and likely harms at both the general and individual patient levels. The possibility of drug causation of an AE should not be dismissed when dealing with limited evidence [115]. A full discussion of ethics in pharmacovigilance can be found in Chap. 14.

17 Future Challenges

Identifying and analysing suspected ADRs are likely to remain the bedrock of pharmacovigilance for the foreseeable future—recent reviews have continued to show the dominance of spontaneous reporting as a source of signals. As we move to more of a 'big data' world [116], connecting, enriching, and contextualizing AEs with other data streams, leveraging emerging technologies like large language models [117], and other new AI developments will all remain critical. However, understanding the concerns of patients and health-care professionals [118] about the adverse effects of medicinal products, and communicating useful information to ensure appropriate benefit–harm profiles of medicines, and prevent and mitigate harms in individual patients must remain at the heart of all that we do.

Many of the pharmacovigilance practices have evolved over time with drivers such as legislative requirements. Differences, internationally, have led to complex processes and activities with sometimes limited evidence, if any, for a significant positive impact on patient safety, e.g. submission and exchange of ICSRs to multiple recipients. There is much activity in pharmacovigilance, which is critical, however, and we must as a field strive to ever better focus on those activities that will most positively impact patient safety. Better patient engagement and personalized safety are key future directions.

18 Summary and Conclusions

As medicines are one of the key interventions in health care, ensuring that a positive balance of benefits and harms exists for medicines at the population level is essential. The science of pharmacovigilance is constantly evolving with the incorporation of new methodologies, data sources, and technologies such as pharmacogenomics and AI. However, the clinical suspicions of health-care professionals will remain important for the detection of ADRs, and, increasingly, there will be more involvement of patients in individual decision-making as well as in regulatory settings. At the individual level, the burden of ADRs can be reduced by ensuring the rational evidence-based use of drugs and by performing regular reviews of prescribed medicines. A key component of pharmacovigilance is communication, which can be complex, particularly in evolving situations—both at the individual level and when addressing the wider public.

Disclosure Statement Andrew Bate is an employee of GSK and holds stock and stock options.

References

1. Rawlins MD. Pharmacovigilance: paradise lost, regained or postponed? The William Withering Lecture 1994. J R Coll Physicians Lond. 1995;29(1):41–9.
2. Mann R, Andrew E. The Basis of pharmacovigilance: introduction. In: Mann R, Andrews E, editors. Pharmacovigilance. 2nd ed. Chichester: John Wiley and Sons Ltd; 2007. p. 3–11.
3. World Health Organization. Regulation and prequalification. 2023. Available at: https://www.who.int/teams/regulationprequalification/regulation-and-safety/pharmacovigilance. Accessed 9 Nov 2023.
4. Council for International Organisations of Medical Sciences. WHO Working Group on Vaccine Pharmacovigilance. Definition and application of terms for vaccine pharmacovigilance. 2012. https://cioms.ch/wp-content/uploads/2017/01/report_working_group_on_vaccine_LR.pdf. Accessed 1 Dec 2023.
5. Fornasier G, Francescon S, Leone R, Baldo P. An historical overview over Pharmacovigilance. Int J Clin Pharm. 2018;40:744–7.

6. Routledge P. 150 years of pharmacovigilance. Lancet (London, England). 1998;351(9110):1200–1. https://doi.org/10.1016/S0140-6736(98)03148.
7. Stephens MD. The dawn of drug safety. Hampshire: George Mann; 2010.
8. Van Grootheest K. The dawn of pharmacovigilance: an historical perspective. Int J Pharm Med. 2003;17(5–6):195–200.
9. Geiling EMK, Cannon PR. Pathogenic effects of elixir of sulfanilamide (diethylene glycol) poisoning. JAMA. 1938;111:919.
10. World Health Organization. WHO urges action to protect children from contaminated medicines. 23 Jan 2023b. Available at: https://www.who.int/news/item/23-01-2023-who-urges-action-to-protect-children-from-contaminated-medicines. Accessed 13 Nov 2023.
11. Shafique S. Thalidomide—an overview and the species-specific teratogenicity. Res J Congenit Dis. 2019;2:1.
12. McBride WG. Thalidomide and congenital abnormalities. Lancet. 1961;2(1358):90927–8.
13. Mohamed IN. Pharmacovigilance and reporting adverse drug reactions. Med Health. 2014;9(2):92–102.
14. Edwards IR. An agenda for UK clinical pharmacology: pharmacovigilance. Br J Clin Pharmacol. 2012;73(6):979–82.
15. Mann RD. An instructive example of a long-latency adverse drug reaction—sclerosing peritonitis due to practolol. Pharmacoepidemiol Drug Saf. 2007;16(11):1211–6.
16. Goldkind L, Laine L. A systematic review of NSAIDs withdrawn from the market due to hepatotoxicity: lessons learned from the bromfenac experience. Pharmacoepidemiol Drug Saf. 2006;15(4):213–20.
17. Solomon DH, Avorn J. Coxibs, science, and the public trust. Arch Intern Med. 2005;165(2):158–60.
18. Platt R, Brown JS, Robb M, McClellan M, Ball R, Nguyen MD, Sherman RE. The FDA sentinel initiative—an evolving national resource. N Engl J Med. 2018;379(22):2091–3.
19. Syrowatka A, Song W, Amato MG, Foer D, Edrees H, Kuznetsova M, Dulgarian S, Seger DL, Simona A, Bain PA, Jackson GP. Key use cases for artificial intelligence to reduce the frequency of adverse drug events: a scoping review. Lancet Digital Health. 2022;4(2):e137–48.
20. Freidman MA, et al. The safety of newly marketed approved medicines: do recent market removals mean there is a problem? JAMA. 1999;281(18):1728–34.
21. Santoro A, Genov G, Spooner A, Raine J, Arlett P. Promoting and protecting public health: how the European Union pharmacovigilance system works. Drug Saf. 2017;40:855–69.
22. Park JE, Yi J, Kwon O. Twenty years of traditional and complementary medicine regulation and its impact in Malaysia: achievements and policy lessons. BMC Health Serv Res. 2022;22(1):1–3.
23. Tsintis P, La Mache E. CIOMS and ICH initiatives in pharmacovigilance and risk management: overview and implications. Drug Saf. 2004;27:509–17.
24. Aronson JK, Ferner RE. Clarification of terminology in drug safety. Drug Saf. 2005;28(10):851–70. https://doi.org/10.2165/00002018-200528100-00003.
25. World Health Organization. International drug monitoring: the role of national centres. Technical report series no. 498. Geneva: WHO; 1972.
26. Council for International Organizations of Medical Sciences (CIOMS). CIOMS cumulative pharmacovigilance glossary, Geneva, Switzerland. 2021. https://cioms.ch/wp-content/uploads/2021/03/CIOMS-Cumulative-PV-Glossary-v1.0.pdf. Accessed 12 Aug 2022.
27. International Council for Harmonisation of Technical Requirements for Pharmaceuticals for Human Use. ICH Topic E 2 A clinical safety data management: definitions and standards for expedited reporting. 1995. Available at: https://www.ema.europa.eu/en/documents/scientific-guideline/international-conference-harmonisation-technical-requirements-registration-pharmaceuticals-human-use_en-15.pdf. Accessed 3 Aug 2022.
28. European Medicine Agency. Eudravigilance—European database of suspected adverse drug reaction reports. 2001. https://www.adrreports.eu/en/glossary.html#. Accessed 28 Nov 2023.
29. US Food and Drug Administration. CFR—Code of Federal Regulations Title 21. 2023. https://www.accessdata.fda.gov/scripts/cdrh/cfdocs/cfcfr/cfrsearch.cfm?fr=201.57. Accessed 28 Nov 2023.
30. Health Canada—Canada Vigilance Program. The guidance document for industry—reporting adverse reactions to marketed health products. 2009. https://publications.gc.ca/collections/collection_2009/sc-hc/H164-33-2009E.pdf. Accessed 28 Nov 2023.
31. American Society of Hospital Pharmacy. ASHP guidelines on adverse drug reaction monitoring and reporting. Am J Health Syst Pharm (AJHP). 1995;52(4):417–9. https://doi.org/10.1093/ajhp/52.4.417.
32. Schatz SN, Weber RJ. Adverse drug reactions. PSAP. 2015. Available at: https://www.accp.com/docs/bookstore/psap/2015B2.SampleChapter.pdf. Accessed 3 Aug 2022.
33. Krska K, Cox AR. Adverse drug reactions. In: Whittlesea K, Hodson K, editors. Clinical pharmacy and therapeutics. 6th ed. Oxford: Elsevier; 2019.
34. European Medical Writers Association. Pharmacovigilance glossary. 2017. https://www.emwa.org/media/2640/pv-sig-glossary-august-2017.pdf. Accessed 22 Aug 2022.
35. European Medicine Agency. Clinical safety data management: definitions and standards for expedited reporting. 1995. https://www.ema.europa.eu/en/documents/scientific-guideline/international-conference-harmonisation-technical-requirements-registration-pharmaceuticals-human-use_en-15.pdf.

36. World Health Organization. Safety monitoring of medicinal products—reporting system for the general public. 2012. 9789241503198-eng.pdf (who.int). Accessed 12 Nov 2023.
37. World Health Organization. Serious AEFI. 2018. https://www.who.int/groups/global-advisory-committee-on-vaccine-safety/topics/aefi/serious-aefi#cms. Accessed 1 Dec 2023.
38. National Coordinating Council for Medication Error Reporting and Prevention. Medication errors. 2023. Available at: https://www.nccmerp.org/about--medication-errors. Accessed 13 Nov 2023.
39. Rawlins MD. Adverse reactions to drugs. Br Med J. 1981;282:974–6.
40. Edwards IR, Aronson JK. Adverse drug reactions: definitions, diagnosis, and management. Lancet (London, England). 2000;356(9237):1255–9. https://doi.org/10.1016/S0140-6736(00)02799-9.
41. Aronson JK, Ferner RE. The law of mass action and the pharmacological concentration-effect curve: resolving the paradox of apparently non-dose-related adverse drug reactions. Br J Clin Pharmacol. 2016;81(1):56.
42. Aronson JK, Ferner RE. Joining the DoTS: new approach to classifying adverse drug reactions. BMJ (Clinical research ed). 2003;327(7425):1222–5. https://doi.org/10.1136/bmj.327.7425.1222.
43. Dipiro CV. Obesity. In: Schwinghammer TL, Dipiro JT, Ellingrod VL, Dipiro CV, editors. Dipiro's pharmacotherapy handbook. 12th ed. McGraw Hill; 2023. p. 657–6.
44. Lee SJ, Kavanaugh A. Adverse reactions to biologic agents: focus on autoimmune disease therapies. J Allergy Clin Immunol. 2005;116(4):900–5. https://doi.org/10.1016/j.jaci.2005.03.028.
45. Pichler WJ. Adverse side-effects to biological agents. Allergy. 2006;61(8):912–20. https://doi.org/10.1111/j.1398-9995.2006.01058.
46. Ditto AM. Drug allergy part A: introduction, epidemiology, classification of adverse reactions, immunological basis, risk factors, evaluation of patients with suspected drug allergy, patient management considerations. In: Grammer LC, Greenberger PA, editors. Patterson's allergic diseases. 6th ed. Philadelphia: Lippincott, Williams & Wilkins; 2002. p. 295–334.
47. Greenberger PA. Drug allergy. J Allergy Clin Immunol. 2006;117(2 Suppl Mini-Primer):S464–70. https://doi.org/10.1016/j.jaci.2005.11.002.
48. European Commission Enterprise and Industry Directorate-General. A guideline on summary of product characteristics. Revision 2. 2009. https://health.ec.europa.eu/system/files/2016-1/smpc_guideline_rev2_en_0.pdf. Accessed 12 Nov 2023.
49. International Council for Harmonisation of Technical Requirements for Pharmaceuticals for Human Use. Medical dictionary. 2023. https://www.meddra.org/about-meddra/history. Accessed Aug 2022.
50. Uppsala Monitoring Centre. WHO-ART legacy service. 2023. https://who-umc.org/vigibase/vigibase-services/who-art/. Accessed 19 Nov 2023.
51. World Health Organisation. International Statistical Classification of Diseases and Related Health Problems (ICD). https://www.who.int/standards/classifications/classification-of-diseases. Accessed on 24 th February 2024.
52. SNOMED International. SNOMED CT. 2022. Available at: https://www.snomed.org/. Accessed 5 Aug 2022.
53. Council for International Organizations of Medical Sciences (CIOMS). Reporting adverse drug reactions. Definition of terms and criteria for their use. 1999. https://cioms.ch/wp-content/uploads/2017/01/reporting_adverse_drug.pdf. Accessed 5 Aug 2022.
54. Lagerlund O, Strese S, Fladvad M, Lindquist M. WHODrug: a global, validated and updated dictionary for medicinal information. Ther Innov Regul Sci. 2020;54(5):1116–22. https://doi.org/10.1007/s43441-020-00130-6.
55. Uppsala Monitoring Centre. WHO-drug global. 2022. Available at: https://who-umc.org/whodrug/whodrug-global/. Accessed 5 Aug 2022.
56. European Medicine Agency. Electronic submission of medicinal product information by marketing-authorisation holders Article 57 (2) of Regulation (EC) No 726/2004. Available at https://www.ema.europa.eu/en/documents/other/electronic-submission-medicinal-product-information-marketing-authorisation-holders_en.pdf. Accessed on 14 th May 2024.
57. Pirmohamed M, Breckenridge AM, Kitteringham NR, Park BK. Adverse drug reactions. BMJ (Clin Res Ed). 1998;316(7140):1295–8. https://doi.org/10.1136/bmj.316.7140.1295.
58. European Medicine Agency. Guideline on key aspects for the use of pharmacogenomics in the pharmacovigilance of medicinal products. 2015. https://www.ema.europa.eu/en/documents/scientific-guideline/guideline-key-aspects-use-pharmacogenomics-pharmacovigilance-medicinal-products_en.pdf. Accessed 22 Aug 2022.
59. Schwab M, Schaeffeler E. Pharmacogenomics: a key component of personalized therapy. Genome Med. 2012;4(11):93. https://doi.org/10.1186/gm394.
60. Dere WH, Suto TS. The role of pharmacogenetics and pharmacogenomics in improving translational medicine. Clin Cases Miner Bone Metab. 2009;6(1):13–6.
61. Rawlins M. De Testimonio: on the evidence for decisions about the use of therapeutic interventions. Clin Med (Lond). 2008;8(6):579–88.
62. Borgerson K. Valuing evidence: bias and the evidence hierarchy of evidence-based medicine. Perspect Biol Med. 2009;52(2):218–33. https://doi.org/10.1353/pbm.0.0086.

63. Solomon M. Just a paradigm: evidence-based medicine in epistemological context. Eur J Philos Sci. 2011;1(3):451–66.
64. Stegenga J. Down with the hierarchies. Topoi. 2013;33(2):313–22.
65. Bluhm R. From hierarchy to network: a richer view of evidence for evidence-based medicine. Perspect Biol Med. 2005;48(4):535–47.
66. Baron JA, Sandler RS, Bresalier RS, Lanas A, Morton DG, Riddell R, Iverson ER, DeMets DL. Cardiovascular events associated with rofecoxib: final analysis of the APPROVe trial. Lancet. 2008;372(9651):1756–64.
67. Pitrou I, Boutron I, Ahmad N, Ravaud P. Reporting of safety results in published reports of randomized controlled trials. Arch Intern Med. 2009;169(19):1756–61. https://doi.org/10.1001/archinternmed.2009.306.
68. Onakpoya IJ, Heneghan CJ, Aronson JK. Post-marketing withdrawal of 462 medicinal products because of adverse drug reactions: a systematic review of the world literature. BMC Med. 2016;14:10. https://doi.org/10.1186/s12916-016-0553-2.
69. Aronson JK, Hauben M. Anecdotes that provide definitive evidence. BMJ. 2006;2006(333):1267. https://doi.org/10.1136/bmj.39036.666389.94.
70. Scheife RT, Hines LE, Boyce RD, Chung SP, Momper JD, Sommer CD, Abernethy DR, Horn JR, Sklar SJ, Wong SK, Jones G, Brown ML, Grizzle AJ, Comes S, Wilkins TL, Borst C, Wittie MA, Malone DC. Consensus recommendations for systematic evaluation of drug-drug interaction evidence for clinical decision support. Drug Saf. 2015;38(2):197–206. https://doi.org/10.1007/s40264-014-0262-8.
71. Ventola CL. Big data and pharmacovigilance: data mining for adverse drug events and interactions. P T. 2018;43(6):340–51.
72. Dimbil M, Kyle R, Brown JS, Aldairy W. Using real-world data for rapid safety investigations: value of near-real-time clinical data querying. Drug Saf. 2022;45(10):1251–2.
73. Lieu TA, Kulldorff M, Davis RL, Lewis EM, Weintraub E, Yih K, Yin R, Brown JS, Platt R, Vaccine Safety Datalink Rapid Cycle Analysis Team. Real-time vaccine safety surveillance for the early detection of adverse events. Med Care. 2007;45:S89–95.
74. Bate A, Hornbuckle K, Juhaeri J, et al. Hypothesis-free signal detection in healthcare databases: finding its value for pharmacovigilance. Ther Adv Drug Saf. 2019;10:2042098619864744.
75. Gatto NM, Sobel RE, Geier J, Mo J, Bate A, Reynolds RF. The role of pharmacoepidemiology in industry. In: Pharmacoepidemiology. Wiley; 2019. p. 98–125.
76. Talbot JC, Nilsson BS. Pharmacovigilance in the pharmaceutical industry. Br J Clin Pharmacol. 1998;45(5):427.
77. Hartford CG, Petchel KS, Mickail H, Perez-Gutthann S, McHale M, Grana JM, Marquez P. Pharmacovigilance during the pre-approval phases: an evolving pharmaceutical industry model in response to ICH E2E, CIOMS VI, FDA and EMEA/CHMP risk-management guidelines. Drug Saf. 2006;29:657–73.
78. Bahri P. Public pharmacovigilance communication: a process calling for evidence-based, objective-driven strategies. Drug Saf. 2010;33:1065–79.
79. Ricci JR, et al. Prescriber compliance with black box warnings in older adult patients. Am J Manag Care. 2009;15(11):e103–883.
80. Forbes N, Cooray M, et al. Changes in domperidone prescribing practices after a "Black Box" warning: are we exposing inpatients to unnecessary cardiac risk? Am J Gastroenterol. 2013;108:S476.
81. Hollingsbee D, Maskrey N, Hutchinson A, Underhill J, Bowes A. Changing current practice—the prescribing of NSAIDs. Prescriber. 2011;22:45–8. https://doi.org/10.1002/psb.795.
82. Chinchilla K, Matos C, Hall V, van Hunsel F. Patient organizations' barriers in pharmacovigilance and strategies to stimulate their participation. Drug Saf. 2021;44(2):181–91. https://doi.org/10.1007/s40264-020-00999-0.
83. Dal Pan GJ. Ongoing challenges in pharmacovigilance. Drug Saf. 2014;37(1):1–8. https://doi.org/10.1007/s40264-013-0123-x.
84. Seselja Perisin A, Bukic J, Rusic D, Leskur D, Bozic J, Mihanovic A, Vilovic M, Cohadzic T, Modun D. Teaching pharmacovigilance to healthcare students: identifying gaps and opportunities for improvement. Pharmacy (Basel, Switzerland). 2021;9(3):147. https://doi.org/10.3390/pharmacy9030147.
85. Beckmann J, Hagemann U, Bahri P, Bate A, Boyd IW, Dal Pan GJ, Edwards BD, Edwards IR, Hartigan-Go K, Lindquist M, McEwen J, Moride Y, Olsson S, Pal SN, Soulaymani-Bencheikh R, Tuccori M, Vaca CP, Wong IC. Teaching pharmacovigilance: the WHO-ISoP core elements of a comprehensive modular curriculum. Drug Saf. 2014;37(10):743–59. https://doi.org/10.1007/s40264-014-0216-1.
86. Cox AR, Marriott JF, Wilson KA, Ferner RE. Adverse drug reaction teaching in UK undergraduate medical and pharmacy programmes. J Clin Pharm Ther. 2004;29:31–5.
87. Comoglio RH. Undergraduate and postgraduate pharmacovigilance education: a proposal for appropriate curriculum content. Br J Clin Pharmacol. 2020;86(4):779–90. https://doi.org/10.1111/bcp.14179.
88. Hartman J, Härmark L, van Puijenbroek E. A global view of undergraduate education in pharmacovigilance. Eur J Clin Pharmacol. 2017;73(7):891–9. https://doi.org/10.1007/s00228-017-2237-z. Epub 2017 Mar 17.
89. Jose J, van Eekeren R, Jimmy B. Medication safety education through games: a potential approach to

educate healthcare students on adverse drug reactions. Int J Pharm Pract. 2021;29(1):91–2. https://doi.org/10.1111/ijpp.12657.
90. Schutte T, Tichelaar J, Reumerman MO, van Eekeren R, Rolfes L, van Puijenbroek EP, Richir MC, van Agtmael MA. Feasibility and educational value of a student-run pharmacovigilance programme: a prospective cohort study. Drug Saf. 2017;40(5):409–18. https://doi.org/10.1007/s40264-016-0502-1.
91. Reumerman M, Tichelaar J, Piersma B, Richir MC, van Agtmael MA. Urgent need to modernize pharmacovigilance education in healthcare curricula: review of the literature. Eur J Clin Pharmacol. 2018;74(10):1235–48. https://doi.org/10.1007/s00228-018-2500-y.
92. van Eekeren R, Rolfes L, Koster AS, Magro L, Parthasarathi G, Al Ramimmy H, Schutte T, Tanaka D, van Puijenbroek E, Härmark L. What future healthcare professionals need to know about pharmacovigilance: introduction of the WHO PV core curriculum for university teaching with focus on clinical aspects. Drug Saf. 2018;41(11):1003–11. https://doi.org/10.1007/s40264-018-0681-z.
93. Jose J. Communication on drug safety-related matters to patients: is it even more significant in this digital era? Ther Adv Drug Saf. 2020;11:2042098620915057. https://doi.org/10.1177/2042098620915057.
94. Steurbaut S, Hanssens Y. Pharmacovigilance: empowering healthcare professionals and patients. Int J Clin Pharm. 2014;36(5):859–62. https://doi.org/10.1007/s11096-014-0004-0.
95. Panagioti M, Khan K, Keers R N, Abuzour A, Phipps D, Kontopantelis E et al. Prevalence, severity, and nature of preventable patient harm across medical care settings: systematic review and meta-analysis BMJ 2019;366:l4185. https://doi.org/10.1136/bmj.l4185.
96. Reeve E, Gnjidic D, Long J, Hilmer S. A systematic review of the emerging definition of 'deprescribing' with network analysis: implications for future research and clinical practice. Br J Clin Pharmacol. 2015;80(6):1254–68. https://doi.org/10.1111/bcp.12732.
97. Swen JJ, van der Wouden CH, Manson LE, Abdullah-Koolmees H, Blagec K, Blagus T, Böhringer S, Cambon-Thomsen A, Cecchin E, Cheung KC, Deneer VH, Dupui M, Ingelman-Sundberg M, Jonsson S, Joefield-Roka C, Just KS, Karlsson MO, Konta L, Koopmann R, Kriek M, et al. A 12-gene pharmacogenetic panel to prevent adverse drug reactions: an open-label, multicentre, controlled, cluster-randomised crossover implementation study. Lancet (London, England). 2023;401(10374):347–56. https://doi.org/10.1016/S0140-6736(22)01841-4.
98. World Health Organization. Medication without harm. 2017. https://www.who.int/initiatives/medication-without-harm. Accessed 8 Nov 2023.
99. Seden K, Kirkham JJ, Kennedy T, et al. Cross-sectional study of prescribing errors in patients admitted to nine hospitals across North West England. BMJ Open. 2013;3:e002036. https://doi.org/10.1136/bmjopen-2012-002036.
100. Nuckols TK, Smith-Spangler C, Morton SC, Asch SM, Patel VM, Anderson LJ, et al. The effectiveness of computerized order entry at reducing preventable adverse drug events and medication errors in hospital settings: a systematic review and meta-analysis. Syst Rev. 2014;3:56. https://doi.org/10.1186/2046-4053-3-56.
101. Schwartzberg D, Ivanovic S, Patel S, Burjonrappa SC. We thought we would be perfect: medication errors before and after the initiation of computerized physician order entry. J Surg Res. 2015;198(1):108–14.
102. Jose J. Pharmacovigilance: basic concepts and application of pharmacoinformatics. In: Gasmelseid TG, editor. Pharmacoinformatics and drug discovery technologies: theories and applications. 1st ed. Pennsylvania: IGI Global; 2012. p. 322–43.
103. Frontiers in Pharmacology. Pharmacoinformatics: new developments and challenges in drug design. Available at: https://www.frontiersin.org/research-topics/50433/pharmacoinformatics-new-developments-and-challenges-in-drug-design. Accessed 23 Sept 2023.
104. Lewis DJ, McCallum JF. Utilizing advanced technologies to augment pharmacovigilance systems: challenges and opportunities. Ther Innov Regul Sci. 2020;54(4):888–99.https://doi.org/10.1007/s43441--019-00023-3. Epub 2019 Dec 28.
105. Ball R, Dal Pan G. "Artificial intelligence" for pharmacovigilance: ready for prime time? Drug Saf. 2022;45(5):429–38. https://doi.org/10.1007/s40264-022-01157-4.
106. Hauben M. The potential of artificial intelligence in pharmacovigilance. J Faculty Pharm Med. 2020. Available at: https://www.fpm.org.uk/journals/the-potential-of-artificial-intelligence-in-pharmacovigilance/. Accessed 21 Sept 2023.
107. Google Cloud. Artificial intelligence (AI) vs. machine learning (ML). https://cloud.google.com/learn/artificial-intelligence-vs-machine-learning. Accessed 24 Sept 2023.
108. Bate A, Stegmann J. Artificial intelligence and pharmacovigilance: what is happening, what could happen and what should happen? Health Policy Technol. 2023;12(2):2023.
109. Painter JL, Raymond K, Bate A. An industry perspective on the use of machine learning in drug and vaccine safety. Front Drug Saf Regul. 2023b;3:1110498. https://doi.org/10.3389/fdsfr.2023.1110498.
110. Comfort S, Dorrell D, Meireis S, Fine J. MOdified NARanjo Causality Scale for ICSRs (MONARCSi): a decision support tool for safety scientists. Drug Saf. 2018;41(11):1073–85. https://doi.org/10.1007/s40264-018-0690-y.

111. Ghosh R, Kempf D, Pufko A, Barrios Martinez LF, Davis CM, et al. Automation opportunities in pharmacovigilance: an industry survey. Pharmaceut Med. 2020;34:7–18.
112. Salas M, Petracek J, Yalamanchili P, Aimer O, Kasthuril D, Dhingra S, Junaid T, Bostic T. The use of artificial intelligence in pharmacovigilance: a systematic review of the literature. Pharm Med. 2022;36(5):295–306. https://doi.org/10.1007/s40290-022-00441-z.
113. Alowais SA, Alghamdi SS, Alsuhebany N, Alqahtani T, Alshaya AI, Almohareb SN, Aldairem A, Alrashed M, Bin Saleh K, Badreldin HA, Al Yami MS, Al Harbi S, Albekairy AM. Revolutionizing healthcare: the role of artificial intelligence in clinical practice. BMC Med Educ. 2023;23(1):689. https://doi.org/10.1186/s12909-023-04698-z.
114. Smith MJ, Komparic A, Thompson A. Deploying the precautionary principle to protect vulnerable populations in Canadian post-market drug surveillance. Can J Bioethics. 2020;3(1):110–8.
115. Edwards IR. The future of pharmacovigilance: a personal view. Eur J Clin Pharmacol. 2008;64(2):173–81.
116. Trifirò G, Sultana J, Bate A. From big data to smart data for pharmacovigilance: the role of healthcare databases and other emerging sources. Drug Saf. 2018;41:143–9.
117. Painter JL, Mahaux O, Vanini M, Kara V, Roshan C, Karwowski M, Chalamalasetti VR, Bate A. Enhancing drug safety documentation search capabilities with large language models: a user-centric approach. In: 2023 International conference on computational science and computational intelligence (CSCI). IEEE CPS proceedings; 2023a. (in press).
118. Edwards IR. Spontaneous reporting—of what? Clinical concerns about drugs. Br J Clin Pharmacol. 1999;48(2):138.

An Overview of Immunological Reactions to Drugs

2

Sowmya Nagarajan, Bernard Yu-Hor Thong, Rashmeet Bhogal, and Mamidipudi Thirumala Krishna

Abstract

Drug hypersensitivity reactions (DHRs) are immunologically mediated responses and a part of the spectrum of adverse drug reactions (ADRs). ADRs account for about 5–7% of all hospital admissions, and DHRs constitute about <10% of all ADRs. Detailed history, physical examination, and review of hospital records relating to an index episode are key to DHR workup. Skin tests and in vitro tests for immediate and non-immediate DHRs are useful although positive and negative predictive values have not been elucidated for the majority of drugs. Hence, these tests must be carefully interpreted by an experienced specialist in drug allergy in the context of clinical presentation. Drug eruptions may resemble viral exanthemata, making diagnosis particularly challenging in children. A drug provocation test is the "gold standard" in the diagnosis of DHRs although this intervention is mainly employed to demonstrate clinical tolerance and is undertaken after performing a careful risk–benefit analysis. Management of DHRs involves immediate cessation of exposure to possible culprit/s and supportive management. When an alternative drug is under consideration for clinical use, potential cross-reactivity needs to be considered. Rapid drug desensitization is an intervention employed to induce temporary immunological tolerance in patients with an immediate DHR and where there are no suitable alternatives. This procedure must only be undertaken under the guidance of a specialist allergist in a safe clinical environment with immediate access to critical care management.

Keywords

Desensitization · Drug allergy · Drug hypersensitivity reaction · Drug provocation test · Immunological reactions

S. Nagarajan (✉)
Paediatric Allergy and Immunology, Sanjeevini Specialist Clinic and Kanagaroo Care Hospitals, Bangalore, India
e-mail: dr.sowmya.nagaraj@gmail.com

B. Y.-H. Thong
Division of Medicine, Department of Rheumatology, Allergy and Immunology, Tan Tock Seng Hospital, Singapore, Singapore

R. Bhogal
Clinical Pharmacy, Institute of Clinical Sciences, Robert Aitken Institute for Clinical Research, College of Medical and Dental Sciences, Birmingham, UK

M. T. Krishna
Allergy, Clinical Immunology and Global Health, Institute of Immunology and Immunotherapy, University of Birmingham, Birmingham, UK

University Hospitals Birmingham NHS Foundation Trust, University of Birmingham, Birmingham, UK

J. Jose et al. (eds.), *Principles and Practice of Pharmacovigilance and Drug Safety*,
https://doi.org/10.1007/978-3-031-51089-2_2

Learning Objectives

- To provide an overview of drug hypersensitivity reactions, including classification, mechanism, clinical manifestations, and diagnosis.
- To understand the clinical implications of true and inaccurate drug allergy labels.
- To offer an understanding of the clinical approach applied to a patient with a suspected drug hypersensitivity reaction.

Key Points

- Skin manifestations are the common clinical presentation of a drug hypersensitivity reaction.
- Diagnosis is dependent on a robust clinical history and scrutiny of clinical records, and there are limitations surrounding drug allergy tests.
- The gold standard of establishing clinical tolerance involves a supervised drug provocation test (a challenge test) and must be conducted only after performing a careful risk–benefit analysis and in a safe clinical environment. This intervention is usually employed when "true" drug hypersensitivity is the most unlikely.

1 Introduction

Adverse drug reactions (ADRs) are a burden to patients and health-care systems as they are associated with increased health-care costs and delays in delivering treatment. Depending on the severity, they are also associated with an enhanced risk of morbidity and mortality [1–5]. In addition, ADRs may potentially affect the relationship between prescribers and patients, thus impacting future adherence [3].

Pharmacovigilance, patient safety, and governance policies have helped raise awareness among health-care professionals and patients regarding ADRs and have guided the former to document ADRs on prescribing systems, e.g., electronic medical records (EMRs) [6]. EMRs may be linked to electronic decision support systems to prevent accidental prescribing of the same or potentially cross-reacting medications that patients with drug allergies should avoid.

Drug allergy labels are often challenging in any health-care setting and require the prescriber's expertise to source a suitable alternative medication, which will meet the criteria of good therapeutic benefit, availability, safety profile, and minimal drug interactions.

Beta-lactam antibiotics are the most common drugs involved in drug hypersensitivity reactions (DHRs). Penicillin "allergy labels" enhance the risk of antimicrobial resistance (AMR). Research conducted in high-income countries have reported that 90–95% of penicillin allergy labels are inaccurate. The global increase in AMR is a threat to public health, as it accounts for nearly 5 million deaths every year [7]. Penicillin and other antibiotic allergy labels adversely impact the global campaign to improve antimicrobial stewardship and tackle AMR. Furthermore, antibiotic allergy labels increase the risk of infections resistant to broad-spectrum antibiotics, increase health-care costs, and result in the use of expensive third- or fourth-line antibiotics to treat AMR [8–10].

2 Classification

ADRs can be broadly classified into type A (predictable) and B (unpredictable, idiosyncratic) reactions [1–4, 6, 11]. Table 2.1 outlines the main classification of ADRs.

The initial classification was suggested by Rawlins and Thompson in 1977. The letters A and B in these reactions represent "augmented" and "bizarre," respectively.

Up to 20% of ADRs are type B reactions [1], which can be subcategorized into immunological and non-immunological [1, 6]. Immunological reactions are often referred to as hypersensitive reactions or drug allergy, affect approximately 10% of all ADRs, and are a growing public health concern [6]. Patient factors that increase the likelihood of a type A reaction include age, gender, genetics, concomitant diseases, nutrition, immunological status, level of physical activity, and concomitant medications [11]. The properties of a drug that increase the likelihood of a type B reaction include the drug metabolism pathway and the presence of toxic metabolites [11].

DHRs or drug allergies are usually either immunoglobulin E (IgE)- or T-cell-mediated [2]. These are categorized as per the Gell and Coombs classification into types I–IV reactions [2, 12]. A type I reaction is immediate and IgE-mediated, and a type IV hypersensitivity reaction is non-immediate or delayed (usually 48–72 h after exposure) and is mediated by T cells. Type IV DHRs are subclassified as per T-cell subtype involvement by Pichler [2, 12, 13]. While types I and IV DHRs lend themselves to skin tests, types II and III DHRs remain a clinical diagnosis and require a high index of clinical suspicion.

Table 2.2 summarizes the characterization of types I–IV DHRs.

Table 2.1 Classification of adverse drug reactions (type A and type B)

ADR	Mechanism	Examples: clinical presentation
Type A: Predictable	Related to the drugs' mechanism of action Dose-dependent	Infections as a result of immunosuppressant treatment Alopecia with chemotherapy
Type B: Unpredictable	Independent of the drugs' mechanism of action and dose	Anaphylaxis with penicillin antibiotics Stevens–Johnson syndrome with allopurinol, phenytoin, phenobarbitone, and sulfamethoxazole

Table 2.2 Characterization of various types of drug hypersensitivity reactions [2, 12, 13]

Hypersensitivity reaction	Mechanism of reaction	Clinical presentation
Type I	IgE-mediated	Urticaria, angioedema, bronchospasm, anaphylaxis
Type II	IgG-/IgM-mediated	Anemia, cytopenia, thrombocytopenia
Type III	IgG-/IgM-mediated	Vasculitis, lymphadenopathy, fever, arthropathy, rashes, serum sickness
Type IV(a)	Th1 cells rely on IFN and TNF pathways to activate monocytes and macrophages	Contact dermatitis, bullous exanthema
Type IV(b)	Th2 cells rely on activation of IL-5, IL-4, IL-13, and eotaxin to facilitate eosinophilic inflammation	Maculopapular and bullous rashes
Type IV(c)	CD4/CD8 cytotoxic T cells use perforin, granzyme B, and FasL pathways to kill targets	Contact dermatitis, maculopapular, pustularand bullous exanthemata
Type IV(d)	Neutrophil activation via T cells by CXCL and GM-CSF pathways	Pustular exanthemata

Abbreviations: *IFN* interferon, *TNF* tumor necrosis factor, *IgG* immunoglobulin G, *IgM* immunoglobulin M, *Th1* T helper cell type 1, *Th2* T helper cell type 2, *IL* interleukin, *CD4/8* cluster of differentiation 4/8, *CXCL* chemokine (C–X–C motif) ligand 1, *GM-CSF* granulocyte macrophage colony-stimulating factor

3 The Mechanism of Reaction

IgE-mediated reactions are a consequence of drug antigen antibody cross-linking on the surface of mast cells followed by activation and degranulation, resulting in the release of histamine, cytokines, and other vasoactive amines [14]. Mast cell activation may also occur without involvement of allergen-specific IgE, i.e., non-IgE-mediated mast cell degranulation caused by activation of the members of the Mas-related G-protein coupled receptors (MRGPRs) [14–18].

4 Diagnosis

4.1 History

A diagnosis of a DHR is underpinned by a careful and detailed evaluation of the temporal association based on the chronology of symptoms and signs following exposure to culprit drug/s. This involves scrutiny of the clinical, prescription, and laboratory records related to the index episode. This may be particularly challenging in low- and middle-income countries where there may be limited or no EMRs. The important principles in the diagnosis of a DHR are as follows [19–23]:

1. A DHR usually occurs in the context of previous exposure resulting in sensitization. It remains to be established why only some patients become sensitized, whereas the vast majority is not.
2. Most DHRs are relatively mild, non-immediate, or delayed and are limited to the cutaneous compartment.
3. Life-threatening systemic DHRs are relatively rare events and include severe immediate DHRs (anaphylaxis) or severe systemic delayed reactions such as Stevens–Johnson syndrome (SJS) and toxic epidermal necrolysis (TEN).

Table 2.3 summarizes the characterization of DHRs based on the time of presentation while Tables 2.4 and 2.5 list tips for history taking and early warning signs of DHRs, respectively.

Table 2.3 Classification of common drug hypersensitivity reactions based on time of presentation

Immediate DHRs (IgE-mediated)	Non-immediate severe systemic DHRs (non-IgE-mediated)
Urticaria	Stevens–Johnson syndrome
Bronchospasm	Toxic epidermal necrolysis
Hypotension	Drug reaction with eosinophilia and systemic symptoms (DRESS)
Angioedema	Acute interstitial nephritis
	Pulmonary/hepatic/renal involvement
	Vasculitis
	Hemolytic anemia
	Thrombocytopenia
	Eosinophilia
	Lymphocytosis

Table 2.4 Useful clinical tips for history taking in the evaluation of drug hypersensitivity reactions

History and extraction of clinical information from patient records
1. Capture information regarding names, dose, time, and route of administration of drugs used prior to the onset of the reaction
2. Note the temporal association between administration of the drug and the onset of reaction
3. Can other drugs administered concurrently contribute to the reaction?
4. Is there a history of similar reaction previously? What treatment was given?
5. Did the patient have concurrent infection during or prior to the suspected reaction?
6. Does the patient have a genetic predisposition to non-immediate or delayed systemic DHRs?

4.2 Physical Examination

Physical examination is an important step in the evaluation of an acute episode, specifically describing characteristics of skin lesions alongside systemic involvement. The majority of cutaneous lesions are usually benign and relatively mild, with generalized maculopapular exanthema being the most common manifestation. Therefore, it is prudent to consider a differential diagnosis of an underlying infection in all cases of a suspected DHR.

It is important to evaluate (consider) for systemic involvement, specifically the liver, kidneys, lungs, and heart with relevant laboratory workup, including a complete hemogram, liver/renal

Table 2.5 Early warning signs in drug hypersensitivity reactions

Reactions	Manifestations
Immediate	Pruritis around the mouth and on the palms and soles Erythema, urticaria, angioedema Rhinoconjunctivitis Respiratory distress Gastrointestinal manifestations such as vomiting and diarrhea
Non-immediate or delayed	Fever, malaise Lymphadenopathy Mucosal involvement Maculopapular or exanthematous rash Bullous lesions, epidermal separation (Nikolsky's sign) Confluent lesions in extensive skin areas Angioedema and diffuse erythematous swelling Eosinophilia (>1.5 × 10^9/L) Hepatic involvement Renal involvement Lung involvement Cardiac involvement Peripheral and/or central nervous system involvement

function, urine dipstick examination, skin biopsy (including direct immunofluorescence for complement and immunoglobulin deposition), and, where deemed necessary, imaging and electrophysiological studies for lung and cardiac involvement.

Table 2.6 describes the systemic manifestations of DHRs [2, 24–26].

4.2.1 Differential Diagnosis

The common differentials to consider include viral infection, allergic contact dermatitis, chronic urticaria, erythema nodosum, lymphoproliferative disorder, and clonal mast cell disorders based on the clinical scenario. Contact dermatitis has a predilection to the areas of direct contact with the drug and resolves following cessation of exposure. Chronic spontaneous urticaria is characterized by a history of recurrent "hives," usually associated with angioedema, and systemic involvement is rare.

Table 2.6 Systemic manifestations of drug hypersensitivity reactions

S. No.	Manifestations	Clinical symptoms	Drugs commonly involved
1.	DRESS syndrome	DRESS syndrome is an acronym for drug reaction with eosinophilia and systemic symptoms. It is also known as drug-induced pseudo-lymphoma and drug hypersensitivity syndrome. The symptoms of DRESS syndrome usually begin 1–8 weeks after exposure to the offending drug Symptoms: Fever, extensive rash (morbilliform, erythroderma), lymphadenopathy, hepatocellular injury, acute kidney injury, peripheral blood eosinophilia, atypical lymphocytes, other hematological abnormalities, cardiac involvement (myocarditis, pericarditis), neurological involvement (meningitis, encephalitis, polyneuritis), pneumonitis, myositis, etc.	Carbamazepine, phenobarbital, phenytoin, terbinafine, and valproic acid

(continued)

Table 2.6 (continued)

S. No.	Manifestations	Clinical symptoms	Drugs commonly involved
2.	Stevens–Johnson syndrome (SJS)	Severe and occasionally fatal form of erythema multiforme, accompanied by any or all of the following: – Fever, myalgia, malaise, headache, arthralgia, and ocular involvement, with bullae (positive Nikolsky's sign) and erosions covering less than 10% of the body surface – Painful stomatitis is an early and conspicuous symptom. Hemorrhagic bullae may appear over the lips, mouth, and genital mucous membranes. Patients are often acutely ill with high fever. The course from eruption to the healing of the lesions may extend up to 6 weeks – Peripheral blood eosinophilia and atypical lymphocytes absent (in comparison to DRESS)	Allopurinol, barbiturates, carbamazepine, estrogens/progesterone, gold, lamotrigine, non-steroidal anti-inflammatory drugs (NSAIDs), penicillamine, phenytoin, sulfonamides, tetracycline, tolbutamide, and valproic acid
3.	Toxic epidermal necrolysis (TEN)	Also known as Lyell's syndrome, it is a rare and serious acute exfoliative, bullous eruption of the skin and mucous membranes that usually develops as a reaction to diverse drugs. TEN can also be the result of a bacterial or viral infection and can develop after radiation therapy or vaccinations. Skin biopsy shows cleavage of the epidermis from the dermal layer and is associated with necrosis. The clinical picture resembles an extensive second-degree burn; the patient is acutely ill. Fatigue, vomiting, diarrhea, and angina are prodromal symptoms. In a few hours, the condition becomes grave. TEN is a medical emergency and unless the offending agent is discontinued immediately, the outcome may be fatal in the course of a few days.	Allopurinol, ampicillin, amoxicillin, carbamazepine, phenobarbital, pentamidine, phenytoin, pyrazolones, sulfonamides, NSAIDs
4.	Fixed drug eruption (FDE)	Fixed drug eruption is an unusual hypersensitivity reaction characterized by one or more well-demarcated erythematous plaques that recur at the same cutaneous (or mucosal) site/s following each one's exposure to the offending drug. The size of the lesions vary from a few millimeters to 20 cm in diameter. It usually develops 30 min to 8 h following the administration of a drug and mainly affects the hands, legs, and groin.	Ampicillin, aspirin, barbiturates, NSAIDs, oral contraceptives, phenytoin, quinine, sulfonamides, and tetracyclines
5.	Lupus erythematosus	A reaction, clinically and pathologically resembling idiopathic systemic lupus erythematosus (SLE), has been reported in association with a large variety of drugs. These symptoms recede within days or weeks following discontinuation of the drug responsible.	Beta-blockers, carbamazepine, chlorpromazine, estrogens, isoniazid, lithium, minoxidil, and oral contraceptives

4.2.2 Diagnostic Tests

Tests used for the assessment of DHRs are limited and must be employed and interpreted in conjunction with the clinical situation. Table 2.7 lists the points to be considered prior to a DHR evaluation.

Peripheral blood eosinophilia is a characteristic feature of DRESS and may be associated with

Table 2.7 Points to be considered prior to a drug hypersensitivity reaction evaluation [27–29]

The history of the DHR and the implicated drug is required. An equally effective, structurally unrelated alternative drug is not available.
A risk benefit assessment is favorable for investigation if the patient can benefit from de-labeling
The patient (where relevant, the carer) has the capacity to give informed consent

atypical lymphocytes. Biopsy and histopathological evaluation is useful in the assessment of severe skin lesions. Coombs test is employed in the diagnosis of immune-mediated hemolytic anemia. A negative test, however, does not exclude the diagnosis. Liver function tests are useful for evaluating the presence of hepatocellular damage and urine examination and renal function tests for acute kidney injury, in all cases of suspected systemic DHRs.

Serial serum total tryptase measurements are indicated in the assessment of anaphylaxis. Three samples are recommended: the first one as soon as possible following clinical stabilization of the patient, the second within 1–2 h after the onset of the reaction, and the third comprising a baseline sample at ≥24 h. A threshold for a significant rise to indicate mast cell degranulation has been proposed and validated as ≥2 mcg/L + 1.2 × baseline serum total tryptase [30]. A baseline serum total tryptase ≥20 mcg/L indicates a diagnosis of systemic mastocytosis.

Skin Tests

The same diagnostic algorithms and techniques are employed in children and adults, assuming that the immune system reacts in the same way at any given point in life. Skin tests include prick tests and intradermal tests. Skin tests remain the main tool for evaluation of immediate (type I) and non-immediate (type IV) DHRs. It is important to note that positive and negative predictive values of skin tests have not been established for most drugs, although nonirritant concentrations have been published for commonly evaluated drugs [31]. These data must be interpreted in conjunction with clinical presentation, and the yield of these tests is superior in experienced hands when a pretest probability has been duly considered prior. It is not within the scope of this chapter to provide details of the practical steps involved in conducting and interpreting skin tests.

Patch Tests

Patch tests are an alternative to intradermal tests in the evaluation of type IV DHRs. However, they are less frequently employed in routine clinical practice, as they are less sensitive than intradermal tests. They may be preferred to intradermal tests in the context of severe cutaneous adverse reactions such as DRESS and TEN.

In Vitro Tests

A basophil activation test (BAT) involves assessment of activation markers such as CD63 and CD203c on the surface of basophils by flow cytometry, following incubation of peripheral blood with the relevant drug. A lymphocyte transformation test (LTT) might serve as a useful adjunct in the assessment of type IV DHRs. Both BAT and LTT are resource-dependent, expensive, and require a specialist laboratory and personnel. Further research is needed to validate the performance characteristics of these tests for various drug classes before their place is considered in the routine investigation pathway for DHRs.

Drug Provocation Tests

A drug provocation test (DPT) is the gold standard in the diagnosis of DHRs. However, in routine clinical practice, it is mainly employed to exclude DHRs and demonstrate clinical tolerance rather than clinical reactivity. The decision to conduct a DPT therefore requires careful assessment by an experienced specialist in allergy. A DPT is conducted when the likelihood of a DHR is extremely low based on clinical presentation with or without undertaking skin tests (a direct DPT). There is mounting evidence regarding the utility and safety of a direct DPT for de-labeling patients with inaccurate penicillin allergy labels [32–34]. A direct DPT is undertaken in "low-risk" patients, i.e., in those where the clinical presentation and/or prescription records suggest that a DHR to penicillin is most unlikely. A number of protocols, including single and graded challenges, have been proposed for DPTs, although none has been validated [35]. A prolonged DPT is undertaken to exclude type IV DHRs in those where the index clinical episode is either indeterminate or suggestive of a delayed or non-immediate reaction. A DPT is conducted in a hospital setting with immediate access to management of anaphylaxis and critical care facility. Details regarding patient selection for a DPT are

Table 2.8 Common clinical scenarios and contraindications for a drug provocation test

Common clinical scenarios
To exclude an allergy: history suggests that it is unlikely
Examples: local anesthesia-related reactions, vague childhood penicillin reactions, vasovagal episode, benign skin rash, etc.
Confirm/exclude allergy: skin tests negative, inconclusive or not available, and clinical presentation suggests "drug DHR unlikely"
Exclude an allergy in simultaneous exposures
Perioperative reactions, skin tests negative (not to be undertaken for neuromuscular blocking drugs or other general anesthetic agents)
Exclude cross-reactivity after demonstrating negative skin tests
Example: Beta-lactams
Contraindications
Index episode suggestive of severe life-threatening DHRs
Index episode suggestive of severe cutaneous reactions, e.g., SJS, TEN, DRESS, vasculitis, acute generalized exanthematous pustulosis (AGEP)
Patient declines to give informed consent for the procedure
Safe alternatives and comparable efficacious options are available
Severe concurrent illness or pregnancy (unless the drug is essential for the concurrent illness or required during pregnancy or delivery)

summarized in Table 2.8 [25, 26, 36, 37]. A case report of a DPT is provided separately in a clinical scenario under the section of case studies.

5 Drug Desensitization

Rapid drug desensitization (RDD) is a therapeutic intervention undertaken to induce temporary immunological tolerance, usually in the context of type I DHRs. It is also undertaken in patients with aspirin-exacerbated respiratory disease (AERD) and recurrent nasal polyps, and in those requiring dual antiplatelet therapy following coronary stent procedure in the context of AERD or aspirin intolerance. There is also some evidence regarding use of desensitization in patients with a relatively mild-type IV DHR. Desensitization should only be considered in the absence of suitable therapeutic alternatives and after undertaking a careful risk–benefit analysis [38–42]. As desensitization is a means of inducing temporary immunological tolerance, the allergy label must not be removed. This is in contrast to "de-labeling" for an inaccurate allergy label and negative DPT [43].

RDD requires one-to-one clinical supervision of patients, preferably in an intensive care unit or a high dependency unit where there is immediate access to critical care management. This procedure must be carried out only under expert supervision and with input from a clinical pharmacist for preparing drug dilutions. It can be delivered via intravenous or oral routes, with the latter being relatively safer. In principle, it involves 12–16 steps, starting at an extremely minute dose with dose escalations at an interval of 15–30 min in between steps. An important caveat is that immunological tolerance lasts as long as the patient is receiving regular daily therapy and that tolerance status is lost following cessation of treatment or if there is a break in the treatment schedule [44–46].

A written informed consent must be obtained in all cases after counseling the patient regarding the possibility of allergic reactions, including anaphylaxis. The common indications for desensitization are summarized in Table 2.9 [27, 43–53].

Table 2.9 Common indications for rapid drug desensitization (drugs involved)

Bacterial endocarditis (penicillin)
Syphilis in pregnancy (penicillin)
Neurosyphilis (penicillin)
Tuberculosis
Chemotherapeutic drugs
Biologics
Cystic fibrosis (penicillin, cephalosporins, carbapenems)
Aspirin-sensitive asthma
AERD with recurrent nasal polyposis (aspirin)
Coronary stent procedure in a patient with aspirin-induced allergic reaction

AERD aspirin-exacerbated respiratory disease

6 Future Directions in Drug Hypersensitivity Reaction Diagnosis and Management

Precision and personalized medicine is already being practiced in drug allergy in the following way:

- Human leukocyte antigen (HLA) genotyping prior to initiation of drugs at "high risk" of causing severe cutaneous adverse reactions, e.g., HLA-B*1502 (carbamazepine), HLA-B*5701 (abacavir), and HLA-B*5801(allopurinol) [54].
- Drug allergy "alert cards" and applications to empower individual patients to be aware of their drug allergies and potentially cross-reactive drugs to avoid [55].
- Clinical decision support within EMR systems at the point of medication orders to prevent accidental prescription [56, 57].
- Medication safety tools and enablers at the point of medication administration and dispensing.
- "Direct" DPT in "low-risk" patients with an inaccurate penicillin allergy label to improve antimicrobial stewardship and reduce the risk of AMR.
- Education of health-care professionals and patients regarding drug allergies. A list of drugs to be avoided should be given to patients/parents (To Whom It May Concern Letter), including medications that can be used as safe alternatives.
- Pathways for referral to an allergy specialist.

The following e-tools for predicting drug allergy remain investigational:

- Phenotyping and endotyping DHRs according to the different patterns of biomarkers/cytokines released [28, 58].
- Multidimensional approaches including predictive analytics, artificial intelligence techniques, and "point-of-care" clinical decision tools [29].
- Machine learning (e.g., artificial neural networks) to predict beta-lactam DHRs [59], nonsteroidal anti-inflammatory drug-exacerbated respiratory disease [60], and diagnosis of early SJS/TEN [61].

7 Summary and Conclusions

DHRs are mediated by the immune system. Broadly, they are classified as either immediate or non-immediate reactions. Most reactions are relatively mild and involve the skin, although rarely, serious multisystem presentations can occur. Prompt recognition is paramount to keeping patients safe. Evaluation of suspected drug hypersensitivity involves a thorough clinical history, scrutiny of clinical/prescription records, skin tests, and DPTs to establish clinical tolerance and insert appropriate "allergy alerts" in clinical records. DPTs must be carried out by an experienced clinician, in a safe clinical environment, and after a careful risk–benefit analysis. Rapid drug desensitization is a specialist intervention employed to induce temporary immune tolerance in a patient with type I hypersensitivity to a certain drug and is undertaken when there are no suitable alternatives.

8 Case Studies

8.1 Case Study 1: Case Report of a Drug Provocation Test

A 45-year-old male patient with a label of penicillin allergy requires penicillin prophylaxis prior to a dental procedure. He has a prosthetic mitral valve and hence requires penicillin prophylaxis to prevent bacterial endocarditis.

The index history dates back to his childhood. He was informed by his parents that he had a mild "whole body rash" when he took a penicillin antibiotic for glandular fever, although this did not require hospitalization. The family physician advised avoiding exposure to penicillin in future.

1. *What investigations can be conducted for evaluation of this patient?*

   A skin prick test, an intradermal test for penicillin major and minor determinants, benzyl penicillin, and amoxicillin, and a serum-specific IgE for penicillin V, penicillin G, and amoxicillin can be conducted.

The skin prick test and intradermal tests for penicillin major and minor determinants, benzylpenicillin, and amoxicillin were negative for immediate and non-immediate hypersensitivity response. Serum-specific IgE was also negative for penicillin V, penicillin G, and amoxicillin.

2. *What further investigation can be conducted in the index patient?*

   A drug provocation test with oral amoxicillin can be carried out.

The patient underwent a supervised DPT with a single oral dose of amoxicillin (500 mg) followed by 250 mg twice daily for 3 days. There was no evidence of type I and type IV hypersensitivity reaction.

3. *How would you proceed after the patient passed the drug provocation test?*

   He was counseled regarding the de-labeled status, and his family physician was informed accordingly. His clinical records were updated regarding the de-labeled status as follows:

   (a) Communicate the outcome of the DPT to the patient and provide written communication in relation to this. Counsel the patient about which antibiotics the patient can now receive and check the patient's understanding of this.
   (b) Tell the patient to inform all health-care professionals that are responsible for their care, e.g., their general practitioner, local pharmacy, cardiologist or secondary care clinical team, nurse, etc.
   (c) Send written communication to primary and secondary care or equivalent to inform them of the outcome of the DPT and to encourage them to update the patient's allergy status.
   (d) Encourage the patient to inform their next of kin in case of an emergency.
   (e) It is also advisable to follow-up the patient after a period of time to check that all the above was understood and that all relevant records have been updated (helps prevent relabeling).

References

1. Thong BY, Tan TC. Epidemiology and risk factors for drug allergy. Br J Clin Pharmacol. 2011;71(5):684–700.
2. Mirakian R, Ewan PW, Durham SR, Youlten LJ, Dugué P, Friedmann PS, English JS, Huber PA, Nasser SM. BSACI guidelines for the management of drug allergy. Clin Exp Allergy. 2009;39(1):43–61.
3. Coleman JJ, Pontefract SK. Adverse drug reactions. Clin Med. 2016;16(5):481.
4. Montané E, Santesmases J. Adverse drug reactions. Med Clín (Engl Ed). 2020;154(5):178–84.
5. Pirmohamed M, James S, Meakin S, Green C, Scott AK, Walley TJ, Farrar K, Park BK, Breckenridge AM. Adverse drug reactions as cause of admission to hospital: prospective analysis of 18 820 patients. BMJ. 2004;329(7456):15–9.
6. Tanno LK, Torres MJ, Castells M, Demoly P, Joint Allergy Academies. What can we learn in drug allergy management from World Health Organization's international classifications? Allergy. 2018;73(5):987–92.
7. World Health Organisation. WHO strategic priorities on antimicrobial resistance: preserving antimicrobials for today and tomorrow. World Health Organisation; 2021. Available from: 9789240041387-eng(1).pdf. Accessed 7/8/22.
8. Krishna MT, Huissoon AP, Li M, Richter A, Pillay DG, Sambanthan D, et al. Enhancing antibiotic stewardship by tackling "spurious" penicillin allergy. Clin Exp Allergy. 2017;47(11):1362–73.
9. Blumenthal KG, Lu N, Zhang Y, Li Y, Walensky RP, Choi HK. Risk of meticillin resistant Staphylococcus aureus and Clostridium difficile in patients with a documented penicillin allergy: population based matched cohort study. Br Med J. 2018;361:k2400.
10. Bermingham WH, Hussain A, Bhogal R, Balaji A, Krishna MT. The adverse impact of penicillin Allergy labels on antimicrobial stewardship in sepsis and associated pharmacoeconomics—an observational cohort study (IMPALAS). J Allergy Clin Immunol Pract. 2020;5:1747–9.
11. Iasella CJ, Johnson HJ, Dunn MA. Adverse drug reactions: type a (intrinsic) or type B (idiosyncratic). Clin Liver Dis. 2017;21(1):73–87.
12. Gell PGH, Coombs RRA. Clinical aspects of immunology. 3rd ed. Oxford: Blackwell Scientific Publications; 1975. p. 6.
13. Pichler WJ. Delayed drug hypersensitivity reactions. Ann Intern Med. 2003;139:683–93.

14. Meixiong J, Anderson M, Limjunyawong N, Sabbagh MF, Hu E, Mack MR, Oetjen LK, Wang F, Kim BS, Dong X. Activation of mast-cell-expressed mas-related G-protein-coupled receptors drives non-histaminergic itch. Immunity. 2019;50(5):1163–71.
15. Schrijvers R, Gilissen L, Chiriac AM, Demoly P. Pathogenesis and diagnosis of delayed-type drug hypersensitivity reactions, from bedside to bench and back. Clin Transl Allergy. 2015;5(1):1.
16. Adam J, Pichler WJ, Yerly D. Delayed drug hypersensitivity: models of T-cell stimulation. Br J Clin Pharmacol. 2011;71(5):701–7.
17. Yun J, Cai F, Lee FJ, Pichler WJ. T-cell-mediated drug hypersensitivity: immune mechanisms and their clinical relevance. Asia Pac Allergy. 2016;6(2):77–89.
18. Pichler WJ. The pi concept: pharmacological interaction of drugs with immune receptors. World Allergy Organ J. 2008;1(6):96–102.
19. Khan DA, Solensky R. Drug allergy. J Allergy Clin Immunol. 2010;125(2 Suppl 2):S126–37. https://doi.org/10.1016/j.jaci.2009.10.028.
20. Lazarou J, Pomeranz BH, Corey PN. Incidence of adverse drug reactions in hospitalized patients: a meta-analysis of prospective studies. JAMA. 1998;279(15):1200–5.
21. Gandhi TK, Weingart SN, Borus J, Seger AC, Peterson J, Burdick E, Seger DL, Shu K, Frank Federico R, Leape LL, Bates DW. Adverse drug events in ambulatory care. N Engl J Med. 2003;348:1556–64.
22. Vervloet D, Durham S. Adverse reactions to drugs. BMJ. 1998;316(7143):1511–4.
23. Sylvia LM. Drug allergy, pseudo allergy and cutaneous diseases. In: Tisdale JE, Miller DA, editors. Drug-induced diseases: prevention, detection and management. 2nd ed. Bethesda: American Society of Health System Pharmacists; 2010.
24. Nagarajan S, Whitaker P. Management of adverse reactions to first-line tuberculosis antibiotics. Curr Opin Allergy Clin Immunol. 2018;18(4):333.
25. Eric M, et al. Practical management of antibiotic hypersensitivity. J Allergy Clin Immunol Pract. 2017;5(3):577–86.
26. Wesley Burks A, et al. Middleton's allergy: principles and practice. 9th ed. Elsevier; 2020.
27. Bermingham WH, Bhogal R, Arudi Nagarajan S, Mutlu L, El-Shabrawy RM, Madhan R, Krishnaswamy UM, Murali MR, Kudagammana ST, Shrestha R, Sumantri S, Christopher DJ, Mahesh PA, Dedicoat M, Krishna MT. Practical management of suspected hypersensitivity reactions to anti-tuberculosis drugs. Clin Exp Allergy. 2022;52(3):375–86. https://doi.org/10.1111/cea.14084. Epub 2022 Jan 20.
28. Castells MC. Drug Allergy: phenotypes, endotypes, and biomarkers. J Allergy Clin Immunol Pract. 2017;5(3):626–7. https://doi.org/10.1016/j.jaip.2017.03.026.
29. Ramsey A, Sheikh A. Innovations in health care delivery: drug allergy. J Allergy Clin Immunol Pract. 2019;7(7):2143–50. https://doi.org/10.1016/j.jaip.2019.04.050. Epub 2019 May 17.
30. Baretto RL, Beck S, Heslegrave J, Melchior C, Mohamed O, Ekbote A, Huissoon AP, Krishna MT. Validation of international consensus equation for acute serum total tryptase in mast cell activation: a perioperative perspective. Allergy. 2017;72(12):2031–4. https://doi.org/10.1111/all.13226. Epub 2017 Jul 12.
31. Brockow K, Garvey LH, Aberer W, Atanaskovic-Markovic M, Barbaud A, Bilo MB, Bircher A, Blanca M, Bonadonna B, Campi P, Castro E, Cernadas JR, Chiriac AM, Demoly P, Grosber M, Gooi J, Lombardo C, Mertes PM, Mosbech H, Nasser S, Pagani M, Ring J, Romano A, Scherer K, Schnyder B, Testi S, Torres M, Trautmann A, Terreehorst I, ENDA/EAACI Drug Allergy Interest Group. Skin test concentrations for systemically administered drugs—an ENDA/EAACI Drug Allergy Interest Group position paper. Allergy. 2013;68(6):702–12.
32. Krishna MT, Misbah SA. Is direct oral amoxicillin challenge a viable approach for 'low-risk' patients labelled with penicillin allergy? J Antimicrob Chemother. 2019;74(9):2475–9.
33. Savic L, Ardern-Jones M, Avery A, et al. BSACI guideline for the set-up of penicillin allergy de-labelling services by non-allergists working in a hospital setting. Clin Exp Allergy. 2022;52:1–7.
34. Shenoy ES, Macy E, Rowe T, Blumenthal KG. Evaluation and management of penicillin allergy: a review. JAMA. 2019;321(2):188–99. https://doi.org/10.1001/jama.2018.19283.
35. Bhogal R, Hussain A, Balaji A, et al. The role of a clinical pharmacist in spurious penicillin allergy: a narrative review. Int J Clin Pharm. 2021;43:461–75.
36. Macy E. Optimizing penicillin allergy delabeling: one big step forward and several small steps sideways. J Allergy Clin Immunol Pract. 2019;7(7:2171–2. https://doi.org/10.1016/j.jaip.2019.06.018.
37. Mustafa SS, Conn K, Ramsey A. Comparing direct challenge to penicillin skin testing for the outpatient evaluation of penicillin allergy: a randomized controlled trial. J Allergy Clin Immunol Pract. 2019;7:2163–70.
38. Yang BC, Castells MC. The who, what, where, when, why, and how of drug desensitization. Immunol Allergy Clin N Am. 2022;42(2):403–20. https://doi.org/10.1016/j.iac.2021.12.004. Epub 2022 Mar 31.
39. Kang SY, Seo J, Kang HR. Desensitization for the prevention of drug hypersensitivity reactions. Korean J Intern Med. 2022;37(2):261–70. https://doi.org/10.3904/kjim.2021.438. Epub 2022 Feb 28.
40. Cernadas JR, Brockow K, Romano A, Aberer W, Torres MJ, Bircher A, Campi P, Sanz ML, Castells M, Demoly P, Pichler WJ, European Network of Drug Allergy and the EAACI Interest Group on Drug Hypersensitivity. General considerations on rapid desensitization for drug hypersensitivity—a consensus statement. Allergy. 2010;65(11):1357–66. https://doi.org/10.1111/j.1398-9995.2010.02441.x. Epub 2010 Aug 17.
41. Scherer K, Brockow K, Aberer W, Gooi JH, Demoly P, Romano A, Schnyder B, Whitaker P, Cernadas JS,

Bircher AJ, ENDA, the European Network on Drug Allergy and the EAACI Drug Allergy Interest Group. Desensitization in delayed drug hypersensitivity reactions—an EAACI position paper of the Drug Allergy Interest Group. Allergy. 2013;68(7):844–52. https://doi.org/10.1111/all.12161. Epub 2013 Jun 7.
42. Krishna MT, Huissoon AP. Clinical immunology review series: an approach to desensitization. Clin Exp Immunol. 2011;163:131–46.
43. Reichel A, Röding K, Stoevesandt J, Trautmann A. De-labelling antibiotic allergy through five key questions. Clin Exp Allergy. 2020;50(4):532–5. https://doi.org/10.1111/cea.13576. Epub 2020 Feb 3.
44. Brennan PJ, Rodriguez Bouza T, Hsu FI, Sloane DE, Castells MC. Hypersensitivity reactions to mAbs: 105 desensitizations in 23 patients, from evaluation to treatment. J Allergy Clin Immunol. 2009;124(6):1259–66. https://doi.org/10.1016/j.jaci.2009.09.009.
45. Castells MC, Tennant NM, Sloane DE, Hsu FI, Barrett NA, Hong DI, Laidlaw TM, Legere HJ, Nallamshetty SN, Palis RI, Rao JJ, Berlin ST, Campos SM, Matulonis UA. Hypersensitivity reactions to chemotherapy: outcomes and safety of rapid desensitization in 413 cases. J Allergy Clin Immunol. 2008;122(3):574–80. https://doi.org/10.1016/j.jaci.2008.02.044. Epub 2008 May 27.
46. Diaferio L, Giovannini M, Clark E, Castagnoli R, Caimmi D. Protocols for drug allergy desensitization in children. Expert Rev Clin Immunol. 2020;16(1):91–100. https://doi.org/10.1080/1744666X.2019.1698294. Epub 2019 Dec 8.
47. Madrigal-Burgaleta R, Steering Committee Authors, Review Panel Members. Standards for practical intravenous rapid drug desensitization & delabeling: a WAO committee statement. World Allergy Organ J. 2022;15(6):100640. https://doi.org/10.1016/j.waojou.2022.100640.
48. Stevens WW, Jerschow E, Baptist AP, Borish L, Bosso JV, Buchheit KM, Cahill KN, Campo P, Cho SH, Keswani A, Levy JM, Nanda A, Laidlaw TM, White AA. The role of aspirin desensitization followed by oral aspirin therapy in managing patients with aspirin-exacerbated respiratory disease: a work group report from the Rhinitis, Rhinosinusitis and Ocular Allergy Committee of the American Academy of Allergy, Asthma & Immunology. J Allergy Clin Immunol. 2021;147(3):827–44. https://doi.org/10.1016/j.jaci.2020.10.043. Epub 2020 Dec 9.
49. Rossini R, Iorio A, Pozzi R, Bianco M, Musumeci G, Leonardi S, Lettieri C, Bossi I, Colombo P, Rigattieri S, Dossena C, Anzuini A, Capodanno D, Senni M, Angiolillo DJ. Aspirin desensitization in patients with coronary artery disease: results of the multicenter ADAPTED registry (aspirin desensitization in patients with coronary artery disease). Circ Cardiovasc Interv. 2017;10(2):e004368. https://doi.org/10.1161/CIRCINTERVENTIONS.116.004368.
50. Vega A, Peña MI, Torrado I. Use of rapid drug desensitization in delayed hypersensitivity reactions to chemotherapy and monoclonal antibodies. Front Allergy. 2022;2:786863. https://doi.org/10.3389/falgy.2021.786863.
51. Pyle RC, Butterfield JH, Volcheck GW, Podjasek JC, Rank MA, Li JT, Harish A, Poe KL, Park MA. Successful outpatient graded administration of trimethoprim-sulfamethoxazole in patients without HIV and with a history of sulfonamide adverse drug reaction. J Allergy Clin Immunol Pract. 2014;2(1):52–8. https://doi.org/10.1016/j.jaip.2013.11.002.
52. Castells M. Rapid desensitization for hypersensitivity reactions to medications. Immunol Allergy Clin N Am. 2009;29(3):585–606. https://doi.org/10.1016/j.iac.2009.04.012.
53. Krishna MT, Huissoon AP. Clinical immunology review series: an approach to desensitization. Clin Exp Immunol. 2011;163(2):131–46. https://doi.org/10.1111/j.1365-2249.2010.04296.x. Epub 2010 Dec 22.
54. Wang CW, Preclaro IAC, Lin WH, Chung WH. An updated review of genetic associations with severe adverse drug reactions: translation and implementation of pharmacogenomic testing in clinical practice. Front Pharmacol. 2022;13:886377. https://doi.org/10.3389/fphar.2022.886377.
55. Brockow K, Aberer W, Atanaskovic-Markovic M, Bavbek S, Bircher A, Bilo B, Blanca M, Bonadonna P, Burbach G, Calogiuri G, Caruso C, Celik G, Cernadas J, Chiriac A, Demoly P, Oude Elberink JN, Fernandez J, Gomes E, Garvey LH, Gooi J, Gotua M, Grosber M, Kauppi P, Kvedariene V, Laguna JJ, Makowska JS, Mosbech H, Nakonechna A, Papadopolous NG, Ring J, Romano A, Rockmann H, Sargur R, Sedlackova L, Sigurdardottir S, Schnyder B, Storaas T, Torres M, Zidarn M, Terreehorst I. Drug allergy passport and other documentation for patients with drug hypersensitivity—an ENDA/EAACI drug Allergy interest group position paper. Allergy. 2016;71(11):1533–9. https://doi.org/10.1111/all.12929. Epub 2016 Aug 14.
56. Wright A, Rubins D, Shenoy ES, Wickner PG, McEvoy D, Wolfson AR, Carballo VA, Blumenthal KG. Clinical decision support improved allergy documentation of antibiotic test dose results. J Allergy Clin Immunol Pract. 2019;7(8):2919–21. https://doi.org/10.1016/j.jaip.2019.04.052. Epub 2019 May 25.
57. Elkhalifa S, Bhana R, Blaga A, Joshi S, Svejda M, Kasilingam V, Garcez T, Calisti G. Development and validation of a mobile clinical decision support tool for the diagnosis of drug allergy in adults: the drug allergy app. J Allergy Clin Immunol Pract. 2021;9(12):4410–4418.e4. https://doi.org/10.1016/j.jaip.2021.07.057. Epub 2021 Sep 8.
58. de Las Vecillas Sánchez L, Alenazy LA, Garcia-Neuer M, Castells MC. Drug hypersensitivity and desensitizations: mechanisms and new approaches. Int J Mol Sci. 2017;18(6):1316. https://doi.org/10.3390/ijms18061316.
59. Moreno EM, Moreno V, Laffond E, Gracia-Bara MT, Muñoz-Bellido FJ, Macías EM, Curto B, Campanon

MV, de Arriba S, Martin C, Davila I. Usefulness of an artificial neural network in the prediction of β-lactam allergy. J Allergy Clin Immunol Pract. 2020;8(9):2974–2982.e1. https://doi.org/10.1016/j.jaip.2020.07.010. Epub 2020 Jul 21.
60. Tyrak KE, Pajdzik K, Konduracka E, Ćmiel A, Jakieła B, Celejewska-Wójcik N, Trąd G, Kot A, Urbańska A, Zabiegło E, Kacorzyk R, Kupryś-Lipińska I, Oleś K, Kuna P, Sanak M, Mastalerz L. Artificial neural network identifies nonsteroidal anti-inflammatory drugs exacerbated respiratory disease (N-ERD) cohort. Allergy. 2020;75(7):1649–58. https://doi.org/10.1111/all.14214. Epub 2020 Mar 3.
61. Fujimoto A, Iwai Y, Ishikawa T, Shinkuma S, Shido K, Yamasaki K, Fujisawa Y, Fujimoto M, Muramatsu S, Abe R. Deep neural network for early image diagnosis of Stevens-Johnson syndrome/toxic epidermal necrolysis. J Allergy Clin Immunol Pract. 2022;10(1):277–83. https://doi.org/10.1016/j.jaip.2021.09.014. Epub 2021 Sep 20.

3 Predisposing Factors for Adverse Drug Reactions

Jimmy Jose and Francisco J. de Abajo

Abstract

Adverse drug reactions (ADRs) are multifactorial phenomena, and predisposing factors for ADRs can be considered components of a constellation of causes, including the drug, needed for an ADR to be induced. The identification of the predisposing factors for ADRs is an important task of pharmacovigilance, as it may contribute to prevent the occurrence of ADRs. There are four types of predisposing factors: (1) those related to patient characteristics (e.g., age, sex, ethnicity, genetics); (2) those related to the underlying diseases or comorbidities (e.g., renal failure, liver disorders, metabolic disorders); (3) those related to environmental and lifestyle factors (e.g., smoking, alcohol consumption, caffeine use); and (4) those related to the concomitant use of other drugs (e.g., drug–drug interactions, polypharmacy). Predisposing factors interact with the drug to increase the risk of presenting an ADR, and the best tools to identify them are analytical epidemiological studies. Through them, it is possible to estimate the measures of a drug–event association and then assess which factors may strengthen such an association. Once a predisposing factor has been identified, it is necessary to translate this information into appropriate regulatory measures in order to minimize the risk of ADRs. In this context, health-care professionals play a crucial role in implementing risk minimization measures, informing patients, and monitoring the results.

Keywords

Adverse drug reactions · Predisposing factors · Risk factors · Multicausality · Effect modifiers · Risk management · Risk minimization · Interactions · Clinical practice · Regulatory

Learning Objectives

- To understand the concept and importance of predisposing factors for adverse drug reactions (ADRs).
- To learn the main types of predisposing factors for ADRs.
- To learn how researchers can identify predisposing factors for ADRs.

J. Jose (✉)
Pharmacy Practice, School of Pharmacy, College of Health Sciences, University of Nizwa, Nizwa, Oman
e-mail: jimmy.jose@unizwa.edu.om

F. J. de Abajo
Department of Biomedical Sciences (Pharmacology), University of Alcalá (IRYCIS),
Alcalá de Henares, Madrid, Spain

Unit of Clinical Pharmacology, University Hospital Príncipe de Asturias,
Alcalá de Henares, Madrid, Spain

J. Jose et al. (eds.), *Principles and Practice of Pharmacovigilance and Drug Safety*,
https://doi.org/10.1007/978-3-031-51089-2_3

- To know how predisposing factors for ADRs are managed in both drug regulation and clinical practice settings.

Key Points

- Predisposing factors for ADRs can be conceptualized as components of a sufficient cause that, along with the drug, can lead to an adverse event.
- Identification of predisposing factors is important to reduce the burden of ADRs.
- Predisposing factors can be grouped into four categories: (1) those related to patient characteristics; (2) those related to the underlying diseases; (3) those related to environmental factors; and (4) those that are drug-related.
- Analytical epidemiological studies are the main tool for the identification and evaluation of predisposing factors for ADRs.
- Predisposing factors should be managed at both regulatory and clinical practice levels to effectively minimize the risk posed by ADRs to patients.

1 Introduction

The ultimate objective of pharmacovigilance is to prevent or minimize the risks associated with the use of drugs. To this end, it is important to know that not only the drug's effects and its pharmacological characteristics but also the factors that interact with it can increase the risk of a specific adverse drug reaction (ADR). Broadly speaking, these are called "predisposing factors." Many risk minimization measures address such predisposing factors, and their prompt identification is crucial to adopt regulatory measures to optimize the benefit–harm ratio of the drug. At the clinical level, a better understanding of predisposing factors will facilitate more individualized drug use and thereby improve patient safety. As the amount of information available on drug safety is limited when first introduced in the market, information regarding the predisposing factors for ADRs increases with general use of the drugs. Various tools are available to obtain and increase the knowledge database of the predisposing factors for individual drug use. This chapter will introduce to the readers the concept of predisposing factors, their different types, the available methods to identify them, and, finally, how they are managed in pharmacovigilance and clinical practice.

2 Conceptual Framework and Definition

It is a common observation that, fortunately, not all patients who use a drug present a specific ADR. In addition, among those presenting the same ADR, not all experience it with the same seriousness, the same intensity (severity), at the same time, or with the same drug posology (dose, frequency, duration). This variability occurs regardless of the type of ADR, either type A (related to the pharmacological action of the drug) or type B (unrelated to the pharmacological action), though it is often stated that all patients could experience an ADR of type A provided that the drug used is over a certain dose threshold. However, the dose threshold can vary between patients. What is the reason for such variability? The answer comes from the consideration of ADRs as multifactorial or multicausal phenomena. Following the "causal pie model" proposed by Rothman [1] (Fig. 3.1), we can accept that drugs never behave as a "sufficient cause" of a disease or an event and other components have to be present. In other words, an event is set off when the "causal pie" is complete and the drug is just a piece of that pie. In a few cases, the event only occurs when the drug is present; in this sense, the drug can be considered as a "necessary cause" of such an event. Some examples include oculomucocutaneous syndrome, a disease that has only been described to be associated with the use of practolol [2], malignant neuroleptic syndrome, or serotonin syndrome induced by serotonergic drugs. Much more often, nevertheless, a

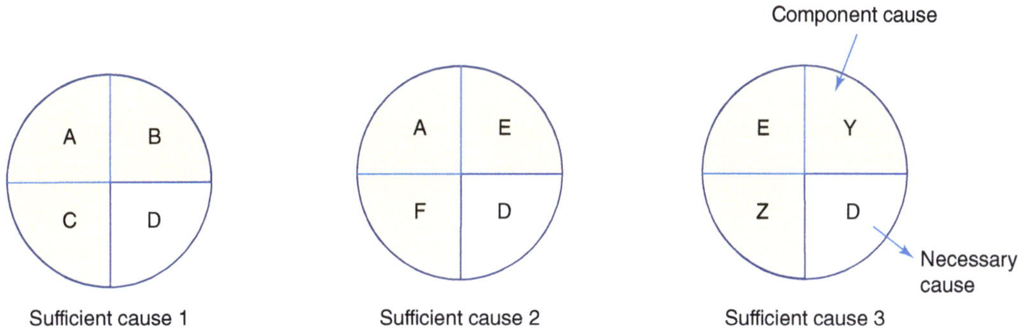

Fig. 3.1 The "causal pie model" proposed by Rothman [1]. A disease or event can be developed by different "sufficient causes," which are made up of different "component causes." When a component cause is present in all sufficient causes, it can be considered as a "necessary cause" (D, in this example)

drug is just a "component cause" and the event may occur even in its absence (e.g., myocardial infarction and coxibs). Irrespective of whether the drug is a necessary or a component cause, an event is not triggered until all the components conforming to the "sufficient cause" are present, often appearing at different points in time. Admittedly, an ADR is a special type of event because, by definition, a drug should always be present and, in this sense, drugs can always be considered as the necessary causes of ADRs, but it is just a terminology question with no biological substrate because, biologically speaking, as mentioned above, a drug is rarely a necessary cause of a disease and, likely, is never a sufficient cause.

Once the sufficient cause is completed, the disease (the ADR, in our case) starts, and, after a latency or subclinical period, the disease turns up clinically. This latency period may last for minutes, as in the case of immediate allergic reactions, or for years, as in the case of breast cancer associated with hormone replacement therapy. The latency period is conceptually different from the induction period, with the latter being the time span since the exposure to a particular cause until the start of the disease, but often they are erroneously mixed up. The induction period is not an attribute of the disease, but it is specific to each cause and can differ considerably from one component cause to another: for instance, diethylstilbestrol taken by pregnant women had a long induction period (around 15 years) for the vaginal cancer that developed in their daughters, whereas the hormonal explosion in puberty, among other component causes, showed a much shorter induction period (a few years) for the same event. Therefore, the presence of causal components, different from the drug itself, actually determines whether the ADR appears or not, and when, being actually the reason for the observed interindividual variability. Obviously, the features of the drug (pharmacological actions, dose, duration, pharmaceutical form, route of administration, etc.) also count, but they are not enough.

The set of component causes of an ADR, different from the drug itself, can be considered, broadly speaking, as "predisposing factors." Depending on the timing of the causal components with respect to the drug administration, we can classify them into three categories: (1) **pure predisposing factors**, when they precede the drug administration; (2) **triggering factors**,[1] when they are subsequent to the drug administration; and (3) **co-inducers or cooperators** when they are simultaneous with the drug use (co-inducers having an independent effect, whereas cooperators do not). An explanatory depiction is shown in Fig. 3.2, and examples are described in Table 3.1. Finally, the factors that block or reduce

[1]Sometimes these factors are also referred to as "catalysts," as they shorten the induction time of the disease to occur or be diagnosed. Drugs may act as catalysts themselves (some drugs with some antidopaminergic activity may unmask the diagnosis of Parkinson's disease rather inducing parkinsonism).

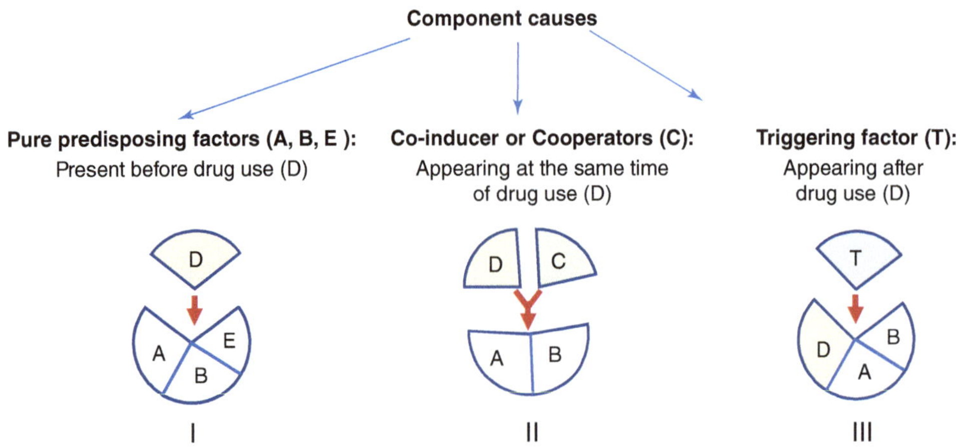

Fig. 3.2 Depiction of the conceptual framework for pure predisposing factors, co-inducers/cooperators, and triggering factors. (I) When the drug use (D) is the last component cause that completes the pie, all others (A, B, and E) precede the drug and can be considered as pure predisposing factors. (II) When the component cause (C) occurs at the same time as the drug use (D), it can be considered a co-inducer (if it has an independent effect) or a cooperator (if it has no independent effect per se and only acts as a cause when the drug is present). (III) The drug (D) and other component causes (A and B) are present, but the disease does not start until T shows up

the expression of the component causes, different from the drug itself, would act as **preventive or minimizing factors** of the ADR, whereas those blocking the action of the drug itself can be specifically considered as **antagonists** (though, practically speaking, they also behave as preventive factors).

Putting the timing aside, we can pragmatically define a predisposing factor for a specific ADR as "*a third variable, different from the drug itself and the indication for which the drug is taken that, when present, increases the risk of suffering an ADR, including the probability of its occurrence, its seriousness or its severity (understood as intensity).*" In other words, a predisposing factor is a "component cause" of a constellation of causes that, along with the drug, conform to the sufficient cause that induces the event that we consider an ADR. As we will explain later on, a predisposing factor may have an independent effect (given other component causes), which is added to the drug effect (given other component causes) or, more often, its combination with the drug may give rise to an overall effect that is stronger than the mere addition of their independent effects. When the latter occurs, we call such a phenomenon "effect modification" or "interaction" (see Sect. 5).

Table 3.1 Categories of predisposing factors based on timing of causal components with respect to drug administration

	Pure predisposing factors	Co-inducers	Cooperators	Triggering factors
Timing with respect to the drug use	Usually before	At the same time	At the same time	After
Capability of inducing the adverse event (in the absence of the drug)	Usually but not necessarily	Always	Never	Usually but not necessarily
Examples	– Old age is a pure predisposing factor for upper gastrointestinal bleeding induced by aspirin – HLA-B*15:02 is a pure predisposing factor for the Stevens–Johnson syndrome/toxic epidermal necrolysis induced by carbamazepine in South Asian populations – Renal failure is a pure predisposing factor for type A ADRs induced by drugs eliminated unaltered by urine when it exists before the drug intake (for chronic treatments, an impairment of renal function may increase the risk of type A ADRs, but, in this case, it would behave as a triggering factor)	– Nonsteroidal anti-inflammatory drugs (NSAIDs) and anticoagulants are co-inducers of upper gastrointestinal bleeding if administered simultaneously (if the NSAID is administered in a patient already anticoagulated, then the anticoagulant may be considered a pure predisposing factor for the upper gastrointestinal bleeding induced by the NSAID, and vice versa) – Most drug–drug pharmacodynamic interactions usually fall under this category	– Potent inhibitors of CYP450 3A4, like macrolides, are cooperators of the toxicity provoked by colchicine overdose, but they are not an independent cause of such toxicity (in the absence of colchicine). If the patient is already treated with a macrolide before using colchicine, then the former can also be viewed as a pure predisposing factor for colchicine toxicity – Most drug–drug or food–drug pharmacokinetic interactions fall under this category	– Estrogen explosion in puberty was presumed to be the triggering factor of vaginal cancer observed in young women whose mothers used diethylstilbestrol during pregnancy (after around 15 years) – Dental intervention is a triggering factor for osteonecrosis of the jaw induced by bisphosphonates

3 The Importance of Predisposing Factors in Pharmacovigilance and Clinical Practice

The identification of predisposing factors is of utmost importance in pharmacovigilance as they are the target of minimization measures such as the restriction of indications or the addition of contraindications or warnings on the drug label. Often, these measures are concerned with predisposing factors like age, sex, the presence of a disease that impairs the elimination of the drug (e.g., renal failure) or increases its effect (e.g., previous peptic ulcer that increases the risk of experiencing an upper gastrointestinal complication in patients using nonsteroidal anti-inflammatory drugs (NSAIDs)), ethnic origin, carrier of a genetic biomarker, etc. The evaluation of causal relationships at the individual level may be beneficial when the ADR report contains information on potential predisposing factors. Some causality algorithms include the existence of predisposing factors as an item to assess such as the one by the Spanish Pharmacovigilance System [3] and others [4].

Knowledge of predisposing factors is also important for the individual care of patients, as a physician could individualize the pharmacological treatment in a better way. For instance, the prescription of a drug, which is eliminated unaltered by urine from a patient with moderate or severe renal insufficiency without dose adjustment, could lead to drug accumulation and dose-dependent ADRs (e.g., metformin and lactic acidosis, or dabigatran and bleeding). Actually, these cases can be categorized as medication errors, with legal consequences to both the practitioner and the health system. In this line, drug utilization studies often use the presence of well-known predisposing factors to assess the quality of the prescription. Finally, patients should be informed by their health-care professionals (physicians, pharmacists, and nurses) on the well-known predisposing factors (e.g., anticoagulated patients should be advised to not use NSAIDs, including those dispensed over the counter (OTC), without informing their doctors first). Health education programs focused on therapy should include the information on the predisposing factors for ADRs as an essential part.

Table 3.2 provides a summary of how the knowledge of predisposing factors may contribute positively to pharmacovigilance and clinical practice.

Table 3.2 Examples on how the knowledge of predisposing factors may help improve pharmacovigilance and clinical practice

Pharmacovigilance practice
Individual causality assessment of ADRs (some algorithms include predisposing factors as an item). To this end, ADR reporting should include information on potential predisposing factors
Changes in the drug label (e.g., inclusion of contraindications, warnings, interactions)
Proposing risk minimization measures in risk management plans
Assessing the quality of prescription through drug utilization studies
Assessing medication errors (the presence of a well-known predisposing factor may be the basis for considering an ADR as a medication error)
Clinical practice
Selecting an alternative drug for the patient with a predisposing factor
Selecting the most appropriate dose schedule for the patient with a predisposing factor
Closer monitoring of patients with predisposing factors (e.g., request of serum levels of the drug)
Intervening on modifiable predisposing factors (e.g., alcohol intake, drug–drug interactions, and food–drug interactions)
Patient education to avoid or minimize the influence of modifiable predisposing factors
Collectively, adequate consideration of predisposing factors contributes to the preventability of ADRs

The burden of disease due to ADRs is considerable, as many studies have pointed out [5, 6], and the identification of certain predisposing factors can help reduce such a burden when effective measures are implemented at the population level. An extraordinary example is the 87.1% reduction of the risk of Stevens–Johnson syndrome/toxic epidermal necrolysis (SJS/TEN) induced by carbamazepine in Taiwan after the implementation of a national program of screening for HLA-B*15:02 in patients who are candidates to receive the drug and selection of an alternative drug in carriers of that trait [7]. Similar trends have also been observed in other Asian countries [8], so that genotyping to prevent these ADRs is now considered the standard of care. Another example is the reduction of hospitalizations (from 54.6 to 25.8 per 100,000 person-years) due to peptic ulcer bleeding (many of which were caused by drugs such as NSAIDs, low-dose aspirin, and anticoagulants) detected in Spain [9], due to the increasing eradication of *Helicobacter pylori* from the population and the wide use of proton pump inhibitors in patients at a high risk of experiencing such complications (e.g., the elderly, antecedents of peptic ulcer, concomitant use of NSAIDs with low-dose aspirin, anticoagulants, or other interacting drugs).

4 Types of Predisposing Factors

There is much information available on the general predisposing factors for ADRs as well as specific information on the predisposing factors for ADRs to specific drugs and specific types of reactions. Pharmacokinetic and pharmacodynamic factors may lead to toxic or exaggerated responses to normal drug doses, thereby leading to adverse events. It could be due to altered pharmacokinetics, resulting in excessively high concentrations of the unbound drug or metabolite at the site of action. Alternatively, a response to a given concentration of drug or metabolite at the site of the action may be exaggerated or unusual because of pharmacodynamic factors, including changes in the number and/or binding affinity of the target receptors as well as alternations in the signal transduction pathways [10]. The pharmacokinetic and pharmacodynamic behaviors of drugs may be influenced by various factors related to patient demographics, disease state, physiological status, drug interactions, and lifestyle. There are essentially four types of predisposing factors: those related to patient characteristics, those related to the underlying diseases, those related to environmental and lifestyle factors, and those related to the use of other drugs.

4.1 Factors Related to Patient Characteristics

4.1.1 Age

Age is a well-identified, significant predisposing factor for the development of adverse drug effects to which geriatric and pediatric populations are more prone.

The Elderly

The International Conference on Harmonization considers older people a "special population," as they differ from younger adults in terms of comorbidity, polypharmacy, and pharmacokinetics and thereby have a higher predisposition to ADRs [11]. The increase in the number of diseases in older people leads to polypharmacy, which naturally increases the risk of drug interactions and adverse events [12]. Aging is associated with physiological changes that affect an individual's medicine-handling capacity, including alterations to body composition, causing changes in volumes of drug distribution and alterations in organ mass, and to blood circulation, causing changes in metabolism and clearance [13, 14].

The majority of ADRs in older people are type A reactions; i.e., they are attributable to a predictable known pharmacological effect of a drug but an exaggerated response resulting in an adverse effect [13]. Age-related decline in renal function and hepatic metabolism may lead to toxicity through excess drug accumulation. Reduced hepatic size and blood flow also contribute to reduced first-pass metabolism, which is especially relevant for drugs with high hepatic extraction that undergo significant first-pass metabolism, e.g., propranolol. In the elderly, the glomerular filtration rate (GFR) is significantly affected due to age-related reductions in renal function and disease states that are common. This can affect the clearance of drugs predominantly eliminated by the kidneys, e.g., penicillin, diuretics, and digoxin. The relative decrease in total body water seen in the elderly may result in a smaller volume of distribution and therefore in higher serum concentrations for water-soluble drugs (e.g., alcohol, gentamicin). On the other hand, the higher proportion of body fat seen in aging can prolong the half-lives of fat-soluble drugs like diazepam and amitriptyline [13, 15]. Elderly patients may have altered pharmacodynamic responses, e.g., the risk of orthostatic hypotension is greater in older people who are prescribed vasodilators because of attenuated baroreceptor responses [13]. Of the many transporters expressed at the blood–brain barrier (BBB) endothelium, several have been implicated in influx and/or efflux of drugs into the central nervous system (CNS). Decreased expression and/or defective function of these transporters leads to increased BBB permeability and thereby toxic effects of drugs [16].

The main risk factors or predictors of ADR-related admissions among older people are advanced age, polypharmacy, comorbidity, longer duration of treatment, and potentially inappropriate medications [17–19]. In the systematic review conducted by Alhawassi et al. [20] for assessing the prevalence and risk factors for ADRs in the elderly in an acute care setting, it was noticed that at least 1 in 10 elderly patients experienced an ADR, leading to or during their hospital stay.

Children

There are multiple factors that influence the different responses of children to drugs compared with adults. The prevalence and nature of ADRs may differ depending on the age of children. For example, neonates are more likely to be sensitive to the adverse effects of morphine, whereas drugs like sodium valproate are associated with an increased risk of problems in children of any age [21]. The risk of specific ADRs may be increased by neonatal differences in body composition, metabolism, and other physiological parameters. With regard to body composition, higher body water content can increase the volume of distribution for water-soluble drugs, and reduced albumin and total protein may result in a higher concentration of highly protein-bound drugs. The immature BBB in neonates can increase sensitivity to drugs acting on the CNS, such as morphine [21, 22]. Chloramphenicol, digoxin, and ototoxic antibiotics such as streptomycin are examples of drugs that have a higher risk of toxicity in the first weeks of life [22]. Although case reports of chloramphenicol toxicity have also been reported in children and adolescents, premature infants and neonates are at highest risk of the gray baby syndrome from chloramphenicol exposure due to their decreased hepatic and renal function [23].

Compared to the available information on the benefits/risks in individual adults, the currently existing information to enable informed decisions to identify and quantify ADRs in neonates and infants is much more limited. Infants commonly receive drugs used off-label, at dosages extrapolated from those in older children or adults. Besides the lack of labeling, inappropriate formulations, polypharmacy, immature organ function, and multiple illnesses further raise the risk of ADRs in neonates and infants [24]. Drugs administered to the mother in the perinatal period also constitute a major route of exposure to ADRs [25].

It is not only neonates, infants, and young children who exhibit increased susceptibility to ADRs but older children and young adults may also do so. A classic example is the increased risk of extrapyramidal effects associated with metoclopramide in children and young adults (15–19 years of age) [26]. The heightened probability of dosing errors due to dose calculations using body weight can also contribute to potential harms [22]. When drugs are newly introduced to the market, they usually do not possess adequate safety information related to children, as this group is under-represented in clinical trials. Moreover, children may present specific ADRs related to maturity, growth, and development that are nonexistent in adults. An example is the growth retardation observed with systemic corticosteroids [27].

In a focused analysis on adverse drug events as reported in the MedWatch adverse event reports system, Moore et al. identified 7111 reports (1.5% of the total dataset) in infants and children under 2 years of age over a period of 3 years, with a high mortality rate in the first month of life [25]. All reports of suspected ADRs with a fatal outcome in children received by the UK Committee on Safety of Medicines through its Yellow Card Scheme from 1964 until December 2000 were reviewed. It was identified that there were 331 deaths with 390 suspected medicines reported for children aged 16 years or less. The medicines most frequently mentioned were anticonvulsants, cytotoxics, anesthetic agents, and antibiotics, and the individual drug most frequently mentioned was sodium valproate. Hepatic failure was the most frequently occurring serious ADR [28].

4.1.2 Sex

In general, women may be more susceptible to ADRs and the female sex is considered as a risk factor for the development of ADRs in a variety of drug groups [10, 22, 29]. It is postulated that women are more at risk of developing ADRs due to differences in pharmacokinetics, pharmacodynamics, toxicokinetics, toxicodynamics, and drug use compared to men [10, 22, 29, 30]. Women generally have a lower lean body mass, reduced hepatic clearance, differences in the activity of cytochrome P450 (CYP) enzymes, and metabolize drugs at different rates compared to men [10]. Furthermore, hormonal status, body composition (the relative proportions of muscular and adipose tissues), amount of drug-binding proteins, renal blood flow, and sex-specific differences in the immune system could influence drug responses [30, 31]. Sex-dependent activity of clinically relevant CYP families is present, with evidence suggesting that CYP2E1 and CYP1A2 activities are higher in males than in females, whereas CYP3A, one of the most clinically relevant CYP isoforms, appears to exhibit greater activity in females [32]. In addition, important factors such as conjugation, absorption, protein binding, and renal elimination may all have some sex-based differences [10]. Furthermore, sex-specific hormonal effects or interaction with signaling molecules that can affect drug safety are important [30]. Men and women also show different pharmacodynamic responses to a variety of drugs, particularly with cardiac and psychotropic medications [10, 30].

Unique issues in women, such as menopause, pregnancy, oral contraceptive use, and physiological and hormonal changes during the menstrual cycle, can also have significant effects on drug metabolism, which can be clinically important [30, 31]. It is likely that a variety of physiological changes that occur during pregnancy may affect the pharmacokinetics of drugs. Drug distribution and protein binding are changed by pregnancy. While some drug-metabolizing enzymes demonstrate an increase in activity, others exhibit an apparent decrease in activity. Pregnancy alters the apparent activities of multiple drug transporters, resulting in changes in the net renal secretion of drugs. The higher serum concentrations of digoxin reported in pregnant patients may be caused by increased bioavailability due to decreased gastric emptying time during pregnancy [33].

Sex can influence the amount and type of medications used. Women use a significantly different range of drugs than do men, particularly drugs associated with oral contraception, menopause, and pregnancy. Oral contraceptives can both affect the metabolism of and be affected by a wide range of other therapeutic drugs. For example, paracetamol is conjugated more in women taking an oral contraceptive compared with controls [34]. A number of conditions, including urinary tract infections, arthritis, depression, and anxiety disorders, are also more prevalent in women, and, accordingly, the use of medications for managing these conditions differs [10]. In general, not only do women use more sex-specific drugs, they may also use more general medications [35]. Additionally, factors such as the difference, if any, in the promptness in seeking medical attention when medical complications arise, and the importance placed on illness between sex have been suggested to be responsible for the possible difference in the prevalence of ADRs based on sex [36].

There are certain ADRs that appear to be more common in women. It is generally established that women experience more severe ADR outcomes compared to men, such as hepatic ones [30]. Impairment of concentration and psychiatric adverse events associated with mefloquine are more common in females [22]. Females are more susceptible to drug-induced torsade de pointes, a ventricular arrythmia, which is considered to be due to their longer QTc interval (duration of ventricular electrical systole (QT) corrected for heart rate) compared to men [22]. Estrogen seems to reduce the density of I_{Kr} potassium channels (I_{Kr} type; inward rectifier potassium current), which results in slower repolarization and prolongation of the QT interval [37].

Rodenburg et al. conducted a large study in the Netherlands to understand the sex-related differences in hospital admissions attributed to ADRs. In all different drug classes, significant differences existed between the sexes in ADR-related hospital admissions, with cardiovascular drugs accounting for the most pronounced differences. Overall, the number of ADR-related hospital admissions confirmed the higher risk of women to be hospitalized due to an ADR. Instead, the risk of ADR-related hospitalizations attributed to antirheumatic drug use was higher in men. Diabetes due to glucocorticoids and hypoglycemic coma due to insulin and antidiabetic agents were more frequent in men. Men were more frequently hospitalized for ADRs following antibiotic use. Admission for osteoporosis due to adrenal cortical steroids was more frequent in women [29].

4.1.3 Ethnicity

Ethnicity may be associated with a higher prevalence of certain genetic variants of human leukocyte antigens (HLAs), crucial for some hypersensitivity reactions (see Sect. 4.1.4), and may also be associated with polymorphisms affecting some drug metabolic routes, such as cytochrome P450, which can explain the greater susceptibility to ADRs of some ethnic groups [22]. Moreover, social behaviors and lifestyle factors can be linked to ethnicity. Although the study results were limited by multiple factors, a systematic review conducted by Baehr et al. [38] to assess the racial and ethnic disparities in ADRs identified the following findings. Asians may be at particular risk of anticoagulant-related ADRs, Blacks may be at increased risk of diabetic agent-related ADRs, and Whites may be at increased risk of opioid-related ADRs. It was reported in a pharmacogenomic study by Takahashi et al. that *VKORC1* and CYP2C9 polymorphisms contribute to interpopulation differences in warfarin doses among the three studied populations: Caucasians, Japanese, and African Americans [39].

McDowell et al. [40] systematically reviewed the evidence for increased susceptibility to adverse reactions to cardiovascular drugs in certain ethnic groups. Although their study had reported limitations, it provided valuable details as presented below. The relative risk (RR) of angioedema associated with angiotensin-converting enzyme (ACE) inhibitors was higher in Black patients compared with White patients, and the risk of cough was enhanced in patients from East Asia (i.e., China, Korea, or Japan), compared with White patients. In Black patients, thrombolytic therapy was associated with an increased risk of moderate or severe bleeding and also with intracranial hemorrhage [40]. Individual studies of hypertensive therapy reported an increased risk of depression with hydrochlorothiazide and with all hypertensive therapy in Blacks compared with Whites. Digitalis therapy was also associated with an increased risk of hospital admission for ADRs in Black patients compared with White patients [41]. Pharmacokinetic studies suggest greater plasma concentrations of some statins or their active metabolites in subjects of East Asian ethnicity compared with Whites due to differences in the prevalence of variant alleles coding for statin-metabolizing enzymes and membrane transporters. Chinese patients appear to be more susceptible to myopathy induced by simvastatin [42]. The most obvious difference in statin pharmacokinetics in East Asians is in terms of rosuvastatin [43].

4.1.4 Genetic Factors

Most pharmacokinetic processes are mediated by proteins, such as drug-metabolizing enzymes or membrane drug transporters. Moreover, many drug targets are proteins themselves such as ion channels, enzymes, or receptors. Thus, their functionality is genetically determined and a variation in the genes that encode them may increase the probability of experiencing an ADR of type A or, on the other hand, it may reduce the efficacy of the drug [44, 45]. Moreover, some ADRs of type B can be genetically mediated, such as those linked to some enzymatic deficits that control critical physiological processes (e.g., hemolytic anemia induced by oxidative drugs in patients with a glucose-6-phosphatase dehydrogenase deficiency) or those triggered by immunogenic mechanisms in susceptible populations (e.g., hypersensitivity reactions) [46–48]. Depending on the underlying mechanism, we can envision five categories of genetically determined ADRs: (1) variant drug-metabolizing enzymes;

(2) variant drug transporters; (3) variant drug targets (enzymes, channels, receptors); (4) variant human leukocyte antigens (HLAs); and (5) variant enzyme-governing processes not related to the drug's own pharmacokinetics or pharmacodynamics (which predispose to the so-called idiosyncratic reactions). The first three induce ADRs of type A and the last two ADRs of type B. Table 3.3 provides some examples in which there is consistent information of a genetic basis. The identification of a genetic variation as a predisposing factor for some ADRs may lead to the clinical use of biomarkers to predict the ADR and help minimize the risk in the population. However, showing an association between an ADR and a genetic variation is not enough. For a predictive genetic test to be included in clinical practice, the following criteria should be consid

Table 3.3 Types and examples of genetic variants as predisposing factors for ADRs

Drug	Mechanism	Genetic factor	ADR (type)	Genotyping included in drug label (FDA)[a] or SmPC (EU)
Abacavir[b,c,d]	Hypersensitivity reaction	HLA-B*57:01	Hypersensitivity reactions, DRESS syndrome (type B)	Yes, mandatory to all patients before treatment
Allopurinol[b,c,d]	Hypersensitivity reaction	HLA-B*58:01	SJS/TEN (type B)	Yes, for information (in Han Chinese, Thai, Korean)
Amoxicillin–clavulanic acid[e,f]	Hypersensitivity reaction	HLA-DRB1*15:01 HLA-DQB1*06:02 HLA-A*02:01 HLA-B*18:01	DILI (type B)	No
Antiarrhythmic classes IA and III[e]	Variant drug target (cardiac K channel)	KCNQ1 KCNH2	Arrhythmias (TdP) in patients with cLQTS (type A)	No
Azathioprine[c]	Variant drug-metabolizing enzyme	TPMT NUDT15	Myelosuppression (type A)	Yes, mandatory or highly recommended. Alternatively, consider phenotype testing for TPMT
Carbamazepine[b,c]	Hypersensitivity reaction	HLA-B*15:02	SJS/TEN (type B)	Yes, highly recommended in Han Chinese and Thai populations (Malaysian and Indian)
Carbamazepine[b,c]	Hypersensitivity reaction	HLA-B*31:01	DRESS, SJS/TEN (type B)	Yes, for information (in European descendants and Japanese populations)
Flecainide[e]	Variant drug target (cardiac Na channel)	SCN5A	Brugada syndrome (type A)	No
Flucloxacillin[d,e,f]	Hypersensitivity reaction	HLA-B*57:01	DILI (type B)	No
Irinotecan[c,d]	PK-drug-metabolizing enzyme (UGT1A1)	UGT1A1	Neutropenia, severe diarrhea (type A)	Yes, for information
Oxidant drugs (sulfonamides, chloroquine, quinolones)[d,e]	Idiosyncratic reaction In patients with G6PDH deficiency	G6PDH	Hemolytic anemia (type B)	No

(continued)

Table 3.3 (continued)

Drug	Mechanism	Genetic factor	ADR (type)	Genotyping included in drug label (FDA)[a] or SmPC (EU)
Simvastatin[b]	Variant drug transporter (OATP1B1)	SLCO1B1	Myopathy (type A)	Yes, for information (recommended if high doses)
Warfarin[c,d]	Variant drug-metabolizing enzyme	CYP2C9	Bleeding (type A)	Yes, for information
Warfarin[b,c,d]	Variant drug target (enzyme)	VKORC1	Bleeding (type A)	Yes, for information

Abbreviations: *cLQTS* congenital long QT syndrome, *CYP* cytochrome P450, *DILI* drug-induced liver injury, *DRESS* drug reaction with eosinophilia and systemic symptoms, *G6PDH* glucose-6-phosphate dehydrogenase, *K* potassium, *EMA* European Medicines Agency, *FDA* Food and Drug Administration, *Na* sodium, *OATP1B1* organic anion transporter polypeptide family member 1B1, *SLCO1B1* solute carrier organic anion transporter family member 1B1, *SmPC* summary of product characteristics, *SSJ/TEN* Stevens–Johnson syndrome/toxic epidermal necrolysis, *TdP* torsade de pointes, *TPMT* thiopurine methyltransferase, *UGT1A1* UDP glucuronosyltransferase family one member A1, *VKORC1* vitamin K epoxide reductase complex type 1

[a] A updated list can be found at https://www.fda.gov/drugs/science-and-research-drugs/table-pharmacogenomic-biomarkers-drug-labeling

[b] EMA/CHMP/281371/2013: A guideline on the key aspects of the use of pharmacogenomics in the pharmacovigilance of medicinal products, 2015

[c] Pratt et al., Medical Genetics Summaries, National Center for Biotechnology Information (US), 2021

[d] Wang et al. [44]

[e] Micaglio et al. [46]

[f] Böhm and Cascorbi [48]

ered [49]: (1) medical need; (2) clinical validity and utility of testing (low probability of false-positive and false-negative results and a low number of patients needed to screen to prevent the event); (3) relative ease of use; and (4) existing choice of treatments. It is advisable to refer to Chap. 23 for further details on the influence of genetics on drug safety.

4.1.5 Immunological Considerations

ADRs that involve a specific drug-induced immune response are referred to as drug hypersensitivity reactions. Although induction of a drug-induced immune response is the main event involved in drug hypersensitivity, induction of an antibody response alone is not the pathological process. Taking into consideration that many patients with antidrug antibodies or drug-induced autoantibodies remain asymptomatic, it is highly likely that there are individual risk factors associated with the translation of an immune response into tissue damage. All drug hypersensitivity reactions involve several sequential steps, each of which may provide sources of interindividual variation [15].

4.2 Factors Related to the Underlying Diseases

Concomitant host disease or comorbidities may influence susceptibility to ADRs. The best example is human immunodeficiency virus (HIV) disease, which increases the frequency of toxicity with co-trimoxazole. It is reported that adverse reactions to co-trimoxazole increase from approximately 2–8% in the general population to more than 43% among HIV-positive individuals to approximately 69% in subjects with acquired immunodeficiency syndrome (AIDS) [50]. The reasons behind this increased frequency of ADRs with co-trimoxazole are likely to be more complex than only changes in drug-metabolizing capacity; immune dysregulation may also play a part [51]. Another classical example of the influence of specific disease is infectious mononucleosis (due to Epstein–Barr virus), which greatly increases the risk of rash in patients administered amoxicillin [21].

Usual doses of drugs produce higher-than-normal serum drug concentrations in patients with kidney or liver disease, especially for drug or drug metabolites that are highly dependent on the kidneys or liver for elimination. This requires special consideration, particularly for drugs with a narrow therapeutic index, which might result in an exaggerated response [10]. Reductions in renal and hepatic function can alter drug handling, and this has implications for practical therapeutics, including an increased risk of ADRs [21]. Reduction in hepatic blood flow as a consequence of acute myocardial infarction or heart failure may decrease the elimination of drugs that are normally highly extracted by the liver. Hypothyroidism may be associated with a decrease in both hepatic and renal drug clearances, resulting in an exaggerated response [10]. Table 3.4 provides examples of few specific drug–disease interactions, which increase the risk of ADRs.

4.3 Factors Related to Environmental Factors

4.3.1 Lifestyle Factors

Both the pharmacokinetics and pharmacodynamics of drugs may be altered by lifestyle factors such as alcohol and caffeine consumption. Alcohol can exaggerate the CNS depressant effects of drugs, including benzodiazepines, phenothiazines, tricyclic antidepressants, opiates, and some antihistamines. Caffeine has a potentially dangerous stimulant effect when taken with ephedrine in herbal weight loss and athletic performance-enhancing supplements [55]. Cigarette smoking is known to increase the metabolism of many drugs via inducing CYP1A2 (e.g., clozapine, olanzapine, caffeine, R-warfarin, erlotinib) [56, 57], CYP2B6 (e.g., methadone) [56], and uridine diphosphate (UDP)-glucuronyltransferase (UGT) (e.g., clozapine, mirtazapine) [57].

4.3.2 Food–Drug Interactions

Food–drug interactions can also have negative outcomes. The salt, protein, or vitamin content of a diet may affect the renal excretion of drugs. An

Table 3.4 Disease effects on drug pharmacokinetics and pharmacodynamics and influence on safety

Drug–disease interaction	End effect	Mechanism
Cefepime and kidney disease [52]	Life-threatening cefepime induced neurotoxicity in patients with acute kidney failure	Cefepime is highly dependent on the kidneys for elimination, and, hence, dose reductions are highly critical in patients with severe kidney disease
Opioids and liver [53]	Patients with liver disease have an unusual sensitivity to opioids such that even small doses can precipitate encephalopathy	Increased density and affinity to opioid receptors in the brain is the proposed explanation
Digoxin and hypothyroidism [54]	Increased risk of digoxin toxicity	Hypothyroidism increases serum digoxin concentration by decreasing the glomerular filtration rate and volume of distribution of digoxin. The myocardium of patients with myxoedema may have a reduced tolerance to digoxin
Digoxin and electrolyte imbalance (hypokalemia) [54]	Increased risk of digoxin toxicity	Potassium competes with digoxin for myocardial receptor-binding sites, and hypokalemia results in an increase in myocardial digoxin uptake, a decrease in sodium–potassium pump activity (increased digoxin binding to the sodium potassium pump), and a decrease in tubular secretion of digoxin

example is when a patient taking lithium initiates a low-salt diet for treatment of hypertension or heart failure, he/she excretes less lithium, which may result in higher serum lithium concentrations and potential toxicity [58]. A further example is a low-protein diet that is associated with decreased renal clearance of oxypurinol (the active metabolite of allopurinol) [59].

Concomitant administration of grapefruit juice can increase the plasma concentration of numerous drugs in humans, and such elevations of drug plasma concentrations have, on occasion, resulted in adverse clinical effects. Increased concentrations are primarily mediated by chemicals in grapefruit juice, which inhibit the CYP 3A4 drug-metabolizing enzyme in the small intestines [60]. A classic example is the interaction between grapefruit juice and cyclosporine, which has been shown to cause an increase in both parent and metabolite profiles, indicating an alteration in the disposition of cyclosporine and metabolites. This interaction is of potential clinical importance in terms of mechanism, side effects, and dosing [61]. Similarly, a sudden decrease in vitamin K intake from dark-green vegetables can increase the risk of bleeding in patients using warfarin [62].

4.4 Drug-Related Factors

It is important to note that while the dose and duration of treatment are, obviously, factors linked to ADRs (in particular to type A), they are dimensions of the drug itself and thus cannot be formally considered predisposing factors. According to the definition provided in Sect. 2, a predisposing factor should be "a third variable, different from the drug itself and the indication for which the drug is taken." Thus, in this section, we will consider other factors that may modify the effect of the drug such as interactions, polypharmacy, and pharmaceutical factors that may alter its bioavailability.

4.4.1 Drug–Drug Interactions

Altered pharmacokinetics or pharmacodynamics as a result of drug–drug interactions may contribute to ADRs. The most frequent contributing factors are those drug interactions that affect bioavailability and drug elimination. Most commonly, drug-induced inhibition of cytochrome P450 enzymes can result in the reduced metabolism of certain drugs, resulting in increased concentration of the affected drugs and resultant ADRs. P-glycoprotein, a protein expressed on the luminal surface of intestinal epithelial cells, biliary hepatocytes, and renal tubular cells transports the drug from within the cell to the intestine, bile, or urine, respectively. Inhibition of P-glycoprotein by certain drugs can increase the bioavailability and decrease the renal and biliary excretion of their substrates, thus increasing their serum concentrations [63].

Displacement of a drug from plasma proteins by another drug results in only transient increases in the free and active drug and hence does not generally result in adverse effects [64, 65]. However, there may be significant interactions when the affected drugs have a narrow therapeutic margin; an example is drug interactions with warfarin, which can result in displacement of warfarin from the protein-binding site and in an increase in free warfarin plasma concentration.

Pharmacodynamic mechanisms could also be behind drug–drug interactions. They arise when the pharmacological effect of one drug is affected by that of another. Pharmacodynamic drug–drug interactions are typically categorized as synergistic, additive, or antagonistic [66]. Examples include serotonin syndrome caused by adding tramadol to a selective serotonin reuptake inhibitor (SSRI) [67] or excessive reduction in blood pressure and symptomatic hypotension by addition of ACE inhibitors in patients who have been sodium and/or volume depleted by thiazide or loop diuretics [68].

The information available regarding drug interactions from various resources has certain limitations. The value of these tools could be diminished if too many minor or clinically insignificant interactions are included, which leads to the phenomenon of alert fatigue where practitioners ignore the alerts provided by the system due to the total volume of the generated alerts [69, 70]. Furthermore, there is a lack of consistency and standardization in the information provided by different resources. The availability of drug–drug interaction evidence in a standardized format with adequate literature support and inclusion of clinical management options can improve prescribing decisions [71]. The use of the number needed to treat to have a clinical interaction, as suggested by Martín-Pérez et al., would be a helpful tool for clinicians [72].

4.4.2 Polypharmacy

The probability of ADRs increases as the number of medications increases in a patient. The risk may be higher due to the basic increase in the probability of any ADR as more drugs are included as well as the increased risk of drug–drug interactions. The effects of multiple drug use are not simply additive but are rather likely to be synergistic. At the same time, the concept of confounding by multiple disease states must be borne in mind [21].

The likelihood of a serious ADR increases with multiple drug exposures/the number of drugs received, and this relationship becomes statistically significant when patients are exposed to four or more drugs [64]. In a systematic review conducted by Saedder et al. to evaluate the evidence of the relationship between patient-related risk factors and the risk of serious ADRs, the total number of drugs was the most consistent correlated risk factor found in both univariate and multivariate analyses in both the general adult population and the elderly [73].

4.4.3 Pharmaceutical Factors

The pharmaceutical aspects of a particular dosage form can lead to predictable ADRs because of alterations in the quantity of the drug present or of its release characteristics [21]. For example, a rate-controlled preparation of indomethacin was withdrawn after reports of localized intestinal bleeding and perforation that occurred as a consequence of the delayed-release mechanism [28].

5 Tools to Identify Predisposing Factors

As previously discussed, a predisposing factor is a component of a constellation of causes, in addition to the drug, which constitutes the sufficient cause inducing the ADR. Such predisposing factors may be biologically acting independently of the drug, simply summing its contribution, or, often, may interact with the drug, resulting in an overall effect different than the addition of their independent effects. In the latter case, epidemiologists say that there is an "interaction of causes" or "an effect modification." Both terms are essentially synonyms [74], but "effect modification" is more appealing when, according to the hypothetical causal model, it is clear which variable is the main exposure of interest and which is the potential effect modifier. Using this terminology, many predisposing factors of drug safety problems can be conceived as effect modifiers.

In drug safety, an effect modifier is a third variable, distinct from both the drug and the event, which modifies the magnitude of the drug–event association when present (for dichotomous effect modifiers) or when it changes its category (for polytomous effect modifiers) or level (for ordinal and quantitative effect modifiers). For simplicity's sake, we will consider the example of a dichotomous effect modifier in the discussion that follows. When the modification moves the effect measure (or more properly the measure of association[2]) away from its null value, the effect modifier strengthens the association (either positive or negative). This situation is also called "synergistic interaction". When the effect modifier brings the measure of association closer to its null value, the effect modifier weakens the asso-

[2]When the causality is not yet established, the term "association" or "measure of association" is more appropriate than the term "effect" or "effect measure," as the latter always implies a causal relationship. For this reason, we consider it preferable to use "association" throughout this chapter. However, the term "effect modifier" or "effect modification factor" is commonly used in the epidemiological textbooks and literature, and, for the sake of consistency, we follow this terminology, but the reader should have this caveat present.

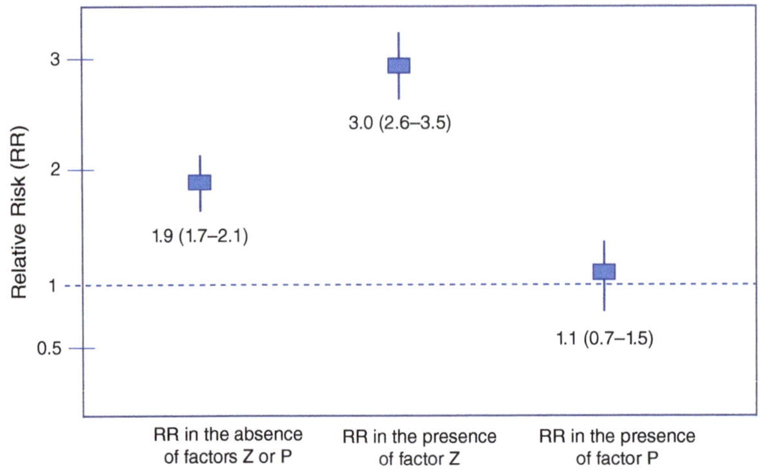

Fig. 3.3 Graphical representation of the two types of effect modifiers that are of special interest in pharmacovigilance: a predisposing factor (*Z*) and a preventive factor (*P*). A hypothetical example. The effect of a drug on an event is estimated through the relative risk (the ratio of the incidence among the exposed divided by the incidence among the nonexposed). In people who have neither factor *Z* nor factor *P*, the exposure to the study drug (as compared to those nonexposed) increases by 90% the risk of the event (a relative risk of 1.9, with a 95% confidence interval (95% CI) of 1.7–2.1). Among people who have factor *Z* (but not factor *P*), the exposure to the drug further increases the risk of the event up to a relative risk of 3.0 (with a 95% CI of 2.6–3.5), whereas among people who have factor *P* (but not factor *Z*), the effect of the drug weakens or practically disappears (showed by a relative risk of 1.1, with a 95% CI of 0.7–1.5). A predisposing factor would operatively act as factor *Z*. A preventive factor, a minimization measure, or an antagonist would operatively act as factor *P*. In this representation, for simplicity's sake, both factors *Z* and *P* are assumed to be dichotomous

ciation (either positive or negative). This is usually called "antagonistic interaction".

On the additive scale, a positive association is operatively defined when the risk difference between the exposed and the unexposed is >0 (in this case, the risk difference is usually known as attributable risk) and is negative when it is <0 (usually called absolute risk reduction).[3] On the multiplicative scale, a positive association is defined when the measure of association (relative risk [RR], rate ratio, hazard ratio [HR], or odds ratio [OR]) is >1 and is negative when it is below (i.e., between >0 and <1). From a conceptual point of view, a positive association means that the probability (or risk[4]) of presenting an event increases in the presence of the drug, whereas a negative association means that the probability (or risk) of presenting an event decreases when a drug is present. An ADR, by definition, implies that the risk of presenting the event increases, and, then, in pharmacovigilance, we usually deal with positive associations, unless we are evaluating the effectiveness of a risk minimization measure, in which case a negative association is expected. In this context, a predisposing factor for experiencing an ADR induced by a certain drug is an effect modifier that strengthens a positive association. On the contrary, a preventive factor or a risk minimization measure weakens a positive association (see Fig. 3.3 for a graphical representation of these concepts).

According to this conceptual framework, a predisposing factor can only be formally identified through study designs that allow estimating valid measures of association (usually called "analytical" studies). In "nonanalytical" or "defective" study designs, the existence of a predisposing factor can be suggested but not formally assessed.

[3]The measures of association on the additive scale (attributable risk and absolute risk reduction) are more frequently denominated as "impact measures" or "population impact measures."

[4]Risk always implies causality.

5.1 Identifying Predisposing Factors Through Analytical Study Designs

An analytical design is a study that allows computing measures of association that, under optimal conditions of comparability (validity), can be interpreted as causal effects. The most reliable of all analytical methods is the randomized clinical trial, actually the paradigm of clinical research, but its interventional nature makes it hard to be used in drug safety assessment (unless the outcome is a surrogate variable, as the area under the curve in the case of pharmacokinetic drug–drug interactions), also their limited sample size and usually short duration make the clinical trials inefficient to detect ADRs of low frequency and long induction periods. For this reason, in the pharmacovigilance arena (as well as in public health in general), we rely on observational methods and, among them, cohort and case–control studies are the most widely used (the so-called traditional designs). Notwithstanding, in the last two decades, case-only designs have been increasingly used in pharmacoepidemiology to assess drug safety issues, provided that events are sudden and transient and, importantly, that drug exposure varies over time [75, 76].

For assessing effect modifiers, the measures obtained on the multiplicative scale (relative risk [RR], rate ratio [RR], hazard ratio [HR], or odds ratio [OR]) are by far the most widely used. The reason is twofold: (1) the relative measures can be estimated in all analytical epidemiological studies and (2) the regression models, which are the most commonly used methods for confounding control are built on the multiplicative scale and allow directly assessing the effect modification by including a multiplicative term in the model. However, it may happen that an effect modifier is only detected on the additive scale, and, from a pharmacovigilance standpoint, it is, certainly, of interest. In the following, we will review both.

5.1.1 Assessing Effect Modifiers on the Multiplicative Scale

The simplest way to assess an effect modifier on the multiplicative scale is through a stratified analysis in which the population is divided in two strata: those who present the potential effect modifier and those who do not. In each stratum, the drug–event association is assessed and, then, the differences between the two measures of association obtained are compared using an interaction test. A practical way to do this is by using the interaction test described by Altman and Bland [77] in which the ratio of relative risks (RRRs) is calculated along with their respective 95% CIs. When the 95% CI does not embrace the null value, the difference between the two RRs is considered statistically significant. Based on this method, Hutchon [78] developed an offline calculator that easily allows estimating the RRR and its 95% CI (see the example provided in Table 3.5). In case–control studies, we would compute the ratio of ORs instead of RRRs. Alternatively, researchers may opt to assess the presence of potential interactions on the multiplicative scale by introducing a product term in the regression models [74, 79].

5.1.2 Assessing Effect Modifiers on the Additive Scale

Assuming *A* to be the drug and *Z* to be the potential predisposing factor, the *expected* absolute risk in patients who used *A* and had factor *Z*, assuming no effect modification, would be as follows [79]:

$$\text{Expected}\,R_{A+Z} = R_A + R_Z - R_{\text{No}A-\text{No}Z} \qquad (3.1)$$

where Expected R_{A+Z} = expected absolute risk of the drug *A* in patients with the predisposing factor *Z*; R_A = observed absolute risk of the drug itself (in the absence of *Z*); and R_Z = observed absolute risk of the predisposing factor *Z* itself (in the absence of *A*). As R_{NoANoZ} is the background risk and is counted twice, in both R_A and R_Z, it is necessary to be subtracted once.

Table 3.5 Assessment of a predisposing factor on the multiplicative scale. In this hypothetical example, a cohort study was carried out to evaluate the risk of upper gastrointestinal bleeding (UGIB) in patients using nonsteroidal anti-inflammatory drugs (NSAIDs). The researchers examined whether the antecedents of previous UGIB were a predisposing factor for having a new episode. To do this, they grouped patients into two strata: those with UGIB antecedents and those without, estimated the rate ratios in each stratum, and compared them using the interaction test described by Altman and Bland [77]. The results show that having a history of UGIB significantly increases by almost three times the rate ratio of presenting a new episode when exposed to NSAIDs (from 2.47 to 7.14)

	Current users of NSAIDs	Nonusers of NSAIDs	Rate ratio (95% CI)
All patients			
UGIB cases	100	32	–
Person-years (p-y)	10,000	10,000	–
Incidence rate	10.0 per 1000 p-y	3.2 per 1000 p-y	3.13 (2.08–4.81)
Stratum 1: Patients with a history of UGIB[a]			
UGIB cases	50	14	–
Person-years	1000	2000	–
Incidence rate	50.0 per 1000 p-y	7.0 per 1000 p-y	7.14 (3.89–13.99)
Stratum 2: Patients with no history of UGIB			
UGIB cases	50	18	–
Person-years	9000	8000	–
Incidence rate	5.6 per 1000 p-y	2.3 per 1000 p-y	2.47 (1.42–4.50)
Ratio of rate ratios (95% CI) (RR of stratum 1/RR of stratum 2)			**RRR = 2.89 (1.22–6.84)**[b] *Z*-score: 2.4151 *p*-value = 0.016

[a] Having antecedents of UGIB has an independent effect for a new episode to occur and can be estimated in the cohort of nonusers by dividing the rate of patients with antecedents by the rate of patients without, that is, 7.0 per 1000 p-y/2.3 per 1000 p-y = 3.04. Thus, having an antecedent of UGIB increases the risk of a new one by 3 times (from 2.3 to 7.0 per 1000 person-years), but if the patient uses an NSAID, then his/her risk increases by 21 times (from 2.3 to 50 per 1000 person-years)

[b] RRR, ratio of rate ratios (or ratio of relative risks) calculated using the Hutchon calculator [78]

We may express Eq. (3.1) as attributable risks (ARs), by subtracting the baseline risk (when neither *A* nor *Z* is present) from each absolute risk, as follows:

$$\text{Expected}\left(R_{A+Z} - R_{\text{No}A\text{No}Z}\right) = \left[R_A - R_{\text{No}A\text{No}Z}\right] + \left[R_Z - R_{\text{No}A\text{No}Z}\right] \quad (3.2)$$

which may be simplified as follows:

$$\text{Expected}\,\text{AR}_{A+Z} = \text{AR}_A + \text{AR}_Z \quad (3.3)$$

Then, the *expected* effect[5] of the combination of *A* and *Z* is simply the sum of their independent effects, under the assumption of no effect modification (or no interaction).

Now, the *observed* AR_{A+Z} (the result found in the study) is compared with the *expected* AR_{A+Z}. A difference >0 would denote the presence of an effect modification and would allow us to conclude that factor *Z* is an effect modifier.

Table 3.6 shows the results using the data from Table 3.5. The *observed* AR of NSAIDs in patients with antecedents of UGIB is 47.7, whereas the *expected* AR of NSAIDs in these patients is 8 (the sum of the independent ARs of NSAIDs and antecedents of UGIB). As AR is a measure of the effects of the respective factors studied on UGIB, the interpretation is that the

[5] Attributable risk can be considered an estimation of the effect of the exposure concerned, assuming that there is no bias.

Table 3.6 Assessment of a predisposing factor on the additive scale. Data were obtained from Table 3.5. The predisposing factor assessed is the antecedents of UGIB, and the drugs of interest is NSAIDs. To calculate the attributable risks, we subtract the corresponding incidence rate from the incidence rate of reference (that of nonusers who had no UGIB antecedents)

	NSAIDs users	Nonusers
(a) Incidence rates		
Antecedents of UGIB	50.0	7.0
No antecedents of UGIB	5.6	2.3
(b) Attributable risks		
Antecedents of UGIB	47.7	4.7
No antecedents of UGIB	3.3	0.0

AR_A (independent effect of NSAIDs when there are no antecedents of UGIB) = 5.6 − 2.3 (per 1000 person-years) = 3.3 (per 1000 person-years)
AR_Z (independent effect of antecedents of UGIB when NSAIDs are not present: nonusers) = 7.0 − 2.3 (per 1000 person-years) = 4.7 (per 1000 person-years)
Expected $AR_{A+Z} = 3.3 + 4.7 = 8.0$
Observed $AR_{A+Z} = 47.7$

NSAIDs' effect (on UGIB) is much greater when the patients had antecedents of UGIB than when they did not. Then, it is demonstrated that having an antecedent of UGIB is a predisposing factor for presenting a new one when the patient is exposed to NSAIDs.

The assessment on the additive scale can also be carried out using relative measures, which is highly convenient as ARs cannot be derived from all analytical studies, but all of them do provide relative measures. The method is described by Rothman [79] and consists of estimating the "relative excess risk due to interaction" (RERI), with the equation to assess the interaction between two factors *A* (the drug in our case) and *Z* (the potential predisposing factor) as follows:

$$\text{RERI} = \text{Observed}\,\text{RR}_{A+Z} - \left(\text{Observed}\,\text{RR}_{A} + \text{Observed}\,\text{RR}_{Z} - 1\right) \quad (3.4)$$

where Observed RR_{A+Z} is the observed risk in patients having the two factors (users of NSAIDs with UGIB antecedents) relative to the reference (situation in which none of the two factors are present) and RR_A and RR_Z are the observed independent risks of factors *A* and *Z*, respectively, relative to the reference (Eq. (3.4) derives from Eq. (3.1) when we divide all terms by $R_{NoA-NoZ}$ to obtain the respective relative risks).[6] To apply this equation, it is necessary to build a variable with four categories (for two dichotomous variables): neither *A* nor *Z*, *A* alone, *Z* alone, and *A* + *Z*, and obtain the RR of each category as compared to the reference (No*A*–No*Z*). The sum of the observed RR_A and RR_Z would be the expected RR_{A+Z}, assuming that there is no interaction or effect modification, but as the null value of the RR is 1 and it is summed two times, we should subtract 1 to avoid duplication. An RERI >0 means that the observed relative effect of the combination of the two factors is greater than the sum of the independent relative effects, denoting that there is an interaction or an effect modification on the additive scale between *A* and *Z*. In other words, assuming that *A* is the drug and *Z* is the potential predisposing factor, an RERI >0 means that the potential predis-

[6]Expected $R_{A+Z}/R_{NoA-NoZ} = (R_A/R_{NoA-NoZ}) + (R_Z/R_{NoA-NoZ}) - (R_{NoA-NoZ}/R_{NoA-NoZ})$; then,
Expected RR_{A+Z} = Observed RR_A + Observed RR_Z − 1;
RERI = Observed RR_{A+Z} − Expected RR_{A+Z} = Observed RR_{A+Z} − (Observed RR_A + Observed RR_Z − 1).

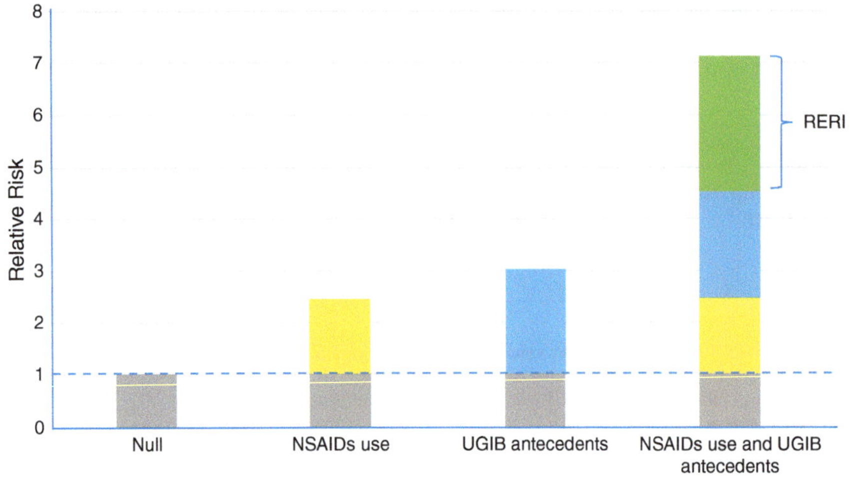

Fig. 3.4 Assessing the antecedents of UGIB as a potential predisposing factor for presenting a new episode of UGIB associated with NSAIDs using relative measures on an additive scale. The data were obtained from Table 3.5. The null value of the relative risk (value = 1) is presented in gray, the excess relative risk associated with NSAID use (RR-1 = 1.47) in yellow, the relative excess risk associated with the antecedents of UGIB (RR-1 = 2.13) in blue, and the relative excess risk due to the interaction (RERI = 2.54) in green. The last bar represents the RR observed in NSAID users with UGIB antecedents, which is 2.54 units greater than the sum of the independent relative effects of NSAIDs and antecedents of UGIB

posing factor *Z* modifies the relative effect of *A* beyond the mere additivity of effects. The equation can be adapted to the particular case of a potential predisposing factor (PPF) as follows:

$$\text{RERI} = \text{RR}_{\text{drug used by patients with the PPF}} - \left(\text{RR}_{\text{drug used by patients without the PPF}} + \text{RR}_{\text{PPF itself}} - 1\right)$$

Applying this to the case study shown in Table 3.5:

$$\text{RERI} = 7.14 - (2.47 + 3.13 - 1) = 2.54$$

This result suggests that having an antecedent of UGIB increases the risk of presenting a new episode associated with NSAID use, and it can be considered a predisposing factor for this drug–event association. The result can be graphically represented as shown in Fig. 3.4.

With the help of the figure, the effect of the combination of *A* + *Z* would be as follows:

$$\begin{aligned}\text{Observed}\,\text{RR}_{A+Z} &= 1\ (\text{null value})(\text{gray}) + \text{Observed excess}\,\text{RR}_A(\text{yellow}) \\ &+ \text{Observed excess}\,\text{RR}_Z(\text{blue}) + \text{RERI}(\text{green})\end{aligned}$$

Obtaining the 95% CI for RERI is not straightforward, but Richardson and Kaufman [80] have developed a program in SAS and STATA that can provide it.

In case–control studies, the computed OR can be used to estimate the RR and the formula can be applied to this design by simply replacing RR by OR

$$\text{RERI} = \text{Observed}\,\text{OR}_{A+Z} - \left(\text{Observed}\text{OR}_A + \text{Observed}\,\text{OR}_Z - 1\right) \tag{3.5}$$

5.1.3 The Case–Control Study Nested in a Cohort of Drug Users: A Special Design to Directly Estimate Predisposing Factors

In pharmacogenetics, a special case–control study is often used to identify genetic susceptibility factors involved in acute ADRs, like hypersensitivity reactions. The particularity of this case–control study is that both cases and controls are exposed to the drug of interest (both are "nested" in a cohort of drug-exposed subjects): cases are those who took the drug and experienced the event (and the drug is considered the culprit of the reaction) and controls are patients who were exposed to the drug over a sufficient period of time to have presented the ADR but they did not ("tolerant controls"). Analytically, researchers proceed as in any case–control study: they identify the carriers of the genetic factor among the cases and controls and, then, compute the odds ratio. When the odds ratio is over 1 and statistically significant, it can be interpreted as the times the odds of presenting the ADR induced by the drug increases in the presence of the genetic biomarker as compared to its absence. Conceptually speaking, with this design, we can directly estimate the effect of the effect modification factor (assuming causality). In other words, the computed OR (actually, OR_{A+Z}) estimates the RERI explained before (Eq. 3.4) because the odds ratio of the drug (OR_A) is 1, as all patients are exposed, and the odds ratio of the genetic factor (OR_Z) is also 1, as it has no effect per se on the absence of the drug:

$$\text{RERI} = \text{Observed}\,\text{OR}_{A+Z} - \left(\text{Observed}\text{OR}_A + \text{Observed}\,\text{OR}_Z - 1\right) \tag{3.6}$$

$$\text{RERI} = \text{Observed}\,\text{OR}_{A+Z} - 1$$

Applications of this method can be found in Ramírez et al. [81] and Bellón et al. [82]. In Table 3.7, an example is presented, in which this method was used to assess whether the HLA-A*32:01 was a predisposing factor for experiencing a drug reaction with eosinophilia and systemic symptoms (DRESS) syndrome with vancomycin. The results showed that HLA-A*32:01 was 13 times more frequent among DRESS cases

Table 3.7 Example of the use of the case–control approach to assess HLA-A*32:01 as a predisposing factor for DRESS (drug reaction with eosinophilia and systemic symptoms) syndrome in patients treated with vancomycin. All patients were exposed to vancomycin. Data were obtained from Bellón et al. [82]

HLA-A*32:01	DRESS cases ($N = 14$)	Tolerant controls ($N = 25$)	OR (95% CI)
Yes	5	1	13.33
No	9	24	(1.36–130.3)

exposed to vancomycin than among tolerant controls, which strongly suggests that it is a relevant predisposing factor and could be a potential biomarker (to be assessed in future studies).

This method can be used in other contexts. For instance, Martín-Pérez et al. [83] used it to identify predictors of over-anticoagulation in a cohort of warfarin users. They compared patients presenting an International Normalized Ratio (INR) $\geq$4 (cases) with patients presenting an INR $\leq$3 (controls) and identified renal failure (30–44 mL/min/1.73 m^2, OR = 1.45; 1.14–1.85; and <30 mL/min/1.73 m^2, OR = 1.85; 1.23–2.78) as a predisposing factor for over-anticoagulation in warfarin users (assuming that renal failure has no effect per se on the INR).

5.2 Identifying Predisposing Factors Through Defective Study Designs

When a study design does not allow deriving effect measures (or measures of association) that can be interpreted as causal effects under optimal conditions of comparability, it may be called "defective" (or nonanalytical), that is, a design that is faulty because something is missing. In a series of exposed people (also called a "registry of exposed" when the series is exhaustive in a certain geographical area) and in a series of cases (or a "registry of cases" when the series of cases is exhaustive in a certain geographical area), they are both defective because the reference control group is lacking (the unexposed group or unexposed person-time in the former and the non-case group in the latter). However, with complementary information from the underlying source population, it is possible to convert a registry of cases in a case-population study that allows estimating measures of association and assessing potential effect modifiers [84, 85]. Moreover, in a series of exposed people, it is also possible to apply a nested case–control study to identify potential predisposing factors among the exposed people, as shown in Sect. 5.1.3.

Prescription event monitoring is an example of a series (or cohort) of exposed people that merits additional comments. Although in this method, there is no formal unexposed group, researchers have managed to identify potential predisposing factors. First, they use a case/non-case evaluation within the cohort of exposed people (equivalent to a case–control nested in a cohort of drug users, as described in Sect. 5.1.3) to detect associations between potential predisposing factors and the event. Once a factor is identified, researchers compute the incidence rate of the event of interest in people with such a factor in the cohort (for instance, males) and compare it with the incidence rate among people not having such a factor (e.g., females), adjusting for other covariates in the multivariate analyses. With this methodological approach, Layton et al. identified that a history of peripheral edema was the most important predictor of having peripheral edema associated with vildagliptin [86]. Moreover, they found that among those with such antecedents, the elderly males had a much higher hazard ratio than elderly women. The problem of this approach is that the independent effect of the predisposing factor cannot be estimated (as there is no unexposed cohort), and, then, it is not possible to disentangle which part is due to the predisposing factor per se and which one is due to the interaction between the drug and the predisposing factor. If we can reasonably assume that the predisposing factor has no effect per se, then the estimations are entirely imputable to the interaction.

Spontaneous reporting schemes continue to be the cornerstone of pharmacovigilance to identify new potential risks. However, its simplicity is also its Achilles' heel to formally assess drug–event associations and to identify potential predisposing factors because it is the most defective of all study designs. Expressing the data from spontaneous reporting in a two-by-two table, we can easily observe that the information from three out of four cells is lacking and, from the one that we do have information, the data are incomplete and probably biased (due to both underreporting and selective reporting) (Table 3.8). Bearing this in mind, the limitation of spontaneous reporting to assess the presence of any potential predisposing factor is obvious. For this reason, this method can only be used for

Table 3.8 A two-by-two table showing the information known through spontaneous reporting schemes

	Cases	Non-cases	Total
Exposed	a (only those suspected and reported)	b (unknown)	a + b
Nonexposed	c (unknown)	d (unknown)	c + d
Total	a + c	b + d	a + b + c + d

hypothesis-generating purposes, either with a qualitative interpretation (e.g., there are more ADR reports in patients having a certain factor such as sex, age, underlying disease, etc., though this sole information may be misleading without using the distribution of such factors in the population who uses the drug) or, better, through a quantitative approach (using subgroup analysis with measures of disproportionality or using drug consumption data to calculate reporting rates by subgroups) [87, 88].

Finally, the potential for big data and artificial intelligence to assist in identifying new ADRs and predisposing factors is a growing area that, in the years to come, may be an important new source of information for pharmacovigilance practice [89].

6 Management of Predisposing Factors

Once a predisposing factor has been identified using any of the methods discussed in the previous sections, it is time to use such information for ADR prevention or minimization. This can be done at two levels: (1) public health and drug regulation and (2) clinical practice.

6.1 Management of Predisposing Factors at Public Health and Regulatory Levels

The identified predisposing factors must be mentioned in the appropriate sections of the drug label (the Summary of Product Characteristics in the European Union) in order to inform physicians and in patient information leaflets (to inform patients) on which circumstances, situations, or conditions, or in which special populations, an important ADR is most probable to occur and which measures should be checked before the drug is used (e.g., renal function, liver function, ion concentration in serum, and genetic susceptibility biomarkers) and during treatment (e.g., the introduction of a new drug, which may interact with the ones that the patient already uses). For this reason, it is of utmost importance that the marketing authorization holders and regulatory authorities alike are diligent in including new information in the drug label concerning potential predisposing factors and informing about the measures that can be applied to reduce their impact (dose adjustment, monitoring of certain parameters, etc.). When the ADR is serious enough, it should appear specifically in the section of Warnings and Precautions, especially when it has been identified as a risk minimization measure that should be applied in all patients or in certain groups. The ADR may also be the origin of a formal contraindication to avoid the risk (e.g., use of the drug in patients with an antecedent of a serious allergic reaction caused by the drug).

Sometimes, the inclusion of the information in the drug label is not enough and more proactive measures are needed to prevent the impact of predisposing factors. This is the aim of the additional risk minimization measures included in the Risk Management Plans of the European Union [90] and the Risk Evaluation and Mitigation Strategies of the United States [91]. However, when the risk minimization measures fail to prevent a serious safety concern, restrictive regulatory measures should be implemented, including the market withdrawal of the drug. A striking example of this is the withdrawal of cerivastatin from the world market in August 2001, due to a risk of rhabdomyolysis. The risk was 16 times higher than the one estimated with other statins, which was worsened by concomitant use with gemfibrozil, another cholesterol-lowering drug, which was contraindicated. The implemented risk minimization methods failed to prevent co-prescribing of the two drugs, leading to the withdrawal of cerivastatin, showing the difficulties of changing clinical practice [92].

6.2 Management of Predisposing Factors in Clinical Practice

Taking into account that ensuring safe outcomes is the primary goal of drug use in patients, predisposing factors for ADRs require careful consideration at various steps of drug use in clinical practice. Accordingly, the various stakeholders have a significant role to play and a multidisciplinary approach is critical. Appropriate knowledge of providers, clinicians, pharmacists, and nurses about the general and specific predisposing factors for ADRs, is extremely essential to promote safer use of drugs by avoiding preventable ADRs to the maximum.

6.2.1 Prescription/Selection of Drug Therapy

Clinicians must review the details from patient records, patient interviews, and other sources to identify the presence of predisposing factors before making a decision of prescribing a specific medication. In situations where dysfunctions such as renal, hepatic, and blood abnormalities could be a predisposing factor, specific laboratory investigations should be conducted before using the particular medication in the patient. If the patient has a specific predisposing factor, then the possibility of selecting alternative drugs that may be safer to the patient should be considered. Physicians should avoid inappropriate prescribing and unnecessary polypharmacy [93].

Careful consideration should be given to special groups such as the elderly and children. Older patients are often more sensitive to the effects of medications than are their younger counterparts because of altered pharmacodynamic responses such as excessive sedation and confusion with morphine and increased anticoagulant effect with warfarin when used at "standard" treatment doses. Such pharmacodynamic responses are generally predictable and can be minimized by starting at the lowest possible dose and titrating to response. Good clinical practice for detecting and predicting ADRs in vulnerable patients includes detailed documentation and regular review of prescribed and OTC medications through standardized medication reconciliation. Deprescribing should occur at an individual level when drugs are no longer beneficial or indicated or when safer alternatives exist [93]. Understanding the different effects of patient factors on ADRs enables health-care professionals to give the best advice to their patients to prevent or minimize these ADRs. Pharmacogenomic principles and facilities should be utilized in clinical practice, wherever they have shown to be useful and practically possible, to help appropriate drug selection or dose titration. Information technology such as computer physician order entry with decision support helps check for problems such as drug allergies and drug–drug interactions, providing dosage adjustment calculations, checking for appropriate baseline laboratory results, updating the prescriber with the latest drug information, and thereby helping use of medications safely with careful consideration of predisposing factors [94].

Patient involvement is required for making decisions on the safe use of medications through appropriate discussions with the patient or caregiver. It should be borne in mind that, though the predisposing factors for specific ADRs may not be present at the time of prescribing, there is a possibility of its development during drug use, especially for chronic medications. For instance, development of renal dysfunction in a patient on digoxin during the course of drug use can increase the risk of digoxin toxicity. Prescribers should be knowledgeable and vigilant for ADRs and their contributory risk factors, to give the best advice to their patients.

6.2.2 Dispensing and Counseling

Pharmacists should, before dispensing medications, carefully consider the presence of any predisposing factors for ADRs in the patient, the need for any specific requirement according to the drug label, and the presence of safer alternatives (to be discussed with the prescriber). Appropriate counseling should be provided to the patient, which ensures avoidance or minimizing ADRs in relation to the predisposing factors, wherever possible.

Special attention must be paid to potential drug–drug interactions (including interaction with OTC drugs and herbal medicines) and food–drug interactions. Pharmacists should inform the prescriber of any potential safety issues with the drugs prescribed.

6.2.3 Administration of the Drug

Predisposing factors need to be carefully considered when the drug is administered by the clinician or nurse. Necessary precautions should be taken to avoid ADRs and immediate management to be instituted if it occurs. An appropriate review of the patient, disease, and drug details before administration will help minimize or prevent the occurrence of ADRs.

6.2.4 Use by Patients

Patient education and understanding will increase the chance of safer medication use with careful consideration of predisposing factors. Support for the patient should be provided during the entire drug use process.

6.2.5 Monitoring/Follow-Ups

There might be specific monitoring parameters for individual drugs to check the presence or development of predisposing factors. These monitoring steps should be informed to the patient at the time of prescribing and their involvement in adhering to these steps. Appropriate action should be taken wherever required based on the results of these monitoring parameters.

7 Summary and Conclusions

The existence of predisposing factors for ADRs explains why not all patients who use a drug develop a specific ADR and those who develop do not experience it with the same seriousness, severity, at the same time, or with the same drug posology. Predisposing factors for ADRs can be considered as components of a sufficient cause that, along with the drug, can lead to an adverse event. The identification of predisposing factors is important to reduce the burden of ADRs and is of importance in pharmacovigilance as they are the target of risk minimization measures such as the restriction of indications or the addition of contraindications or warnings on the drug label. The knowledge of predisposing factors is also imperative to the individual care of patients, as physicians could individualize the pharmacological treatment in an effective way, and patients could be better informed, thereby preventing and managing ADRs in a more useful manner. Predisposing factors can be grouped into four categories, including those related to patient characteristics, those related to the underlying diseases, those related to environmental factors, and those that are drug-related. Among the various tools available for identification and evaluation of predisposing factors, analytical epidemiological studies are the main one. Predisposing factors should be managed at public health, regulatory, and clinical practice levels. At the public health and regulatory levels, management involves updating of the drug label, active implementation of additional risk minimization measures by marketing authorization holders, and/or adoption of restrictive regulatory measures. Predisposing factors for ADRs require careful consideration at various steps of drug use in clinical practice, which highlights the unique role of various stakeholders and the need for a multidisciplinary approach.

8 Case Studies

8.1 Case Study 1: A Pharmacovigilance Signal Suggesting a Predisposing Factor

The pharmacovigilance center, at which you are working, has received 40 spontaneous reports of acute liver injury associated with the use of drug *A* after 6 months of its marketing. Most cases were serious enough to require hospitalization, but no fatalities were reported. Remarkably, in 32 out of the 40 reports (80%), the patients were females.

1. *With this information, might you consider that the female sex is a predisposing factor for acute liver injury?*

   Not necessarily. Such distribution of cases may reflect the actual use of drug *A* (it may occur that around 80% of users are women).

2. *Which additional data will you look for, and what assessment will you make depending on the results?*

   At least, drug consumption by sex in the same geographical area or country from where the ADR reports are obtained must be looked for. If the distribution of use by sex is similar to that found in the ADR reporting series, then it will rule out that female sex was actually a predisposing factor for this ADR. However, if the distribution by sex is extremely different in the series of the ADR reports compared to that of the population, then the next step would be to assess how likely selective reporting is in females. For instance, it would be important to look at the indication for which the drug was administered, the dose, the duration, and the concomitant medications. It may happen that the ADR would occur more often when the drug is used for a certain disease, at a certain dose, or duration, or when used with certain medications (potential pharmacological interaction) that may be specific or more frequent in females. Moreover, it could happen that women treated with the drug are older than men, and, then, age may be the real predisposing factor behind the greater frequency of the ADR among women; in this case, we would say that age is a "confounding factor" that leads us to observe a spurious association between the ADR and female sex.

3. *If a study is judged necessary, which kind of study would you propose to carry out and how would you determine whether the female sex is a predisposing factor?*

   The type of study to be carried out would be an analytical study, for instance, a cohort study, or a case–control study, in which it would be possible to properly assess the potential epidemiological interaction between drug exposure and sex to induce liver injury while controlling for the confounding factors. If female sex is a predisposing factor for liver injury induced by drug *A*, then the measure of association between drug and liver injury will be much greater among females than among males. Such a difference can be assessed through an interaction test (like the Altman and Bland test). Alternatively, relative excess risk due to interaction (RERI) can be estimated and, if greater than 0, it would suggest that the female sex is a predisposing factor for liver injury associated with drug *A*.

   If the ADR was detected in premarketing clinical trials, it would be interesting to request the marketing authorization holder to explore the clinical database and make a subgroup analysis by sex.

4. *If the whole available evidence confirms that female sex is a predisposing factor, then how would you manage the issue at the regulatory level? How will you manage the issue at the clinical practice level?*

   At the regulatory level, it would be necessary to perform an overall benefit–risk assessment in females. Depending on this and the seriousness of the ADR, the risk minimization measures would range from including a warning on the drug label up to including a contraindication to avoid the use of drug *A* in women. The possibility of applying additional risk minimization measures should also be considered, such as educational material for physicians and patients, or the possibility of implementing clinical or analytical monitoring (e.g., liver enzymes) to prevent or, at least, to detect the safety issue as soon as possible. It will also be necessary to communicate the safety issue to the health-care professionals and patients, recommending specific actions to prevent or minimize the risk (such as analytical monitoring).

   At the clinical practice level, physicians should apply regulatory decisions. If drug *A* is contraindicated in women, then the physician should abstain from prescribing this drug to them. If not contraindicated, then the physicians should inform the female patients and discuss with them the benefits and risks of this drug and also the possible alternatives. If the drug is finally prescribed, then the clinical team (including nurses and pharmacists) will ensure that the risk minimization measures are correctly implemented.

8.2 Case Study 2: The Hazard of Ignoring an Important Predisposing Factor

An 81-year-old patient is admitted to a hospital for pancytopenia. He had myasthenia gravis (an autoimmune disease) treated with azathioprine since 3 years at a dose of 75 mg/day and pyridostigmine (a cholinesterase inhibitor) at a dose of 60 mg four times daily, with good response. The thiopurine methyltransferase (TPMT) activity performed before prescribing azathioprine was 21.4 U/mL, which indicates a normal function. Among the antecedents, the patient reports that the primary care physician found hyperuricemia in an analytical test (8.4 mg/dL) and decided to initiate treatment with allopurinol (300 mg/day) to reduce this level.

1. *Pancytopenia is a well-known ADR of azathioprine. What type of ADR is it? Can you identify any predisposing factor in this case?*

   Bone marrow toxicity is an ADR resulting from the augmentation of the pharmacological action of azathioprine (a type A ADR). Old age and, presumably, an impaired renal function can be considered as predisposing factors. However, in this particular case, the most important risk factor seems to be a drug–drug interaction with allopurinol (a triggering factor, actually). Allopurinol is a xanthine oxidase inhibitor and, by this mechanism, inhibits the formation of uric acid, but this enzyme also contributes partly to metabolize azathioprine. So, its inhibition by allopurinol increases the pharmacological action of azathioprine and predisposes patients to bone marrow toxicity. It is a well-known pharmacokinetic interaction described in the drug labels of both drugs.

2. *Could this health problem have been prevented? How should it have been managed in clinical practice?*

   As the bone marrow toxicity of azathioprine is a dose-dependent ADR, it can be minimized with an appropriate dose. Physicians should take into account factors that can increase the pharmacological action of azathioprine, such as renal function and the concomitant use of xanthine oxidase inhibitors. In the latter case, the recommended daily dose should be reduced to 25% of the usual one.

   On the other hand, it seems that allopurinol has been prescribed to treat an asymptomatic hyperuricemia, and this is an inappropriate use. Allopurinol is indicated to prevent acute gout flares (by maintaining the uricemia level below 6 mg/dL). Thus, as the patient had no antecedents of gout attacks, allopurinol should not have been prescribed. It can be considered as a medication error.

3. *What is TMPT activity, and why is it important to know its value before prescribing azathioprine?*

   Azathioprine is metabolized by the enzyme thiopurine methyltransferase (TPMT), which is polymorphic. When its activity is below 5 U/mL, patients are at high risk of presenting bone marrow toxicity, so it is better to avoid its use for nonmalignant indications. Alternatively, if TPMT can be genotyped, azathioprine should be avoided for nonmalignant indications in patients who are poor metabolizers (carriers of two nonfunctional alleles) or the starting dose should be reduced (30–80% of normal dose) in case of intermediate metabolizers [95].

References

1. Rothman KJ. Causes. Am J Epidemiol. 1976;104:587–92.
2. Wright P. Untoward effects associated with practolol administration: oculomucocutaneous syndrome. BMJ. 1975;1:595–8.

3. Aguirre C, García M. Evaluación de la causalidad en las comunicaciones de reacciones adversas a medicamentos. Algoritmo del Sistema Español de Farmacovigilancia. Med Clin (Barc). 2016;147(10):461–4. https://doi.org/10.1016/j.medcli.2016.06.012.
4. García-Cortés M, Stephens C, Lucena MI, Fernández-Castañer A, Andrade RJ. Causality assessment methods in drug induced liver injury: strengths and weaknesses. J Hepatol. 2011;55(3):683–91. https://doi.org/10.1016/j.jhep.2011.02.007.
5. Lazarou J, Pomeranz BH, Corey PN. Incidence of adverse drug reactions in hospitalized patients: a meta-analysis of prospective studies. JAMA. 1998;279(15):1200–5. https://doi.org/10.1001/jama.279.15.1200.
6. Pirmohamed M, James S, Meakin S, Green C, Scott AK, Walley TJ, Farrar K, Park BK, Breckenridge AM. Adverse drug reactions as cause of admission to hospital: prospective analysis of 18,820 patients. BMJ. 2004;329(7456):15–9. https://doi.org/10.1136/bmj.329.7456.15.
7. Lin CW, Huang WI, Chao PH, Chen WW, Hsiao FY. Temporal trends and patterns in carbamazepine use, related severe cutaneous adverse reactions, and HLA-B*15:02 screening: a nationwide study. Epilepsia. 2018;59(12):2325–39. https://doi.org/10.1111/epi.14599.
8. Sung C, Tan L, Limenta M, Ganesan G, Toh D, Chan CL. Usage pattern of carbamazepine and associated severe cutaneous adverse reactions in Singapore following implementation of HLA-B*15:02 genotyping as standard-of-care. Front Pharmacol. 2020;11:527. https://doi.org/10.3389/fphar.2020.00527.
9. Lanas A, García-Rodríguez LA, Polo-Tomás M, Ponce M, Quintero E, Perez-Aisa GJP, Bujanda L, Castro M, Muñoz M, Del Pino MD, García S, Calvet X. The changing face of hospitalisation due to gastrointestinal bleeding and perforation. Aliment Pharmacol Ther. 2011;33:585–91. https://doi.org/10.1111/j.1365-2036.2010.04563.x.
10. Rademaker M. Do women have more adverse drug reactions?. Am J Clin Dermatol 2001;2(6), 349–351. https://doi.org/10.2165/00128071-200102060-00001.
11. ICH Final Guideline on special populations: Geriatrics (E7). Released, Jun 1993.
12. Field TS, Gurwitz JH, Avorn J, McCormick D, Jain S, Eckler M, Benser M, Bates DW. Risk factors for adverse drug events among nursing home residents. Arch Intern Med. 2001;161(13):1629–34. https://doi.org/10.1001/archinte.161.13.1629.
13. Davies EA, O'Mahony MS. Adverse drug reactions in special populations—the elderly. Br J Clin Pharmacol. 2015;80(4):796–807. https://doi.org/10.1111/bcp.12596.
14. Mangoni AA, Jackson SH. Age-related changes in pharmacokinetics and pharmacodynamics: basic principles and practical applications. Br J Clin Pharmacol. 2004;57(1):6–14. https://doi.org/10.1046/j.1365-2125.2003.02007.
15. Park BK, Pirmohamed M, Kitteringham NR. Idiosyncratic drug reactions: a mechanistic evaluation of risk factors. Br J Clin Pharmacol. 1992;34(5):377–95. https://doi.org/10.1111/j.1365-2125.1992.tb05647.
16. Erdő F, Denes L, de Lange E. Age-associated physiological and pathological changes at the blood-brain barrier: a review. J Cerebral Blood Flow Metab. 2017;37(1):4–24. https://doi.org/10.1177/0271678X16679420.
17. Kojima T, Matsui T, Suzuki Y, Takeya Y, Tomita N, Kozaki K, Kuzuya M, Rakugi H, Arai H, Akishita M. Risk factors for adverse drug reactions in older inpatients of geriatric wards at admission: multicenter study. Geriatr Gerontol Int. 2020;20(2):144–9. https://doi.org/10.1111/ggi.13844.
18. Mandavi, D'Cruz S, Sachdev A, Tiwari P. Adverse drug reactions & their risk factors among Indian ambulatory elderly patients. Indian J Med Res. 2012;136(3):404–10.
19. Parameswaran Nair N, Chalmers L, Peterson GM, Bereznicki BJ, Castelino RL, Bereznicki LR. Hospitalization in older patients due to adverse drug reactions—the need for a prediction tool. Clin Interv Aging. 2016;11:497–505. https://doi.org/10.2147/CIA.S99097.
20. Alhawassi TM, Krass I, Bajorek BV, Pont LG. A systematic review of the prevalence and risk factors for adverse drug reactions in the elderly in the acute care setting. Clin Interv Aging. 2014;9:2079–86. https://doi.org/10.2147/CIA.S71178.
21. Beard K, Lee A. Introduction. In: Lee A, editor. Adverse drug reactions. 2nd ed. London: Pharmaceutical Press; 2006. p. 1–22.
22. Krska J, Cox AR. Adverse drug reactions. In: Whittlesea C, Hodson K, editors. Clinical pharmacy and therapeutics. 6th ed. Amsterdam: Elsevier; 2018. p. 66–80.
23. Cummings ED, et al. Gray baby syndrome [updated 2022 Jun 8]. In: StatPearls. Treasure Island, FL: StatPearls Publishing; 2022. Available from: https://www.ncbi.nlm.nih.gov/books/NBK448133/?report=classic.
24. Allegaert K, van den Anker JN. Adverse drug reactions in neonates and infants: a population-tailored approach is needed. Br J Clin Pharmacol. 2015;80(4):788–95. https://doi.org/10.1111/bcp.12430.
25. Moore TJ, Weiss SR, Kaplan S, Blaisdell CJ. Reported adverse drug events in infants and children under 2 years of age. Pediatrics. 2002;110(5):e53. https://doi.org/10.1542/peds.1110.5.e53.
26. Royal Pharmaceutical Society. British National Formulary. 73rd ed. Royal Pharmaceutical Society; 2019.
27. Aljebab F, Choonara I, Conroy S. Long-course oral corticosteroid toxicity in children. Arch Dis Child. 2016;101:e2.
28. Clarkson A, Choonara I. Surveillance for fatal suspected adverse drug reactions in the UK. Arch Dis Child. 2002;87(6):462–6. https://doi.org/10.1136/adc.87.6.462.

29. Rodenburg EM, Stricker BH, Visser LE. Sex-related differences in hospital admissions attributed to adverse drug reactions in The Netherlands. Br J Clin Pharmacol. 2011;71(1):95–104. https://doi.org/10.1111/j.1365-2125.2010.03811.
30. Amacher DE. Female gender as a susceptibility factor for drug-induced liver injury. Hum Exp Toxicol. 2014;33(9):928–39. https://doi.org/10.1177/0960327113512860.
31. Fletcher CV, Acosta EP, Strykowski JM. Gender differences in human pharmacokinetics and pharmacodynamics. J Adolesc Health. 1994;15(8):619–29. https://doi.org/10.1016/s1054-139x(94)90628-9.
32. Scandlyn MJ, Stuart EC, Rosengren RJ. Sex-specific differences in CYP450 isoforms in humans. Expert Opin Drug Metab Toxicol. 2008;4(4):413–24. https://doi.org/10.1517/17425255.4.4.413.
33. Tasnif Y, Morado J, Hebert MF. Pregnancy-related pharmacokinetic changes. Clin Pharmacol Ther. 2016;100(1):53–62. https://doi.org/10.1002/cpt.382.
34. Allegaert K, Peeters MY, Beleyn B, Smits A, Kulo A, van Calsteren K, Deprest J, de Hoon J, Knibbe CA. Paracetamol pharmacokinetics and metabolism in young women. BMC Anesthesiol. 2015;15:163. https://doi.org/10.1186/s12871-015-0144-3.
35. Al-Windi A, Elmfeldt D, Svärdsudd K. The relationship between age, gender, well-being and symptoms, and the use of pharmaceuticals, herbal medicines and self-care products in a Swedish municipality. Eur J Clin Pharmacol. 2000;56(4):311–7. https://doi.org/10.1007/s002280000152.
36. Ajayi FO, Sun H, Perry J. Adverse drug reactions: a review of relevant factors. J Clin Pharmacol. 2000;40(10):1093–101.
37. Drici MD, Clément N. Is gender a risk factor for adverse drug reactions? The example of drug-induced long QT syndrome. Drug Saf. 2001;24(8):575–85. https://doi.org/10.2165/00002018-200124080-00002.
38. Baehr A, Peña JC, Hu DJ. Racial and ethnic disparities in adverse drug events: a systematic review of the literature. J Racial Ethn Health Disparities. 2015;2(4):527–36. https://doi.org/10.1007/s40615-015-0101-3.
39. Takahashi H, Wilkinson GR, Nutescu EA, Morita T, Ritchie MD, Scordo MG, Pengo V, Barban M, Padrini R, Ieiri I, Otsubo K, Kashima T, Kimura S, Kijima S, Echizen H. Different contributions of polymorphisms in VKORC1 and CYP2C9 to intra- and inter-population differences in maintenance dose of warfarin in Japanese, Caucasians and African-Americans. Pharmacogenet Genomics. 2006;16(2):101–10. https://doi.org/10.1097/01.fpc.0000184955.08453.a8.
40. McDowell SE, Coleman JJ, Ferner RE. Systematic review and meta-analysis of ethnic differences in risks of adverse reactions to drugs used in cardiovascular medicine. BMJ (Clin Res Ed). 2006;332(7551):1177–81. https://doi.org/10.1136/bmj.38803.528113.55.
41. Walling A. Does ethnicity influence adverse reactions to drugs? Am Fam Physician. 2006;74(8):1410–1.
42. Newman CB, Preiss D, Tobert JA, Jacobson TA, Page RL 2nd, Goldstein LB, Chin C, Tannock LR, Miller M, Raghuveer G, Duell PB, Brinton EA, Pollak A, Braun LT, Welty FK, American Heart Association Clinical Lipidology, Lipoprotein, Metabolism and Thrombosis Committee, a Joint Committee of the Council on Atherosclerosis, Thrombosis and Vascular Biology and Council on Lifestyle and Cardiometabolic Health, Council on Cardiovascular Disease in the Young, Council on Clinical Cardiology, and Stroke Council. Statin safety and associated adverse events: a scientific statement from the American Heart Association. Arterioscler Thromb Vasc Biol. 2019;39(2):e38–81. https://doi.org/10.1161/ATV.0000000000000073.
43. Tomlinson B, Chan P, Liu ZM. Statin intolerance-an Asian perspective. J Atheroscler Thromb. 2020;27(5):485–8. https://doi.org/10.5551/jat.50435.
44. Wang CW, Preclaro IAC, Lin WH, Chung WH. An updated review of genetic associations with sever adverse drug reactions: translation and implementation of pharmacogenomics testing in clinical practice. Front Pharmacol 2022;13:886377; https://doi.org/10.3389/fphar.2022.886377.
45. Nakamura Y. Pharmacogenomics and drug toxicity. N Engl J Med 2008;359(8):856–8. https://doi.org/10.1056/NEJMe0805136.
46. Micaglio E, Locati ET, Monasky MM, Romani F, Heilbron F and Pappone C. Role of Pharmacogenetics in adverse drug reactions: an update towards personalized medicine. Front Pharmacol, 2021;12:651720. https://doi.org/10.3389/fphar.2021.651720.
47. Ingelman-Sundberg M. Pharmacogenomic biomarkers for prediction of severe adverse drug reactions. N Engl J Med 2008;358(6):637–9. https://doi.org/10.1056/NEJMe0708842.
48. Böhm R, Cascorbi I. Pharmacogenetics and predictive testing of drug hypersensitivity reactions. Front Pharmacol. 2016;7:396. https://doi.org/10.3389/fphar.2016.00396.
49. Shah J. Criteria influencing the clinical uptake of pharmacogenomics strategies. BMJ. 2004;328:1482–6. https://doi.org/10.1136/bmj.328.7454.1482.
50. Hoosen K, Mosam A, Dlova NC, Grayson W. An update on adverse cutaneous drug reactions in HIV/AIDS. Dermatopathology (Basel, Switzerland). 2019;6(2):111–25. https://doi.org/10.1159/000496389.
51. Pirmohamed M, Breckenridge AM, Kitteringham NR, Park BK. Adverse drug reactions. BMJ (Clin Res Ed). 1998;316(7140):1295–8. https://doi.org/10.1136/bmj.316.7140.1295.
52. Chatellier D, Jourdain M, Mangalaboyi J, Ader F, Chopin C, Derambure P, Fourrier F. Cefepime-induced neurotoxicity: an underestimated complication of antibiotherapy in patients with acute renal failure. Intensive Care Med. 2002;28(2):214–7. https://doi.org/10.1007/s00134-001-1170-9.
53. Bergasa NV, Rothman RB, Mukerjee E, Vergalla J, Jones EA. Up-regulation of central mu-opioid recep-

tors in a model of hepatic encephalopathy: a potential mechanism for increased sensitivity to morphine in liver failure. Life Sci. 2002;70(14):1701–8. https://doi.org/10.1016/s0024-3205(02)01487-x.
54. Bhatia SJ. Digitalis toxicity—turning over a new leaf? West J Med. 1986;145(1):74–82.
55. Haller CA, Jacob P 3rd, Benowitz NL. Enhanced stimulant and metabolic effects of combined ephedrine and caffeine. Clin Pharmacol Ther. 2004;75(4):259–73. https://doi.org/10.1016/j.clpt.2003.11.375.
56. Lucas C, Martin J. Smoking and drug interactions. Aust Prescr. 2013;36(13):102–104a.
57. Maideen NMP. Tobacco smoking and its drug interactions with comedications involving CYP and UGT enzymes and nicotine. World J Pharmacol. 2019;8(2):14–25. https://doi.org/10.5497/wjp.v8.i2.14.
58. Bettinge TL, Crimson ML. Lithium. In: Burton ME, Shaw LM, Schentag JJ, et al., editors. Applied pharmacokinetics and pharmacodynamic: principles of therapeutic drug monitoring. 4th ed. Baltimore, MD: Lippincott, Williams and Wilkins; 2006. p. 798–812.
59. Ensom MHH, Blouin RA. Dietary influences on drug disposition. In: Burton ME, Shaw LM, Schentag JJ, et al., editors. Applied pharmacokinetics and Pharmacodynamic: principles of therapeutic drug monitoring. 4th ed. Baltimore, MD: Lippincott, Williams and Wilkins; 2006. p. 242–56.
60. Bressler R. Grapefruit juice and drug interactions. Exploring mechanisms of this interaction and potential toxicity for certain drugs. Geriatrics. 2006;61(11):12–8.
61. Ioannides-Demos LL, Christophidis N, Ryan P, Angelis P, Liolios L, McLean AJ. Dosing implications of a clinical interaction between grapefruit juice and cyclosporine and metabolite concentrations in patients with autoimmune diseases. J Rheumatol. 1997;24(1):49–54.
62. Johnson MA. Influence of vitamin K on anticoagulant therapy depends on vitamin K status and the source and chemical forms of vitamin K. Nutr Rev. 2005;63(3):91–7. https://doi.org/10.1111/j.1753-4887.2005.tb00126.x.
63. MacKichan JJ, Lee MWL. Factors contributing to drug induced diseases. In: Tisdale JE, Miller DA, editors. Drug induced diseases—prevention, detection and management. 2nd ed. Bethesda: American Health System Pharmacists; 2010. p. 23–30.
64. Macedo AF, Alves C, Craveiro N, Marques FB. Multiple drug exposure as a risk factor for the seriousness of adverse drug reactions. J Nurs Manag. 2011;19(3):395–9. https://doi.org/10.1111/j.1365-2834.2011.01216.x.
65. McElnay JC, D'Arcy PF. Protein binding displacement interactions and their clinical importance. Drugs. 1983;25(5):495–513. https://doi.org/10.2165/00003495-198325050-00003.
66. Niu J, Straubinger RM, Mager DE. Pharmacodynamic drug-drug interactions. Clin Pharmacol Ther. 2019;105(6):1395–406. https://doi.org/10.1002/cpt.1434.
67. Spies PE, Pot JLWH, Willems RPJ, Bos JM, and Kramers C. Interaction between tramadol and selective serotonin reuptake inhibitors: are doctors aware of potential risks in their prescription practice?. European journal of hospital pharmacy: science and practice. 2017;24(2):124–7. https://doi.org/10.1136/ejhpharm-2015-000838.
68. Mignat C, Unger T. ACE inhibitors. Drug interactions of clinical significance. Drug Saf. 1995;12(5):334–47. https://doi.org/10.2165/00002018-199512050-00005.
69. Greenberg M, Ridgely MS. Clinical decision support and malpractice risk. JAMA. 2011;306(1):90–1. https://doi.org/10.1001/jama.2011.929.
70. Phansalkar S, van der Sijs H, Tucker AD, Desai AA, Bell DS, Teich JM, Middleton B, Bates DW. Drug-drug interactions that should be non-interruptive in order to reduce alert fatigue in electronic health records. J Am Med Inform Assoc (JAMIA). 2013;20(3):489–93. https://doi.org/10.1136/amiajnl-2012-001089.
71. Kontsioti E, Maskell S, Bensalem A, Dutta B, Pirmohamed M. Similarity and consistency assessment of three major online drug-drug interaction resources. Br J Clin Pharmacol. 2022;88(9):4067–79. https://doi.org/10.1111/bcp.15341.
72. Martín-Pérez M, Gaist D, de Abajo FJ, García Rodríguez LA. Population impact of drug interactions with warfarin: a real-world data approach. Thromb Haemost. 2018;118(3):461–70. https://doi.org/10.1055/s-0038-1627100.
73. Saedder EA, Lisby M, Nielsen LP, Bonnerup DK, Brock B. Number of drugs most frequently found to be independent risk factors for serious adverse reactions: a systematic literature review. Br J Clin Pharmacol. 2015;80(4):808–17. https://doi.org/10.1111/bcp.12600.
74. Szklo M, Nieto FJ. Epidemiology—beyond the basics. 4th ed. Burlington: Jones and Barttlett Learning; 2019. p. 209–54.
75. Maclure M, Mittleman MA. Should we use a case-crossover design? Annu Rev Public Health. 2000;21:193–221. https://doi.org/10.1146/annurev.publhealth.21.1.193.
76. Whitaker HJ, Farrington CP, Spiessens B, Musonda P. Tutorial in biostatistics: the self-controlled case series method. Stat Med. 2006;25(10):1768–97.
77. Altman DG, Bland JM. Interaction revisited: the difference between two estimates. BMJ. 2003;326(7382):219. https://doi.org/10.1136/bmj.326.7382.219.
78. Hutchon DR. Calculations for comparing two estimated relative risks. 2005. Available in: http://www.hutchon.net/CompareRR.htm.
79. Rothman KJ. Interactions between causes, in modern epidemiology. 1st ed. Boston: Little Brown and Company; 1986. p. 311–26.
80. Richardson DB, Kaufman JS. Estimation of the relative excess risk due to interaction and associated confi-

dence bounds. Am J Epidemiol. 2009;169(6):756–60. https://doi.org/10.1093/aje/kwn411.
81. Ramírez E, Bellón T, Tong HY, Borobia AM, de Abajo FJ, Lerma V, Moreno Hidalgo MA, Castañer JL, Cabañas R, Fiandor A, González-Ramos J, Herranz P, Cachafeiro L, González-Herrada C, González O, Aramburu JA, Laosa O, Hernández R, Carcas AJ, Frías J. Significant HLA class I type associations with aromatic antiepileptic drug (AED)-induced SJS/TEN are different from those found for the same AED-induced DRESS in the Spanish population. Pharmacol Res. 2017;115:168–78. https://doi.org/10.1016/j.phrs.2016.11.027.
82. Bellón T, Lerma V, Guijarro J, Ramírez E, Martínez C, Escudero C, Fiandor A, Barranco R, de Barrio M, de Abajo F, Cabañas R, for the PIELenRed Study Group. LTT and HLA testing as diagnostic tools in Spanish vancomycin-induced DRESS cases: a case-control study. Front Pharmacol. 2022;13:959321. https://doi.org/10.3389/fphar.2022.959321.
83. Martín-Pérez M, Gaist D, de Abajo FJ, García Rodríguez LA. Predictors of over-anticoagulation in warfarin users in the UK general population: a nested case-control study in a primary health care database. Thromb Haemost. 2019;119(1):66–76. https://doi.org/10.1055/s-0038-1676519.
84. Rodríguez-Martín S, Martín-Merino E, Lerma V, Rodríguez-Miguel A, González O, González-Herrada C, Ramírez E, Bellón T, de Abajo FJ. Active surveillance of severe cutaneous adverse reactions: a case-population approach using a registry and a health care database. Pharmacoepidemiol Drug Saf. 2018;27(9):1042–50. https://doi.org/10.1002/pds.4622.
85. Rodríguez-Martín S, Martín-Merino E, Lerma V, Rodríguez-Miguel A, González O, González-Herrada C, Ramírez E, Bellón T, de Abajo FJ. Incidence of Stevens-Johnson syndrome/toxic epidermal necrolysis among new users of different individual drugs in a European population: a case-population study. Eur J Clin Pharmacol. 2019;75:237–46. https://doi.org/10.1007/s00228-018-2569-3.
86. Layton D, Coughtrie AL, Qayum N, Shakir SAW. Pattern of onset and risk factors for peripheral oedema during vidagliptin use: analysis from the Vildagliptin prescription-event monitoring in England. Drug Saf. 2016;39:1093–104. https://doi.org/10.1007/s40264-016-0451-8.
87. Dubrall D, Leitzen S, Toni I, et al. Descriptive analysis of adverse drug reaction reports in children and adolescents from Germany: frequently reported reactions and suspected drugs. BMC Pharmacol Toxicol. 2021;22(1):56. Published 2021 Oct 7. https://doi.org/10.1186/s40360-021-00520-y.
88. Seabroke S, Candore G, Juhlin K, Quarcoo N, Wisniewski A, Arani R, Painter J, Tregunno P, Norén GN, Slattery J. Performance of stratified and subgrouped disproportionality analyses in spontaneous databases. Drug Saf. 2016;39(4):355–64. https://doi.org/10.1007/s40264-015-0388-3.
89. Hussain, R. Big data, medicines safety and pharmacovigilance. J of Pharm Policy and Pract. 2021;14(48). https://doi.org/10.1186/s40545-021-00329-4.
90. EMA/838713/2011 Rev 2*. Guideline on good pharmacovigilance practices (GVP). Module V—risk management systems (Rev 2), 28 Mar 2017. Available at: https://www.ema.europa.eu/en/documents/scientific-guideline/guideline-good-pharmacovigilance-practices-module-v-risk-management-systems-rev-2_en.pdf.
91. Food and Drug Administration. Risk evaluation and mitigation strategies / REMS. Available at: https://www.fda.gov/drugs/drug-safety-and-availability/risk-evaluation-and-mitigation-strategies-rems. Accessed: 9 Februabry, 2024.
92. Davidson MH. Controversy surrounding the safety of cerivastatin. Expert Opin Drug Saf. 2002;1(3):207–12. https://doi.org/10.1517/14740338.1.3.207.
93. Lavan AH, Gallagher P. Predicting risk of adverse drug reactions in older adults. Ther Adv Drug Saf. 2016;7(1):11–22. https://doi.org/10.1177/2042098615615472.
94. Agrawal A. Medication errors: prevention using information technology systems. Br J Clin Pharmacol. 2009;67(6):681–6. https://doi.org/10.1111/j.1365-2125.2009.03427.
95. Relling MV, Schwab M, Whirl-Carrillo M, Suarez-Kurtz G, Pui CH, Stein CM, Moyer AM, Evans WE, Klein TE, Antillon-Klussmann FG, Caudle KE, Kato M, Yeoh AEJ, Schmiegelow K, Yang JJ. Clinical pharmacogenetics implementation consortium guideline for thiopurine dosing based on TPMT and NUDT15 genotypes: 2018 update. Clin Pharmacol Ther. 2019;105(5):1095–105. https://doi.org/10.1002/cpt.1304.

Drug Interactions and Their Management

4

Suzanne McCarthy and Aoife Fleming

Abstract

With the increasing prevalence of polypharmacy, it is more important than ever to consider the possibility of drug–drug interactions. A drug–drug interaction occurs when the way in which a drug works is altered by the presence of another drug. Interactions can also occur between drugs and other substances contained in herbs, supplements, food, and smoking. Further drug interactions can include drug–disease and drug–laboratory test interactions. Drug–drug interactions can be classified into two main categories: pharmacokinetic and pharmacodynamic. Pharmacokinetic drug interactions occur when one drug alters the rate or extent of absorption, distribution, metabolism, or excretion of another drug. Many drug interactions that occur in practice are pharmacokinetic in nature, for example, those interactions affecting the metabolism of a drug through the involvement of cytochrome P450 enzymes in the liver. Pharmacodynamic drug interactions occur when the action of a drug in the body is altered by a coadministered drug. In this chapter, we will consider the mechanisms by which drug interactions occur, examine some clinically relevant drug interactions, outline how drug interactions can be managed and prevented in practice by healthcare professionals, and consider the future research needs relating to drug interactions.

Keywords

Drug interactions · Pharmacokinetic · Pharmacodynamic · Cytochrome P450 enzymes

Learning Objectives
By the end of this chapter, readers should be able to:

- Discuss the prevalence of drug interactions and the factors that increase the risk of their occurrence.
- Categorize drug interactions according to their mechanisms of action.
- Describe the different mechanisms by which pharmacokinetic drug interactions occur and their effects.
- Describe the different types of pharmacodynamic drug interactions and their effects.

S. McCarthy (✉)
School of Pharmacy, University College Cork, Cork, Ireland
e-mail: s.mccarthy@ucc.ie

A. Fleming
School of Pharmacy, University College Cork, Cork, Ireland

Pharmacy Department, Mercy University Hospital, Cork, Ireland

J. Jose et al. (eds.), *Principles and Practice of Pharmacovigilance and Drug Safety*,
https://doi.org/10.1007/978-3-031-51089-2_4

- Appreciate various clinically relevant drug interactions.
- Discuss drug–herb, drug–food, drug–disease, and drug–laboratory test interactions.
- Describe ways in which pharmacists and health-care professionals can prevent and manage drug interactions in practice.

Key Points

- Drug interactions can occur between two or more medications or between a medication and another substance, including foods, supplements and herbs, diseases, and laboratory tests.
- Drug interactions can lead to reduced efficacy of the medication, increased side effects, or unexpected adverse reactions.
- Types of drug interactions based on mechanism include pharmacokinetic interactions that affect the absorption, distribution, metabolism, and excretion of drugs and pharmacodynamic interactions that occur when the pharmacological effect of one drug is altered by that of the other.
- Health-care professionals must consider a patient's medical history, current medications, and individual characteristics to predict and manage potential interactions.
- Patients also play a pivotal role in preventing interactions by informing their health-care providers about all medications and supplements they are taking.
- Some interactions are well-documented and studied, whereas others may be less understood, emphasizing the importance of continuous research and vigilance in the field. Overall, awareness of drug interactions is essential for ensuring safe and effective patient care.

1 Introduction

Globally, people are living longer, with the average life expectancy at 73.4 years in 2019 up from 66.8 years in the year 2000 [1]. This demographic change results in an increase in older people living with chronic medical conditions requiring medical and medication interventions. The use of multiple medications is frequently observed in practice where single conditions may require several medications such as in the case of type 2 diabetes mellitus or hypertension and, in addition, where patients present with multiple conditions, thus requiring many more medications. We often consider the term "polypharmacy," commonly defined as the use of five or more medicines [2], as synonymous with inappropriate prescribing, and, while this is not the case, it is important to consider that the more medications a patient is prescribed, the higher the risk of adverse drug reactions and harm [3]. One of the mechanisms by which this can occur is through drug interactions. In this chapter, we will examine in detail the different types of drug interactions that exist, the mechanism by which they occur, and how to prevent and manage them.

2 An Overview of Drug Interactions

2.1 What Are Drug Interactions?

A drug interaction occurs when the effects of one drug are altered by the coadministration of another drug, food, or substance [4]. We often think of drug interactions occurring when the way in which a drug works is altered by the presence of another drug (drug–drug interaction (DDI)), which may be a prescribed medication or a medication purchased over the counter (OTC) at a pharmacy. However, drug interactions can also occur when a drug is altered by the presence of excipients in medications, by the presence of food, herbs, or dietary supplements, or other environmental chemical agents [4].

Drug interactions can be classified in several ways. They can be classified according to their mechanisms of action, e.g., pharmacokinetic or pharmacodynamic (Sect. 3), classified as actual or potential interactions, and classified according to the risk of harm for the patient. "Potential drug–drug interaction" is the term that is used to refer to the possibility that a drug can alter the effects of another drug when they are administered simultaneously [5]. Actual drug–drug interactions are when we consider that the interactions have occurred in the patient. The drug interaction resource Lexicomp® provides definitions of drug interactions based on the risk to the patient as follows: Major-Severity Major, which are potentially severe or life-threatening interactions, the significance of which is supported by the primary literature; Moderate-Severity Moderate, which are interactions that may cause deterioration in the patient's clinical status, the significance of which is supported by the primary literature; Moderate-Severity Major, which are interactions that although may cause major effects, the literature to support their significance is highly limited; Minor-Suspected, which are interactions that are unlikely to be clinically relevant, the significance of which is supported by the limited primary literature; Doubtful/Unknown, which are interactions that are unlikely to be clinically significant and in addition are only supported by limited or conflicted data [6].

2.2 Prevalence of Drug–Drug Interactions

Determining how prevalent DDIs are can be difficult. First, many DDIs may not be recognized by health-care professionals and adverse drug reactions that may occur as a result may be attributed to a new medical condition. Second, even when DDIs are identified, they may be underreported by health-care professionals. A systematic review examining factors associated with under-reporting of adverse drug reactions reported that ignorance of the need to report, diffidence, lethargy, indifference to the benefit of reporting, insecurity in determining causation, and complacency that all drugs that are available on the market are safe were attributed to health-care professional reporting [7]. Finally, studies that investigate the epidemiology of DDIs lack standardization in terms of classifying DDIs and the methods used (for example, considering actual DDI occurrence or the potential for DDI based on medications prescribed), all leading to heterogeneity among studies and huge variability in the reported figures [8]. A systematic review and meta-analysis in hospitalized patients reported the prevalence of potential DDIs among 33% of general patients and 67% of intensive care patients [9]. A systematic review of the prevalence of drug interactions in hospitalized elderly patients reported the prevalence of DDIs to be between 8.34% and 100% [8]. Studies in the community-dwelling population also report high levels of DDIs among older people; a study by Hughes et al. in Ireland reported that approximately one-quarter of people aged 70 years and older were potentially exposed to at least one severe DDI affecting the cardiovascular or central nervous system [10]. Although there is certainly variability across the studies, it is evident that even at the lowest end of this range, DDIs are a significant patient safety issue.

2.3 Risk Factors Associated with Drug–Drug Interactions

The risk factors associated with DDIs are numerous; increasing age, multimorbidity, and polypharmacy are frequently reported in studies [10, 11]. The involvement of multiple prescribers has also been reported as a risk factor for DDIs [12, 13]. This is important to consider in light of a study conducted by Dumbreck et al. who examined the potential for DDIs within UK National Clinical Guidelines for type 2 diabetes mellitus, heart failure, and depression [14]. This study identified many serious interactions between drugs recommended by guidelines in each of the three index conditions and drugs recommended for 11 other conditions. Therefore, clinicians who may be prescribing within the recommendations of a condition-specific guideline may be unintentionally putting their patients at risk of DDIs.

3 Types of Drug–Drug Interactions

DDIs can be classified based on their mechanisms of action as either pharmacokinetic or pharmacodynamic.

3.1 Pharmacokinetic Drug Interactions

Pharmacokinetics describes what the body does to a drug; pharmacokinetic DDIs occur when one drug alters the rate or extent of absorption, distribution, metabolism, or excretion (ADME) of another drug. Pharmacokinetic DDIs can alter drug concentrations, thus affecting clinical response [15]. We will review how DDIs occur at each of the stages of ADME and some common examples.

3.1.1 Absorption

The oral route is the most common route of administration as it is a noninvasive, convenient route for drug delivery [16, 17]. However, many factors can influence the absorption of drugs administered orally, including gastric pH, volume and composition of gastric fluids, and gastric emptying time, leading to variability in drug absorption [17]. This variability can occur due to physiological causes (e.g., in pediatrics and the elderly), due to medical conditions (e.g., post-bariatric surgery), and due to the presence of drug interactions [17]. We will now consider the mechanism by which some of these absorption drug interactions can occur. It should be noted that for drugs administered via the intravenous route, absorption is complete.

Change in Gastric pH

Most drugs are administered orally and thus need to be absorbed through the gastrointestinal (GI) mucosa. The movement of drugs by simple passive diffusion relies on the extent to which they exist in the non-ionized lipid-soluble form, which, in turn, depends on factors such as the drug pK_a and the pH of the GI tract [4]. If a drug alters the gastric pH, for example, in the case of proton pump inhibitors (PPIs), which reduce acid secretion and increase gastric pH, then this has the potential to change the kinetics of the coadministered drugs. An example of this is the interaction between PPIs and certain tyrosine kinase inhibitors, used in the treatment of solid and hematological malignancies [18].

Adsorption and Other Complex Mechanisms

Certain drugs such as cholestyramine, ions such as calcium (found in dairy products), aluminum and magnesium (often found in antacids), and iron compounds can affect absorption by binding to and forming complexes with medications. This can then reduce the absorption of the medication. This pharmacokinetic interaction is the basis of using activated charcoal as an adsorbing agent in case of an overdose. These types of interactions can often be overcome by separating the administration time of the doses by 2–3 hours [4], and, so, patient education is an important aspect of managing and minimizing the potential effects of such interactions.

Inhibition or Induction of Drug Transporter Proteins

Drug transporter proteins serve to transport drugs into and out of cells, which affect systemic drug concentration [19]. One of the key drug transporter proteins is the permeability glycoprotein or P-gp, a member of the adenosine triphosphate (ATP)-binding cassette (ABC) family of transporters, which is located in various parts of the body, including the luminal membrane of the small intestine and blood–brain barrier, and the apical membranes of excretory cells of the liver and kidneys [20]. P-gp plays a role in intestinal absorption of drugs, in addition to limiting the entry of drugs into the central nervous system, and in biliary and urinary excretion of drugs [20]. Drugs can be substrates of P-gp and are thus transported by P-gp across membranes, can act as inhibitors of P-gp and thus impair the actions of P-gp, and can act as inducers of P-gp and thus enhance P-gp activity [19].

Examples of drugs that are P-gp substrates are digoxin, losartan, ciclosporin, tacrolimus, diltiazem, verapamil, ondansetron, morphine, phenytoin, doxorubicin, ritonavir, erythromycin, dabigatran, apixaban, rivaroxaban, and edoxaban [21]. If two of these drugs are prescribed together, then they can compete for the P-gp transporters and lead to an alteration in their absorption, excretion, and tissue distribution at sites where the P-gp transporter is expressed.

Drugs that inhibit P-gp can cause DDIs, for example, the cardiovascular drug verapamil, a calcium antagonist, inhibits the activity of P-gp, which can increase concentrations of P-gp substrates such as digoxin [4]. Clarithromycin inhibits P-gp and may reduce the renal clearance of digoxin, thus increasing the risk of digoxin toxicity [21]. The expression of P-gp can be induced by drugs such as the antituberculosis drug rifampicin, which, in the presence of digoxin, reduces its plasma concentration [4]. Many of the drugs that are affected by P-gp interactions are also affected by interactions affecting the cytochrome P450 system, in particular CYP3A4, which we will look at later in this chapter.

Changes in Gastric Motility

The movement of drugs through the gastrointestinal tract to the main site of absorption, the small intestine, can be altered by drugs that alter gastric motility. One such drug is the prokinetic agent metoclopramide, which exhibits activity on dopamine and 5-hydroxytryptamine (5-HT) receptors in the gastrointestinal tract [22]. By accelerating gastric emptying, metoclopramide can increase the rate of absorption of several drugs, including paracetamol (acetaminophen), an interaction which is taken advantage of when the two drugs are used in combination for the treatment of migraine, a condition often accompanied by delayed gastric emptying [22].

3.1.2 Distribution

The next step in the process is the distribution of the drug through the body's blood and tissues.

Displacement from Protein-Binding Sites

Several factors can impact drug distribution, including plasma-binding proteins, particularly the albumins. Some drugs are highly protein-bound meaning that a large proportion of the drug is reversibly bound to the protein and only the unbound molecule is available for passive diffusion to extravascular or tissue sites where it can exert its pharmacological action [4]. Drug interactions may arise from displacement from plasma protein-binding sites, but such effects are typically of limited clinical significance since the metabolism of the displaced drug generally increases alongside the increased concentration of unbound drug. However, it may have importance and should be considered for highly bound drugs having a narrow therapeutic window, a high hepatic extraction ratio (if administered intravenously), or a high renal extraction ratio [23]. Awareness of this interaction with narrow therapeutic drugs is important as it can alter the interpretation of therapeutic drug monitoring. This is the information provided in the reference included. For example, if the antiepileptic drug phenytoin was displaced from its binding site, then the amount of free phenytoin would initially increase, but, through metabolism and excretion, the amount of free phenytoin would reduce back to the original level. However, the total amount of phenytoin would be reduced as a result, and, thus, interpretation of this reduced level, without consideration of the interaction, may lead a clinician to incorrectly increasing the dose of phenytoin [4].

Inhibition or Induction of Drug Transporter Proteins

In addition to their role in drug absorption, drug transporter proteins, including P-gp, influence drug distribution by limiting penetration into several sensitive tissues such as the brain [24]. DDIs that inhibit or induce drug transporter proteins could therefore affect the uptake of drug substrates to areas such as the brain.

3.1.3 Metabolism

Drug metabolism is the process by which a drug is chemically changed so as to facilitate its excretion from the body. The liver is the primary site for drug metabolism, although metabolism can occur in other areas of the body, including the skin, lungs, intestines, kidneys, and plasma [4, 25]. In the liver, drugs are metabolized through either phase I reactions (oxidation, reduction, hydrolysis reactions) or phase II reactions (glucuronidation, acetylation, sulfation reactions) or both, with the aim of converting lipid-soluble to more water-soluble compounds for excretion [25]. Phase I reactions are catalyzed by a family of enzymes within the liver microsomes called cytochrome P450, comprising 18 families and 44 subfamily members [26]. However, the most clinically relevant CYP isoenzymes for drug metabolism are CYP1A2, CYP2C9, CYP2C19, CYP2D6, CYP2E1, and CYP3A4/5, which account for 90% of metabolic activity [27]. The liver is also a key site for DDIs to occur, notably through induction and inhibition of CYP enzymes.

Induction

Drugs that are inducers increase the synthesis of a CYP450 enzyme, resulting in increases in enzymatic activity. This leads to a decrease in serum concentrations of other drugs metabolized by the same isoenzyme. Induction reactions tend to be delayed in their onset and their resolution, the effects dependent on the half-life of the inducing drug, the dose of the inducing drug, and the rate of turnover of the enzyme being induced [4, 28]. Examples of inducers include the antiepileptic drugs carbamazepine and phenytoin and the antituberculosis drug rifampicin [4]. Induction reactions can often be overcome by increasing the dose of the affected drug; however, this requires careful monitoring, including ensuring that the dose is modified if the interacting drug is stopped.

Inhibition

The most common mechanism leading to DDIs is inhibition of the CYP450 system [29]. This occurs when a drug (precipitant drug) inhibits the CYP450 isoenzyme that is responsible for the metabolism of another drug (object drug), resulting in an increase in the plasma concentration of the object drug. There are several ways in which inhibition can occur: reversible inhibition, which includes competitive and noncompetitive inhibition, and irreversible or mechanism-based inhibition [29]. Competitive inhibition occurs when two drugs that are substrates for the same enzyme compete for the same active site of the CYP450 enzyme. A substrate with a stronger affinity to the binding site can displace the weaker substrate from the active site, thus resulting in increased plasma concentration and the potential for an adverse event to occur [29]. The effect of this type of competitive inhibition is almost immediate in contrast to induction interactions, which are slower at onset. Noncompetitive inhibition occurs when the precipitant drug binds to the allosteric site of the enzyme and thus does not prevent the object drug from also binding to the enzyme at the active site. However, by binding to the allosteric site, a conformational change occurs at the active site, and it loses its affinity toward the object drug. Similar to competitive inhibition, the effect of noncompetitive inhibition is almost immediate [29]. There are also examples of mixed inhibition, whereby a drug can act in both a competitive and noncompetitive way, binding at the active site and at the allosteric site of the enzyme; these drugs, such as the azoles, tend to be potent inhibitors [29]. Irreversible and quasi-irreversible inhibitions are together known as mechanism-based inhibition; this involves the metabolism of the inhibitor drug into a reactive metabolite, which modifies the CYP enzyme, leading to irreversible loss of enzymatic activity [30]. Examples of drugs that interact in this way include the macrolides, clarithromycin and erythromycin, and the proton pump inhibitor omeprazole [4, 29]. Health-care professionals should recognize when an inhibition interaction has occurred or has the potential to occur and take appropriate steps to avoid adverse effects to the patient.

The CYP3A4 enzymes are also expressed in the intestine, with their expression level varying across the intestine, with high levels in the duodenum. These enzymes are responsible for a significant number of DDIs as they are involved in the metabolism of many drugs. Determining specific DDIs with 3A4 enzymes can be challenging as they are also present in the liver. An example of such a DDI is the inhibition of intestinal 3A4 by itraconazole, which leads to increased gut oral bioavailability of midazolam [31].

Table 4.1 presents some common CYP450-mediated drug–drug interactions.

3.1.4 Excretion

The final step in the pharmacokinetic pathway is the removal of drugs from the body. Excretion of drugs can occur through different mechanisms, including the lungs, sweat, saliva, and milk; however, the main routes of excretion are through involvement of the kidneys (which accounts for more than two-thirds of drug excretion) and the liver through excretion via the bile [32]. Hydrophilic drugs are typically excreted directly by the kidneys, whereas hydrophobic drugs require biotransformation (most often by the liver) before excretion by the kidneys.

Urinary pH

Urinary pH can impact excretion of drugs by the kidneys. If a drug exists in its ionized lipid-insoluble form, it cannot undergo passive reabsorption into the tubule cells and so will be removed from the body in the urine. For drugs that are weak acids with a pK_a between 3 and 7.5, this situation will arise at high pH values, whereas for drugs that are weakly basic with a pK_a between 7.5 and 10.5, this situation arises at low pH values. Changes in

Table 4.1 Examples of substrates, inducers, and inhibitors of cytochrome P450 enzymes

Substrates	Inducers	Inhibitors
CYP3A4: Apixaban, rivaroxaban, atorvastatin, simvastatin, calcium channel blockers, ciclosporin, codeine, benzodiazepines, oral contraceptives, verapamil, R-warfarin	CYP3A4: Barbiturates, carbamazepine, dexamethasone, rifampicin, St. John's wort	CYP3A4: Amiodarone, diltiazem, clarithromycin, erythromycin, cimetidine, fluconazole, itraconazole, fluoxetine, sertraline, venlafaxine, grapefruit juice, tamoxifen, tricyclic antidepressants
CYP2D6: Beta-blockers, codeine, donepezil, flecainide, tricyclic antidepressants, tolterodine, risperidone	CYP2D6: Carbamazepine, rifampicin	CYP2D6: Amiodarone, chlorpheniramine, fluoxetine, paroxetine, sertraline, tricyclic antidepressants, venlafaxine, ketoconazole, haloperidol
CYP2C9: Aspirin, most NSAIDs, diazepam, selective serotonin reuptake inhibitors, S-warfarin, statins	CYP2C9: Barbiturates, rifampicin, phenytoin	CYP2C9: Cimetidine, fluoxetine, omeprazole, metronidazole, fluconazole, voriconazole
CYP1A2: Caffeine, clozapine, imipramine, olanzapine, theophylline, tricyclic antidepressants, R-warfarin, duloxetine	CYP1A2: Omeprazole, lansoprazole, phenytoin, tobacco smoke	CYP1A2: Amiodarone, cimetidine, quinolones, fluvoxamine
CYP2C19: Citalopram, clopidogrel, diazepam, lansoprazole, omeprazole, voriconazole	CYP2C19: Carbamazepine, rifampicin, omeprazole	CYP2C19: Cannabidiol, esomeprazole, fluconazole, fluoxetine

Disclaimer: This table is not exhaustive

urinary pH can alter the amount of drug excreted; however, this interaction appears to be only clinically significant in a small number of cases [4]. One such example is urine alkalinization with methotrexate. Methotrexate is poorly soluble at an acidic pH, which can result in it and its metabolites precipitating in the renal tubules, leading to acute kidney injury. Administration of urine alkalinizers, such as sodium bicarbonate, to achieve a urinary pH of 7 increases the solubility of methotrexate and reduces the risk of crystal formation [33].

The Role of Drug Transporters

Various drug transporters, including P-gp, organic anionic transporters (OATs), and organic cationic transporters (OCTs), are predominantly expressed in the renal proximal tubules and function to eliminate drugs into the urine from the circulation [34]. Drugs that inhibit renal drug transporters can decrease renal clearance, which can lead to increased plasma drug concentrations and consequent adverse effects. The interaction can also lead to drug-induced nephrotoxicity due to accumulation of the drug in the proximal tubule cells [34]. An example of this interaction occurs with the drug probenecid, a uricosuric agent used in the treatment of gout, which inhibits OATs. Probenecid inhibits OAT1 and OAT3, leading to the inhibition of renal excretion of methotrexate, which can lead to toxic effects of methotrexate [4].

Biliary Excretion

Biliary excretion occurs when drugs, either unchanged or conjugated, are excreted into bile, ready for removal from the body. The hepatobiliary elimination process is complex involving multiple processes and many different transporter proteins, including P-gp, OATs, and OCTs [4]. Drugs that induce or inhibit the activity of these transporter proteins can alter the pharmacokinetics of the victim drug [35]; however, the clinical relevance of these drug interactions is unclear [4].

3.2 Pharmacodynamic Drug Interactions

Pharmacodynamics is concerned with what a drug does to the body to elicit a physiological response [32]. Pharmacodynamic DDIs occur when the pharmacodynamics of one drug is altered by that of a coadministered drug. Pharmacodynamic DDIs can be classified as additive, synergistic, or antagonistic [36]. In addition, pharmacodynamic DDIs can be used intentionally for beneficial effects (e.g., combinations of drugs to lower blood pressure) or can be unintended and lead to adverse effects (e.g., selective serotonin reuptake inhibitors [SSRIs] in combination with the analgesic tramadol with the potential to cause serotonin syndrome [SS]).

3.2.1 Additive Pharmacodynamic Drug Interactions

An additive pharmacodynamic DDI occurs when the interaction produces an effect equal to the sum of the pharmacological effects of each drug involved [36]. An example of this interaction is the coadministration of the antidiabetic medications liraglutide and insulin detemir, which produce an additive glucose-lowering effect [37].

3.2.2 Synergistic Pharmacodynamic Drug Interactions

A synergistic pharmacodynamic DDI occurs when the combination of two drugs results in an effect, which is greater than the sum of the effects of each drug individually [32]. An example of this is the synergism between volatile anesthetics and opioids in which the dose requirements of various anesthetics, including desflurane, propofol, and thiopental, might be lower after opioid use [4]. Another example involves the combination of the antibacterial drugs sulfamethoxazole and trimethoprim, as the preparation co-trimoxazole, in which both drugs work synergistically to inhibit steps along the folic acid biosynthetic pathway [38].

3.2.3 Antagonistic Pharmacodynamic Drug Interactions

Antagonistic pharmacodynamic DDIs occur when one drug, the perpetrator, inhibits the effect of the second drug, the victim drug. An example of this interaction for beneficial purposes is the use of naloxone and flumazenil to counteract the effects of opioids and benzodiazepines, respectively. An unwanted antagonistic DDI occurs if a non-cardioselective beta-blocker can oppose the bronchodilator effects of beta-agonist bronchodilators, which can lead to serious bronchospasm [4].

4 Clinically Relevant Drug–Drug Interactions

The following section provides an overview of commonly encountered, clinically relevant DDIs. It should be noted that this is not an exhaustive list.

4.1 Antimicrobial Drug–Drug Interactions

Antimicrobial stewardship, which aims to ensure that antibiotics and antifungal therapies are used appropriately and responsibly, can be negatively impacted by antimicrobial–drug interactions. The risk of patient toxicity increases if they are prescribed medications that can interact with antimicrobial therapy. Some antibacterial medications interact with many other medications, and the increasing burden of chronic disease and polypharmacy increases the risk of DDIs involving antimicrobials. Macrolides (e.g., clarithromycin, erythromycin, azithromycin) interact with statins, potentially leading to life-threatening rhabdomyolysis and resulting in acute kidney injury. Macrolides are CYP3A4 inhibitors and statins are CYP3A4 substrates; concomitant use of both medications can increase the systemic exposure to statins [39].

Fluoroquinolones (e.g., ciprofloxacin, levofloxacin) interact with some antiarrhythmic agents, resulting in torsade de pointes, due to QT (the duration of ventricular electrical systole) interval prolongation [4]. Multivalent cations (e.g., antacids, supplements, or feeds containing calcium, iron, magnesium, zinc, sucralfate, bismuth) bind to fluoroquinolones and reduce their absorption from the gastrointestinal tract. If used together, administration times must be spaced apart [4].

Antifungal medications pose a particular challenge with a high degree of risk and serious drug interactions, which can occur between antifungal medications and many other medications [40, 41]. Most of these interactions occur due to CYP450 interactions, with some new interaction pathways, e.g., organic anion-transporting polypeptide 1B1 (OATP1B1) and breast cancer resistance protein pathways (BCRPs). Interactions with antifungals can lead to life-threatening adverse effects, e.g., QT interval prolongation, neuromuscular toxicity, and death [42]. Antifungal agents inhibit key metabolizing cytochrome P450 enzymes (e.g., CYP3A4) and membrane-bound transport systems (e.g., P-gp), thus affecting the absorption, metabolism, and excretion of coadministered drugs. DDIs may preclude the use of first-line antifungal agents (e.g., anti-mold azoles may be problematic in patients on concurrent chemotherapy or antiretrovirals due to unpredictable drug interactions). Azole antifungals and phenytoin can interact in a bidirectional manner; azole first inhibits the CYP-mediated metabolism of phenytoin, which is followed by the phenytoin-induced, CYP-mediated metabolism of azoles. This can result in phenytoin toxicity and/or treatment failure with the azole antifungal [43].

The Antifungals Interaction Database is a single central resource, which holds interactions data, and is a useful source of information for health-care professionals on drug interactions with antifungal agents [44]. Some commonly encountered drug and antifungal interactions are outlined in Table 4.2 [45].

4.2 Antiretroviral Drug–Drug Interactions

Antiretrovirals (ARVs) have complicated and unpredictable DDIs, leading to toxicity and treatment failure, including human immunodeficiency virus (HIV) treatment failure. There is an increasing number of ARVs available for treating HIV and coupled with the increasing life expectancy of patients living with HIV, the risk of DDIs increases. Absorption of ARVs can be impacted

Table 4.2 Examples of drug interactions with antifungal medications

Antifungal agent	Interacting drug	Comment
Fluconazole, Miconazole (oral gel)	Statins (simvastatin, atorvastatin)	Increased risk of myopathy and rhabdomyolysis. Check statin summary of product characteristics for detailed information
	Direct anticoagulants (apixaban, dabigatran, rivaroxaban, edoxaban)	Fluconazole can increase bleeding risk
	Warfarin	Increased risk of bleeding due to raised International Normalized Ratio (INR); also risk with miconazole oral gel
	Clopidogrel	Reduced antiplatelet activity; increased bleeding risk
	Domperidone	QT interval prolongation
Fluconazole, itraconazole	Benzodiazepines	Increased and prolonged sedative effects
	Ciclosporin, tacrolimus	Increased risk of toxicity; renal impairment
Caspofungin	Rifampicin Phenytoin Carbamazepine Dexamethasone	Reduced caspofungin plasma concentration
	Tacrolimus	Increase in tacrolimus levels. Monitor levels and adjust as needed.

Disclaimer: This table is not an exhaustive list of all drug interactions with antifungal agents. Please check product summary of product characteristics for comprehensive information

by gastric pH; for example, lansoprazole and omeprazole can reduce the absorption of atazanavir and rilpivirine. Drugs that increase or slow the rate of gastric emptying can impact ARV absorption. Polyvalent cations (e.g., calcium, iron, magnesium, zinc) can chelate with integrase inhibitors (e.g., dolutegravir, raltegravir) and reduce absorption.

Most ARVs are hepatically metabolized by the CYP450 system or by glucuronidation via uridyl-diphosphate-glucuronosyl-transferase 1A1 (UGT1A1) (dolutegravir and raltegravir) [46]. CYP3A4 has a significant impact on ARV metabolism. From a clinical perspective, treatment of other conditions in HIV is challenging. For example, rifampicin, which is a potent CYP450 enzyme inducer and UGT1A1 inducer, and indicated for treating tuberculosis, poses challenges in HIV patients, resulting in reduced levels of ARVs such as raltegravir [47].

Prescribing and reviewing of ARV medications is a specialized area, and health-care professionals should seek expert advice in this area before changing medication regimens. ARVs can be substrates, inhibitors, and inducers of CYP450 and drug transporter systems. DDIs with ARVs can impact HIV treatment and treatment of other conditions. Caution should be exercised when managing patients on drugs with a narrow therapeutic index and interactions with ARVs. Further information can be sourced online at www.hiv--druginteractions.org [48] and https://clinicalinfo.hiv.gov/en/guidelines/hiv-clinical-guidelines-adult-and-adolescent-arv/drug-interactions-overview?view=full provided by the Office of AIDS Research in the National Institutes of Health in the United States [49].

4.3 Anti-Seizure Medication Drug–Drug Interactions

Interactions between Anti-Seizure Medications (ASMs) are complex and can increase the risk of side effects and toxicity, usually as a result of hepatic enzyme inhibition or induction. Patients with epilepsy are often prescribed a number of medications, including other ASMs, which increases the risk of DDIs. The potent enzyme inducers phenytoin and carbamazepine carry a risk of DDIs with many drug classes, including statins, antidepressants, and neuroleptics [50].

Sodium valproate is an inhibitor of CYP450 enzymes and contributes to several pharmacokinetic interactions. When co-prescribed with lamotrigine, it can increase its half-life and lead to reduced lamotrigine clearance. Adjustment of the existing lamotrigine dose may be required if it is co-prescribed with sodium valproate.

Carbamazepine is a potent CYP450 inducer, which leads to significant drug interactions. One interaction of note is with the estrogen and progestogen components of the contraceptive pill, which can result in contraceptive failure [4]. Levetiracetam is an ASM with fewer interactions and is often chosen for this reason, if clinically appropriate.

ASMs are at risk of DDIs due to antimicrobials in the fluoroquinolone and macrolide class (CYP3A4 inhibition). Phenytoin and carbamazepine are older ASMs, which are enzyme inducers, and may reduce the levels of antimicrobials, thus reducing their therapeutic effect. An example of bidirectional DDI exists between the antifungal voriconazole and several ASMs. Voriconazole is metabolized and is a strong inhibitor of CYP3A4, CYP2C9/10, and CYP2C19. Phenytoin has been shown to induce voriconazole metabolism with possible loss of its efficacy, whereas voriconazole increases the levels of phenytoin [51].

In the process of prescribing medications for patients taking ASMs, care should be taken to screen for DDIs, adjust the medication dose as appropriate, conduct therapeutic drug monitoring, and carry out clinical monitoring to reduce patient adverse consequences [52]. It should be noted that some antimicrobials (e.g., fluoroquinolones, monobactams, cephalosporins, isoniazid) have epileptogenic properties due to disturbing gamma-aminobutyric acid (GABA) neurotransmission [52].

4.4 Drug Interactions and QT Prolongation

QT interval prolongation can be caused by congenital and acquired causes, common of which is drug-induced QT interval prolongation [53]. QT prolongation is a risk factor for torsade de point and ventricular arrhythmias and results in cardiac death. DDIs can increase the risk of QT interval prolongation, a) if more than one QT-prolonging medication is prescribed (pharmacodynamic interaction), b) if its metabolism is inhibited by another medication (pharmacokinetic interaction), c) if a medication, which disturbs electrolytes, is prescribed, then this increases the risk of QT prolongation [54].

When prescribing a drug that may cause QT prolongation, it is important to assess the risks and benefits for the patient, and their individual factors should be considered. Individual patient factors such as female sex, age over 65 years, thyroid disease, cardiac disease, bradycardia, congenital long QT syndrome, and electrolyte disturbances can increase the risk of QT interval prolongation [54].

An extensive list of medications associated with QT prolongation is available on www.crediblemeds.org [55]. The list is frequently updated and categorizes the medications according to the risk of QT prolongation. There is a particular section of this online resource, which highlights clinically relevant, common drug–drug interactions, e.g. amiodarone and quinolones.

The risks and benefits of QT-prolonging medications must be evaluated on a case-by-case basis. If a QT-prolonging medication is recommended, then an electrocardiogram (ECG) at baseline and regular monitoring could be considered [53, 54]. As it would not be practical to request an ECG each time a QT-prolonging drug is prescribed, an algorithm is presented in Fig. 4.1 [53]. Patients prescribed QT-prolonging medications who present with palpitations, light-headedness, and dizziness should be investigated.

A systematic review summarizing and comparing tools for assessing safety risks with QT interval-prolonging medications reported on nine risk assessment tools, mostly applying risk scores, with risk assessment included in a clinical decision support system or computerized physician order entry [56]. Most studies were conducted in hospital in-patient settings, and risk assessments were primarily designed for use by physicians and pharmacists. An intervention study conducted in 20 community pharmacies in the Netherlands introduced a clinical decision support (CDS) prediction tool to support the risk management of QT interval DDIs [57]. The study did not report a statistically significant difference in the proportion of QT interval DDIs where a pharmacist intervention was conducted after implementation of the CDS; however, phar-

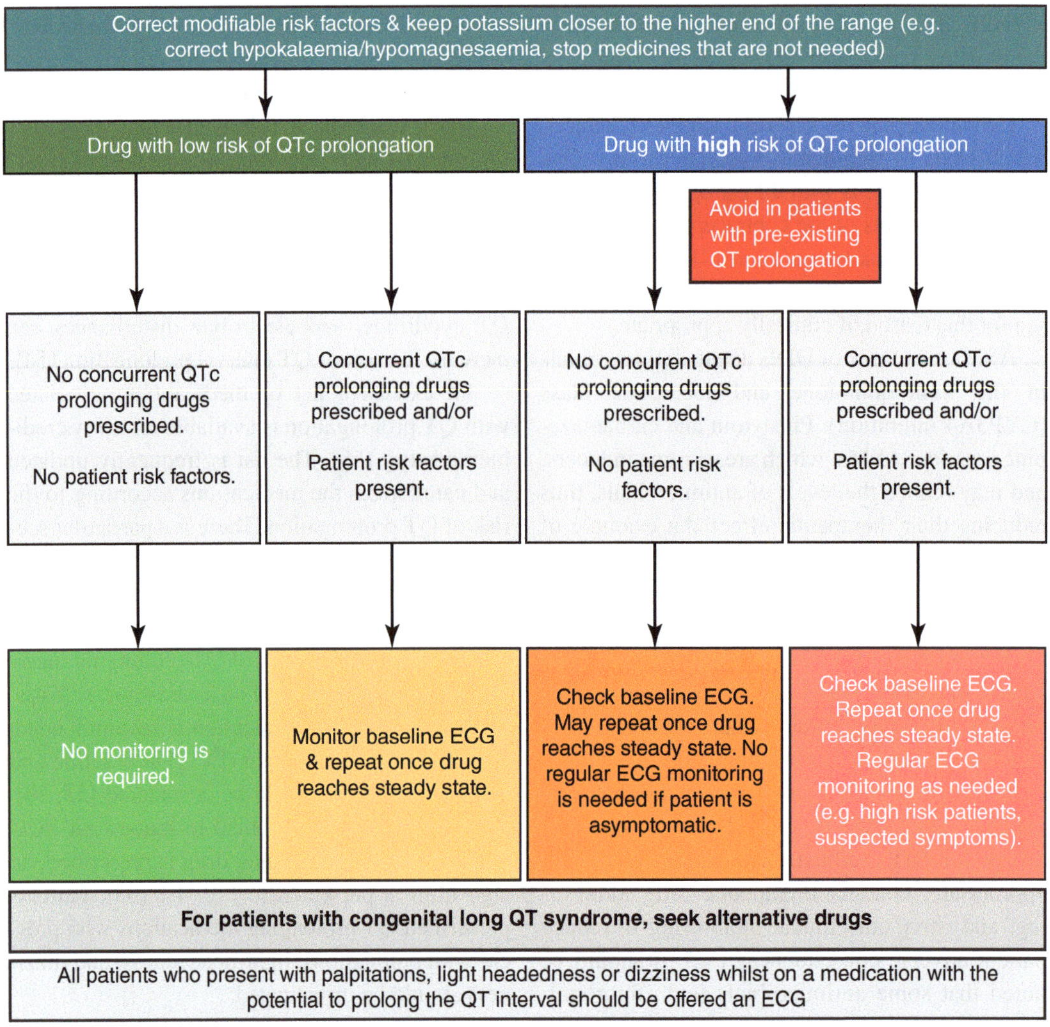

Fig. 4.1 Management of QT prolongation in practice. (Reproduced with permission from Khatib et al. [53])

macists reported that less time was spent on the management of these DDIs when tool was used.

4.5 Drug Interactions and Serotonin Syndrome

Serotonin syndrome (SS) is the clinical manifestation of excess serotonin in the body, resulting from therapeutic use or overdose of serotonergic medications. The clinical features of SS range on a spectrum from minor symptoms to death and present as neuromuscular excitation (e.g., shivering, tremor, tooth-grinding, myoclonus, hyperreflexia), autonomic effects (e.g., diarrhea, sweating, flushing, tachycardia, hyper- or hypotension), and altered mental status (e.g., agitation, confusion, delirium); however, not all are present in all cases [58]. There are a wide range of drugs that contribute to SS (Table 4.3), and over-the-counter, herbal medicines, and drugs of abuse can also contribute [59] to it. Many cases occur due to the use or combined use of serotonergic medications or when one serotonergic medication is stopped and another is started. CYP3A4 and CYP2D6 inhibitors may also contribute by inhibiting the metabolism of serotonergic medications, leading to SS [60]. Table 4.3 presents examples of drugs contributing to SS [59].

Table 4.3 Drugs causing serotonin syndrome

Mechanism	Drugs involved
Increase in serotonin production	L-Tryptophan
Inhibition of serotonin metabolism	Monoamine oxidase inhibitors (e.g., phenelzine, moclobemide) Selegiline Linezolid
Increase in serotonin release	Amphetamines Aminoindanes (e.g., MDAI (5,6-methylenedioxy-2-aminoindane)) Benzofurans (e.g., benzofury) 3,4-Methylenedioxy-methamphetamine (MDMA—"Ecstasy") Methylphenidate
Inhibition of serotonin reuptake	Selective serotonin reuptake inhibitors (e.g., escitalopram) Tricyclic antidepressants (e.g., amitriptyline, imipramine) Serotonin norepinephrine reuptake inhibitors (e.g., venlafaxine, duloxetine) Opioid analgesics (e.g., fentanyl, pethidine, tramadol) St. John's wort (*Hypericum perforatum*)
Serotonin receptor agonism	Buspirone Sumatriptan Lithium Tryptamines (e.g., alpha-methyltryptamine—AMT)

Disclaimer: This table is not exhaustive

Prevention of SS requires clinical awareness of the toxic potential of serotonergic medications and avoiding combined use of these medications. Patients should be educated about taking their medications as prescribed and to be aware of the signs of SS. Prescribers should minimize the unnecessary use of serotonergic medications and observe safe wash-out periods when transitioning patients between antidepressant medications to prevent overlap [61]. Taking particular care to follow the manufacturer's summary of product characteristics is needed when changing from an SSRI to a monoamine oxidase inhibitor (MAOI), and vice versa. SSRIs with a long half-life, e.g., fluoxetine, need to have an appropriate wash-out period before another serotonergic medication is started.

5 Drug–Herb Interactions

Health-care professionals must be alert to the potential of herb–drug interactions. There can be misperceptions that herbs are harmless, as they are perceived to be natural. However, there is potential for significant clinical impact, for example, traditional Chinese medicine herbs or herbal products may exhibit steroidal activity [62]. Herbal medicinal products and supplements are largely unregulated by medicinal products regulators. Studies have found that up to one-third of patients do not disclose complementary, herbal, or supplement use to health-care professionals [63, 64]. Drugs with a narrow therapeutic index (e.g., warfarin) raise a safety concern when taken concomitantly with herbal products. Pharmacokinetic herb–drug interactions can occur via mechanisms affecting drug absorption, induction and inhibition of metabolic enzymes, and transport proteins, which can be countered by changing the drug dose [64]. For example, ginseng (*Panax ginseng*) can increase/decrease/have no effect on warfarin efficacy and, as such, extreme caution is needed. Less common pharmacodynamic herb–drug interaction mechanisms due to the intrinsic pharmacological properties of herbal supplements acting on drug sites/receptors can result in synergistic, additive, and/or antagonistic effects of the concomitant drug without alteration of its level and are also unlikely to be countered by a change in drug dosage [64]. Of interest in recent years has been the increasing use of cannabis-based medicinal products containing cannabidiol (CBD) and tetrahydrocannabinol (THC). Both THC and CBD have been found to inhibit CYP1A1, CYP1A2, and CYP1B1 enzymes in in vitro studies [65]. CBD is a potent inhibitor of CYP2C19 and CYP3A4 [66]. Concurrent use of other medications that induce, inhibit, or are metabolized by CYP3A4 may require a dose adjustment to avoid treatment failure or increased risk of adverse effects. There may be enhanced sedation with central nervous system depressants such as benzodiazepines, opioids, and phenobarbital.

Several other commonly used herbal medicines with the potential for pharmacokinetic and pharmacodynamic drug interactions are saw palmetto, echinacea, feverfew, kava, goldenseal, and turmeric. Concomitant use of any herbal medication with regular or short-term prescribed medications should involve screening for drug–herb interactions.

6 Drug–Food Interactions

Drug–food interactions typically result from reduced gastrointestinal absorption or motility. Chelation between some drugs and foods (e.g., iron-, calcium-, magnesium-containing foods and certain medications) can reduce GI absorption and is usually countered by spacing out administration times by a specified period of time. Grapefruit juice inhibits intestinal CYP3A4 and can increase levels of CYP3A4 substrates (e.g., simvastatin). It is a CYP3A4 inhibitor (mainly intestinal) and a drug transporter protein inhibitor and can interact with felodipine and some statins. MAOIs (e.g., tranylcypromine, selegiline) inhibit the breakdown of tyramine. When MAOIs are taken with foods high in tyramine content (e.g., chocolate, red wine, cheese, smoked fish/meat, fermented foods), tyramine accumulation can occur, resulting in hypertensive crisis (symptoms include severe headache, dizziness, flushing, sweating, nausea, vomiting). Cranberry juice has been reported to increase International Normalized Ratio (INR) levels when taken with warfarin. Warfarin is a vitamin K antagonist, which inhibits the enzyme vitamin K epoxide reductase, thus reducing the synthesis of vitamin K-dependent blood clotting factors by the liver. Fluctuations in dietary intake of vitamin K_1 (e.g., cruciferous vegetables such as broccoli, brussels sprouts, cabbage) may impact warfarin levels. If the intake of dietary vitamin K_1 increases, then the synthesis of the blood clotting factors begins to return to normal [4].

Table 4.4 lists some examples of herb–drug and food–drug interactions, which may have clinical significance [67–72].

Table 4.4 Examples of reported drug–herb and drug–food interactions

Herb	Drug	Mechanism	Effect
Black cohosh (*Actaea racemosa, Cimicifuga racemosa*)	Statins	CYP3A4 inhibition	Elevated statin levels, resulting in raised liver enzymes
Garlic (*Allium sativum*)	Paracetamol Warfarin Saquinavir	P-gp induction	Changes in pharmacokinetic variable Increased INR Decreased concentration
Ginkgo (*Ginkgo biloba*)	Warfarin Amiodarone	Antiplatelet effect CYP3A4 inhibition	Increased bleeding risk Increased toxicity risk
Ginseng (*Panax ginseng*)	Some chemotherapy, antiretrovirals, antidepressants, antihypertensives, statins	CYP3A4 induction	Reduced effectiveness of the drug
St. John's wort (*Hypericum perforatum*)	Oral contraceptive pill, warfarin, digoxin, tacrolimus, benzodiazepines, statins	CYP3A4 induction P-gp induction	Reduced effectiveness of the drug
Liquorice (*Glycyrrhiza glabra*)	Monoamine oxidase inhibitors (MAOI)	MAOI activity	MAOI toxicity
	Diuretics	Sodium and water retention	Exacerbated hypokalemia
Glucosamine	Warfarin, anticoagulants, direct anticoagulants, antiplatelets	Anticoagulant effect	Increased bleeding risk
Cannabidiol	Anticonvulsants		Increase in drug concentration; increase in liver function tests of some anticonvulsants
	Phenytoin	CYP2 C19 inhibition	Increased plasma phenytoin concentration
	Antiplatelets/anticoagulants	Inhibition of platelet aggregation	Increased bleeding risk

Table 4.4 (continued)

Food	Drug	Mechanism	Effect
Grapefruit/grapefruit juice	Digoxin	P-gp induction	Reduced effectiveness of digoxin
	Dihydropyridine calcium channel blockers, amiodarone, simvastatin, tacrolimus	CYP3A4 inhibition	Increased effectiveness of the drug
Green vegetables (e.g., cabbage, broccoli, brussels sprouts)	Warfarin	High vitamin K content interferes with warfarin action	Reduced anticoagulant effect of warfarin
Milk and dairy products	Ciprofloxacin, tetracycline, levothyroxine, bisphosphonate	Chelation with the drug	Reduced absorption and effectiveness of the drug
Hard cheese	MAOIs, linezolid	Accumulation of monoamine oxidase	Increase in blood pressure, headaches

7 Drug–Disease Interactions

Drug–disease interactions are situations where the pharmacotherapy used to treat a disease causes a worsening of another preexisting disease or condition in a patient [73]. Similarly, the presence of a particular disease condition could influence the action of a specific drug, altering its ADME or pharmacodynamic response and resulting in altered effectiveness and/or safety. Older patients are particularly at risk of drug–disease interactions due to the coexistence of comorbidities and risk of polypharmacy. The American Geriatrics Society has identified drug–disease interactions as a key element of care for older persons with multimorbidity [74].

A systematic examination of recommendations in 12 United Kingdom national clinical guidelines reported a number of potentially serious drug–disease interactions between drugs recommended for type 2 diabetes mellitus, depression, and heart failure, particularly when a patient has comorbid chronic kidney disease [14].

Patients with diabetes mellitus are at risk of hypoglycemia, polypharmacy, and drug–drug and drug–disease interactions [74]. This risk is exacerbated or results in potentially greater clinical risk when the patient has multimorbidity.

Examples of drug–disease interactions with potential clinical consequences include the following:

- Beta-blockers taken for heart disease or hypertension can worsen a patient's asthma [73].
- Metformin and heart failure: Metformin should be avoided in patients with heart failure and renal impairment due to the risk of lactic acidosis [74].
- Bisphosphonates and renal impairment: The patient's renal function and bisphosphonate dose and duration of therapy due to the risk of further renal impairment should be reviewed [74].
- Anticholinergic drugs and dementia can result in delirium [75].
- Aspirin taken when a patient has peptic ulcer disease could result in gastrointestinal bleeding [76].
- Nonsteroidal anti-inflammatory drugs (NSAIDs) can worsen heart failure [77].

It must also be noted that drug-induced renal or hepatic impairment may impact the elimination of another drug. Liver and cardiac diseases that affect hepatic blood flow can affect drug metabolism. In some cases, patients present with conditions that are exacerbated by drug–disease interaction. For example, a patient with fatigue may feel more fatigued if they are prescribed a beta-blocker to slow the heart rate or if they experience unstable blood glucose levels (e.g., risk of hypoglycemia with sulfonylureas).

When prescribing for patients with multimorbidity and polypharmacy and for older patients, a comprehensive assessment of the patient's risk factors (e.g., comorbidities, renal function, hepatic function, concomitant medications) must be conducted. The use of clinical decision support tools and guidelines developed for patients with multimorbidity is recommended to support safe prescribing for patients with multimorbidity and polypharmacy [78]. Screening tools such as the Beers criteria, Screening Tool of Older Persons' Prescriptions (STOPP) and Screening Tool to Alert to Right Treatment (START) criteria, and the Screening Tool of Older Persons' Prescriptions in Frail Adults with Limited Life Expectancy (STOPP-FRAIL) are supportive tools to improve appropriate and safe prescribing for older persons [79–81]. In the Netherlands, pharmacies use clinical decision support implemented in their pharmacy information system that generates alerts for drug-related problems, such as drug hypersensitivity, drug–drug interactions, and drug–disease interactions [82]. This system was first developed by a multidisciplinary expert panel who created a panel of recommendations for drug–disease interactions for 57 diseases, which were embedded into the clinical decision support system [83]. This system supports pharmacists and physicians as a point-of-care signal to support medication safety.

8 Drug–Laboratory Test Interactions

Drugs may impact the interpretation of laboratory test results. Drug–laboratory test interactions (DLTIs) represent a source of diagnostic and/or therapeutic errors; this is a well-recognized and well-evidenced issue in clinical practice [84]. DLTIs are categorized as either physiological (pharmacological, biological, in vivo) or analytical (methodological, in vitro) [84]. Analytical drug–test interactions occur when a drug alters the test specimen or interferes with the test reagent. Laboratory testing and diagnostic methodologies are continuously being improved in terms of accuracy and sensitivity; however, a margin of error exists for all tests, with drugs presenting a source of error [85]. DLTIs may result in the need for an additional test, inaccurate diagnosis, and inaccurate treatment, potentially resulting in morbidity or mortality. A review of all the US Food and Drug Administration (FDA)-approved drug labels found that 134/1368 (9.8%) single-ingredient prescription drugs interfere with at least 1 clinical laboratory test, 31 drug labels (2.3%) listed that the drug did not interfere with laboratory tests, and 4 drug labels listed that there was no available information [85]. The review reported that antibacterial agents, psychotropic drugs, and contrast media were the classes of drugs reported as most likely to lead to DLTIs. Despite DLTIs being an important clinical issue, many drug monographs do not include information on them [86].

One of the most common examples of DLTIs are with urine specimens due to drugs interfering with the chemical components of the urine, e.g., cephalosporins may interfere with urine glucose and ketone tests [86].

Other examples of drugs and DLTIs are the following [84]:

- Fluoxetine leads to increased reported triglyceride levels.
- Simvastatin, atorvastatin, and rosuvastatin lead to increased reported glucose levels.
- Daptomycin can falsely prolong or elevate reported prothrombin time and the INR [87].

Measures to prevent and minimize the clinical impact of DLTIs include reminder or notification systems on laboratory test programs to screen for DLTIs based on a patient's prescription medications. Other recommendations include the reporting of DLTI studies during post-marketing surveillance and in clinical practice to improve the recording and awareness of DLTIs. There are online databases that contain DLTI information such as the DailyMed website, where FDA-approved drug interactions with laboratory or diagnostic testing are listed [88]. A review of the licensed drug monograph is recommended in the event that a laboratory result is not congruent with the clinical picture. However, in the event of no information being included in the monograph, healthcare and laboratory professionals should consider a repeat test or testing using another assay method [86].

9 Prevention and Management of Drug Interactions in Practice

Prescribing and medicine management is increasing in complexity, with an ever-growing number of medications on the market, and rising polypharmacy. It must be acknowledged that it is not possible to remember all DDIs that are clinically relevant. DDIs are the responsibility of all health-care professionals involved in the prescribing, dispensing, and administration of medications, which includes doctors, dentists, pharmacists and pharmacy staff, and nurses, in all health-care settings.

The risk of a DDI becoming clinically significant can depend on both patient and medication factors. A recent point prevalence study (n = 1466 patients) of Irish data has found that one-quarter of older adults (≥70-years-old) were potentially exposed to one "severe" cardiovascular or central nervous system DDI. Those prescribed warfarin, escitalopram, atorvastatin, furosemide, or clarithromycin had the highest burden of potential exposure to DDIs [10]. The therapeutic index of the drug, the concentration of the interacting drug, and the clearance of the drug all have an impact on the clinical significance of an interaction; this is variable from patient to patient. Recommendations on how to reduce the risk of DDIs occurring are presented in Table 4.5.

When co-prescribing medications, the impact of one on the other, additive clinical effect (pharmacodynamic interaction), and the risks and benefits to patients should all be considered. Patients should be monitored for signs of DDIs or toxicity, and patient involvement and education to support this is important [90]. Certain DDIs that have been associated with negative clinical outcomes include the following:

- Warfarin and aspirin/other interacting medications: GI bleeding [91]
- NSAIDs and aspirin: GI adverse effects [91]
- Diuretic combinations: Renal failure [92]
- Diuretics and angiotensin-converting enzyme inhibitor (ACEIs): Renal failure [92]
- Digoxin and interacting medications: Digoxin toxicity [93]

Table 4.5 Interventions to minimize the risk of potential drug–drug interactions

Factor	Action
High-risk patients	Carefully monitor older patients, patients with polypharmacy, comorbidities, renal/hepatic disease, and impact on pharmacokinetics and pharmacodynamics
Medication history	Conduct a thorough and detailed medication history (include prescribed regular and as required medications, OTC medications, herbal medications, supplements, certain foods (e.g., grapefruit juice, calcium-containing foods). Conduct thorough medication reconciliation at transitions of care
Drugs with a narrow therapeutic index	Monitor drugs in this class (e.g., warfarin, phenytoin, antiepileptics, direct oral anticoagulants, digoxin, antineoplastic drugs). Consider the impact when prescribing other medications for patients on narrow therapeutic index medications
High-risk medications	Be aware of commonly prescribed enzyme inducers (e.g., phenytoin, carbamazepine, rifampicin) and enzyme inhibitors (e.g., azole antifungals, HIV protease inhibitors, macrolide antibiotics, selective serotonin reuptake inhibitors)
Combinations of medications	Be aware of the potential risks of combining high-risk medications, and consider the potential for increased risk of pharmacodynamic interactions
Genetic polymorphisms	Pharmacogenetic testing can guide individualized dosing for patients with gene mutations impacting drug metabolism and increasing DDI risk (e.g., CYP2C19 testing for patients on venlafaxine requiring co-trimoxazole treatment) [89]
Patient monitoring	Where medications that have the potential for DDI are being used, ensure that patient monitoring is conducted to ensure appropriate clinical response and any signs of adverse effects or toxicity

Anticoagulants, including warfarin and direct oral anticoagulants (DOACs), have a narrow therapeutic index and are susceptible to DDIs, increasing the risk of bleeding or thrombosis [94]. Particular care must be given when co-prescribing other medications with these agents, especially CYP450 inducers (e.g., CYP3A4 inducer rifampicin) or inhibitors (e.g., CYP3A4 inhibitor clarithromycin). DOACs are P-gp substrates and at risk of DDI with P-gp inducers (e.g., carbamazepine, phenytoin) and P-gp inhibitors (e.g., clarithromycin, fluconazole).

Lithium, prescribed for mood disorders, has a narrow therapeutic index and is susceptible to several clinically relevant interactions, mainly due to an interacting drug altering renal function, particularly glomerular filtration rate and tubular reabsorption. ACEIs, angiotensin receptor blockers, nonsteroidal anti-inflammatory drugs, and diuretics have a high risk of reducing lithium excretion, resulting in clinical toxicity [95]. Prescribers and pharmacists must be alert to the potential for interaction and patient harm, and increased monitoring of lithium blood levels is required if an interacting drug is prescribed. A change in patients' status (e.g., renal or hepatic function) may necessitate a medication review, which should consider the potential for any clinically relevant DDIs [96].

Patient education and highlighting the importance and risk of drug–drug, drug–herb, and, in some cases, drug–food interactions are vital to inform patients about the risks of taking new medications, especially nonprescription over-the-counter/herbal medications or supplements.

When a drug interaction occurs, there are several courses of action that may be taken. In all cases, clinical judgment and knowledge of the patient's medical and medication history are advised as well as discussion with the patient's physician as appropriate. Some possible actions to take to avoid negative clinical consequences for a patient with a potential or actual DDI include the following [4, 73]:

- Discontinue one or both of the interacting agents (including food, herbal, supplementary medicines, etc.).
- Consider an alternative medication.
- Carefully monitor the patient without changing therapy.
- Adjust the dose or dosing schedule of one or both drugs.
- Change the route of administration.

Preventive measures and system processes to identify and prevent DDIs from occurring are essential. Electronic prescribing systems and pharmacy dispensing software systems with DDI alerts are an important measure to alert healthcare professionals to DDIs. Sources of medication information such as the British National Formulary and Stockley's Drug Interactions (book or online subscription via Medicines Complete), manufacturers' licensed product information, and various online sources are available to screen for DDIs and assess the clinical risk of a DDI. Examples of specific online sources of DDI information are listed below:

- Lexicomp Drug Interactions: Available with subscription
- Micromedex: Available freely online at https://www.merckmanuals.com/professional/druginformation/drug-interactions
- CredibleMeds: Information on medications that prolong the QT interval
- Medscape Drug Interaction Checker: Primarily based on medications licensed in the United States
- HIV Drug Interactions Checker: Operated by the University of Liverpool
- Cancer Drug Interactions: Operated by the University of Radboud, The Netherlands, and the University of Liverpool
- Hepatitis C Drug Interactions: Operated by the University of Liverpool

Health-care professionals, including doctors, nurses, and pharmacists, should be encouraged to report drug–drug/drug–herb/drug–food interactions, which result in patient adverse events to their national medicinal products regulator, e.g., USFDA, United Kingdom Medicines and Healthcare Products Regulatory Agency (MHRA), etc.

9.1 Patient Involvement

Patients frequently request information on their medications, including any interactions that their medications may have with each other. DDI management involves a complex risk–benefit assessment, in which patient preferences should be considered [97]. Patient empowerment is important for patients to feel confident in managing their medications. It is important to provide appropriate medicine information to patients to support their understanding and medication adherence [98]. Online information for patients to explain what DDIs are and how to avoid them is available; however, there is less guidance on how to provide tailored information at an individual patient level [99, 100]. A recent scoping review of providing DDI services for patients has found that there are numerous online and digital DDI services available; however, large variations in quality have been reported, which could potentially lead to safety issues [101]. Although there is a demand for online DDI checkers, the use of these by patients poses a safety risk and could undermine the patient's confidence in their medications or result in patients changing their regime without first consulting with a health-care professional [98]. A focus group with patients exploring their preferences for the management of DDIs found that emotional, cognitive, situational, and personal factors such as fear, trust, risk perception, and openness to change influenced their needs [97]. Shared decision-making involves more than just information provision, and patient values and preferences must be considered in the health-care professional–patient communication on DDIs. Future research should investigate the impact of communication models and tools to provide DDI information on patient outcomes, such as their levels of confidence and risk perception, and on clinical outcomes, such as medication adherence.

10 Areas for Future Research

Identifying DDIs is a key area for researchers and practitioners alike. For any newly approved drug, the post-marketing phase is key to identifying any potential DDIs. In this phase, the new drug is taken by many more patients, with multiple comorbidities and medications and thus previously unknown interactions may occur. A challenge for the pharmaceutical industry and researchers is the ability to detect any new DDIs in a timely manner. More recent research has focused on the ability of machines to detect DDIs in large real-world datasets and to predict DDIs that may occur before a drug comes to the market [102]. This area of research, which is progressing rapidly with more powerful and sophisticated models utilizing the power of artificial intelligence to detect and predict DDIs, holds tremendous potential to advance drug safety assessment, facilitate proactive risk mitigation strategies, and ultimately contribute to the safe use of medicines.

11 Summary and Conclusions

This chapter provides health-care professionals with an overview of drug interactions, the mechanisms by which they occur, and the impact they can have on treatment efficacy and patient safety.

- The first step for health-care professionals is prevention, and, thus, when starting a medication for a patient, a thorough history should be obtained, which should include all medications (including all prescribed, OTC, and herbal or alternative medicines). It is important to be aware of any drugs with a narrow therapeutic index (e.g., warfarin).
- Health-care professionals should be aware of medications that are commonly associated with drug interactions such as antimicrobials (macrolides, azoles) and ASMs (e.g., carbamazepine, sodium valproate). Health-care professionals should consider the possibility that any new symptom a patient presents with could be due to a DDI and manage it appropriately. This is particularly relevant for patients at high risk of DDI, including older patients, patients with polypharmacy, and patients with comorbidities such as renal and hepatic disease. Providing patients with information on their medications and the potential for interactions could help empower them to identify and avoid DDIs.
- Finally, health-care professionals should be aware of reference resources available to review DDIs, which can support them when making clinical decisions on the management of DDIs in patients.

12 Case Studies

12.1 Case Study 1

A 73-year-old male was experiencing symptoms of cough and sputum production. On a Friday evening, he phoned an out-of-hours physician service and discussed with the physician (not his regular physician) his symptoms. The patient is usually fit and well. His medical history included high blood pressure and type 2 diabetes; his current medications included ramipril, amlodipine, bendroflumethiazide, spironolactone, metformin, and atorvastatin.

The physician made a diagnosis of bronchitis and considered appropriate antibiotics, given the patient's age and comorbidities. The physician prescribed clarithromycin 500 mg twice a day orally for 5 days.

The prescription was sent to the late-night pharmacy (not his regular pharmacy), and the patient's daughter collected the prescription for him that night. The patient started the antibiotic on Saturday morning. On Monday morning, the patient felt dizzy and faint. He visited his regular physician who noted his blood pressure as 92/38 mmHg and pulse rate as 43 bpm. His physician arranged for the patient to be transferred to a hospital.

In the emergency department, the patient was assessed for septic shock, cardiogenic shock, and hypovolemic shock; however, all parameters linked to these diagnoses were normal. On conducting a medication reconciliation, the pharmacist determined that the patient had recently started a course of clarithromycin and, therefore, the hypotension was likely drug-induced. Following supportive treatment at the hospital, the patient's condition stabilized and he was discharged 6 days later.

1. *What is the pharmacokinetic basis for the drug–drug interaction(s) in this case?*

   Clarithromycin and amlodipine:

   (a) Clarithromycin is a macrolide antibacterial, which is commonly used for the treatment of various infections, including lower respiratory tract infections.

   (b) As discussed earlier in this chapter, clarithromycin is a potent inhibitor of CYP3A4, the enzyme largely responsible for the metabolism of the calcium channel blocker amlodipine.

   (c) It can also inhibit the organic anion-transporting polypeptides OATP1B1 and OATP1B3 [103].

   Clarithromycin and atorvastatin:

   (d) Another possible interaction could have occurred between clarithromycin and atorvastatin.

   (e) Clarithromycin, through not only its effects on CYP3A4 but also its effect as an inhibitor of hepatic statin uptake transporters, increases the systemic exposure to most statins, the extent to which varies depending on the type of statin used [104].

2. *What clinical impact does this interaction have on the patient?*

   Clarithromycin and amlodipine:

   (a) In this case, inhibition of CYP3A4 led to increased concentration of amlodipine and increased blood pressure-lowering effect.

   (b) This situation arose for this patient because of the interaction between clarithromycin and amlodipine, the effects of which were likely enhanced by the multiple antihypertensives prescribed.

   Clarithromycin and atorvastatin:

   (c) In this patient's case, it is considered that an interaction and adverse effects, such as myopathy and rhabdomyolysis, are possible with atorvastatin and clarithromycin coadministration [4].

3. *How could a situation like the one experienced by this patient be avoided?*

   We need to consider the factors that contributed to this case.

   (a) Both the physician and the pharmacist who dispensed the medication were unfamiliar with the patient, likely did not have access to the patient's medical/medication records, and therefore may not have had an accurate picture of the patient's risk factors.

   (b) The patient was an older man and had significant medical comorbidities and polypharmacy.

   To prevent this from occurring again:

   (c) Therefore, the first step when prescribing or dispensing medication is to ensure that an accurate history of all medications is known.

   (d) This includes all prescribed medications (considering that multiple prescribers may be involved in the care of a patient), medication recently started or stopped, medication that the patient may purchase over the counter, herbal, or other preparations, and also consider whether patients are taking all medications prescribed, as issues with adherence, if not considered, may lead to additional medications being prescribed.

   (e) The perpetrator drug in this case is clarithromycin, a drug well-documented for causing DDIs. Although it is impossible for health-care professionals to know every single potential DDI, they should be familiar with some of the commonly implicated drugs, such as clarithromycin. If clarithromycin is indicated for a patient, then a thorough check for possible interactions should be undertaken.

4. *What action should be taken when these interactions occur?*

   (a) How to deal with an interaction will depend on the nature of the interaction and the potential for harm to the patient, and the long-term impact of the action chosen, and the decision and action taken should involve the patient's doctor.

   (b) In some cases, a drug–drug combination will be contraindicated and an alternative will be required, e.g., changing clarithromycin to another, appropriate, antimicrobial agent.

   (c) A temporary discontinuation of a drug may be a suitable course of action and should be discussed with the patient's doctor (e.g., putting atorvastatin on hold when taking clarithromycin). The clinical impact of this needs to be carefully considered.

   (d) Sometimes a change in dose or change in administration timing may be sufficient to avoid adverse effects.

   (e) There are many reputable sources available to support health-care professionals to determine the best course of action to take to minimize the risk of harm from DDIs, as discussed above, such as those listed previously.

12.2 Case Study 2

A 78-year-old lady presents to a hospital emergency department following referral by her family physician. She presents with a history of increasing disorientation, tremor, and drowsiness, and she also says that she has been experiencing "racing heart beat" or palpitations. She has a history of chronic lower back pain for which she takes morphine 10 mg twice daily and amitriptyline 10 mg once daily. She recently had a fall at home and her back pain has worsened, for which she was prescribed a combined analgesic with paracetamol 325 mg and tramadol 37.5 mg, one tablet four times a day, 5 days ago.

She was admitted, and, over the course of her initial day in hospital, she became increasingly unwell, with sweating, fever, worsening confusion, and muscular rigidity. There was no evidence of infection upon examination, and blood samples were sent to the laboratory for investigation.

Her laboratory results reported elevated serum creatinine kinase and transaminases.

Following review of her medications, history, and assessment, the multidisciplinary team stopped all medications and administered supportive care. Within 24 h, her condition stabilized and her symptoms were resolving. The team diagnosed SS as a result of the interaction between amitriptyline and the newly prescribing tramadol.

1. *What is the basis for the drug–drug interaction(s) in this case?*

   Amitriptyline and tramadol:

   (a) Amitriptyline is a tricyclic antidepressant, often prescribed for pain, which increases noradrenergic or serotonergic neurotransmission by blocking the noradrenaline or serotonin transporter at presynaptic terminals.

   (b) Tramadol is an atypical opioid analgesic with weak μ-receptor agonism and central reuptake inhibition of serotonin and noradrenaline. Although it is a less potent opioid analgesic than morphine, it poses safety risks of its own.

   (c) Tramadol has been reported to contribute to a significant number of cases of SS, either when prescribed by itself or in combination with other serotonergic medications [105].

   (d) Patients with comorbidities, those taking high doses of tramadol, and those taking other serotonergic medications are at an increased risk of SS.

   (e) SSRIs, serotonin noradrenaline reuptake inhibitors (SNRIs), MAOIs, and tricyclic antidepressants have all been shown to cause or contribute to SS. Other medications such as tramadol, diphenhydramine (a first-generation antihistamine that may also inhibit serotonin reuptake), and linezolid (a weak, reversible, nonselective monoamine oxidase A and B inhibitor) have also been implicated in cases of SS [106].

2. *What clinical impact does this interaction have on the patient?*

   (a) SS can be diagnosed using Sternbach's criteria or Hunter Serotonin Toxicity criteria [59].

   (b) Sternbach's criteria diagnoses SS on presentation of at least three of the following:
      - Mental status changes (confusion, hypomania)
      - Agitation
      - Myoclonus
      - Hyperreflexia
      - Diaphoresis
      - Tremor
      - Diarrhea
      - Incoordination/ataxia
      - Fever

   (c) Hunter Serotonin Toxicity criteria are a presentation of any of the following:
      - Spontaneous clonus
      - Inducible or ocular clonus and agitation or diaphoresis
      - Tremor and hyperreflexia
      - Hypertonia and hyperpyrexia (temperature exceeding 38 °C) and ocular/inducible clonus

3. *How could a situation like the one experienced by this patient be avoided?*

   We need to consider the factors that contributed to this case.

   (a) The patient was at risk as she was an older patient and was prescribed a combination of medications posing a risk of DDI.

   (b) She was prescribed a combination of medications, several of which had a central nervous system effect and a serotonergic effect.

   To prevent this from occurring again:

   (c) The first step when prescribing or dispensing medication is to ensure that an accurate history of all medications is known.

   (d) A risk–benefit assessment to consider the risk and potential clinical consequences of a DDI should be conducted by the prescriber, supported by information from DDI information checkers.

(e) When the acute phase has passed, the patient should be informed about what occurred and the risks of DDIs explained clearly and how to avoid them. The patient should be informed of the risk of combining any medications with her long-term amitriptyline medication, and all medication decisions should be made with her physician and/or pharmacist. She should ensure in the future that all health-care providers are aware of her medications.

(f) In some patient groups, the risk of SS posed by combining medications with recreational drugs such as ecstasy and LSD (lysergic acid diethylamide) should be highlighted.

(g) Patients on medications with a serotonergic effect should be taught how to recognize the signs and symptoms of SS, which is at an increased risk if a medication dose is being increased or a new medication is prescribed.

(h) Useful information is provided for patients such as an infographic developed by Foong et al. [107].

4. *What action should be taken when these interactions occur?*

   (a) The management of SS involves discontinuation of serotonergic medications and implementing supportive care.

   (b) Vital signs (blood pressure, temperature, pulse) and renal function should be monitored.

   (c) Intravenous fluids may be required to replace fluid loss or correct hypotension.

   (d) Diazepam or lorazepam may be administered for convulsions or agitation. In most mild cases, symptoms usually resolve within 24 h of discontinuing the serotonergic medication(s); however, symptoms may persist in cases involving medications with long half-lives.

   (e) High-dependency unit care may be needed for more severe cases.

   (f) Cyproheptadine (a histamine-1 receptor antagonist with nonspecific 5-hydroxytryptamine (5-HT)1A and 5-HT2A antagonistic properties) has been used in certain cases, but definitive evidence of its effectiveness is lacking [58].

References

1. World Health Organization. Life tables. Global Health Observatory; 2022. https://www.who.int/data/gho/data/themes/mortality-and-global-health-estimates/ghe-life-expectancy-and-healthy-life-expectancy.
2. Masnoon N, Shakib S, Kalisch-Ellett L, Caughey GE. What is polypharmacy? A systematic review of definitions. BMC Geriatr. 2017;17(1):230. https://doi.org/10.1186/s12877-017-0621-2.
3. Maher RL, Hanlon J, Hajjar ER. Clinical consequences of polypharmacy in elderly. Expert Opin Drug Saf. 2014;13(1):57–65. https://doi.org/10.1517/14740338.2013.827660.
4. Baxter K, Preston CL. Stockley's drug interactions [Online]. London: Pharmaceutical Press; 2022. https://www-medicinescomplete-com.ucc.idm.oclc.org/#/content/stockley/x01-3201?hspl=additive&hspl=or&hspl=synergistic&hspl=interactions.
5. Alvim MM, da Silva LA, Leite ICG, Silvério MS. Adverse events caused by potential drug-drug interactions in an intensive care unit of a teaching hospital. Revista Brasileira de Terapia Intensiva. 2015;27(4):353–9. https://doi.org/10.5935/0103-507X.20150060.
6. Lexicomp Online. 2023. https://online.lexi.com.
7. Lopez-Gonzalez E, Herdeiro MT, Figueiras A. Determinants of under-reporting of adverse drug reactions. Drug Saf. 2009;32(1):19–31. https://doi.org/10.2165/00002018-200932010-00002.
8. de Oliveira LM, do Amaral Carneiro Diel J, Nunes A, da Silva Dal Pizzol T. Prevalence of drug interactions in hospitalised elderly patients: a systematic review. Eur J Hosp Pharm. 2021;28(1):4–9. https://doi.org/10.1136/ejhpharm-2019-002111.
9. Zheng WY, Richardson LC, Li L, Day RO, Westbrook JI, Baysari MT. Drug-drug interactions and their harmful effects in hospitalised patients: a systematic review and meta-analysis. Eur J Clin Pharmacol. 2018;74(1):15–27. https://doi.org/10.1007/s00228-017-2357-5.

10. Hughes JE, Russo V, Walsh C, Menditto E, Bennett K, Cahir C. Prevalence and factors associated with potential drug-drug interactions in older community-dwelling adults: a prospective cohort study. Drugs Aging. 2021;38(11):1025–37. https://doi.org/10.1007/s40266-021-00898-8.
11. Guthrie B, Makubate B, Hernandez-Santiago V, Dreischulte T. The rising tide of polypharmacy and drug-drug interactions: population database analysis 1995–2010. BMC Med. 2015;13(1):74. https://doi.org/10.1186/s12916-015-0322-7.
12. Bjerrum L, Gonzalez Lopez-Valcarcel B, Petersen G. Risk factors for potential drug interactions in general practice. Eur J Gen Pract. 2008;14(1):23–9. https://doi.org/10.1080/13814780701815116.
13. Obreli Neto PR, Nobili A, Marusic S, Pilger D, Guidoni CM, de Oliveira Baldoni A, Cruciol-Souza JM, da Cruz AN, Gaeti WP, Cuman RKN. Prevalence and predictors of potential drug-drug interactions in the elderly: a cross-sectional study in the Brazilian primary public health system. J Pharm Pharm Sci. 2012;15(2):344–54. https://doi.org/10.18433/J37K5W.
14. Dumbreck S, Flynn A, Nairn M, Wilson M, Treweek S, Mercer SW, Alderson P, Thompson A, Payne K, Guthrie B. Drug-disease and drug-drug interactions: systematic examination of recommendations in 12 UK national clinical guidelines. BMJ. 2015;350:h949. https://doi.org/10.1136/bmj.h949.
15. Mallet L, Spinewine A, Huang A. The challenge of managing drug interactions in elderly people. Lancet. 2007;370(9582):185–91. https://doi.org/10.1016/S0140-6736(07)61092-7.
16. Liu F, Ranmal S, Batchelor HK, Orlu-Gul M, Ernest TB, Thomas IW, Flanagan T, Tuleu C. Patient-centered pharmaceutical design to improve acceptability of medicines: similarities and differences in paediatric and geriatric populations. Drugs. 2014;74(16):1871–89. https://doi.org/10.1007/s40265-014-0297-2.
17. Vinarov Z, Abdallah M, Agundez JAG, Allegaert K, Basit AW, Braeckmans M, Ceulemans J, Corsetti M, Griffin BT, Grimm M, Keszthelyi D, Koziolek M, Madla CM, Matthys C, McCoubrey LE, Mitra A, Reppas C, Stappaerts J, Steenackers N, et al. Impact of gastrointestinal tract variability on oral drug absorption and pharmacokinetics: an UNGAP review. Eur J Pharm Sci. 2021;162:105812. https://doi.org/10.1016/j.ejps.2021.105812.
18. van Leeuwen RWF, Jansman FGA, Hunfeld NG, Peric R, Reyners AKL, Imholz ALT, Brouwers JRBJ, Aerts JG, van Gelder T, Mathijssen RHJ. Tyrosine kinase inhibitors and proton pump inhibitors: an evaluation of treatment options. Clin Pharmacokinet. 2017;56(7):683–8. https://doi.org/10.1007/s40262-016-0503-3.
19. Wessler JD, Grip LT, Mendell J, Giugliano RP. The P-glycoprotein transport system and cardiovascular drugs. J Am Coll Cardiol. 2013;61(25):2495–502. https://doi.org/10.1016/j.jacc.2013.02.058.
20. Giacomini KM, Huang S-M, Tweedie DJ, Benet LZ, Brouwer KLR, Chu X, Dahlin A, Evers R, Fischer V, Hillgren KM, Hoffmaster KA, Ishikawa T, Keppler D, Kim RB, Lee CA, Niemi M, Polli JW, Sugiyama Y, Swaan PW, et al. Membrane transporters in drug development. Nat Rev Drug Discov. 2010;9(3):215–36. https://doi.org/10.1038/nrd3028.
21. Kennedy C, Brewer L, Williams D. Drug interactions. Medicine. 2020;48(7):450–5. https://doi.org/10.1016/j.mpmed.2020.04.001.
22. Litou C, Effinger A, Kostewicz ES, Box KJ, Fotaki N, Dressman JB. Effects of medicines used to treat gastrointestinal diseases on the pharmacokinetics of coadministered drugs: a PEARRL review. J Pharm Pharmacol. 2019;71(4):643–73. https://doi.org/10.1111/jphp.12983.
23. European Medicines Agency. Guideline on the investigation of drug interactions; 2012. https://www.ema.europa.eu/en/documents/scientific-guideline/guideline-investigation-drug-interactions-revision-1_en.pdf.
24. Elmeliegy M, Vourvahis M, Guo C, Wang DD. Effect of P-glycoprotein (P-gp) inducers on exposure of P-gp substrates: review of clinical drug–drug interaction studies. Clin Pharmacokinet. 2020;59(6):699–714. https://doi.org/10.1007/s40262-020-00867-1.
25. McDonnell AM, Dang CH. Basic review of the cytochrome p450 system. J Adv Pract Oncol. 2013;4(4):263–8. https://doi.org/10.6004/jadpro.2013.4.4.7.
26. Wang Y, Wang C, Wang S, Zhou Q, Dai D, Shi J, Xu X, Luo Q. Cytochrome P450-based drug-drug interactions of vonoprazan in vitro and in vivo. Front Pharmacol. 2020;11. https://www.frontiersin.org/articles/10.3389/fphar.2020.00053.
27. Wijnen PAHM, Op Den Buijsch RAM, Drent M, Kuipers PMJC, Neef C, Bast A, Bekers O, Koek GH. Review article: The prevalence and clinical relevance of cytochrome P450 polymorphisms. Aliment Pharmacol Ther. 2007;26(s2):211–9. https://doi.org/10.1111/j.1365-2036.2007.03490.x.
28. Lynch T, Price A. The effect of cytochrome P450 metabolism on drug response, interactions, and adverse effects. Am Fam Physician. 2007;76(3):391–6.
29. Deodhar M, Al Rihani SB, Arwood MJ, Darakjian L, Dow P, Turgeon J, Michaud V. Mechanisms of CYP450 inhibition: understanding drug-drug interactions due to mechanism-based inhibition in clinical practice. Pharmaceutics. 2020;12(9) https://doi.org/10.3390/pharmaceutics12090846.
30. Lee J-Y, Lee SY, Oh SJ, Lee KH, Jung YS, Kim SK. Assessment of drug–drug interactions caused by metabolism-dependent cytochrome P450 inhibition. Chem Biol Interact. 2012;198(1):49–56. https://doi.org/10.1016/j.cbi.2012.05.007.
31. Templeton I, Peng C-C, Thummel KE, Davis C, Kunze KL, Isoherranen N. Accurate prediction of dose-dependent CYP3A4 inhibition by itraconazole and its metabolites from in vitro inhibition data. Clin

Pharmacol Ther. 2010;88(4):499–505. https://doi.org/10.1038/clpt.2010.119.
32. Roberts A, Gibbs M. Mechanisms and the clinical relevance of complex drug–drug interactions. Clin Pharmacol. 2018;10:123–34.
33. Howard SC, McCormick J, Pui C-H, Buddington RK, Harvey RD. Preventing and managing toxicities of high-dose methotrexate. Oncologist. 2016;21(12):1471–82. https://doi.org/10.1634/theoncologist.2015-0164.
34. Yin J, Wang J. Renal drug transporters and their significance in drug–drug interactions. Drug Metab Pharmacokinet. 2016;6(5):363–73. https://doi.org/10.1016/j.apsb.2016.07.013.
35. Malik MY, Jaiswal S, Sharma A, Shukla M, Lal J. Role of enterohepatic recirculation in drug disposition: cooperation and complications. Drug Metab Rev. 2016;48(2):281–327. https://doi.org/10.3109/03602532.2016.1157600.
36. Niu J, Straubinger RM, Mager DE. Pharmacodynamic drug–drug interactions. Clin Pharmacol Ther. 2019;105(6):1395–406. https://doi.org/10.1002/cpt.1434.
37. Morrow L, Hompesch M, Guthrie H, Chang D, Chatterjee DJ. Co-administration of liraglutide with insulin detemir demonstrates additive pharmacodynamic effects with no pharmacokinetic interaction. Diabetes Obes Metab. 2011;13(1):75–80. https://doi.org/10.1111/j.1463-1326.2010.01322.x.
38. Wambaugh MA, Denham ST, Ayala M, Brammer B, Stonhill MA, Brown JC. Synergistic and antagonistic drug interactions in the treatment of systemic fungal infections. elife. 2020;9:e54160. https://doi.org/10.7554/eLife.54160.
39. Jacobson TA. Comparative pharmacokinetic interaction profiles of pravastatin, simvastatin, and atorvastatin when coadministered with cytochrome P450 inhibitors. Am J Cardiol. 2004;94(9):1140–6. https://doi.org/10.1016/j.amjcard.2004.07.080.
40. Niazi-Ali S. Pharmacists should make themselves familiar with the antifungal drug interactions database. Pharm J. 2020;305(7939):305. https://doi.org/10.1211/PJ.2020.20208143.
41. Lempers VJ, Brüggemann RJ. Antifungal therapy: drug-drug interactions at your fingertips. J Antimicrob Chemother. 2016;71(2):285–9. https://doi.org/10.1093/jac/dkv350.
42. Gupta AK, Versteeg SG, Shear NH. Common drug-drug interactions in antifungal treatments for superficial fungal infections. Expert Opin Drug Metab Toxicol. 2018;14(4):387–98. https://doi.org/10.1080/17425255.2018.1461834.
43. Bellmann R, Smuszkiewicz P. Pharmacokinetics of antifungal drugs: practical implications for optimized treatment of patients. Infection. 2017;45(6):737–79. https://doi.org/10.1007/s15010-017-1042-z.
44. National Aspergillosis Centre and Fungal Infection Trust. Antifungal drug interactions; 2023. https://www.aspergillus.org.uk/antifungal-drug-interactions/.
45. Niazi-Ali S, Atherton GT, Walczak M, Denning DW. Drug–drug interaction database for safe prescribing of systemic antifungal agents. Ther Adv Infect Dis. 2021;8:20499361211010604. https://doi.org/10.1177/20499361211010605.
46. Guidelines Working Groups of the NIH Office of AIDS Research Advisory Council. Guidelines for the use of antiretroviral agents in adults and adolescents living with HIV; 2022. https://clinicalinfo.hiv.gov/en/guidelines/hiv-clinical-guidelines-adult-and-adolescent-arv/overview?view=full.
47. Semvua HH, Kibiki GS, Kisanga ER, Boeree MJ, Burger DM, Aarnoutse R. Pharmacological interactions between rifampicin and antiretroviral drugs: challenges and research priorities for resource-limited settings. Ther Drug Monit. 2015;37(1):22–32. https://doi.org/10.1097/FTD.0000000000000108.
48. University of Liverpool. Liverpool HIV interactions; 2023. https://hiv-druginteractions.org/checker.
49. Panel on Antiretroviral Guidelines for Adults and Adolescents. Guidelines for the use of antiretroviral agents in adults and adolescents with HIV; 2023. https://clinicalinfo.hiv.gov/en/guidelines/hiv-clinical-guidelines-adult-and-adolescent-arv/drug-interactions-overview?view=full.
50. Bosak M, Słowik A, Iwańska A, Lipińska M, Turaj W. Co-medication and potential drug interactions among patients with epilepsy. Seizure. 2019;66:47–52. https://doi.org/10.1016/j.seizure.2019.01.014.
51. Zaccara G, Lattanzi S. A review of pharmacokinetic drug interactions between antimicrobial and antiseizure medications in children. Epileptic Disord. 2021;23(2):229–56. https://doi.org/10.1684/epd.2021.1261.
52. Wanleenuwat P, Suntharampillai N, Iwanowski P. Antibiotic-induced epileptic seizures: mechanisms of action and clinical considerations. Seizure. 2020;81:167–74. https://doi.org/10.1016/j.seizure.2020.08.012.
53. Khatib R, Sabir FRN, Omari C, Pepper C, Tayebjee MH. Managing drug-induced QT prolongation in clinical practice. Postgrad Med J. 2021;97(1149):452–8. https://doi.org/10.1136/postgradmedj-2020-138661.
54. Specialist Pharmacy Service. UKMI QA Drug induced QT prolongation update, Jan 2020. 2022. https://www.sps.nhs.uk.
55. CredibleMeds. Clinically important, common drug-drug interactions; 2022. https://www.crediblemeds.org/index.php/healthcare-providers/common-drug-interactions.
56. Skullbacka S, Airaksinen M, Puustinen J, Toivo T. Risk assessment tools for QT prolonging pharmacotherapy in older adults: a systematic review. Eur J Clin Pharmacol. 2022;78(5):765–79. https://doi.org/10.1007/s00228-022-03285-3.

57. Berger FA, van der Sijs H, van Gelder T, van den Bemt PMLA. The use of a clinical decision support tool to assess the risk of QT drug-drug interactions in community pharmacies. Ther Adv Drug Saf. 2021;12:2042098621996098. https://doi.org/10.1177/2042098621996098.
58. Boyer E, Traub S, Ganetsky M. Serotonin syndrome (serotonin toxicity). UpToDate; 2023. https://www.uptodate.com/contents/serotonin-syndrome-serotonin-toxicity#H12.
59. Thanacoody R. Serotonin syndrome. Medicine. 2015;44(2):95–6.
60. Ables AZ, Nagubilli R. Prevention, recognition, and management of serotonin syndrome. Am Fam Physician. 2010;81(9):1139–42.
61. Caughey GE, Roughead EE, Shakib S, McDermott RA, Vitry AI, Gilbert AL. Comorbidity of chronic disease and potential treatment conflicts in older people dispensed antidepressants. Age Ageing. 2010;39(4):488–94. https://doi.org/10.1093/ageing/afq055.
62. Fung FY, Linn YC. Steroids in traditional Chinese medicine: what is the evidence? Singap Med J. 2017;58(3):115–20. https://doi.org/10.11622/smedj.2017016.
63. Alzahrani AS, Price MJ, Greenfield SM, Paudyal V. Global prevalence and types of complementary and alternative medicines use amongst adults with diabetes: systematic review and meta-analysis. Eur J Clin Pharmacol. 2021;77(9):1259–74. https://doi.org/10.1007/s00228-021-03097-x.
64. Hassen G, Belete G, Carrera KG, Iriowen RO, Araya H, Alemu T, Solomon N, Bam DS, Nicola SM, Araya ME, Debele T, Zouetr M, Jain N. Clinical implications of herbal supplements in conventional medical practice: a US perspective. Cureus. 2022;14(7):e26893. https://doi.org/10.7759/cureus.26893.
65. Stott C, White L, Wright S, Wilbraham D, Guy G. A phase I, open-label, randomized, crossover study in three parallel groups to evaluate the effect of rifampicin, ketoconazole, and omeprazole on the pharmacokinetics of THC/CBD oromucosal spray in healthy volunteers. Springerplus. 2013;2(1):236. https://doi.org/10.1186/2193-1801-2-236.
66. Geffrey AL, Pollack SF, Bruno PL, Thiele EA. Drug-drug interaction between clobazam and cannabidiol in children with refractory epilepsy. Epilepsia. 2015;56(8):1246–51. https://doi.org/10.1111/epi.13060.
67. Asher GN, Corbett AH, Hawke RL. Common Herbal Dietary Supplement-Drug Interactions. Am Fam Physician. 2017;96(2):101–7. Available from: https://www.aafp.org/pubs/afp/issues/2017/0715/p101.html.
68. Chen XW, Sneed KB, Pan SY, Cao C, Kanwar JR, Chew H, Zhou SF. Herb-drug interactions and mechanistic and clinical considerations. Curr Drug Metab. 2012;13(5):640–51. https://doi.org/10.2174/138920021 1209050640. PMID: 22292789.
69. Fasinu PS, Bouic PJ, Rosenkranz B. An Overview of the Evidence and Mechanisms of Herb–Drug Interactions. Frontiers in Pharmacology. 2012;3. https://doi.org/10.3389/fphar.2012.00069.
70. Posadzki P, Watson L, Ernst E. Herb–drug interactions: an overview of systematic reviews. British Journal of Clinical Pharmacology. 2012;75(3):603–18. https://doi.org/10.1111/j.1365-2125.2012.04350.x.
71. Amadi CN, Mgbahurike AA. Selected Food/Herb-Drug Interactions: Mechanisms and Clinical Relevance. Am J Ther. 2018;25(4):e423–e433. https://doi.org/10.1097/MJT.0000000000000705.
72. Mason P. Important drug-nutrient interactions. Proc Nutr Soc. 2010;69(4):551–7. https://doi.org/10.1017/S0029665110001576. Epub 2010 May 28.
73. Whittlesea C, Hodson K. Clinical pharmacy and therapeutics. 6th ed. Elsevier; 2018.
74. American Geriatrics Society Expert Panel on the Care of Older Adults with Multimorbidity. Guiding principles for the care of older adults with multimorbidity: an approach for clinicians. J Am Geriatr Soc. 2012;60(10):E1–E25.
75. Woodford H, Stevenson J. Anticholinergic drugs and dementia: time for transparency in the face of uncertainty. Cochrane Database Syst Rev. 2021;9 https://doi.org/10.1002/14651858.ED000154.
76. Drini M. Peptic ulcer disease and non-steroidal anti-inflammatory drugs. Aust Prescr. 2017;40(3):91–3. https://doi.org/10.18773/austprescr.2017.037.
77. Arfè A, Scotti L, Varas-Lorenzo C, Nicotra F, Zambon A, Kollhorst B, Schink T, Garbe E, Herings R, Straatman H, Schade R, Villa M, Lucchi S, Valkhoff V, Romio S, Thiessard F, Schuemie M, Pariente A, Sturkenboom M, Corrao G. Non-steroidal anti-inflammatory drugs and risk of heart failure in four European countries: nested case-control study. BMJ. 2016;354:i4857. https://doi.org/10.1136/bmj.i4857.
78. Guthrie B, Thompson A, Dumbreck S, Flynn A, Alderson P, Nairn M, Treweek S, Payne K. Better guidelines for better care: accounting for multimorbidity in clinical guidelines—structured examination of exemplar guidelines and health economic modelling. NIHR Journals Library; 2017. http://www.ncbi.nlm.nih.gov/books/NBK426098/.
79. 2023 American Geriatrics Society Beers Criteria(R) Update Expert Panel. American Geriatrics Society 2023 updated AGS Beers Criteria® for potentially inappropriate medication use in older adults. J Am Geriatr Soc. 2023;71(7):2052–81. https://doi.org/10.1111/jgs.18372.
80. Lavan AH, Gallagher P, Parsons C, O'Mahony D. STOPPFrail (screening tool of older persons prescriptions in frail adults with limited life expectancy): consensus validation. Age Ageing. 2017;46(4):600–7. https://doi.org/10.1093/ageing/afx005.
81. O'Mahony D, O'Sullivan D, Byrne S, O'Connor MN, Ryan C, Gallagher P. STOPP/START criteria

for potentially inappropriate prescribing in older people: version 2. Age Ageing. 2015;44(2):213–8. https://doi.org/10.1093/ageing/afu145.
82. Diesveld MME, de Klerk S, Cornu P, Strobach D, Taxis K, Borgsteede SD. Management of drug-disease interactions: a best practice from The Netherlands. Int J Clin Pharm. 2021;43(6):1437–50. https://doi.org/10.1007/s11096-021-01308-0.
83. van Tongeren JMZ, Harkes-Idzinga SF, van der Sijs H, Atiqi R, van den Bemt BJF, Draijer LW, Hiel D, Kerremans A, Kremers B, de Leeuw M, Olthoff MV, Pham TK-L, Valentijn-Robertz R, Tsoi K, Wichers I, de Wit M, Borgsteede SD. The development of practice recommendations for drug-disease interactions by literature review and expert opinion. Front Pharmacol. 2020;11. https://www.frontiersin.org/articles/10.3389/fphar.2020.00707.
84. Katanić J, Stanimirov B, Sekeruš V, Đanić M, Pavlović N, Mikov M, Stankov K. Drug interference with biochemical laboratory tests. Biochem Med (Zagreb). 2023;33(2). https://pubmed.ncbi.nlm.nih.gov/37143715/.
85. Yao H, Rayburn ER, Shi Q, Gao L, Hu W, Li H. FDA-approved drugs that interfere with laboratory tests: a systematic search of US drug labels. Crit Rev Clin Lab Sci. 2017;54(1):1–17. https://doi.org/10.1080/10408363.2016.1191425.
86. Scott G. Which drugs interact with lab tests? 2019. https://www.medscape.com/viewarticle/914303?form=fpf.
87. MSD Ireland (Human Health) Limited. Cubicin 350mg powder for solution for injection or infusion. SPC, Medicines.ie; 2023. https://www.medicines.ie/medicines/cubicin-350mg-powder-for-solution-for-injection-or-infusion-31749/spc.
88. The National Library of Medicine. DailyMed; 2023. https://dailymed.nlm.nih.gov/dailymed/index.cfm.
89. Bahar MA, Setiawan D, Hak E, Wilffert B. Pharmacogenetics of drug-drug interaction and drug-drug-gene interaction: a systematic review on CYP2C9, CYP2C19 and CYP2D6. Pharmacogenomics. 2017;18(7):701–39. https://doi.org/10.2217/pgs-2017-0194.
90. Spinewine A, Schmader KE, Barber N, Hughes C, Lapane KL, Swine C, Hanlon JT. Appropriate prescribing in elderly people: how well can it be measured and optimised? Lancet (London, England). 2007;370(9582):173–84. https://doi.org/10.1016/S0140-6736(07)61091-5.
91. Ho LL, Brighton T. Warfarin, antiplatelet drugs and their interactions. Aust Prescr. 2002;25(4):81–5. https://doi.org/10.18773/austprescr.2002.073.
92. Maideen NMP, Balasubramanian R, Muthusamy S. A comprehensive review of the pharmacologic perspective on loop diuretic drug interactions with therapeutically used drugs. Curr Drug Metab. 2022;23(3):188–99. https://doi.org/10.2174/1389200223666220401092112.
93. GP Notebook. Drug interactions with digoxin—general practice notebook; 2022. https://gpnotebook.com/simplepage.cfm?ID=-1858797543.
94. Chang S-H, Chou I-J, Yeh Y-H, Chiou M-J, Wen M-S, Kuo C-T, See L-C, Kuo C-F. Association between use of non-vitamin K oral anticoagulants with and without concurrent medications and risk of major bleeding in nonvalvular atrial fibrillation. JAMA. 2017;318(13):1250–9. https://doi.org/10.1001/jama.2017.13883.
95. Malhi GS, Bell E, Outhred T, Berk M. Lithium therapy and its interactions. Aust Prescr. 2020;43(3):91–3. https://doi.org/10.18773/austprescr.2020.024.
96. Rochon P. Drug prescribing for older adults. UpToDate; 2022. https://www.uptodate.com/contents/drug-prescribing-for-older-adults?search=drug%20interactions&source=search_result&selectedTitle=2~150&usage_type=default&display_rank=1#H16.
97. Heringa M, Floor-Schreudering A, De Smet PAGM, Bouvy ML. Aspects influencing patients' preferences for the management of drug-drug interactions: a focus group study. Patient Educ Couns. 2018;101(4):723–9. https://doi.org/10.1016/j.pec.2017.11.010.
98. Kusch MK, Haefeli WE, Seidling HM. How to meet patients' individual needs for drug information—a scoping review. Patient Prefer Adherence. 2018;12:2339–55. https://doi.org/10.2147/PPA.S173651.
99. Harvard Health Publishing. 7 things you can do to avoid drug interactions. Harvard Health; 2016. https://www.health.harvard.edu/staying-healthy/7-things-you-can-do-to-avoid-drug-interactions.
100. U.S. Food and Drug Administration. Drug interactions: what you should know. FDA; 2013. https://www.fda.gov/drugs/resources-you-drugs/drug-interactions-what-you-should-know.
101. Hammar T, Hamqvist S, Zetterholm M, Jokela P, Ferati M. Current knowledge about providing drug-drug interaction services for patients—a scoping review. Pharmacy (Basel, Switzerland). 2021;9(2):69. https://doi.org/10.3390/pharmacy9020069.
102. Han K, Cao P, Wang Y, Xie F, Ma J, Yu M, Wang J, Xu Y, Zhang Y, Wan J. A review of approaches for predicting drug–drug interactions based on machine learning. Front Pharmacol. 2022;12. https://www.frontiersin.org/articles/10.3389/fphar.2021.814858.
103. Fleet J, Shariff S, Bailey D, Gandhi S, Juurlink D, Nash D, Mamdani M, Gomes T, Patel A, Garg A. Comparing two types of macrolide antibiotics for the purpose of assessing population-based drug interactions. BMJ Open. 2013;3:e002857. https://doi.org/10.1136/bmjopen-2013-002857.
104. Hougaard Christensen MM, Bruun Haastrup M, Øhlenschlæger T, Esbech P, Arnspang Pedersen S, Bach Dunvald A-C, Bjerregaard Stage T, Pilsgaard

Henriksen D, Thestrup Pedersen AJ. Interaction potential between clarithromycin and individual statins—a systematic review. Basic Clin Pharmacol Toxicol. 2020;126(4):307–17. https://doi.org/10.1111/bcpt.13343.
105. Hassamal S, Miotto K, Dale W, Danovitch I. Tramadol: understanding the risk of serotonin syndrome and seizures. Am J Med. 2018;131(11):1382.e1–6. https://doi.org/10.1016/j.amjmed.2018.04.025.
106. Khan S, Saud S, Khan I, Asif M, Ismail O, Salam A, Yang TJ, Norville KJ. Serotonin syndrome presenting with concomitant tramadol and diphenhydramine use: a case report of an unlikely side-effect. Cureus. 2018;10(4):e2421. https://doi.org/10.7759/cureus.2421.
107. Foong A-L, Grindrod KA, Patel T, Kellar J. Demystifying serotonin syndrome (or serotonin toxicity). Can Fam Physician. 2018;64(10):720–7.

5 Economics of Medication Safety, with a Focus on Preventable Harm

Rachel A. Elliott

Abstract

Adverse drug reactions can be an important cause of morbidity and mortality and may have significant economic consequences, including the increased use of health services and wider societal costs. We can refer to this as 'economic burden'. This chapter defines and explores how to quantify the economic burden of adverse drug reactions. Health economists are particularly interested in the avoidable economic burden caused by medication errors. Therefore, this chapter focuses on the avoidable economic burden caused by medication errors. There are three types of evidence required to understand the economic burden of medication errors: the incidence or prevalence of medication errors, the consequences (health and wider effects) of those medication errors, and the resources consumed due to the consequences associated with those medication errors. The challenges around quantifying harm from medication errors are discussed. Strategies which aim to improve patient safety through interventions such as those that change prescribing or monitoring behaviour are often costly, so we need to know if they are effective or cost-effective. This chapter outlines how different economic evaluation approaches can be carried out alongside randomised controlled trials, non-randomised comparative studies (such as interrupted time series analysis) or as modelling studies. The published evidence around the cost-effectiveness of safety interventions is introduced. The benefits of improved patient safety are not just maximising health, which affects how they are valued by different stakeholders, so this chapter concludes by examining the non-health components of safety intervention outcomes.

Keywords

Economic evaluation · Cost-effectiveness analysis · Cost-utility analysis · Cost of illness · Economics of medication safety · Economic burden of medication errors · Preventable harm · Safety interventions

R. A. Elliott (✉)
Manchester Centre for Health Economics, Division of Population Health, Health Services Research and Primary Care, School of Health Sciences, Faculty of Biology, Medicine and Health, The University of Manchester, Manchester, UK
e-mail: Rachel.a.elliott@manchester.ac.uk; http://research.bmh.manchester.ac.uk/healtheconomics/

Learning Objectives

- Understand how the economic burden of sub-optimal medication safety may be defined and measured.

J. Jose et al. (eds.), *Principles and Practice of Pharmacovigilance and Drug Safety*,
https://doi.org/10.1007/978-3-031-51089-2_5

- Discuss challenges in defining and measuring economic burden.
- Describe and evaluate evidence for economic burden.
- Understand the methods used to assess the cost-effectiveness of strategies to improve medication safety.
- Describe and evaluate evidence for strategies to improve medication safety.
- Discuss challenges in assessing cost-effectiveness of strategies to improve medication safety.

Key Points

- The economic burden of Adverse Drug Reactions (ADRs) can range from the harmful effects on health, quality of life or length of life; the costs incurred by a healthcare provider of having to deal with that harm; to broader effects on society.
- Some medication errors do not cause any harm or incur any costs and we need to focus our efforts on reducing clinically important errors.
- If we want to understand the harm caused by ADRs due to medication errors, we need to be able to link that error to harm outcomes and associated costs.
- Not all harm from medication is preventable, so we are only focused on reducing preventable harm and associated costs.
- The harm and cost from a medication error can extend beyond the initial event, such as the initial hospitalisation.
- When we design interventions to reduce medication errors, we need to quantify the impact on harm and on costs.
- We need to be aware that ADRs can have an impact on non-health outcomes, such as trust, and other costs such as litigation and compensation costs.

1 Introduction

In this chapter, the economic burden of Adverse Drug Reactions (ADRs) is examined. The economic burden of ADRs broadly can be defined as any effects on the person experiencing the harm (such as effects on health, quality of life or length of life); the effects on a healthcare provider of having to deal with that harm (such as treating a gastric bleed); and broader effects on society (such as lost productivity from a person not being able to work or carry out caring activities).

This chapter will look at:

- how economic burden may be measured;
- challenges in defining and measuring economic burden;
- evidence for economic burden.

The cost-effectiveness of strategies to improve medication safety is examined, looking at:

- the methods used to assess cost-effectiveness;
- evidence for strategies to improve patient safety;
- challenges in assessing cost-effectiveness of these strategies.

In 1955, David Barr defined adverse events as 'the price to pay for modern diagnosis and therapy methods' [1]. ADRs, whether preventable or not, negatively affect health and patient experience. If these ADRs occur as a result of an error in the medication use process, this is considered an important cause of avoidable morbidity and mortality [2, 3]. In turn, medication errors may have significant economic consequences, including the increased use of health services such as avoidable medication-related hospital admissions. The potential economic impact of ADRs has been a concern for a long time. In 1965, a Scottish general practitioner estimated that more than a quarter of night and emergency calls were due to 'drug-induced illness' [4]. It has been estimated that approximately 6–7% of hospital admissions appear to be medication-related, with over two-thirds of these considered to be due to medication errors and therefore avoidable [5–7]. A recent meta-analysis of burden of error studies estimated that, globally, around one in 30 patients are exposed to preventable medication harm in medical care, and more than a quarter of this harm is considered severe or life threatening [8]. A recent report suggested that avoidable hospital admissions and increased length of stay due to medication harm cost Organisation for Economic Cooperation and Development (OECD) countries $54 billion annually [9].

The economic impact of medication errors has motivated most health systems to improve patient safety [10]. Strategies aim to improve patient safety through interventions that focus on one or more aspects of the medicines use process, such as those that change prescribing, dispensing, labelling, administration, or monitoring behaviour. These are often costly, with variable evidence of effectiveness or cost-effectiveness [11–13]. The real impact of these interventions is often uncertain, as behaviour may not change as anticipated, or clinical and economic effects of most errors may be minor [14]. In an increasingly financially constrained healthcare environment, it is essential to be clearer about the true (comprehensive) economic impact of interventions to improve patient safety.

2 Economic Burden of Suboptimal Medication Safety

The economic burden of ADRs broadly can be defined as any effects on the person experiencing the harm (such as effects on health, quality of life, or length of life); the effects on a healthcare provider of having to deal with that harm (such as treating a gastric bleed); and broader effects on society (such as lost productivity from a person not being able to work or carry out caring activities).

The 'perspective' is important in determining costs and is discussed in more detail in the subheading 'Perspective' in Sect. 2.1.3.

2.1 How Burden May Be Defined and Measured

Quantifying the economic burden of suboptimal medication safety requires the following types of evidence: the nature and incidence or prevalence of medication errors, the consequences (health and wider effects) of those medication errors, and the resources consumed due to the consequences associated with those medication errors.

2.1.1 Prevalence of Errors

Estimating the prevalence of medication error presents challenges due to varying definitions and classification systems and varying methods of identification and measurement. This topic is covered in more detail in Chap. 15. Errors can be minor, resulting in no patient harm, and range through to major errors causing serious harm and death. Therefore, knowing where and how commonly an error occurs is only the beginning of the story. We need to know how it occurred and what is the impact of that error.

2.1.2 Health Effects of a Medication Error

National Coordinating Council for Medication Error Reporting and Prevention (NCC MERP) defines patient outcomes from medication error in the following way (Table 5.1) [15]:

This is a helpful taxonomy in that it presents the range of severity of harm that can occur due to an error and whether that harm has occurred. However, further information is needed to understand more fully the level of harm that can occur and how it is measured. The harm and associated resource use will be directly related to the specific medication involved in the error, such as amiodarone causing thyrotoxicity or a

Nonsteroidal Anti-inflammatory Drug (NSAID) causing a gastrointestinal (GI) bleed.

Are Medication Errors a Patient Outcome?

Patient outcomes are usually defined as health-related events occurring as the result of an illness or a healthcare intervention. In patient safety, medication errors are measured more often than the effect of that error on a patient's health. The reasons for this are explored in the section 'Quantifying Harm from Medication Errors'. Medication errors are considered to be a 'bad' thing that need to be avoided. However, errors are a process indicator that act as a surrogate for patient outcome, carrying the, not always accurate, assumption that medication errors will have an impact on patient outcome and costs. For example, if a study reports prescribing error rates, an unknown proportion will actually reach the patient because some of those prescribing errors may be picked up at the dispensing or administration stage. Some of those prescribing errors may cause little or no harm if they reach the patient. If harm does occur, the error may be only one of a number of factors (such as patient factors or errors occurring later in the medication use process) leading to a poor outcome.

The value of medication error data is therefore limited as a measure of harm or patient outcome. From an economics perspective, there are limited resources to direct at initiatives to reduce medication errors. Thus, we want to know which medication errors are the ones we should focus on to derive most benefit from finite resources. That means having evidence about the harm from those errors, not just the prevalence of those errors.

The subsequent subsections describe the challenges around quantifying harm from medication errors and then describe the range of methods that have been used to quantify harm, patient outcomes, and cost from a medication error.

Table 5.1 NCC MERP definitions of patient outcome from medication error [15]

NCC MERP code	Category	Patient outcome from medication error
31.1	A	No error
32.1	B	An error occurred but the error did not reach the patient (an 'error of omission' **does** reach the patient)
32.2	C	An error occurred that reached the patient, but did not cause patient harm: 32.2.1 Medication reaches the patient and is administered 32.2.2 Medication reaches the patient but not administered
32.3	D	An error occurred that reached the patient and required monitoring to confirm that it resulted in no harm to the patient and/or required intervention to preclude harm
33.1	E	An error occurred that may have contributed to or resulted in temporary harm to the patient and required intervention
33.2	F	An error occurred that may have contributed to or resulted in temporary harm to the patient and required initial or prolonged hospitalisation
33.3	G	An error occurred that may have contributed to or resulted in permanent patient harm
33.4	H	An error occurred that required intervention necessary to sustain life
34.1	I	An error occurred that may have contributed to or resulted in the patient's death

Quantifying Harm from Medication Errors

There are some significant challenges around directly and robustly estimating patient harm caused by medication errors. One key ethical issue is that once an error has been detected at any point in the medication use process in clinical practice, a research study, or practice audit, it cannot be left uncorrected to reach the patient. Following a known error prospectively through the medication use process to see if it causes harm is unethical. Similarly, a randomised controlled trial (RCT) where one arm of the trial is allocated to receive the error, and the other arm, no error would not be considered ethical.

To directly link errors to harm requires a dataset that has both errors and harm collected within it for an individual patient. This is where routine data collection in health care can be extremely useful, especially if datasets from different sectors of the health system are linked. One example would be a dataset that combines both primary and secondary care data for a cohort of patients. This dataset would allow the identification of a prescribing or monitoring error occurring in primary care and identification of relevant hospitalisations or outpatient visits.

Many types of medication errors cannot currently be detected in routine data records, such as is commonly the case with medication administration errors. This, therefore, restricts the widespread use of this method to areas where data are available.

Challenges with Capturing the Health Effects of a Medication Error

There are increasing numbers of studies that directly link errors to patient harm, primarily around prescribing errors in settings where routinely collected data are available. However, the evidence directly linking errors to patient harm and/or costs is still sparse, with studies using varying methods and having variable quality [16]. Very little data are available that directly measure the link between errors and harm, or what proportion of errors occurring at different stages of the medicines use process reach patients, and what proportion of those errors reaching patients cause actual harm.

Retrospective Linking of Adverse Drug Events to Medication Errors

Researchers have used other methods, in the absence of direct evidence, to link errors to harm.

The first, and most commonly used of these, is via retrospective study, where a known ADR is linked back to a medication error, requiring some form of subjective assumption of causality and preventability. The second of these is to use modelling approaches to link medication errors to ADRs. These are discussed in more detail in this section.

One of the most common ways of capturing the health effects of a medication error is to identify a medication-related adverse event for a cohort of patients and then to look backwards in time to identify a medication error [8, 16, 17]. One of the earlier studies to attempt to identify patient harm from medication errors using this method was Bates et al. (1995) [18]. This US hospital-based study reported that 5 of 530 medication errors (0.9%) resulted in ADRs. This study has been followed by many others who used similar methods that do not directly link medication errors to patient harm and/or costs, but use some form of judgement to attribute the harm or ADR to an error.

A large Dutch study illustrates this approach very clearly [19]. Damen et al. (2017) took a sample of 8071 hospital admissions. Nurses and physicians looked at the notes and decided if a medication-related ADR had occurred leading to hospital admission. They then decided if the ADR was caused by a medication error, and whether the ADR was avoidable. The overall study design is summarised in Fig. 5.1.

This type of design has been used by many other researchers [17, 20, 21]. It raises questions about attributing both causality and preventability to the medication errors and ADRs which are examined in the next two sections.

Did the Error Cause the Harm? (Causality)

Whether the harm, or ADR, has been caused by a medication error is not always clear. These outcomes may or may not be associated with errors in prescribing, dispensing, administration, or monitoring. Not all errors occurring earlier in the medication use process end up reaching the patient and if they do, they may not lead to harm. If harm does occur, the medication error may be only one of many factors leading to a poor outcome. For older, more frail patients, it can be difficult to attribute poor outcomes, such as a hospital admission, directly to the ADR. These patients have higher resource use, including polypharmacy, and are already at greater risk of harm as a result. Furthermore, not all ADRs are avoidable as ADRs can occur when the medicine is used correctly. In studies looking at ADRs retrospectively, causality is usually assessed retrospectively by a group of clinicians. There is variability in how this causality is assigned between studies, making comparison difficult.

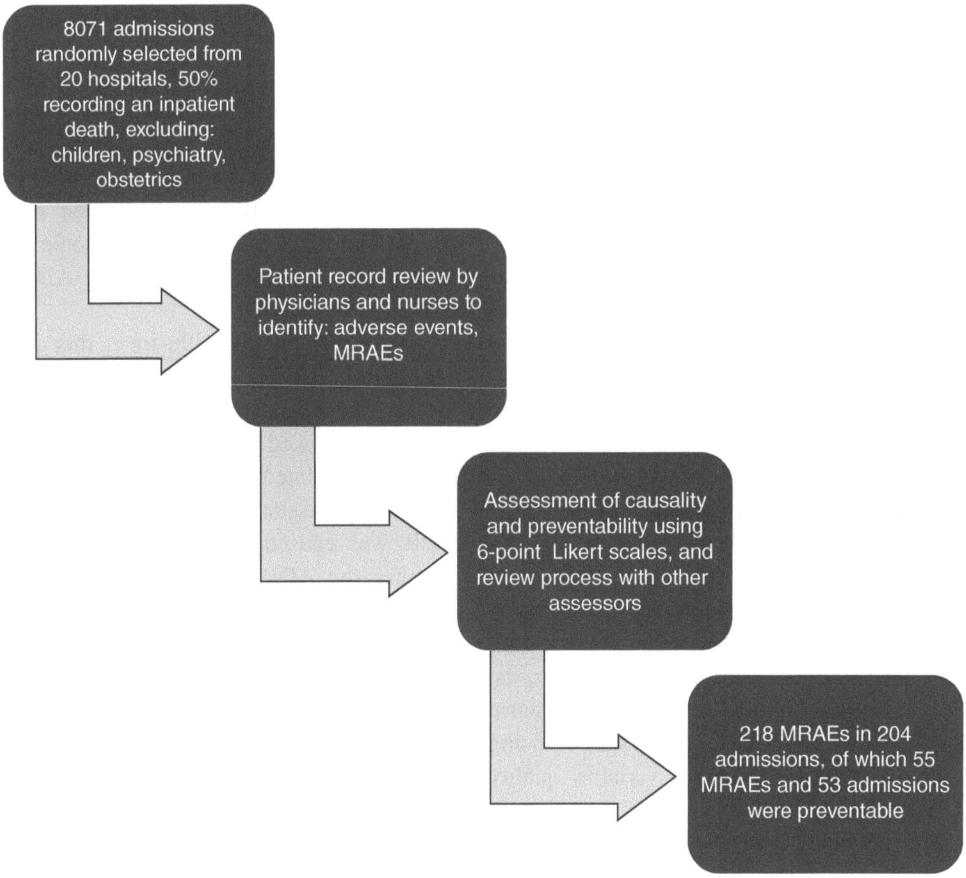

Fig. 5.1 Identification and categorisation of ADRs by Damen et al. [19]. *MRAEs* medication-related adverse events

Could the Harm Have Been Avoided? (Preventability or Avoidability)

Not all ADRs are avoidable. Many ADRs are caused by drugs such as aspirin, warfarin, or diuretics that have potentially significant long-term benefits to patients and are recommended in guidelines due to an evidence base for effect and involve finely balanced decisions about the benefits versus the risks in some categories of patients (e.g. those with multi-morbidity). Therefore, it can often be difficult when retrospectively reviewing prescribing decisions to make a judgement as to the avoidability of the harm. Many ADR studies tend to judge large numbers of ADRs as possibly avoidable [21–23], which are likely to include many cases where hindsight bias might suggest the prescribing decision was wrong, when it had been based on careful balancing of benefits versus harms taking into account evidence-based guidelines and patient preferences. In previous work, we have made the conservative assumption that only definitely avoidable ADRs approximate the harm from medication errors [24], which produces more conservative estimates of avoidable harm, than if both possibly and definitely avoidable ADRs are included, as in the work by the National Patient Safety Agency (NPSA) [25, 26].

Extrapolating Estimates of Harm from Medication Errors

Due to the complexities of linking medication errors to harm, another method that has been used to generate estimates of harm from medication error data is to extrapolate or estimate the harm from medication error data.

Many studies have used the concept of ranking errors by some subjective judgement of harm severity [18, 27–30]. Apart from the NCC MERP system reported earlier in this chapter, many other systems have been developed, a few of which are cited here [31–33]. One system developed by Dean and Barber [31] divides errors into 'minor', 'moderate', or 'severe'. Thirty healthcare professionals from 4 UK hospitals scored 50 medication errors in terms of potential patient outcomes on a scale of 0–10, where 0 represented a case with no potential effect and 10 a case that would result in death. Similarly to the approach used by Damen et al. [19], limitations of this approach lie with the intrinsic subjectivity of the method and the fact that many studies develop their own severity assessment system, limiting the comparability of results from different studies.

Another way to generate estimates of harm from medication error data is to build a model reflecting the types of harm that might occur, and then attach a probability of that harm, and the impact of that harm on health and cost. A model is a simplified version of reality that represents input, process, and outcomes of an event and is used extensively in health economics.

One example of where this has been carried out is the case of NSAIDs. The side effects or adverse events, particularly GI bleeding, renal dysfunction, and impact on cardiovascular function, are well-recognised in NSAIDs [34–36]. We know that an NSAID can cause a range of GI harms when given, ranging from mild intermittent GI discomfort, persistent serious GI discomfort, gastric ulcer to serious or even life-threatening, upper and lower GI bleeding. These events can even occur in people when an NSAID is used appropriately, but are more likely in people with risk factors such as age, a previous GI bleed, long-term use or the use of other medications that increase bleeding risk. Prescribing NSAIDs at all, or in the absence of gastroprotective agents (GPA), in these groups of patients could be seen as a prescribing error. An example of building a Markov model to estimate harm from NSAIDs is presented in Case Study 2.

A key limitation of this approach is that not all medications are associated with the large body of evidence there is around NSAID harm. For example, it might be more difficult to populate such a model with data if one wanted to quantify the harm associated with a drug like amiodarone or lithium.

Measuring Harm and Patient Outcomes from Medication Errors

Medication errors can result in harm. Ideally, a measure of harm would capture all the impacts on health and patient experience, including all effects on morbidity and mortality, over the short and long term. This type of evidence is challenging to collect. It is not routinely available and therefore requires specific research resource. Due to the complexity and cost of following up a cohort of people who have experienced a medication error, other proxies for health or reductions in health are often used to approximate to patient outcomes from a medication error.

The clinical indicator most commonly used to approximate to patient outcomes after primary/ambulatory care errors and secondary care/inpatient errors is increased use of hospital care [16]. Increased use of hospital care due to medication errors can be measured through increased use of emergency departments, hospital admissions, Intensive Care Unit (ICU) admissions, length of hospital stay or readmission to hospital or increased level of intervention during a hospital stay. Hospital admissions and readmissions are the most commonly used clinical indicator to quantify harm from errors in ambulatory/primary care. Hospital length of stay can be used to quantify short-term harm for both inpatient medication errors and also errors in ambulatory/primary care. Admissions to ICU, or other higher-level care, can be used to quantify short-term harm for both inpatient medication errors and also errors in ambulatory/primary care.

Use of hospital care as an outcome measure is problematic because so many other factors affect the supply and use of hospital care, including the specific characteristics embedded in the health system in which the studies are conducted. For example, hospital admissions can be affected by severity of illness, source of referral, case mix, and socioeconomic status and as such all of these confounders require adjustment [37].

Using Mortality to Measure Harm from Medication Errors

Mortality is a useful outcome measure because it is objective and easy to measure. Medical errors in general are suggested to be the third leading cause of death in the USA [38]. However, there are problems associated with mortality as an outcome measure. First of all, people may die from causes other than that of interest to the study, which can mask mortality linked to the medication and thus confound the results. Second, most medication errors reduce quality of life (QoL) rather than mortality. Mortality is a relatively insensitive measure that requires a study with many patients followed up over a long period of time. Finally, people of different ages and sex have a different risk of mortality, so it is important that mortality comparisons correct for age and sex. Everybody dies eventually so it is actually premature mortality we are trying to reduce, such that individuals are able to live out an acceptable lifespan. Therefore, if a premature death is caused by a GI bleeding from an NSAID, or a woman with a family history of stroke prescribed an oral contraceptive dies from a stroke, we have lost years of life for an individual. Therefore, mortality can be converted into life-years lost, or years of life lost (YLL).

Studies of medication error-related harm have attributed deaths to medication errors. For example, in the study conducted by Pirmohamed et al. (2004) [21], the drugs most commonly implicated in causing hospital admissions were low-dose aspirin, diuretics, warfarin, and NSAIDs [21]. GI bleeding was the most common adverse effect, occurring in 157 (72%) of all aspirin-related admissions. Of the 28 deaths which were identified as being a direct result of the ADR (as detailed in either the case notes or on the death certificate), 15 deaths were due to bleeds caused by NSAIDs/aspirin/warfarin. This gave an index hospitalisation death rate of 0.15% due to ADRs (2.3% of ADRs were fatal, 1.25% of ADRs led to fatal GI bleeds). Osanlou et al. also reported that 0.42% of people admitted to hospital due to an ADR died as a result [17].

It is likely that those medication errors leading to the most severe ADRs can lead to death. However, it is important to be able to identify risk of death attributable to the error. In the example of the woman with a family history of a stroke prescribed an oral contraceptive dying from a stroke, she already had an underlying risk of death from a stroke, dependent on age and other risk factors (such as hypertension, cigarette smoking, and migraine). The prescribing of an oral contraceptive increases that risk, rather than introducing a new risk [39]. It should be noted that the quality of evidence in studies around risk can be highly variable. A recent umbrella review (13 meta-analyses of RCTs and 45 meta-analyses of cohort studies) of the association of hormonal contraceptive use with adverse health outcomes concluded that 'Overall, the associations between hormonal contraceptive use and cardiovascular risk, cancer risk, and other major adverse health outcomes were not supported by high-quality evidence' [40].

Using Quality of Life and Utility Measures to Estimate Harm

Using clinical indicators carries the implication that changes in these will extrapolate to an effect on the patient's QoL. However, there is an increasing awareness that it is necessary to measure the impact of health care on an individual's QoL, or health-related quality of life (HRQoL), at least. There are many functional, social, psychological, cognitive, and subjective factors that impact on QoL so measuring QoL is methodologically complex. QoL measures can be disease-specific, such as the Seattle Angina Questionnaire (SAQ) [41], or generic, such as the World Health Organization Quality of Life (WHOQOL) [42]. Disease-specific QoL measures tend to be more sensitive to changes in QoL as they are tailored to disease-specific symptoms. Generic QoL measures can be used to compare QoL in people with different illnesses.

In health economics, utility is the preferred measure, defined as the value attached by an individual to a specific level of health status or a specific health outcome. Different individuals may attach different values to the same health state. For example, some people may be prepared to tolerate a lot of nausea to allow them to be pain free. Other people may prefer to tolerate more pain and reduce the level of nausea. The important concept here is that utility measurement allows patients to value the health state, based on their own preferences.

Like generic QoL measures, utility can be used when looking at groups of patients who may have different illnesses and can be used to compare outcomes in different patient groups. Simply, utility is used to attach a numerical value to the value a person has for a health state, the methods allow individuals to indicate the direction and strength of their preference for a particular health state, where 1.0 indicates perfect health and zero is equivalent to being dead. People can have utility scores below zero, if they value their health state as being worse than being dead. Patients complete a questionnaire describing their health states, upon which a preference-based algorithm is applied to estimate utilities. The EuroQoL five dimensions measure (EQ-5D) is the multi-attribute utility instrument most widely used to measure utilities in clinical trials and related studies and is used most often for cost-utility evaluations in health technology assessments [43]. These utility measures are used to generate quality-adjusted life-years (QALYs). A QALY combines survival periods (quantity of life) with health status valuations (quality of life) to provide a standard unit for measuring health gain. One year in perfect health is one QALY. Less than perfect health states such as surviving with a stroke generate fewer QALYs. Therefore, the harm associated with a medication error can be represented as a QALY decrement, also referred to as disutility.

The disability-adjusted life year (DALY) is a measure of overall disease burden [44]. One DALY represents the loss of the equivalent of 1 year of full health. DALYs for a disease or health condition are the sum of the years of life lost due to premature mortality (YLLs) and the years lived with a disability (YLDs) due to prevalent cases of the disease or health condition in a population. YLL contributes to the mortality aspect of DALY and is the difference between standard life expectancy and age at death. YLD accounts for the morbidity part of DALY and indicates the number of years of life lived in less than full health [45]. In 2017, the total global DALY due to adverse effects from medical care in general was 62.79 (52.09–75.45) per 100,000 population [46].

There are many criticisms around the design and application of QALYs and DALYs, ranging from the appropriateness of combining mortality and morbidity in one measure, equity for different groups of the population (such as older adults, people with disabilities) to tool construction and use [47, 48], which are beyond the scope of this chapter.

Expressing Outcomes Using Monetary Values

Another method of measuring outcome is to convert these benefits into a monetary value. The contingent valuation or 'willingness to pay' method elicits monetary values for health. Contingent valuation accounts for both health and non-health effects and is considered by some to be a more comprehensive measure of the effects of health care. For example, non-health benefits may include patients' preferences for consideration of their dignity, or aspects associated with the process of an intervention, such as location [49]. Willingness to pay has been used to elicit preferences for the avoidance of side effects with antidepressants, identifying those most troublesome to patients [50]. Blurred vision and tremor were the side effects considered most troublesome and were associated with the highest willingness to pay values to avoid them. The primary concern around willingness to pay as a method is its hypothetical nature and the valuation solicited. There are concerns that the values are constructed in response to the questions and that they do not exist before they are measured. This method has not often been used in the area of medication safety.

2.1.3 Resource Use and Costs of Medication Errors and Adverse Drug Reactions

A range of resources are consumed as the result of ADRs and the interventions used to improve safety. Health economics is concerned with identifying and quantifying all the costs incurred, i.e. capturing the true economic cost incurred by a medication error. Calculation of true economic cost is difficult, but it is essential to make sure that cost information reflects true economic cost as closely as possible. This is not usually straightforward in health care because normal markets and pricing mechanisms are not necessarily present. This section introduces key cost concepts and definitions and describes their use in medicines safety. The reader is also directed to Drummond et al. (2015) [51] for further information around these methods.

Costs can be divided into direct and indirect costs.

Direct Costs

Direct costs are the costs associated directly with an illness or healthcare intervention. Direct medical costs are the costs incurred by the healthcare provider and are split into fixed and variable costs. These costs include staff time, medical supplies, hotel costs, capital costs, and overhead costs. Also, there may be direct costs not incurred by the health service (direct non-medical costs). These can include:

- Patients' out-of-pocket expenses (such as travelling or child care costs)
- Costs falling on other parts of the public sector, such as social services (this would include costs like provision of domestic help or disability pension payments)

Fixed costs are those incurred whether patients are treated or not. The two major components of fixed costs are overhead and capital costs. Capital costs are incurred when major capital assets such as counselling rooms are built or equipment is purchased. Overheads are those incurred by the running of the service, such as lighting, heating, and cleaning costs.

Variable costs are incurred from a patient's treatment. This includes disposable equipment, drugs, blood products, investigations, and so on. Drugs and other consumables may have prices that vary between purchasers due to the influence of buying groups, contractual agreements, quantity discounts, and competitive bidding.

If a person has to stay in hospital for longer because of an ADR, the costs associated with that increased length of stay will be a combination of fixed costs incurred by the hospital to make inpatient beds available, allocated top-down to calculate a mean cost for 1 day's stay, and variable costs associated with specific interventions needed to manage the ADR. If a person is admitted to ICU, fixed costs of providing an ICU bed will be much higher than that of a standard inpatient bed, so the fixed costs are correspondingly higher. The interventions carried out on top of that are also likely to be much higher than on a standard ward, so variable costs are also likely to be higher.

How Are Costs Valued?

The two ways of collecting costs are either 'top-down' or 'bottom-up' (also called 'microcosting'). Top-down studies use the total budget to produce average costs per patient. This method is the quicker one, but assumes that all patients have the same diagnosis, severity of illness, and treatment. The costs produced from this method are not sensitive to changes in treatment. Bottom-up studies measure resource use by individual patients so they are able to detect treatment differences between those patients. This method produces much better-quality costs, but can be time consuming and expensive to collect. Also, top-down costs are often available from healthcare accounting systems, whereas bottom-up costs may need to be collected especially for that study.

Resource use is measured in physical units, such as hours of staff time or quantities of drugs given. The next step is to attach costs to that resource use. Most resource use has an associated unit cost, such as cost per hour for staff or cost per dose for drugs. Overheads such as heating and lighting will also have a unit cost, sometimes per hour, or maybe per unit area per year. Market prices for resources are used to approximate to the opportunity cost of that resource.

Costs Versus Charges

It is important to understand the distinction between real cost of a healthcare intervention and the charges that may be used to generate a price for that intervention. The real cost is a reflection of the resources consumed during the intervention, and thus approximates to their opportunity cost. Charges used by healthcare providers often do not reflect true cost. This is because healthcare providers may cross-subsidise losses on some services with profits from others, at the same time running an overall surplus on services to finance new growth. These charges do not reflect the true economic cost of the service, although they have an obvious operational function.

In some settings, including England [52, 53], there are publicly available prices for medicines and some health and social care services. These are the prices charged for specific units of care, so give an approximation of cost. However, many countries, such as the USA, France, Greece, and Cyprus, do not have a lot of readily publicly available cost information.

Litigation Costs

From April 2015 to March 2020, National Health Service (NHS) Resolution received 1420 claims relating to medication errors, of which 487 claims were settled with damages paid, costing the NHS £35 million (excluding legal costs) [54]. Another study estimated total litigation cost to the NHS was £3.6 billion in 2018/2019, a fourfold increase from 2008/9 [55]. Anticoagulants, opioids, antimicrobials, antidepressants, and anticonvulsants were the most common medications to be implicated in incidents. Primary care errors that resulted in litigation quadrupled between 2015 and 2020 with the number of claims and cost per claim increasing every year.

An Irish study of medication-related claims finalised from 2011 to 2016 identified that key medication groups involved were general anaesthetics, opioids, penicillins, antithrombotics, and local anaesthetics [56]. The most commonly pleaded primary injuries in this study were allergic reaction, deterioration in clinical status, and post-traumatic stress disorder. The median total cost of these claims was €60,991, including median damages of €33,858.

Litigation costs may be incurred by healthcare providers as a result of ADRs, so can be considered to come under direct costs, although they are very rarely included in studies of economic impact of medication errors [16].

Indirect Costs

Indirect costs are incurred by the reduced productivity of a patient, and their family, resulting from illness, death, or treatment. These may include time out of work or other unpaid activities (such as caregiving, education); time spent going to healthcare providers; time spent caring for the patient by relatives or paid carers; time forgone from leisure and other non-market activities [57]. The significance of indirect costs depends upon the particular illness and treatment involved. Some indirect costs can be calculated from data (time off work due to sick leave; early retirement; reduced productivity at work) but others are difficult to measure. Also, there are unresolved issues about including indirect costs because this would tend to favour interventions where the individuals are in employment (i.e. not children, 'housewives', the unemployed, and older adults). The alternative to this is to attach a value to unpaid activities, such as attending school or carrying out housework, or informal caregiving. Indirect costs play an important role if the intervention produces benefits that enable the target patient group to return to work or their normal daily activity.

Due to difficulties around identifying, measuring, and valuing indirect costs, they are not often included in economic studies both in general and in patient safety [16]. However, it is likely that serious ADRs will affect indirect costs, so they should always be considered, if not measured.

When indirect costs are included, they can have a dramatic effect on the results of the analysis.

Perspective

When looking at economic burden in general, the costs included depend on the perspective of the analysis. Figure 5.2 summarises the different costs included in different perspectives.

The societal perspective is the widest perspective because it looks at the costs from the viewpoint of society as a whole, including direct and indirect costs. Different studies reporting economic burden often include or exclude some categories of costs, depending on their perspective, and this can contribute to variations in estimates of burden. Due to the methodological challenges associated with collecting and valuing indirect costs described above, many economic studies concentrate on costs from the perspective of the healthcare provider only, most only looking at medication and hospitalisation costs [16]. A good-quality costing study should clearly state the perspective, along with the study population, all relevant costs and their sources included, adjustment for differential timing of costs using discounting (see section 'Discounting Costs and Benefits'), a sensitivity analysis to address parameter or methodological uncertainties [58].

The choice of economic perspective and time horizon are major determinants of the resources and costs measured. A study with an acute care hospital economic perspective and a short time horizon will focus on the direct costs of providing hospital care for the current visit, but will not consider costs of care after hospital discharge, or societal costs of illness resulting from lost productivity. A significant proportion of the cost of ADRs is accrued after discharge from acute care, so this study design will generally underestimate true economic costs [59].

Discounting Costs and Benefits

When determining true economic cost, adjustment of costs for differential timing (discounting) is recommended. Discounting makes current costs worth more than those occurring in the future because individuals would rather spend money later than in the present [60]. This is because any capital held now can be invested, earning interest. Therefore, there is a cost to

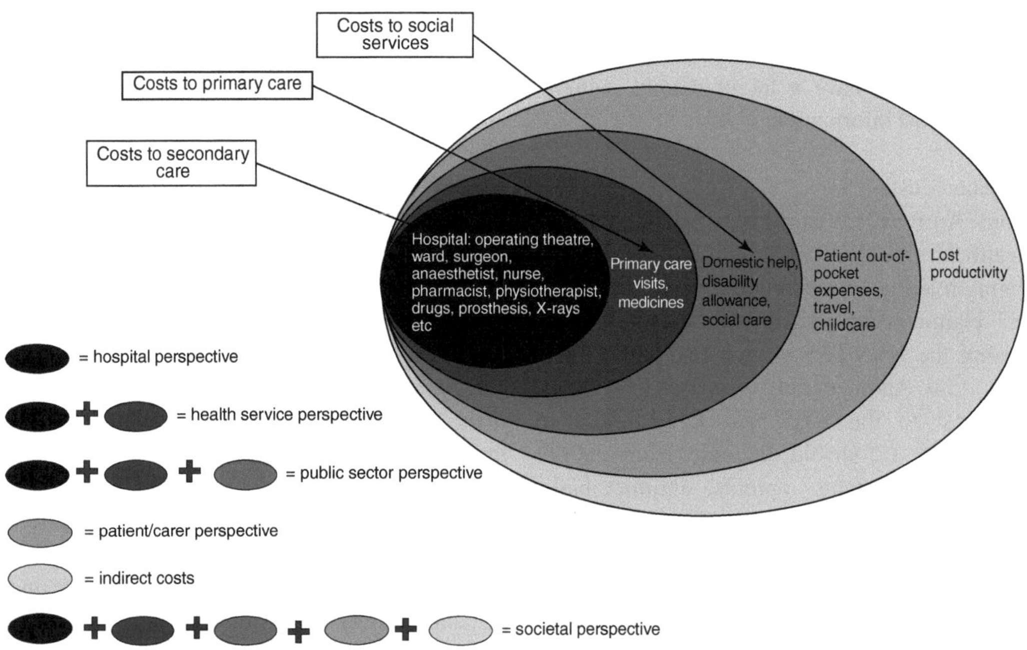

Fig. 5.2 Costs included across different perspectives

spending money in the present. This means that costs incurred now are of greater importance than costs to be incurred in the future. This is known as a 'positive time preference' [61].

Discounting makes current benefits worth more than those occurring in the future because there is desire to enjoy benefits now rather than in the future, also due to the positive time preference. Whether future health benefits should be discounted at the same rate as costs, or at all, and whether discount rates should differ for low middle income countries (LMICs) is under constant debate and the interested reader is directed to Severens et al. [62] and Haackens et al. [63].

2.1.4 Evidence for Economic Burden of Medication Errors

There are many estimates of economic burden of errors, using a mixture of the methods described above. The WHO estimates an annual cost of €4.5–21 billion in Europe [64]. Lim et al. estimate that least 250,000 hospital admissions annually in Australia are medication-related, with an estimated cost of 1.4 billion Australian dollars [65].

However, variations in methodology lead to wide variations in estimates of economic burden of medication errors. A fairly recent systematic review exploring the economic impact of medication errors included 16 studies and reported that the mean cost per error per study ranged from €2.58 to €111,727.08, with most of this variation being due to variation in methods used [16].

In 2007, the NPSA estimated NHS costs of preventable medication errors to be £774 million each year in England, at 2005/6 prices (£954 million at 2015/16 prices) [25, 26]. This sum was derived from costs of admissions (£359 million), costs of increased lengths of admissions from errors occurring whilst in hospital (£411 million), and litigation costs (£4 million). A 2018 study estimated that costs to the NHS in England of definitely avoidable ADRs leading to or extending a hospital admission are £98.5 million (£98,462,582) per annum, consuming 181,626 bed-days and causing or contributing to 704–1708 deaths during the index hospitalisation [24]. The difference between the two estimates of £954 m and £98 m is mostly due to the fact that the NPSA study included harm definitely or probably caused by medication errors and the Elliott et al. study included harm only definitely caused by medication errors. Neither approach is wrong, but illustrates that the numbers in burden of medication safety studies should be viewed with caution.

In conclusion, the results of studies of the economic burden of medication errors are based on a range of methods and are probably not directly comparable. However, they appear to suggest that there is sufficient economic impact to support efforts to reduce medication error rates, associated ADRs, patient harm, and cost. As we move on to look at the economic impact of interventions to improve medication safety in the next section, it is important to remember that not all harm is avoidable. A recent meta-analysis of the types of studies described here suggests that the pooled global prevalence for avoidable medication harm is 3% and for overall medication harm is 9% [8]. This is essential information because any safety intervention can only remove avoidable harm, so in this context, can reduce harm from 9% to 6%, but never to 0%.

3 Economic Evaluation of Interventions to Improve Medication Safety

Interventions to reduce medication errors are not new. In 1972, an educational intervention in digoxin prescribing reduced 'digitalis intoxication' [66]. There have been many reviews of these studies [12, 13, 67, 68]. Until recently, most studies about reducing medication errors had been undertaken in secondary care and tend to be focused on computerised tools, educational strategies, or professional roles [12]. Strategies and initiatives that aim to change prescribing behaviour are generally costly, with little evidence presented around their cost-effectiveness [11, 12]. Economic evaluation allows the decision-maker to see the impact of their decision to fund an intervention, or not, on both costs and patient outcomes and is a useful tool to inform resource allocation decisions.

3.1 What Is an Economic Evaluation?

An economic evaluation is concerned with identifying the differences in costs and outcomes between options. It can be defined as a study that compares the costs and benefits of two or more alternative interventions.

There are two main approaches to economic evaluation: cost-effectiveness analysis (CEA) and cost–benefit analysis (CBA). They differ in the type of outcome measure used. CEA values outcomes in non-monetary terms so the results are presented as incremental changes in cost per unit of outcome. CBA values outcomes in monetary terms so the results are presented as net monetary benefit (NMB). Cost–utility analysis (CUA) is a type of CEA where utility is the outcome. Cost minimisation analysis (CMA) is a special case in CBA or CEA and occurs when the outcomes of different options are equivalent, so the less costly option should be selected.

In CEA (and CUA), the following questions are always asked:

- What is the difference in cost between the interventions?
- What is the difference in outcome between the interventions?

The answers to these questions allow the derivation of the incremental cost-effectiveness ratio (ICER). ICERs may be calculated using the following equation: ICER = $(C_1 - C_0)/(E_1 - E_0)$, where C_1 = cost in intervention group; C_0 = cost in control group; E_1 = effect in intervention group; E_0 = effect in control group.

The ICER expresses the cost required to achieve each extra unit of outcome. When one alternative is more effective, but requires more resources, the ICER must be calculated. In the situation when one alternative is more effective and less costly, this alternative is the dominant therapy. When there is dominance, ICERs do not need to be generated. The generation of the ICER allows us to see how much extra cost is incurred for the extra benefit. It is then left to the decision-maker to make a value judgement as to whether they think that the extra benefit is worth the extra cost. For example, in England, National Institute for Health and Care Excellence (NICE), the decision-making body that recommends technologies for NHS funding, has a cost-effectiveness threshold at £20,000 per QALY. An intervention with an ICER below £20,000 per QALY would be considered a cost-effective use of NHS resources. In other countries, the threshold may not be so explicit and may vary by sector or disease area.

3.2 The Intervention

A key aspect of study design is the definition, description, and clarity of intent of the intervention being carried out, as this will affect both effectiveness and cost aspects of the evaluation, as well as affecting the relevance of the evaluation to other settings. Whether the intervention is in itself grounded in evidence needs to be presented, and as many safety interventions have multiple components, studies should follow the guidelines for complex intervention development [69]. Key questions are as follows:

- At what level does the intervention work (e.g. patient-level, practice-level, hospital level)?
- How long does the intervention last, or is it a 'one-off'?
- Who is delivering the intervention (e.g. a practitioner or a researcher)?
- Is the delivery of the intervention standardised?

3.3 The Comparator

Of similar importance to the intervention being evaluated is the definition, description, and integrity of the comparator as this will also affect both effectiveness and cost aspects of the evaluation. Many studies use 'current practice' as the comparator, but it is not always clear what this is. As such, current practice may differ between settings making comparison or extrapolation of study results difficult.

Some studies do not collect primary data for the comparator, but rather model the counterfactual by making assumptions about (or consulting expert opinion on) what would have happened to the patient [70, 71] or resource consumption [72] in the absence of the intervention. For example, Dooley et al. took ward-based interventions made by pharmacists in eight Australian hospitals and asked an expert panel to estimate the importance of the intervention and any associated treatment and outcomes that may have been averted by that intervention [71]. They then attached unit costs to those data to estimate the costs of the events averted by the intervention. This method is sometimes used in modelling when primary data are not available but presents considerable uncertainty around an effect size.

Given that many interventions are based around pharmacists identifying problems with medicines that have been created or missed by others, the current practice comparator is sometimes non-disclosure of this information to the relevant party in a primary care [73, 74] or secondary care [75] setting. A study of prescriber support described a comparator group where the 'pharmacist proposed recommendations that remained concealed from the physicians' and the physicians were told to 'act as though the pharmacist present in the office is invisible' [74]. However, withholding information that could affect patient outcome is usually perceived to be unethical in healthcare settings where equipoise no longer exists regarding the effect of the intervention. To handle this, some studies have derived comparators where the 'control' was the pharmacist providing written information and the intervention was one of a range of face-to-face interactions between the pharmacist and prescriber [76, 77]. The adaptation of this comparator clearly represents a different evaluation when compared with a comparator that has no input from the pharmacist at all, the latter approach is likely to show a bigger effect of the intervention. For example, Bond et al. compare standard practice with the intervention of giving written medication review feedback to GPs [73]. Interestingly, this intervention was equivalent to the control arm used in other studies that compared written feedback on prescribing with face-to-face meetings or case conferences [76, 77].

3.4 Study Design

An economic evaluation requires a comparative study to provide an estimate of relative effectiveness when comparing one intervention with another, or with current practice. Therefore, economic evaluations are often carried out alongside RCTs. RCTs are considered the gold standard source for effectiveness evidence. It can be a challenge to design and carry out RCTs for complex safety interventions that may function at a practice or hospital level. Contamination between intervention and control arms can be dealt with by clustering at the practice or hospital level [76, 78]. In complex safety interventions, it should be recognised that it is not always possible to carry out an RCT, and therefore other non-randomised comparative study designs can be used. These may use routinely collected data or observational data collected specifically for the study. Study designs tend to be either historical or concurrent controls or both. This type of study will have the possibility of contamination or secular changes, as well leading to the introduction of selection bias through the non-random allocation of intervention and control sites. Estimation of effect sizes in these types of studies need to take account of these potential biases in the data.

A full economic evaluation requires presentation of the costs and outcomes of the intervention and its comparator to allow assessment of the incremental cost and benefit. Some published studies present partial economic evaluations where no incremental analysis is presented, or cost–consequences analyses, which examine costs and consequences without attempting to isolate a single consequence or aggregate consequences into a single measure with no incremental analysis [51]. Budget impact analysis is another related method that focuses on the costs of developing and implementing a safety intervention and over a fixed timescale, often a year, but do not consider longer-term downstream costs, outcomes, or effectiveness. This kind of analysis is usually used instead of, or as a supplement to economic evaluation to reflect the affordability of the intervention.

3.5 Costs

Resource use data should be obtained preferentially from up-to-date locally relevant sources of observation of normal clinical practice, where units of resource use have been reported in a disaggregated manner, to allow attachment of current unit prices. Bottom-up costs allow variation between patients, and thus interventions, to be quantified and are preferable in economic evaluations looking to quantify uncertainty around point estimates of incremental costs. Often in published studies, methods of collecting resource use data are not included, comprehensive or complete costs are not present, some not including cost of the intervention itself [79].

The perspective taken for costs can be the healthcare provider, society, or the consumer. Healthcare provider costs often need to include both primary and secondary care costs incurred. The economic perspective should extend beyond the acute care hospital, as only 22–66% of the economic burden of ADRs in acute care is borne by the acute care hospital, the remaining acute care costs may occur in primary care [59].

3.6 Outcomes

Studies reporting interventions to reduce error reduction often provide information around costs of the intervention, or even the effects of the intervention on prescribing budgets [80] but often do not report evidence around the effect of the intervention on patient outcome or wider, or longer-term costs.

For example, in the study by Kaushal et al., they attempted to quantify the return on investment of a computerised physician order entry (CPOE) system [81]. Between 1993 and 2002, the Boston Women's Hospital (BWH) spent US$11.8 million (2002 prices) to develop, implement, and operate CPOE. Over 10 years, the system saved BWH $28.5 million. Costs were saved through reductions in unnecessary medications, investigations, and staff time utilisation. The authors also determined cost savings from ADR alerts by multiplying the number of averted ADRs by the average cost of an ADR derived from Bates et al. (US$4685 in 1997 dollars) [20].

Another approach reported is the non-standard method of using a 'cost benefit ratio of the intervention', which was apparently calculated by dividing the total costs by the total savings (cost avoidance summed with cost savings) [82]. This approach will provide little relevance outside the immediate research setting and is not recommended.

3.6.1 Use of Error Rates as Outcomes

Economic evaluations of safety interventions that move beyond looking just at savings often rely on errors as the outcome measure, for the reasons discussed earlier in this chapter, and may generate a 'cost per error avoided'. For example, Avery et al. reported that their pharmacist-led intervention to reduce primary care prescribing errors had an ICER of £65 per error avoided, but this ICER included only the costs of delivering the intervention for 6 months and no impact on longer-term costs [76].

3.6.2 Use of Adverse Drug Reactions as Outcomes

Some studies have looked at impact on ADRs. One example used preventable ADRs as a primary outcome and healthcare resource utilisation as secondary outcome at 30 days [83]. Rates of preventable ADRs were significantly lower in the intervention arm compared with the standard care arm, but no significant difference was found in healthcare resource use. No incremental analysis was reported so this was a cost-consequences analysis. Wu et al. examined the impact of an electronic medication ordering and administration system in a Canadian hospital setting and reported that the ICER of the new system was $12,700 (USD) per ADR prevented [84]. This study used primary data collection to generate these results. Another study reporting costs saved by preventing ADRs but used a different method, utilising literature-based estimates of ADR cost and prevalence requiring treatment to inform a model to estimate the potential savings in prevented ADRs overall and per patient [85]. The results reported were US$218 ADR costs avoided per patient who received the intervention.

Those interventions that generate outcomes in a cross-therapeutic area require generic outcomes, and thus rely more on process measures, such as medication errors or ADRs.

Interventions focusing on one therapeutic area can use a patient outcome specific to that disease area, such as GI bleeds in NSAID use. However, the study needs to be powered to detect a difference in outcome, not just the error, and needs to collect outcome data that are linked to the error. One illustrative example is which outcome to measure when looking at the use of psychoactive medications in people with dementia. This is generally considered high-risk prescribing and is generally discouraged unless absolutely necessary. This is partly because of the wide range of ADRs associated with their use in this cohort, including stroke, urinary tract infections, somnolence, abnormal gait [86], and pneumonia [87]. However, evidence suggests no consistent effect on falls [86]. An intervention to reduce the proportion of care home residents taking inappropriate psychoactive medications at 12 months in the intervention homes was shown to be highly effective in terms of reducing prescribing from 50% to 19% (odds ratio = 0.26, 95% confidence interval = 0.14–0.49) after adjustment for clustering within homes [88]. The study examined the impact of the intervention on clinical outcomes, but used falls, and no differences were observed at 12 months in the falls rate between the intervention and control groups. It is possible that if a different clinical outcome was measured, a difference may have been detected.

3.6.3 Use of Utility as an Outcome

Not knowing the impact of the intervention on patient health and wider longer-term costs is an important limitation as the evaluative frameworks in many countries require evidence on impact on patient health and wider longer-term costs to compare the value for money of different healthcare interventions. For example, in England, the NICE requires information presented as a cost per QALY.

One approach to generate cost per QALY has been to attach some hypothetical QALY and cost decrement to error rates to estimate impact [89]. In this study, Karnon et al. [89, 90] used a medication errors model to describe the pathway of errors occurring at hospital admission through to the occurrence of preventable ADRs. The baseline model was populated using literature-based values. Costs were taken from published literature [90]. Probability of harm was divided into significant (resulted in temporary harm to the patient and required intervention without (increase in) hospital stay); serious (resulted in temporary harm and required hospitalisation); and severe, life threatening, or fatal (resulted in permanent patient harm, required intervention to sustain life, or contributed to a patient's death). Utility weights were attached to harm from undetected errors divided into significant, serious, severe, life threatening, or fatal. These hypothetical QALY decrements for errors were derived from discussions within the research team, and a retrospective study estimated that 43% of patients who died following an error defined as definitely or probably preventable would have left the hospital alive given optimal care [91]. This study concluded that the intervention (pharmacist-led medicines reconciliation) dominated standard care. One of the limitations of this approach is the high level of uncertainty around any estimates generated due to the elicitation methods and large numbers of assumptions used.

Another approach has been to model the estimated costs and harm associated with specific types of errors, that is, estimates based on the aggregation of particular harms, using the modelling approach described earlier in this chapter. This approach was used to estimate the QALY decrement and cost associated with six common and clinically significant primary care prescribing and monitoring errors targeted in an error-reducing intervention [92]. Clinical event probability, treatment pathway, resource use, and cost data to populate each of the six models were extracted from published literature and NHS costing tariffs. A composite model was constructed that combined the patient-level error models with practice-level error rates and intervention costs from the trial. One of the limitations of this approach is that it would be a very large task to generate models to cover the huge variety of errors, and there are sometimes very little data to populate these models once specified.

3.6.4 Within-Trial Economic Evaluation or Economic Evaluation Incorporating Modelling?

Economic evaluations of interventions to improve medicines safety can either be within-trial economic evaluations or can incorporate modelling. A within-trial economic evaluation is quicker to do and will generate an ICER using the trial's primary outcome, usually cost-per-error avoided. This can be a very useful metric, but it does not provide evidence on how much harm is avoided, unless ADRs are the primary outcome, in which case cost per ADR avoided can be derived. This also means that the length of follow-up is only the length of the trial. A longer length of follow-up, called a time horizon, would allow us to see the longer-term costs and outcomes associated with an error or ADR. Decision-making bodies such as NICE in England use a lifetime time horizon. This requires metrics like the cost per QALY over a patient's lifetime, which necessitates extrapolating beyond the trial findings by using modelling. Modelling will also be required when there are no RCT data available.

3.7 Quality of Economic Evaluations

Economic evaluations are conducted using widely accepted frameworks and should follow standard quality design and reporting criteria [93, 94]. The sections above describe preferred methodology in economic evaluations, with a specific focus on the challenges associated with evaluating medication safety interventions. A range of aspects of poor study design or data analysis means that some studies of safety interventions may be reported as cost-effective when they are not, or not cost-effective when they are. Furthermore, variation in intervention design, service delivery context, comparator arms, resource use and cost measurement, and lack of standardised outcome measures make comparison between even well-designed studies problematic.

One of the key aspects of an economic evaluation is the level of certainty around the results. A deterministic economic evaluation uses the point estimates of parameters and tests the impact of varying individual parameters on the conclusions. A probabilistic economic evaluation simultaneously varies all parameters, so incorporates all parameter uncertainty. Ideally, a good economic evaluation reports probabilistic results of disaggregated costs, outcomes for each comparator, the incremental cost and outcome, and if appropriate, an ICER. There should also be a series of one- and two-way sensitivity and scenario analyses to illustrate the effect of varying key parameters on the results, along with cost-effectiveness acceptability curves and estimates of net benefit.

3.8 Using Economic Evaluation to Evaluate Safety in Health Care

3.8.1 Challenges

Concerns exist as to what extent standard health economic methods are able to appropriately evaluate interventions to improve safety [95, 96]. In general, the reduction of errors is considered a desirable undertaking, but political support (and willingness to pay) for its implementation may be limited if the errors captured or prevented cannot be robustly linked to an improvement in patient outcomes. There may be barriers to the usefulness of cost-effectiveness to justify the expense associated with the intervention. For example, the costs may be incurred in primary care for the intervention, but the costs saved may occur in secondary care. Also the costs saved and improved outcomes may be downstream from the initial expenditure, a situation not likely to be compatible with return-on-investment calculations carried out on an annual basis.

Preventing errors and adverse events entirely can be argued to be infeasible due to the prohibitive costs involved [68, 97, 98], such that there are diminishing returns associated with increased effort required (or resources consumed) to prevent harm from adverse events [68]. An example of this is the impracticability of testing all patients for allergies to antibiotics [99], suggesting in turn that preventability of ADRs is determined to some extent by affordability [68]. Therefore, the cost-effectiveness of safety interventions should be integral to their development, implementation, and assessment to allow prioritisation of spending on suggested safety improvements [98].

3.8.2 When Is a Safety Intervention 'Efficient'?

The 'efficient' ideal would be achieved if maximum health gain in a defined patient population is attained at the lowest opportunity cost. This may also be viewed as getting the most out of an intervention given a defined budget. Application of the concept of efficiency to healthcare providers infers that decision-makers are striving to reach an optimal situation. A key question is whether decision-makers are health maximisers. What output do decision-makers wish to achieve when using or recommending a healthcare intervention? Clinicians may be entirely concerned with maximising the health of their patient population. Finance managers may want to focus on cost minimisation to control their budget. Patients may want to maximise their satisfaction from the NHS or similar bodies given their budget constraint, which will be a different budget from that of the finance manager. It is important to be aware of the incentives driving decision-makers and their desired objectives in the context of health service provision. By using the methods of economic evaluation where outcomes measured are health, there is an implicit assumption that the main objective is to maximise health gain. Is this appropriate in the context of safety?

3.8.3 Is It Enough to Measure Health in Economic Evaluations of Safety Interventions?

Cost-effectiveness analysis generally includes direct medical costs and some measure of health consequences, such as QALYs. However, this conventional position that all we want from healthcare resources consumed is to produce health is being increasingly challenged [100–103]. Specific examples where health benefits may not drive implementation decisions include diagnostic procedures and interventions with wider social implications. An example of a non-health benefit reflecting the importance of the psychological benefits of 'peace of mind' to patients is that associated with autologous blood donation, an intervention known to show very small health benefits for a substantial increase in cost [104].

If a patient is administered a penicillin in a healthcare setting, is allergic to that penicillin and dies, the health lost is the death and the life years lost of that person. If the patient's notes detail a history of penicillin allergy, then the health lost is the same: the death and the life years lost of that person. However, now that the death was preventable, it feels worse to the family and the healthcare professionals involved, and to society in general. If the outcome is deemed worse because it was avoidable, then it is likely that society is prepared to pay more to reduce this avoidable harm. Recent United Kingdom (UK) research on local and national decision-making shows that considerations of benefits unrelated to health outcomes, such as enhancing patient experiences, greater patient empowerment, improving public trust and confidence, and increasing staff morale, were used to make decisions about implementing services [103].

Attributes suggested to influence the respondents' perceptions of the value of a safety intervention extended beyond health status are the likelihood of the incident and the costs associated with prevention, including preventability, dread, controllability, and trust in the safety intervention [95].

Medical errors in general may be associated with a decreased trust of patients and citizens in healthcare systems and providers, leading to reduced service uptake or political support [95], lost productivity from healthcare professionals blamed for committing an error [105], and litigation and compensation costs [106]. Perceptions of patient safety may affect demand for health care through reduced trust. We know that reduced trust in health care is linked to delay in care-seeking, attendance, and adherence, such as vaccination uptake [107]. There is likely to be an economic impact of reduced trust in healthcare services. Lack of trust increases care avoidance behaviour (reduced care-seeking, attendance, adherence) in so-called silent members [108]. We know that silent members have increased future expenditure risk. This effect may be sociodemographically variable. Ethnic minority consumers may experience inequity in the safety of care and be at higher risk of patient safety events and little has been done to make health care safer for minority ethnic groups [109]. Research suggests that ethnic minorities have significantly increased distrust of health care overall [110].

So, the benefits of improved patient safety are not just maximising health [111]. This suggests that allocating scarce resources to improve medication safety in the most cost-effective way must take account of both the health and non-health components of safety outcomes. However, another study suggests that preventability is not valued highly by the public when assessing importance of interventions, so there is clearly more work to be done before this aspect of safety interventions is understood [112].

4 Summary and Conclusions

It is generally believed that while some medication errors do not lead to harm, others can lead to a range of harms including serious harms and death. Ideally, the data needed to assess impact of medication errors should be sufficient to encompass all effects of error on patient outcomes and societal cost. Methods exist to investigate the economic impact of medication safety interventions. Challenges associated with evaluating these interventions need to be dealt with explicitly. The quality of studies that investigate the economic impact of medication safety interventions is variable and needs to improve to ensure more optimal targeting of resources. Arguments exist to identify and value the non-health outcomes and costs of medication errors and the interventions intended to reduce them.

Future developments in this area include the increased involvement of digital technologies to identify and prevent medication errors at all stages of the medication use process. A related development is increased interoperability between different parts of the health and social care system to allow better transfer of medicines information across care interfaces. The cost of developing these systems needs to be justified by better quantification of impacts on patient safety and workforce costs.

5 Case Studies

5.1 Case Study 1: How to Identify and Estimate Harm and Cost from Prescribing Errors Using Routine Data

The prescribing of NSAIDs in adults receiving oral anticoagulant (OAC) therapy has been identified to be a problem in your healthcare setting. Supporting prescribers to reduce their use of these medicines together requires evidence of the type and quantity of harm caused. You need to design a study to identify and measure those harms.

1. *What study design should you use?*

   RCTs are useful in that they detect ADRs associated with a medicine. However, these could be harms associated with appropriate prescribing, so are not necessarily avoidable, or an error. One example would be the increase in weight associated with some antipsychotic drugs. Whilst undesirable, this is an unfortunate consequence, or side effect that can occur with appropriate prescribing of those drugs. There are specific cases where RCTs have been able to identify the harms associated with prescribing a specific type of medication. One example is the many RCTs that explored the effect of adding GPAs to NSAID therapy to reduce the risk of GI harm. As well as the reduction in risk of harm that might be achieved by prescription of a GPA, the control (or placebo) arms of these studies effectively provide the risk of GI harm when prescribing NSAIDs.

2. *If you can't use an RCT, how could you use routine data to attribute harm to a medication error?*

   If you have routine data collection where both the error and the harm can be measured, you can use these data. One example of this is a recent UK study that examined risk of GI bleeding, major bleeding, stroke, and systemic embolism associated with prescribing NSAIDs in adults receiving OAC therapy [113]. This retrospective cohort study identified patients prescribed OAC therapy and compared the risk of ADRs experienced by new users of NSAIDs with people who were not prescribed NSAIDs. An electronic health record was used that combined routine primary and secondary care data for the cohort. This study matched new users of NSAIDs with people who were not prescribed NSAIDs and generated the increased risk (hazard ratio) of an adverse outcome in the presence of NSAIDs. This analysis suggested that prescribing NSAIDs in adults receiving OAC therapy increased the risk of an adverse outcome by a factor of 2–3. Figure 5.3 summarises the methods and results of this study.

3. *What are the strengths of using routine data to attribute harm to a medication error?*

   A major strength of this approach is the availability of nationally representative linked primary and secondary care data with detailed information on patient demographics and potential confounding variables, such as lifestyle factors, comorbidities, and prescriptions to allow matching and adjustment for confounders.

4. *What are the limitations of using routine data to attribute harm to a medication error?*

   The limitations of this design are that in routinely collected data, if available at all, measurement errors (such as misdiagnosis) cannot be ruled out. Also there may be potential confounders that were not measured in the dataset. For example, in the Penner et al. study, poor INR control is a potential confounder for bleeding events, but this is not routinely collected in the Clinical Practice Research Datalink [113].

   This design only allows measurement of what is recorded which can restrict the information that can be collected. In the example above, it was not possible to obtain data on post-hospital discharge effects or quality of life of the cohort. There is also methodological and measurement complexity. The error needs to happen sufficiently frequently, as does the harm or ADR, to allow measurement. Some error-harm pairs would need impractically large sample sizes and long follow-up times to link the error to the harm.

5.2 Case Study 2: How to Identify and Estimate Harm and Cost from Prescribing Errors Using Economic Modelling

The prescribing of NSAIDs in adults over 65 years of age has been identified to be a problem in your healthcare setting. Supporting prescribers to reduce their use of these medicines in this age group requires evidence of the type and quantity of harm caused. You need to design a study to identify and measure those harms. You already know that there are no routine data to help answer this question, so you need to build an economic model using readily available data.

1. *What is the potential harm (ADRs) that can occur in people who take NSAIDs?*

   The side effects or ADRs, particularly GI bleeding, renal dysfunction, and impact on cardiovascular function, are well recognised

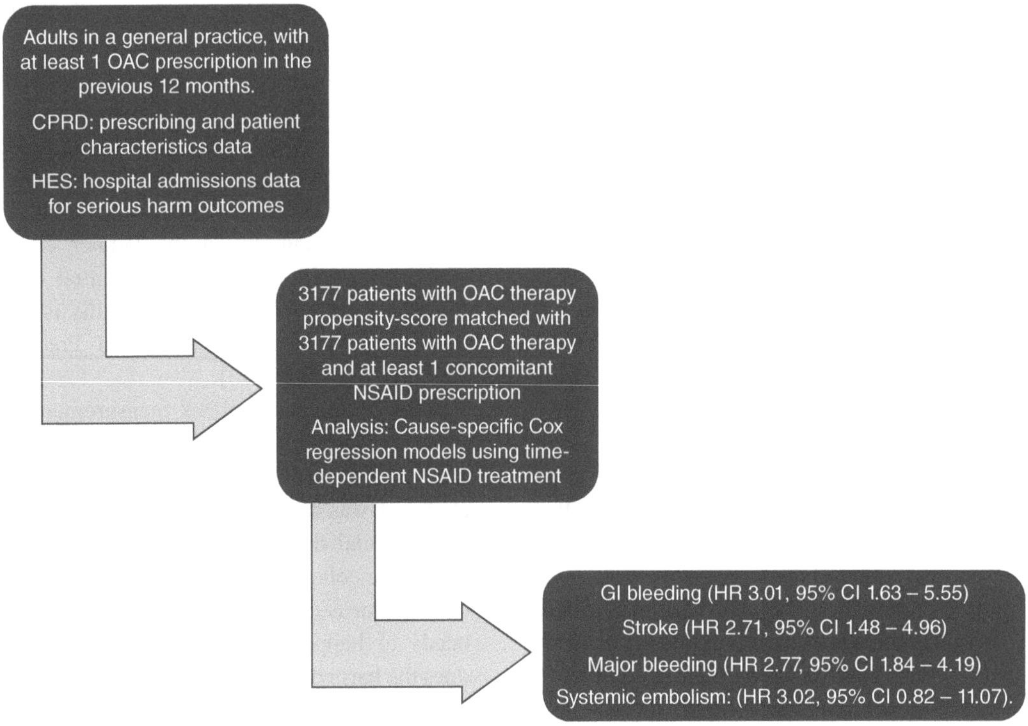

Fig. 5.3 Attribution of harm (ADRs) by Penner et al. [113]. *CI* confidence interval, *CPRD* Clinical Practice Research Datalink, *HES* Hospital Episode Statistics, *HR* hazard ratio, *OAC* oral anticoagulant

in NSAIDs [34–36]. We know that an NSAID can cause a range of GI harms when given, ranging from mild intermittent GI discomfort, persistent serious GI discomfort, gastric ulcer, to serious, or even life-threatening, upper and lower GI bleeding. These events can occur in people when an NSAID is used appropriately, but are more likely in people with risk factors such as age, a previous GI bleed, long-term use, or the use of other medications that increase bleeding risk. Prescribing NSAIDs at all, or in the absence of gastroprotective agents, in these groups of patients could be seen as a prescribing error.

Figure 5.4 presents a simplified representation of the possible events subsequent to prescribing an NSAID in a person over 65 years of age (a 'model' of events). Each of these events is associated with a health state, which can be expressed using health-related quality of life measures, or utility. Note that in these types of models, 'dead' is a health state that is usually included and is given a utility score of zero. This allows the model to include risk of death from events. If the death rate is not affected by an event, such as a minor outcome like dyspepsia, the death rate is assumed to approximate to the general population.

2. *What information do you need to put into a model that estimates the potential harm (ADRs) that can occur in people who take NSAIDs?*

Economic models need three types of data: probabilities of moving from one health state to another, and the utility and costs associated with being in that health state.

Table 5.2 illustrates how a group of health economists have 'populated' this model, with the first category of data, that is, they have attached probabilities to each of the transitions in the model, known as a transition probability. For example, the annual probability of persisting GI discomfort requiring a primary care consultation is 0.648, the probability of a

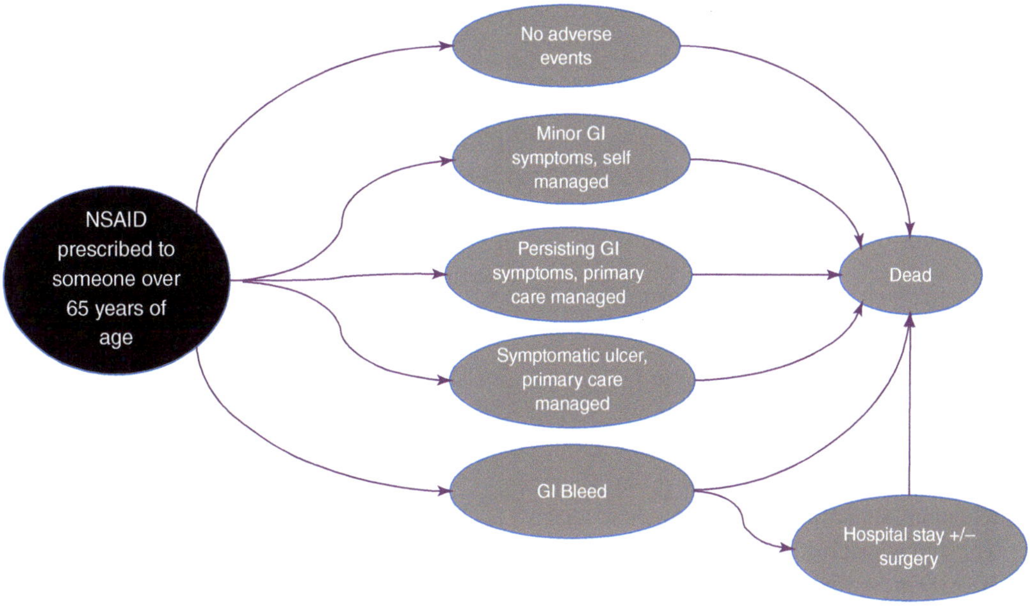

Fig. 5.4 Model of events that can occur after prescribing an NSAID in a person over 65 years of age

Table 5.2 Probability of GI outcomes and mortality in people over 65 taking NSAIDS

Transition probabilities	Estimate (SE/SD/95% CI) and source
Annual persisting GI discomfort rate	0.648 (95% CI: 0.609, 0.688) [114]
Annual symptomatic ulcer rate	0.0112 (95% CI: 0.0066, 0.0169) [115]
Annual serious GI event rate	0.00343 (95% CI: 0.00332, 0.00356) NHS Medication Safety Dashboard (Q1 2015/16–Q3 2019/20) [116]
3-month probability of death from 'no adverse event', GI discomfort, by age group	65–69: 0.0029; 70–74: 0.0046; 75+: 0.0079 [117]
3-month probability of death from symptomatic ulcer by age group	65–69: 0.0157; 70–74: 0.0244; 75+: 0.0429 [118]
3-month probability of death from serious GI event, by age group	65–69: 0.0810; 70–74: 0.1277; 75+: 0.2211 [119]
3-month probability of recurring adverse events (only relevant for first 3 months after event)	0.158 (95% CI: 0.110, 0.205) [120]

symptomatic ulcer is 0.0112, whereas the probability of a serious GI event is 0.00343. It is important to state the period of time over which the probability is being estimated, as probability changes with time of exposure to the error. The cycle length is the length of time spent in one of these health states and can be a week, a month, a year, depending on how quickly disease states change within a specific disease. In this example, the cycle length is 3 months, as this is considered an appropriate length of time over which one event might happen.

Table 5.3 demonstrates the utility associated with the health states in the NSAIDs health states. The utility decrement for the ADR is applied for as long as the health state lasts. For example, a person aged 70–74 years would generate 0.779 QALYs over 1 year in the absence of an ADR. If they have GI discomfort for 6 months of that year, they lose (0.079×2) QALYs and overall now generate 0.621 QALYs over 1 year in the presence of an ADR.

Table 5.3 Utility associated with health states in people over 65 taking NSAIDS

Health state	Utility
No ADR (by age category)	65–69: 0.8041 70–74: 0.7790 75–79: 0.7533 80–84: 0.6985 85–89: 0.6497 [121]
GI discomfort	Decrement (for 3 months): 0.079 [122, 123]
Symptomatic ulcer	Decrement (for 3 months): 0.139 [121]
Serious GI event	Decrement (for 3 months): 0.18 [92]
Dead	0

This study was carried out in the United Kingdom, so routine costs were used to attach a cost to managing the harms associated with NSAID prescribing:

(a) a general practice visit costs £39.23 [53];
(b) a gastroenterology outpatient visit costs £153.12 [52];
(c) and a diagnostic endoscopic upper GI tract procedure costs £396.30 [52].

3. *What are the challenges around finding and using data for this economic model to attribute harm?*

Sources of data vary for different medication errors. In the example above, in England, the prescribing patterns of NSAIDs to people over 65 years of age can be extracted from routine prescribing data and linked to secondary care admissions data [116]. This provides 'real-world' information on the probability of a hospital admission due to a gastric bleed in people over 65 years who are prescribed NSAIDs. However, the routine data do not pick up the other GI outcomes, so different sources have to be used. In the example above, the probability of a symptomatic ulcer has been taken from a cohort study of people over 65 years of age, taking NSAIDs, using routine prescribing data linked to hospital admissions [115]. Sometimes the evidence is not as readily available as for these two parameters. For example, in the example above, the researchers were able to find published evidence that having a gastric ulcer or a GI bleed increased risk of death, but not specifically in a population of people over 65 who were taking an NSAID. It seems clinically plausible that this specific cohort would also have an increased risk of death for these two outcomes, so leaving this aspect of harm out of the model would potentially underestimate the harm associated with NSAIDs in this cohort. However, including the published evidence from a cohort that is not exactly the same as the population of people over 65 who were taking an NSAID means that we have to assume that this evidence can be extrapolated to our cohort of interest. This assumption necessarily increases uncertainty around our estimates of harm that include this other evidence.

In addition, the researchers appear to have assumed that mild GI events do not increase risk of death, so have applied population-level age-adjusted mortality levels to this health state [117]. We would want to know ideally if this assumption were based on observational data of some sort or is it an assumption based on clinically plausibility.

The final aspect of harm included in this example illustrates the likelihood that once someone has experienced an event like a GI bleed, they are at a higher risk of another one occurring, that is, potential likelihood recurrence of the event needs to be included to better estimate harm. For this parameter, a meta-analysis of multiple studies was used to generate estimates of recurrence [120]. When looking at the recurrence rates for individual studies, these ranged from 0% to 31%, suggesting that there is a lot of uncertainty around the evidence for this parameter. This is due to the ranges of definitions used for GI events, measurement methods, follow-up times, sample size, and types of patients included [120]. This meta-analysis concluded that most recurrences occurred within 7 days of the first adverse event, which is why the researchers here have assumed an increased risk of recurrence only for the first 3 months after the initial GI event.

4. *What are the limitations of using economic models to attribute harm to a medication error?*

   One limitation of this method is that the types of harm that are included in the model will affect the harm estimates generated. For example, in the example above, the model presented has not included cardiovascular or renal harms that we know can occur with the use of NSAIDs. Therefore, the model above will underestimate the total harm associated with prescribing NSAIDs to people over 65.

References

1. Barr DP. Hazards of modern diagnosis and therapy: the price we pay. J Am Med Assoc. 1955;159(15):1452–6.
2. Department of Health. An organisation with a memory: report of an expert group on learning from adverse events in the NHS. London: Department of Health; 2000.
3. Kohn L, Corrigan J, Donaldson M. To err is human-building a safer health system. Washington, DC: Institute of Medicine; 1999.
4. Kuenssberg EV. Plenary session on ill-health due to drug-taking. Br Med J. 1965;1:982–3.
5. Patel K, Kedia M, Bajpai D, Mehta S, Kshirsagar N, Gogtay N. Evaluation of the prevalence and economic burden of adverse drug reactions presenting to the medical emergency department of a tertiary referral Centre: a prospective study. BMC Clin Pharmacol. 2007;7(1):8.
6. Pirmohamed M, James S, Meakin S, Green C, Scott AK, Walley TJ, et al. Adverse drug reactions as cause of admission to hospital: prospective analysis of 18,820 patients. Br Med J. 2004;329(7456):15–9.
7. Alexopoulou A, Dourakis SP, Mantzoukis D, Pitsariotis T, Kandyli A, Deutsch M, et al. Adverse drug reactions as a cause of hospital admissions: a 6-month experience in a single center in Greece. Eur J Intern Med. 2008;19(7):505–10.
8. Hodkinson A, Tyler N, Ashcroft DM, Keers RN, Khan K, Phipps D, et al. Preventable medication harm across health care settings: a systematic review and meta-analysis. BMC Med. 2020;18(1):313.
9. de Bienassis K, Esmail L, Lopert R, Klazinga N. The Economics of Medication Safety: improving medication safety through collective, real-time learning. OECD Health Working Papers No. 147; 2022.
10. The Evidence Centre on behalf of The Health Foundation. Research scan: improving safety in primary care. London: The Health Foundation; 2011.
11. Elliott RA. Is QUM an efficient use of healthcare resources? J Pharm Pract Res. 2008;38:172.
12. The Evidence Centre on behalf of The Health Foundation. Evidence scan: reducing prescribing errors. London: The Health Foundation; 2012.
13. Royal S, Smeaton L, Avery AJ, Hurwitz B, Sheikh A. Interventions in primary care to reduce medication related adverse events and hospital admissions: systematic review and meta-analysis. Qual Saf Health Care. 2006;15(1):23–31.
14. Sculpher M. Evaluating the cost-effectiveness of interventions designed to increase the utilization of evidence-based guidelines. Family Pract. 2000;17(Suppl 1):S26–31.
15. National Coordinating Council (NCC) for Medication Error Reporting and Prevention (MERP). Taxonomy of medication errors. 2022. https://www.nccmerp.org/taxonomy-medication-errors-now-available.
16. Walsh EK, Hansen CR, Sahm LJ, Kearney PM, Doherty E, Bradley CP. Economic impact of medication error: a systematic review. Pharmacoepidemiol Drug Saf. 2017;26(5):481–97.
17. Osanlou R, Walker L, Hughes DA, Burnside G, Pirmohamed M. Adverse drug reactions, multimorbidity and polypharmacy: a prospective analysis of 1 month of medical admissions. BMJ Open. 2022;12(7):e055551.
18. Bates DW, Boyle DL, Vander Vliet MB, Schneider J, Leape L. Relationship between medication errors and adverse drug events. J Gen Intern Med. 1995;10(4):199–205.
19. Damen NL, Baines R, Wagner C, Langelaan M. Medication-related adverse events during hospitalization: a retrospective patient record review study in The Netherlands. Pharmacoepidemiol Drug Saf. 2017;26(1):32–9.
20. Bates DW, Spell N, Cullen DJ, Burdick E, Laird N, Petersen LA, et al. The costs of adverse drug events in hospitalized patients. Adverse Drug Events Prevention Study Group. JAMA. 1997;277(4):307–11.
21. Pirmohamed M, James S, Meakin S, Green C, Scott AK, Walley TJ, et al. Adverse drug reactions as cause of admission to hospital: prospective analysis of 18 820 patients. BMJ. 2004;329(7456):15–9.
22. Hallas J, Harvald B, Gram LF, Grodum E, Brosen K, Haghfelt T, et al. Drug related hospital admissions: the role of definitions and intensity of data collection, and the possibility of prevention. J Intern Med. 1990;228(2):83–90.
23. Howard RL, Avery AJ, Slavenburg S, Royal S, Pipe G, Lucassen P, et al. Which drugs cause preventable admissions to hospital? A systematic review. Br J Clin Pharmacol. 2007;63(2):136–47.
24. Elliott RA, Camacho E, Jankovic D, Sculpher MJ, Faria R. Economic analysis of the prevalence and clinical and economic burden of medication error in England. BMJ Qual Saf. 2021;30(2):96–105.
25. National Patient Safety Agency. Safety in doses: medication safety incidents in the NHS. Patient Safety Observatory; 2007.

26. Personal Social Services Research Unit. PSSRU unit costs of health and social care 2016; 2016.
27. Onatade R, Sawieres S, Veck A, Smith L, Gore S, Al-Azeib S. The incidence and severity of errors in pharmacist-written discharge medication orders. Int J Clin Pharm. 2017;39(4):722–8.
28. Avery AJ, Ghaleb M, Barber N, Dean Franklin B, Armstrong SJ, Serumaga B, et al. The prevalence and nature of prescribing and monitoring errors in English general practice: a retrospective case note review. Br J Gen Pract. 2013;63(613):e543–53.
29. Ashcroft DM, Lewis PJ, Tully MP, Farragher TM, Taylor D, Wass V, et al. Prevalence, nature, severity and risk factors for prescribing errors in hospital inpatients: prospective study in 20 UK hospitals. Drug Saf. 2015;38(9):833–43.
30. Haw C, Stubbs J, Dickens G. An observational study of medication administration errors in old-age psychiatric inpatients. Int J Qual Health Care. 2007;19(4):210–6.
31. Dean BS, Barber ND. A validated, reliable method of scoring the severity of medication errors. Am J Health Syst Pharm. 1999;56(1):57–62.
32. Dornan T, Ashcroft D, Heathfield H, Lewis P, Miles J, Taylor D, et al. An in depth investigation into causes of prescribing errors by foundation trainees in relation to their medical education. EQUIP study. Hope Hospital (University of Manchester Medical School Teaching Hospital); 2009.
33. Lesar TS, Lomaestro BM, Pohl H. Medication-prescribing errors in a teaching hospital. A 9-year experience. Arch Intern Med. 1997;157(14):1569–76.
34. Schjerning Olsen A-M, Gislason GH, McGettigan P, Fosbøl E, Sørensen R, Hansen ML, et al. Association of NSAID use with risk of bleeding and cardiovascular events in patients receiving antithrombotic therapy after myocardial infarction. JAMA. 2015;313(8):805–14.
35. Davis A, Robson J. The dangers of NSAIDs: look both ways. Br J Gen Pract. 2016;66(645):172–3.
36. Bhala N, Emberson J, Merhi A, Abramson S, Arber N, Baron JA, et al. Vascular and upper gastrointestinal effects of non-steroidal anti-inflammatory drugs: meta-analyses of individual participant data from randomised trials. Lancet. 2013;382(9894):769–79.
37. Lyratzopoulos G, Havely D, Gemmell I, Cook G. Factors influencing emergency medical readmission risk in a UK district general hospital: a prospective study. BMC Emerg Med. 2005;5(1):1.
38. Makary MA, Daniel M. Medical error—the third leading cause of death in the US. BMJ. 2016;353:i2139.
39. Xu Z, Li Y, Tang S, Huang X, Chen T. Current use of oral contraceptives and the risk of first-ever ischemic stroke: a meta-analysis of observational studies. Thromb Res. 2015;136(1):52–60.
40. Brabaharan S, Veettil SK, Kaiser JE, Raja Rao VR, Wattanayingcharoenchai R, Maharajan M, et al. Association of Hormonal contraceptive use with adverse health outcomes: an umbrella review of meta-analyses of randomized clinical trials and cohort studies. JAMA Netw Open. 2022;5(1):e2143730.
41. Spertus JA, Winder JA, Dewhurst TA, Deyo RA, Prodzinski J, McDonnell M, et al. Development and evaluation of the Seattle Angina Questionnaire: a new functional status measure for coronary artery disease. J Am Coll Cardiol. 1995;25(2):333–41.
42. Organization WH. WHOQOL: measuring quality of life; 2012.
43. EuroQol Group. EuroQol—a new facility for the measurement of health related quality of life. Health Policy. 1990;16:199–208.
44. Organization WH. Disability-adjusted life years (DALYs). Observatory TGH; 2023.
45. Devleesschauwer B, Havelaar AH, Maertens de Noordhout C, Haagsma JA, Praet N, Dorny P, et al. DALY calculation in practice: a stepwise approach. Int J Public Health. 2014;59(3):571–4.
46. Khan MA, Soteriades ES, King J, Govender R, Hashim MJ, Masood-Husain S, et al. Global trends and forecast of the burden of adverse effects of medical treatment: epidemiological analysis based on the global burden of disease study. Cureus. 2020;12(3):e7250.
47. Arnesen T, Nord E. The value of DALY life: problems with ethics and validity of disability adjusted life years. BMJ. 1999;319(7222):1423–5.
48. Nord E. Beyond QALYs: multi-criteria based estimation of maximum willingness to pay for health technologies. Eur J Health Econ. 2018;19(2):267–75.
49. Elliott R, Payne K. Essentials of economic evaluation in healthcare. London: Pharmaceutical Press; 2005.
50. O'Brien BJ, Novosel S, Torrance G, Streiner D. Assessing the economic value of a new antidepressant. A willingness-to-pay approach. Pharmacoeconomics. 1995;8(1):34–45.
51. Drummond MF, Sculpher MJ, Claxton K, Stoddart GL, Torrance GW. Methods for the economic evaluation of health care programmes. 4th ed. Oxford University Press; 2015.
52. Department of Health and Social Care. National schedule of reference costs 2018–2019; 2019.
53. Curtis L, Burns A. Unit costs of health and social care 2019. Kent: PSSRU; 2019.
54. NHS Resolution. Learning from medication errors; 2022.
55. Lane J, Bhome R, Somani B. National trends and cost of litigation in UK National Health Service (NHS): a specialty-specific analysis from the past decade. Scott Med J. 2021;66(4):168–74.
56. McCullagh M, Slattery D. Medication related litigation in Ireland: a 6-year review. Br J Clin Pharmacol. 2019;85(9):2155–62.
57. Hodgson TA. Costs of illness in cost-effectiveness analysis. A review of the methodology. Pharmacoeconomics. 1994;6(6):536–52.
58. Cooper NJ. Economic burden of rheumatoid arthritis: a systematic review. Rheumatology. 2000;39(1):28–33.

59. Etchells E, Koo M, Daneman N, McDonald A, Baker M, Matlow A, et al. Comparative economic analyses of patient safety improvement strategies in acute care: a systematic review. BMJ Qual Saf. 2012;21(6):448–56.
60. Torgerson DJ, Raftery J. Discounting. BMJ. 1999;319(7214):914–5.
61. Robinson R. Costs and cost-minimisation analysis. Br Med J. 1993;307:726–8.
62. Severens JL, Milne RJ. Discounting health outcomes in economic evaluation: the ongoing debate. Value Health. 2004;7(4):397–401.
63. Haacker M, Hallett TB, Atun R. On discount rates for economic evaluations in global health. Health Policy Plan. 2019;35(1):107–14.
64. World Health Organization. The third WHO global patient safety challenge: medication without harm. 2018.
65. Lim R, Ellett LMK, Semple S, Roughead EE. The extent of medication-related hospital admissions in Australia: a review from 1988 to 2021. Drug Saf. 2022;45(3):249–57.
66. Ogilvie RI, Ruedy J. An educational program in digitalis therapy. JAMA. 1972;222(1):50–5.
67. Kaushal R, Shojania KG, Bates DW. Effects of computerized physician order entry and clinical decision support systems on medication safety: a systematic review. Arch Intern Med. 2003;163(12):1409–16.
68. Gray A. Adverse events and the National Health Service: an economic perspective. A report to the National Patient Safety Agency. Oxford: University of Oxford, Health Economics Research Centre; 2003.
69. Medical Research Council. Complex interventions guidance. London: Medical Research Council; 2008.
70. Lowey A, Moore S, Norris C, Wright D, Silcock J, Hammond P. The cost-effectiveness of pharmacist-led treatment of cardiac risk in patients with type 2 diabetes. Pharm World Sci. 2007;29(5):541–5.
71. Dooley MJ, Allen KM, Doecke CJ, Galbraith KJ, Taylor GR, Bright J, et al. A prospective multicentre study of pharmacist initiated changes to drug therapy and patient management in acute care government funded hospitals. Br J Clin Pharmacol. 2004;57(4):513–21.
72. Baqir W, Learoyd T, Sim A, Todd A. Cost analysis of a community pharmacy 'minor ailment scheme' across three primary care trusts in the North East of England. J Public Health. 2011;33(4):551–5.
73. Bond CM, Fish A, Porteous TH, Reid JP, Scott A, Antonazzo E. A randomised controlled trial of the effects of note-based medication review by community pharmacists on prescribing of cardiovascular drugs in general practice. Int J Pharm Pract. 2007;15:39–46.
74. Altavela JL, Jones MK, Ritter M. A prospective trial of a clinical pharmacy intervention in a primary care practice in a capitated payment system. J Manag Care Pharm. 2008;14(9):831–43.
75. Gillespie U, Alassaad A, Henrohn D, Garmo H, Hammarlund-Udenaes M, Toss H, et al. A comprehensive pharmacist intervention to reduce morbidity in patients 80 years or older: a randomized controlled trial. Arch Intern Med. 2009;169(9):894–900.
76. Avery AJ, Rodgers S, Cantrill JA, Armstrong S, Cresswell K, Eden M, et al. A pharmacist-led information technology intervention for medication errors (PINCER): a multicentre, cluster randomised, controlled trial and cost-effectiveness analysis. Lancet. 2012;379(9823):1310–9.
77. Denneboom W, Dautzenberg MGH, Grol R, De Smet PAGM. Treatment reviews of older people on polypharmacy in primary care: cluster controlled trial comparing two approaches. Br J Gen Pract. 2007;57(542):723–31.
78. Tamblyn R, Abrahamowicz M, Buckeridge DL, Bustillo M, Forster AJ, Girard N, et al. Effect of an electronic medication reconciliation intervention on adverse drug events: a cluster randomized trial. JAMA Netw Open. 2019;2(9):e1910756.
79. Elliott R, Putman K, Davies J, Annemans L. A review of the methodological challenges in assessing the cost effectiveness of pharmacist interventions. Pharmacoeconomics. 2014;32:1–15.
80. Niquille A, Ruggli M, Buchmann M, Jordan D, Bugnon O. The nine-year sustained cost-containment impact of Swiss pilot physicians-pharmacists quality circles. Ann Pharmacother. 2010;44(4):650–7.
81. Kaushal R, Jha AK, Franz C, Glaser J, Shetty KD, Jaggi T, et al. Return on Investment for a Computerized Physician Order Entry System. J Am Med Inform Assoc. 2006;13(3):261–6.
82. Wilkes S, Zaal RJ, Abdulla A, Hunfeld NGM. A cost–benefit analysis of hospital-wide medication reviews: a period prevalence study. Int J Clin Pharm. 2022;44(1):138–45.
83. Al-Hashar A, Al-Zakwani I, Eriksson T, Sarakbi A, Al-Zadjali B, Al Mubaihsi S, et al. Impact of medication reconciliation and review and counselling, on adverse drug events and healthcare resource use. Int J Clin Pharm. 2018;40(5):1154–64.
84. Wu RC, Laporte A, Ungar WJ. Cost-effectiveness of an electronic medication ordering and administration system in reducing adverse drug events. J Eval Clin Pract. 2007;13(3):440–8.
85. Fernández EV, Warriner CL, David T, Gordon E, Twigg G, Carroll NV. Potential cost savings by prevention of adverse drug events with a novel medication review program. J Am Pharm Assoc. 2020;60(3):462–469.e464.
86. Schneider LS, Dagerman K, Insel PS. Efficacy and adverse effects of atypical antipsychotics for dementia: meta-analysis of randomized, placebo-controlled trials. Am J Geriatr Psychiatry. 2006;14(3):191–210.
87. Gambassi G, Sultana J, Trifirò G. Antipsychotic use in elderly patients and the risk of pneumonia. Expert Opin Drug Saf. 2015;14(1):1–6.
88. Patterson SM, Hughes CM, Crealey G, Cardwell C, Lapane KL. An evaluation of an adapted U.S. model

of pharmaceutical care to improve psychoactive prescribing for nursing home residents in Northern Ireland (Fleetwood Northern Ireland Study). J Am Geriatr Soc. 2010;58(1):44–53.
89. Karnon J, McIntosh A, Dean J, Bath P, Hutchinson A, Oakley J, et al. Modelling the expected net benefits of interventions to reduce the burden of medication errors. J Health Services Res Policy. 2008;13(2):85–91.
90. Karnon J, Campbell F, Czoski-Murray C. Model-based cost-effectiveness analysis of interventions aimed at preventing medication error at hospital admission (medicines reconciliation). J Eval Clin Pract. 2009;15:299–306.
91. Hayward RA, Hofer TP. Estimating hospital deaths due to medical errors: preventability is in the eye of the reviewer. JAMA. 2001;286(4):415–20.
92. Elliott RA, Putman KD, Franklin M, Annemans L, Verhaeghe N, Eden M, et al. Cost effectiveness of a pharmacist-led information technology intervention for reducing rates of clinically important errors in medicines management in general practices (PINCER). Pharmacoeconomics. 2014;32(6):573–90.
93. Vemer P, Corro Ramos I, van Voorn GAK, Al MJ, Feenstra TL. AdViSHE: a validation-assessment tool of health-economic models for decision makers and model users. Pharmacoeconomics. 2016;34(4):349–61.
94. Husereau D, Drummond M, Augustovski F, de Bekker-Grob E, Briggs AH, Carswell C, et al. Consolidated Health Economic Evaluation Reporting Standards 2022 (CHEERS 2022) statement: updated reporting guidance for health economic evaluations. BMJ. 2022;376:e067975.
95. Steuten L, Buxton M. Economic evaluation of healthcare safety: which attributes of safety do healthcare professionals consider most important in resource allocation decisions? Qual Saf Health Care. 2010;19(5):e6.
96. Mooney GK. What else do we want from our health services? Soc Sci Med. 1994;39(2):151–4.
97. Leape LL, Brennan TA, Laird N, Lawthers AG, Lacolio AR, Barnes BA, et al. The nature of adverse events in hospitalized patients. Results of the Harvard Medical Practice Study II. N Engl J Med. 1991;324(6):377–84.
98. Warburton RN. Patient safety—how much is enough? Health Policy. 2005;71(2):223–32.
99. Brennan TA. The Institute of Medicine report on medical errors—could it do harm? N Engl J Med. 2000;342(15):1123–5.
100. Payne K, McAllister M, Davies LM. Valuing the economic benefits of complex interventions: when maximising health is not enough. Health Econ. 2012;22:258; in print.
101. Barbosa C, Godfrey C, Parrott S. Methodological assessment of economic evaluations of alcohol treatment: what is missing? Alcohol Alcohol (Oxford, Oxfordshire). 2010;45(1):53–63.
102. Berwick DM, Weinstein MC. What do patients value? Willingness to pay for ultrasound in normal pregnancy. Med Care. 1985;23(7):881–93.
103. Shah KK, Praet C, Devlin NJ, Sussex JM, Appleby J, Parkin D. Is the aim of the health care system to maximise QALYs? An investigation of "what else matters" in the NHS. Research paper. London: Office of Health Economics; 2011.
104. Lee SJ, Neumann PJ, Churchill WH, Cannon ME, Weinstein MC, Johannesson M. Patients' willingness to pay for autologous blood donation. Health Policy. 1997;40(1):1–12.
105. Delbanco T, Bell SK. Guilty, afraid, and alone—struggling with medical error. N Engl J Med. 2007;357:1682–3.
106. Rothschild JM, Federico FA, Gandhi TK, Kaushal R, Williams DH, Bates DW. Analysis of medication-related malpractice claims: causes, preventability, and costs. Arch Intern Med. 2002;162(21):2414–20.
107. LaVeist TA, Isaac LA, Williams KP. Mistrust of health care organizations is associated with underutilization of health services. Health Serv Res. 2009;44(6):2093–105.
108. Krause TM, Yay Donderici E, Ganduglia Cazaban C, Franzini L. Future expenditure risk of silent members: a statistical analysis. BMC Health Serv Res. 2016;16:319.
109. Chauhan A, Walton M, Manias E, Walpola RL, Seale H, Latanik M, et al. The safety of health care for ethnic minority patients: a systematic review. Int J Equity Health. 2020;19(1):118.
110. Webb Hooper M, Mitchell C, Marshall VJ, Cheatham C, Austin K, Sanders K, et al. Understanding multilevel factors related to urban community trust in healthcare and research. Int J Environ Res Public Health. 2019;16(18):3280.
111. Payne K, McAllister M, Davies LM. Valuing the economic benefits of complex interventions: when maximising health is not sufficient. Health Econ. 2013;22(3):258–71.
112. Singh J, Lord J, Longworth L, Orr S, McGarry T, Sheldon R, et al. Does responsibility affect the public's valuation of health care interventions? A relative valuation approach to health care safety. Value Health. 2012;15(5):690–8.
113. Penner LS, Gavan SP, Ashcroft DM, Peek N, Elliott RA. Does coprescribing nonsteroidal anti-inflammatory drugs and oral anticoagulants increase the risk of major bleeding, stroke and systemic embolism? Br J Clin Pharmacol. 2022;88:4789.
114. Latimer N, Lord J, Grant RL, O'Mahony R, Dickson J, Conaghan PG. Cost effectiveness of COX 2 selective inhibitors and traditional NSAIDs alone or in combination with a proton pump inhibitor for people with osteoarthritis. BMJ. 2009;339:b2538.
115. Hippisley-Cox J, Coupland C, Logan R. Risk of adverse gastrointestinal outcomes in patients taking cyclo-oxygenase-2 inhibitors or conventional non-steroidal anti-inflammatory drugs: popula-

tion based nested case-control analysis. BMJ. 2005;331(7528):1310–6.
116. NHS Business Services Authority. Catalyst—public insight portal. 2020.
117. Office for National Statistics. Deaths registered in England and Wales (2018). 2019.
118. Malmi H, Kautiainen H, Virta LJ, Farkkila MA. Increased short- and long-term mortality in 8146 hospitalised peptic ulcer patients. Aliment Pharmacol Ther. 2016;44(3):234–45.
119. Crooks CJ, Card TR, West J. Defining upper gastrointestinal bleeding from linked primary and secondary care data and the effect on occurrence and 28 day mortality. BMC Health Serv Res. 2012;12(1):392.
120. Lau JY, Sung J, Hill C, Henderson C, Howden CW, Metz DC. Systematic review of the epidemiology of complicated peptic ulcer disease: incidence, recurrence, risk factors and mortality. Digestion. 2011;84(2):102–13.
121. Ara R, Brazier JE. Using health state utility values from the general population to approximate baselines in decision analytic models when condition-specific data are not available. Value Health. 2011;14(4):539–45.
122. Delaney BC, Qume M, Moayyedi P, Logan RF, Ford AC, Elliott C, et al. Helicobacter pylori test and treat versus proton pump inhibitor in initial management of dyspepsia in primary care: multicentre randomised controlled trial (MRC-CUBE trial). BMJ. 2008;336(7645):651–4.
123. Tai M-LS, Norhatta N, Goh KJ, Moy FM, Sujarita R, Asraff AA, et al. The impact of dyspepsia on symptom severity and quality of life in adults with headache. PLoS One. 2015;10(1):e0115838.

Further Reading

de Bienassis K, Esmail L, Lopert R, Klazinga N. The Economics of Medication Safety: improving medication safety through collective, real-time learning. OECD Health Working Papers No. 147; 2022.

Drummond MF, Sculpher MJ, Claxton K, Stoddart GL, Torrance GW. Methods for the economic evaluation of health care programmes. 4th ed. Oxford University Press; 2015.

Elliott R, Putman K, Davies J, Annemans L. A review of the methodological challenges in assessing the cost effectiveness of pharmacist interventions. Pharmacoeconomics. 2014;32:1–15.

Elliott RA, Putman KD, Franklin M, Annemans L, Verhaeghe N, Eden M, et al. Cost effectiveness of a pharmacist-led information technology intervention for reducing rates of clinically important errors in medicines management in general practices (PINCER). Pharmacoeconomics. 2014;32(6):573–90.

Hodgson TA. Costs of illness in cost-effectiveness analysis. A review of the methodology. Pharmacoeconomics. 1994;6(6):536–52.

Husereau D, Drummond M, Augustovski F, de Bekker-Grob E, Briggs AH, Carswell C, et al. Consolidated Health Economic Evaluation Reporting Standards 2022 (CHEERS 2022) statement: updated reporting guidance for health economic evaluations. BMJ. 2022;376:e067975.

Singh J, Lord J, Longworth L, Orr S, McGarry T, Sheldon R, et al. Does responsibility affect the public's valuation of health care interventions? A rclativc valuation approach to health care safety. Value Health. 2012;15(5):690–8.

Steuten L, Buxton M. Economic evaluation of healthcare safety: which attributes of safety do healthcare professionals consider most important in resource allocation decisions? Qual Saf Health Care. 2010;19(5):e6.

Tamblyn R, Abrahamowicz M, Buckeridge DL, Bustillo M, Forster AJ, Girard N, et al. Effect of an electronic medication reconciliation intervention on adverse drug events: a cluster randomized trial. JAMA Netw Open. 2019;2(9):e1910756.

Vemer P, Corro Ramos I, van Voorn GAK, Al MJ, Feenstra TL. AdViSHE: a validation-assessment tool of health-economic models for decision makers and model users. Pharmacoeconomics. 2016;34(4):349–61.

Principles of Pharmacovigilance and Drug Regulation

6

Lourens T. Bloem, Menno E. van der Elst, and Olaf H. Klungel

Abstract

This chapter aims to establish understanding of the drug regulatory activities that take place to ensure that a drug's benefits outweigh its risks and appreciate how drug regulatory systems support safe and effective use of drugs in clinical practice. First, it discusses the series of historical events that led to the current complex drug regulatory systems. Specifically, the emergence of contemporary drug regulation and pharmacovigilance in response to drug safety crises and European and global drug regulatory harmonisation are addressed. Second, it discusses current principles of pharmacovigilance and drug regulation. Important aspects comprise pharmacovigilance as a drug lifecycle activity, risk management planning, routine pharmacovigilance activities such as periodic safety updates and additional pharmacovigilance activities such as post-authorisation safety studies, as well as post-authorisation efficacy studies and the concept of expedited regulatory pathways. Third, it discusses advanced pharmacoepidemiological approaches in drug regulatory decision-making, including contemporary approaches to signal detection, the use of multi-database observational studies, the use of external control groups to contextualise, for example, single-arm studies, and the target trial emulation approach to facilitate causal inference from observational studies. Although some sections of this chapter focus mostly on the European drug regulatory system, connections to important global activities and developments are made to put the contents in a broad perspective.

Keywords

Pharmacovigilance · Drug regulation · Risk management · Safety specification · Signal detection · Periodic safety update reports · Post-authorisation studies · Pharmacoepidemiology · Multi-database studies · Target trial

L. T. Bloem (✉)
Division of Pharmacoepidemiology and Clinical Pharmacology, Utrecht Institute for Pharmaceutical Sciences, Utrecht University, Utrecht, The Netherlands
e-mail: l.t.bloem@uu.nl

M. E. van der Elst
Dutch Medicines Evaluation Board, Utrecht, The Netherlands

O. H. Klungel
Division of Pharmacoepidemiology and Clinical Pharmacology, Utrecht Institute for Pharmaceutical Sciences, Utrecht University, Utrecht, The Netherlands

Clinical Pharmacology, Pharmacy and Environmental Medicine, Department of Public Health, University of Southern Denmark, Odense, Denmark

J. Jose et al. (eds.), *Principles and Practice of Pharmacovigilance and Drug Safety*,
https://doi.org/10.1007/978-3-031-51089-2_6

Learning Objectives

- To appreciate how drug regulatory systems aim to support safe and effective use of drugs in clinical practice.
- To appreciate the gradual establishment of the complex contemporary frameworks for pharmacovigilance and drug regulation.
- To understand the series of historical events that led to the current drug regulatory systems.
- To recognise efforts aimed at global harmonisation of drug regulatory systems.
- To differentiate between important aspects of pharmacovigilance such as risk management planning, routine pharmacovigilance activities, and additional pharmacovigilance activities.
- To understand the role of post-authorisation efficacy studies and the associated concept of expedited regulatory pathways.
- To appreciate advanced pharmacoepidemiological approaches in drug regulatory decision-making, including for signal detection, the use of multi-database observational studies and external control groups, and the target trial emulation approach for observational studies.

Key Points

- The current drug regulatory systems have gradually evolved over time, often because (series of) historical events required a regulatory response.
- Before a drug can be used in clinical practice, a marketing authorisation needs to be granted by a drug regulator based on sufficient evidence of its quality, safety, and efficacy.
- Essentially, a drug's benefits need to outweigh its risks, at the time of marketing authorisation but also throughout the remainder of the drug's lifecycle.
- Pharmacovigilance contributes importantly to maintaining a positive benefit–risk balance.
- Important aspects of pharmacovigilance and other regulatory decision-making comprise risk management planning, pharmacovigilance activities, periodic safety updates, post-authorisation safety and efficacy studies, and expedited regulatory pathways.
- Advanced pharmacoepidemiological approaches can contribute to drug regulatory decision-making, such as contemporary approaches to signal detection, multi-database observational studies, external control groups that contextualise for example single-arm studies, and the target trial emulation approach that facilitates causal inference from observational studies.

1 Introduction

To provide assurance to society that a drug when it enters the market and is used in daily clinical practice does not cause more harm than it provides benefit to the patients that use it, a marketing authorisation needs to be obtained. Marketing authorisations are granted once a drug regulator such as the European Medicines Agency (EMA) in the European Union (EU), the United States Food and Drug Administration (US FDA), or the Medicines and Healthcare products Regulatory Agency (MHRA) in the United Kingdom (UK) considers that there is sufficient evidence to conclude that the quality aspects of a drug are acceptable and that its benefits outweigh its risks. In other words, the drug's benefit–risk balance is positive. While the US FDA and the MHRA grant marketing authorisations themselves, in the EU, the European Commission (EC) formally grants marketing authorisations after a positive opinion of the EMA for drugs in the centralised authorisation procedure. Such marketing authorisations apply to the entire EU, as well as those in the European Economic Area (EEA), namely, Iceland, Liechtenstein, and Norway. In addition, national regulatory authorities in the EU can also grant national and multinational marketing authorisations through mutual recognition and decentralised procedures. However, drug regulation does not end when a marketing authorisation is granted but extends throughout the entire lifecycle of a drug. One of the most important drug regulatory activities that continues after marketing authorisation is pharmacovigilance: "the science and activities relating to the detection, assessment, understanding and prevention of adverse effects or any other medicine/vaccine related problem" [1, 2]. Pharmacovigilance aims to ensure that the benefit–risk balance of a drug continues to be positive throughout its lifecycle, starting with clinical development and ending when the drug is taken from the market.

This chapter aims to establish understanding of the drug regulatory activities that take place to ensure that a drug's benefits outweigh its risks and appreciate how drug regulatory systems support safe and effective use of drugs in clinical practice. First, it discusses the series of events that led to the current drug regulatory systems. Specifically, the emergence of contemporary drug regulation and pharmacovigilance in response to drug safety crises and European and global drug regulatory harmonisation are addressed. Second, it discusses current principles of pharmacovigilance and drug regulation. Important aspects comprise pharmacovigilance as a drug lifecycle activity, risk management planning, routine pharmacovigilance activities such as periodic safety updates and additional pharmacovigilance activities such as post-authorisation safety studies (PASS), as well as post-authorisation efficacy studies (PAES) and the concept of expedited regulatory pathways. Third, it discusses advanced pharmacoepidemiological approaches in drug regulatory decision-making, including contemporary approaches to signal detection, the use of multi-database observational studies, the use of external control groups to contextualise, for example, single-arm studies, and the target trial emulation approach to facilitate causal inference from observational studies. Although some sections of this chapter focus mostly on the European drug regulatory system, connections to important global activities and developments are made to put the contents in a broad perspective.

2 The Evolution of Drug Regulation

This section explains the need for and important aspects of the complex contemporary frameworks for pharmacovigilance specifically and drug regulation in general. In doing so, the reader is taken along their gradual evolution over time, often as a response to certain historical events in Europe and the US, which ultimately led to the current drug regulatory systems. To illustrate, some compare drug regulatory frameworks with Christmas trees that gradually become more and more decorated with bulbs and other ornaments as years pass, with new items added every year but old ones seldomly removed. The section ends with the establishment of the European Agency for the Evaluation of Medicinal Products (EMEA) in 1995, now known as the EMA.

2.1 Industrial Production of Drugs and Their Early Regulation

Until the nineteenth century, apothecaries were the main discoverers and developers of new drugs. However, when the knowledge of chemistry and pharmacology advanced in the nineteenth century and the industrial revolution took place, the pharmaceutical industry emerged and gradually replaced apothecaries in this role [3–6]. The oldest pharmaceutical company—Merck—was founded as an apothecary in Darmstadt, Germany, in 1668 and was likely the first company to move towards the industrial production of drugs in the first half of the nineteenth century [7, 8]. In the second half of the century, Felix Hoffman at Bayer modified the molecular structure of salicylic acid to reduce its adverse effects. This resulted in acetylsalicylic acid, which was marketed as aspirin in 1899. In 1904, aspirin became available as a tablet rather than loose powder, which allowed exact dosing and prevented adulteration [9]. Aspirin was the first drug to undergo mass advertising activities, with information distributed to over 30,000 physicians worldwide [10]. Also, it received an enormous uptake in daily life, including recognition in popular literature [9].

Increasing proportions of drugs were manufactured by pharmaceutical companies, but there were no agreed methods of assessing clinical efficacy, and these only started to be established after World War II [11]. While (forerunners of) many of our current drugs, including hypnotics, anaesthetics, antipyretics, and analgesics, were produced by those early pharmaceutical companies [5, 7], many other available drugs lacked effectiveness, and some were mainly toxic. Whether efficacious or not, most drugs were commonly known as "patent drugs" (also named "secret" or "proprietary" drugs) and were heavily advertised in medical journals and public press both in Europe and the US [4, 12–15]. In 1905, the American Medical Association (AMA) decided that its journal, the *JAMA*, would only publish advertisements of drugs that had been tested and approved by its newly inaugurated Council on Pharmacy and Chemistry [4, 15]. The Council's tests comprised quality, safety, and basic efficacy evaluations that were published in the *JAMA* [15]—perhaps the earliest form of a more comprehensive and proactive review of drugs. US legislation around that time did not require any proactive review of safety or efficacy, but mainly focused on quality control [16] and aimed to prevent safety crises caused by adulterated and misbranded drugs [15].

2.2 Drug Regulation in Response to Safety Crises

The situation in the United States (US) changed in 1937, when over 100 children and adults died after taking the antibiotic Elixir Sulfanilamide that was produced by S.E. Massengill Co. The AMA received reports of these deaths and analysed samples of Elixir Sulfanilamide to discover that it contained the poisonous liquid diethylene glycol, otherwise used as an antifreeze. They issued a widespread warning but lacked legal authority for enforcement [15, 17–21]. In response, the 1938 Food, Drug, and Cosmetic Act required that for each drug, safety testing "*by all methods reasonably applicable*" should be performed and demonstrated to the US FDA [15, 18]. Thereby, regulatory control in the US shifted from healthcare professionals to the state.

In most of Europe, regulation of drugs was still focused on quality control by healthcare professionals—mainly pharmacists—apart from a few notable exceptions [19, 22]. The German physician and scientist Paul Ehrlich had developed a hypothesis about a "magic bullet" or "chemotherapy"—a drug that could be specifically targeted towards a microorganism and would not harm the human body. These ideas led to his discovery of arsphenamine (branded Salvarsan) as a treatment against syphilis in 1907 [23]. However, during World War I, the German arsphenamine became unavailable to many countries including the UK. After patents and trademarks were suspended, UK companies noticed that it was difficult to control impurities, causing safety and efficacy issues. Considering the biological mechanism of action, chemical tests proved inadequate to ensure a safe and efficacious drug, and clinical data were required. The UK Medical Research Committee (later Medical Research Council) played an important role in regulating arsphenamine in the UK: it ensured clinical data were gathered and approved for every batch before marketing [6, 23, 24]. Moreover, the UK Therapeutic Substances Act 1925 set standards for (testing of) quality, purity, and potency and required a licence to manufacture drugs "of which the purity or potency cannot be adequately tested by chemical means" [20, 24, 25]. Furthermore, Norway (from 1928) and Sweden (from 1934) required that drugs were "medically justified" prior to marketing [19, 26, 27]. France followed in 1946 by installing a committee that evaluated the therapeutic aim and safety of each drug before authorisation for marketing was granted by the Minister of Public Health [28]. Interestingly, the Norwegian regulatory agency only authorised drugs for which there was an unmet need, in order to restrict the number of authorised drugs [27].

However, it would require another major safety crisis before the contours of current regulatory systems were established in most countries. In 1956, thalidomide was first marketed in the

Federal Republic of Germany and thereafter in many other countries across the world, for a variety of indications and under various brand names including Contergan, Softenon, Distaval, Talimol, and Kevadon. Because a single injection did not cause acute toxicity, it was claimed to be safe, also during longer term use. However, in 1959, cases of peripheral neuropathy after thalidomide use were reported, followed in 1961 by cases of infants with significant malformations ("phocomelia"). These teratogenic effects seemed to have occurred after maternal use of thalidomide during pregnancy, often as a hypnotic or an antiemetic [6, 17, 18, 29]. Importantly, physicians that shared their observations of these events and the suspected role of thalidomide helped to stop the tragedy [30, 31]. Worldwide withdrawal of thalidomide-containing drugs followed. The US was spared the disaster because the FDA had concerns about peripheral neuropathy, preventing authorisation [18, 21]. In response to the crisis, in the 1960s and 1970s, countries worldwide founded or changed the mandate of existing regulatory agencies to require evidence of quality, safety, *and efficacy* of a drug before it could be authorised for marketing [18, 21]. Notably, the US FDA also required such evidence for drugs already on the market, which caused many pharmaceutical companies to withdraw them [32].

2.3 The Emergence of Pharmacovigilance

The worldwide thalidomide tragedy did not only result in the common requirement for pre-authorisation evidence of quality, safety, and efficacy but also prompted regulatory follow-up post-authorisation, especially concerning safety. The evolution of clinical trials that aimed to provide robust evidence of efficacy still provided limited evidence of safety. While restricted trial populations allowed identification of adverse drug reactions (ADRs) that occurred frequently and early after a new drug was first used, it limited identification of rare and late-onset ADRs, as well as generalisability to the often-broader clinically interpreted indication, let alone other potential off-label indications [33, 34]. As of 1962, the US FDA required companies to report adverse events in order to establish frequencies of known ADRs and identify new potential ADRs [35]. A few years earlier, after chloramphenicol use had appeared associated with various adverse events including fatal aplastic anaemia, the FDA initiated a pilot study of adverse event reporting in cooperation with, among others, the AMA and the American Society of Hospital Pharmacists that resulted in a spontaneous reporting system with almost 200 participating hospitals [36, 37]. Shortly thereafter, in 1964, the UK started a similar system, the Yellow Card Scheme [38]. Its Committee on Safety of Drugs clearly recognised the need for post-authorisation follow-up: "No drug which is pharmacologically effective is entirely without hazard. The hazard may be insignificant or may be acceptable in relation to the drug's therapeutic action. Furthermore, not all hazards can be known before a drug is marketed; neither tests in animals nor clinical trials will always reveal all the possible side effects of a drug. These may only be known when the drug has been administered to large numbers of patients over considerable periods of time" [39].

In the late 1960s and early 1970s, the World Health Organization (WHO) contributed substantially to the formation of and collaboration between national and international systems for the spontaneous reporting of adverse events, through its Programme for International Drug Monitoring [40]. The thalidomide tragedy was an important driver for this programme since the lack of a worldwide system to share adverse event information had prevented the early recognition of thalidomide-induced phocomelia [41]. Over the years, the programme has expanded extensively, from ten member countries at its inception to over 175 full and associate members in 2023 [42]. Importantly, around the inception of the programme, the use of the term "pharmacovigilance" seems to have started [43].

2.4 European Harmonisation

In 1965, the European Economic Community (EEC) created by the Treaty of Rome in 1957 [44]) issued legislation to harmonise national pharmaceutical legislation and facilitate the establishment of a common European market and the free movement of drugs. Many pieces of legislation followed that ensured further harmonisation and laid the basis for the current European drug regulatory system, including detailed evidence requirements and a slow but steady progress towards EEC-wide regulatory procedures (Table 6.1). The EEC's Committee

Table 6.1 Selection of important developments in the EEC/EU pharmaceutical legislation (1965–1995)

Legislation	Contents
Directive 65/65/EEC [45]	**Definitions and requirements** *"Safeguard public health ... by means which will not hinder the development of the pharmaceutical industry or trade in medicinal products within the Community"* – Definition of "medicinal product" – Requirement for authorisation of drugs before placing on the market – Requirement for submission of quality, pre-clinical and clinical data – Refusal of MA in case of insufficient quality, safety, and efficacy – Five-year validity of MA – Options to revoke or suspend existing MA – Labelling requirements
Directive 75/318/EEC [46]	**Standards and protocols** – Specification of quality, pre-clinical and clinical data required by Directive 65/65/EEC – First mention that benefits ("therapeutic advantages") must outweigh risks – First mention of "comprehensive data" as a requirement for MA – New type of MA: to allow for non-comprehensive data in exceptional circumstances, conditional on supply restrictions and provision of information on lack of data[a]. For drugs: • For rare diseases • For which a lack of scientific knowledge prevents the collection of comprehensive data • For which it is contrary to medical ethical principles to collect comprehensive data
Directive 75/319/EEC [47]	**CPMP, CPMP procedure and further requirements[b]** – Inception of the CPMP for arbitration and the CPMP procedure: mutual recognition of an existing MA by at least five other member states (CPMP opinion not binding) – Option to require additional data during the MA procedure – Requirements for manufacturing, including authorisation and a qualified person – Need for inspections of manufacturers and option to withdraw drugs from the market – Need for a review of MAs granted before Directive 65/65/EEC, within 15 years
Directive 83/570/EEC [48]	**SmPC, assessment reports and revised CPMP procedure** – Requirement for an SmPC, to be kept up to date after MA – Requirement for authorities to draw up assessment reports for drugs containing a "new active substance" – Revised CPMP ("multistate") procedure: at least two other member states – First mention of a "balance" (*"between effectiveness and risk"*)
Directive 87/18/EEC [49]	**Requirement to comply with good laboratory practice**
Directive 87/21/EEC [50]	**Abridged applications for MA** Exceptions for submission of quality, pre-clinical and clinical data[c]

Table 6.1 (continued)

Legislation	Contents
Directive 87/22/EEC [51]	**Concertation procedure for high-technology drugs** – Mandatory for drugs developed through biotechnological processes and optional for other innovative drugs – Required when an MA in more than one member state is sought – Assessment by the CPMP, though opinions not binding
Directive 88/320/EEC [52]	**Verification and inspection of good laboratory practice**
Directive 89/341/EEC [53]	**Package leaflet and good manufacturing practice** – Requirement for a package leaflet – Requirement to comply with good manufacturing practice
Directive 91/507/EEC [54]	**Update of quality, pre-clinical and clinical data requirements**[d] – Adaptation to state-of-the-art science – First mention of "benefit/risk" assessment and profile, including to monitor it post-authorisation[e] – Third condition for MA in exceptional circumstances[f]: post-authorisation studies[g]
Directive 93/39/EEC [55]	**Mutual recognition, pharmacovigilance, and post-authorisation** – Replacement of the multistate procedure with the mutual-recognition procedure, with CPMP opinions now binding – Need to establish national pharmacovigilance systems – Requirements for pharmacovigilance for national MAs, including a qualified person and (periodic) reporting of adverse reactions – First mention of "specific obligations" in the context of MA in exceptional circumstances[f], including post-authorisation studies and notification of adverse reactions – Recognition of potential environmental risks of drugs
Regulation (EEC) No 2309/93 [56]	**EMEA and the centralised procedure**[h] – Establishment of the EMEA: • To house and support the CPMP • To coordinate pharmacovigilance • To coordinate good laboratory, manufacturing, and clinical practice oversight – Replacement of the concertation procedure with the centralised procedure, with binding CPMP opinions – Annual review of specific obligations for MAs in exceptional circumstances – Requirements for pharmacovigilance for MAs through the centralised procedure, including a qualified person and (periodic) reporting of adverse reactions – Need for an environmental risk assessment
Regulation (EC) No 540/95 [57]	**Non-serious, unexpected adverse reactions** – Detailed requirements for periodic reporting – Specification of conditions requiring variation of MA

CPMP Committee for Proprietary Medicinal Products, *EEC* European Economic Community, *EU* European Union, *EMEA* European Agency for the Evaluation of Medicinal Products, *MA* marketing authorisation, *SmPC* Summary of Product Characteristics

[a] Later known as "Authorisation under Exceptional Circumstances"

[b] Not applicable to immunological drugs, radiopharmaceuticals, drugs derived from human blood or human plasma, and homeopathic products, for which separate directives were later issued

[c] For drugs that are "essentially similar" to already authorised drugs (later known as "informed consent" and "generic" applications) and drugs of which the constituents have a "well-established medicinal use"

[d] Now including immunological drugs, radiopharmaceuticals, and drugs derived from human blood or human plasma

[e] "… in order to monitor the benefit/risk assessment after marketing authorisation has been granted, any change to the data in the dossier, any new information not in the original application and all pharmacovigilance reports, shall be submitted to the competent authorities"

[f] See Directive 75/318/EEC

[g] "… an identified programme of studies within a time period specified by the competent authority, the results of which shall form the basis of a reassessment of the benefit/risk profile"

[h] Initially mandatory for certain biological drugs and optional for other innovative drugs

for Proprietary Medicinal Products (CPMP)—instated in 1975—would guide these procedures and act as arbitrator when member states disagreed about safety issues, or as primary assessor when it concerned innovative drugs such as in the concertation and centralised procedures. However, its opinions were not always binding and required regulatory action by the EC or regulatory agencies in individual Member States.

While Table 6.1 lists many important developments that contributed to the EU regulatory harmonisation process, one important regulatory development should be discussed here. In 1983, companies were required to provide a Summary of Product Characteristics (SmPC) together with their application for a marketing authorisation, to be assessed and agreed by the regulatory authorities. This should facilitate the exchange of information between member states [48]. Shortly thereafter, the CPMP published an SmPC guideline that outlined a specific order of information in the SmPC to optimise its relevance as an information source for healthcare professionals [58, 59]. Moreover, legislation about the advertising of drugs to healthcare professionals required that this should be done in line with the SmPC [60]. Thus, the SmPC became an important regulatory means to communicate information about the safe and effective use of drugs to healthcare professionals.

The CPMP considered matters of pharmacovigilance since its inception in 1975 and was supported for this purpose by the Pharmacovigilance Working Party (PhVWP) from 1989 onwards. Their activities comprised for example the establishment of a safety communication system, the organisation of pharmacovigilance hearings, and the incorporation of safety information in the SmPC [61].

The process of regulatory harmonisation in the EEC culminated in 1995 when, following the establishment of the European Single Market and the EU in 1993 [44], the EMEA was established. Along with the EMEA, a "centralised procedure" for regulation of innovative drugs was established [56], and a "mutual recognition procedure" to ensure harmonisation of regulatory decision-making for other drugs [55]. The opinions of the EMEA's main scientific committee, the CPMP, were now binding for all member states. Moreover, pharmacovigilance activities were specified in legislation, including immediate reporting of serious adverse events by companies to the regulatory authorities, and the periodic reporting of all newly available data on adverse events with a scientific evaluation of a potential causal relationship (later known as periodic safety update reports or PSURs) [55–57]. Later, in 2004, the names EMEA and CPMP were changed to EMA and Committee for Medicinal Products for Human Use (CHMP) [62].

2.5 The Drug Regulatory Response to the HIV/AIDS Epidemic

In response to fierce activism for increased availability of and access to drugs to treat HIV/AIDS, the Accelerated Approval pathway for marketing authorisation was introduced in the US in the early 1990s. Together with other regulatory pathways, it enabled the FDA to accept pre-authorisation evidence from fewer trials or based on surrogate rather than clinical endpoints. The benefit–risk balance should then be confirmed by additional evidence from post-authorisation studies. These pathways were aimed at drugs for life-threatening diseases, including HIV/AIDS, and explicitly considered severity of disease and availability of alternative treatments in the benefit–risk assessments [63]. In Europe, a similar regulatory pathway had been available since 1975, for which it was possible to request post-

Table 6.2 Selection of drugs withdrawn for safety reasons

Year	Active substance	Type of drug	Type of adverse events
2004	Rofecoxib	Analgesic	Cardiovascular
2008	Lumiracoxib	Analgesic	Hepatic
2009	Rimonabant	Anorectic	Psychiatric
2010	Benfluorex	Anorectic	Cardiac
2010	Rosiglitazone	Antidiabetic	Cardiac
2010	Sibutramine	Anorectic	Cardiovascular
2010	Sitaxentan	Antihypertensive	Hepatic
2012	Buflomedil	Vasodilator	Cardiac, neurological
2012	Meprobamate	Sedative	Neurological, psychiatric
2013	Nicotinic acid/laropiprant	Hypolipidaemic	Bleeding, myopathy, infections, diabetes
2016	Fusafungine	Antibiotic	Allergic
2017	Gadodiamide, gadopentetic acid, gadoversetamide	Gadolinium contrast agents	Brain deposition
2018	Flupirtine	Analgesic	Hepatic
2018	Daclizumab beta	Immunosuppressant	Immune-related
2019	Cinoxacin, flumequine, nalidixic acid, pipemidic acid	Antibiotics	Involving tendons, muscles, or joints; neurological; psychiatric
2020	Ingenol mebutate	Chemotherapeutic (topical)	Skin cancer

Selected from European Medicines Agency [66–69], Lane et al. [70], McNaughton et al. [71], Onakpoya et al. [72], World Health Organization [73]

authorisation studies as of the early 1990s: the Authorisation under Exceptional Circumstances [46]. This pathway too was used to authorise several drugs to treat HIV/AIDS.

2.6 Global Harmonisation

Many of the early EEC evidence requirements contributed to worldwide evidentiary standards through the International Conference on Harmonisation of Technical Requirements for Registration of Pharmaceuticals for Human Use (ICH). By 1990, the ICH formed an international platform for regulatory authorities and the pharmaceutical industries of Europe, Japan, and the US to formulate guidelines and technical requirements [64]. Further international collaboration between regulatory authorities was effectuated when the International Coalition of Medicines Regulatory Authorities (ICMRA) was established in 2012, an informal group of leaders of global regulatory authorities [65].

2.7 Safety Withdrawals

Despite efforts throughout the more recent history of drug regulation, safety issues have continued to occur, some of which required complete withdrawal from the market (Table 6.2). Therefore, more proactive pharmacovigilance has gradually been developed [74], which is discussed in Sect. 3.

3 Current Principles of Pharmacovigilance and Related Aspects in Drug Regulatory Decision-Making

This section discusses in detail the principles and important aspects of contemporary pharmacovigilance as well as related aspects in drug regulatory decision-making. As highlighted before, these aspects are the result of international developments over decades. Therefore, before diving into these principles and aspects one by one, first the most important developments concerning pharmacovigilance in the twenty-first century are reviewed.

3.1 Pharmacovigilance in the Twenty-First Century

Leading up to the twenty-first century, specifically in the EU, more and more pharmacovigilance procedures were introduced. Important milestones were the establishment of the Pharmacovigilance Working Party (PhVWP) in 1989 [61], which was instigated to support the CPMP—later CHMP—on post-authorisation safety issues. In 1993, the reporting of adverse events was harmonised, including the requirement for a PSUR (see Table 6.1), and in 2001, the EudraVigilance database of suspected adverse reactions became operational [75].

In 2005, the EU Risk Management Plan (RMP) became mandatory for drugs containing a new active substance and regulators could require a PASS as a condition to the marketing authorisation [62, 76, 77]. When the current EU pharmacovigilance legislation came into force in 2012, pharmacovigilance was strengthened with a central role for the EMA's new Pharmacovigilance Risk Assessment Committee (PRAC) that replaced the PhVWP to advise the CHMP on all matters of pharmacovigilance and risk management [78].

Further strengthening of pharmacovigilance was achieved by expanding existing requirements, introducing new ones, establishing new procedures, and developing new pharmacovigilance tools. Requirements for reporting of suspected adverse reactions to EudraVigilance were extended to include all suspected adverse reactions that occur within the EEA and serious adverse reactions outside it. The definition of an adverse reaction was expanded to also include medication errors and effects of off-label use. The submission of an RMP became mandatory for all drugs, the content and focus of the PSUR was revised, and PSURs of drugs authorised in more than one EU member state were now all assessed at the European level through a PSUR single assessment procedure (PSUSA) with a binding outcome for all drugs with the same active substance. For signal detection, a central role was given to EudraVigilance and the PRAC for prioritisation and assessment of signals, leading to a recommendation that is applicable to all affected drugs authorised in the EU [78–80]. The EU pharmaceutical legislation was accompanied with a set of guidelines on Good Pharmacovigilance Practice (GVP) that describe structures and processes of all pharmacovigilance tools and procedures, but also how the EU network operates [81].

3.2 Pharmacovigilance Throughout the Drug Lifecycle

While the decision to allow a new drug to be marketed in short is the answer to the question as to whether there is evidence to demonstrate that the drug's benefits outweigh the anticipated risks, the evaluation of the drug does not end once marketing is granted. The drug's benefit–risk balance continues to be monitored throughout the entire lifecycle of the product. This is needed since at the time of initial authorisation, the knowledge about benefits and risks is usually based on results from clinical trials, as well as data from animal studies. As the clinical trials are relatively short and include relatively few subjects compared to the number of patients that will be exposed to the product once it is placed on the market, these studies are unable to provide information on the occurrence of delayed and uncommon or rare adverse reactions. Moreover, subjects in clinical trials tend to be selected from a more homogeneous and healthier population with fewer comorbidities and less complex disease than the patients that will be exposed in the post-marketing setting and information on relevant subpopulations such as children, elderly, or pregnant women may be lacking at the time of authorisation.

The monitoring of the benefit–risk balance throughout the lifecycle of a drug is mostly focused on safety, i.e. pharmacovigilance, although for some newly authorised drugs, regulators require further confirmation or demonstration of the product's efficacy (see Sects. 3.7 and 3.8 below). Pharmacovigilance aims at preventing harm from adverse reactions in humans arising from the use of authorised medicinal products and promoting the safe and effective use of medicinal products, in particular through providing timely information about the safety of medicinal products to patients, healthcare professionals, and the public [82]. In practice, pharmacovigilance is operationalised with a range of activities such as signal detection, periodic safety reporting, and risk management planning.

3.3 Risk Management Planning

The concept of the EU RMP was devised in 2005 [62, 76, 77]. Since then, both the requirements to the content of the RMP and the situations in which an RMP is required have been revised several times. The RMP enables regulators to proactively monitor and address safety issues throughout the drug's lifecycle by identifying, characterising, and minimising drug's important risks. To achieve this goal, the RMP consists of three main elements. The first part is called the "safety specification" and describes the drug's important identified risks, important potential risks, and missing information. The second part, the "pharmacovigilance plan", describes the pharmacovigilance activities that are needed to further characterise the risks and missing information in the safety specification. For important adverse events for which a causal relationship with the drug has been established, the characterisation would comprise a better understanding of risk factors, severity, or frequency of the adverse reaction, while for the important potential risks this would constitute confirming or refuting of the relations between the adverse events and the drug. The last main part of the RMP provides details of the "risk minimisation measures" that will be taken to reduce the risks associated with respective safety concerns. These measures comprise routine risk minimisation measures, such as the product information, and additional risk minimisation measures, such as educational tools for healthcare professionals and patients, Direct Healthcare Professional Communications (DHPC) or "Dear Doctor" letters, and pregnancy prevention programmes [83]. See the case study on valproate (Case study 1) for some examples.

Internationally, ICH released its Pharmacovigilance Planning E2E Guideline in 2004 [84] and provided a basis for the EU RMP. The ICH E2E Guideline defined two parts of the RMP: the safety specification and the pharmacovigilance plan (not the risk minimisation measures). With this ICH Guideline, the concept of an RMP has also been adopted in other regions worldwide, under different names such as the Risk Evaluation and Mitigation Strategy (REMS) in the US. This REMS also includes specific plans to mitigate known risks, but not the pharmacovigilance activities as in the EU RMP [85]. The Canadian RMP essentially requires the same elements as the EU RMP [86], and the Australian regulator Therapeutic Goods Administration (TGA) requires an EU RMP with an Australia-specific annex [87].

3.4 Pharmacovigilance Activities

For regulatory purposes, pharmacovigilance activities can be divided into routine pharmacovigilance activities and additional pharmacovigilance activities. Routine pharmacovigilance activities are those that are required by the European law for all authorised drugs, and these activities are independent from the safety profile of the drug and any safety concerns in the RMP. Routine pharmacovigilance activities comprise the collection, management, and submission of reports of suspected adverse reactions to the drug; signal detection, analysis, and management; and preparation and submission of PSURs. In contrast, additional pharmacovigilance activities are tailored to specific drugs and their safety concerns and comprise non-clinical studies, clinical trials, or observational studies [83].

Although the analysis of reports of suspected adverse reactions is probably the oldest pharmacovigilance activity, it is still one of the cornerstones of today's pharmacovigilance activities. Even with sophisticated statistical tools for signal detection in large databases being available and well-designed observational studies being performed, the analysis of individual case safety reports (ICSRs) remains an important tool for rapid identification of new safety signals. A relevant example in this regard is the identification of the signal of Thrombosis with Thrombocytopenia Syndrome or Vaccine-induced Immune Thrombotic Thrombocytopenia associated with the coronavirus disease 2019 (COVID-19) adenovector vaccines, which originated from five patients who presented with venous thrombosis and thrombocytopenia 7–10 days after receiving the first dose of the ChAdOx1 nCoV-19 adenoviral vector vaccine against COVID-19 [88].

Apart from the collection and analysis of ICSRs by drug companies and signal detection in their own database, the submission by both drug companies and regulators of all ICSRs to the EudraVigilance database allows for signal detection by the European regulators in a database containing over 25.3 million ICSRs, corresponding to 14.8 million unique suspected ADR case reports, by the end of 2022 [89]. Signal detection in EudraVigilance includes review of ICSRs, statistical analyses, or a combination of both. For signal detection with statistical tools, measures of disproportionality are used and various disproportionality measures are available, such as the Reporting Odds Ratio (ROR), Proportional Reporting Ratio (PRR), the Information Component, or the Empirical Bayes Geometric Mean [90]. For signal detection in the EudraVigilance database, both the ROR and PRR are used, and a signal of disproportionate reporting is then defined with the lower bound of the 95% confidence interval of the ROR greater than one together with a minimum number of cases.

3.5 Periodic Safety Updates

A further routine pharmacovigilance activity is the preparation and submission of PSURs, which are also referred to as periodic benefit–risk evaluation report (PBRER) [91]. The requirement for pharmaceutical companies to submit PSURs in the EU dates back to 1995 [57]. At that time, the focus of the PSUR was to evaluate whether relevant new safety information had emerged that would impact the "reference safety information". Usually, this is the Company Core Safety Information and ultimately the authorised product's product information (the SmPC in the EU). However, with the new EU pharmacovigilance legislation that came into force in 2012 [78–80] and the revision of the ICH Guideline in 2012 [91], the focus shifted from new safety information impacting the product information to new or changed risks that would impact the drug's benefit–risk balance. This also included new evidence that might impact the effectiveness (benefit) of a drug. Other important changes were that the new safety data collected during the period covered by the PSUR should be evaluated in the context of the cumulative data available, and that PSURs for drugs that contained the same active substance were now assessed together, in the PSUSA procedure. Both changes helped to avoid that a bigger picture would be missed due to only pieces of information being considered every time a PSUR was submitted and assessed. The format and content of the current PBRER is described in ICH Guideline E2C (R2) [91], and the PSUR requested by European authorities follows the PBRER format with an EU-specific annex.

Before 2012, the periodicity of submission of a PSUR to European regulatory authorities used to follow standard intervals with a maximum of a three-yearly or five-yearly interval [62, 92]. Since 2012, the submission of PSURs is governed by the so-called EU reference date (EURD) list, and the listed PSUR submission intervals are based on the risk profile of the active substance or combination of active substances contained in the drug [80]. With this, submission intervals range from every 6 months to 28 years although even longer cycles would be possible. While the EURD list is maintained by the EU regulators, regulators in some other regions accept PSUR submissions according to the European cycles.

While the aim of the PSUR may have changed from new safety information and its impact on the product information to a benefit–risk assessment at defined points in time, the impact of new information on the benefit–risk balance continues to translate into an amendment of the product information in 15–20% of the PSUR assessment procedures done at the EU level [89]. These amendments of the product information can vary from addition of a newly recognised ADR to the inclusion of new warnings or recommendations that provide new safeguards to avoid an ADR, decrease its severity, or increase earlier recognition and thereby prevent progression to more serious ADRs. Also, safety data from PSURs can necessitate restricting the use of a drug in certain patients to protect them from harm and in such cases new contraindications may be introduced or the drug's indication for use is restricted. Ultimately, if no measures can be envisaged that would adequately protect patients in clinical practice, the drug should be removed from the market. Although such decision can be a result of the evaluation of PSUR data, in the EU, this is normally taken forward in another type of regulatory procedure, the so-called pharmacovigilance referral, to allow an in-depth evaluation of both data on benefits and on risks, with input from clinical experts and patients as appropriate.

3.6 Post-authorisation Safety Studies

While routine pharmacovigilance activities are applicable to all authorised drugs and are independent from the safety profile of the drug, additional pharmacovigilance activities are tailored to specific drugs and their safety concerns. Additional pharmacovigilance activities can be non-clinical studies, clinical trials, or observational studies. In Europe, such studies are referred to as PASS. Outside Europe, similar studies are requested by regulators or proposed by drug companies, with different terminology used such as post-market studies or post-marketing surveillance studies.

Although the prime purpose of all PASS is to investigate the safety of a drug that received authorisation to be placed on the market, they vary with regard to their precise aim and methodology. Most PASS are performed to contribute to the understanding of the safety profile of a drug. This can be the identification of new ADRs, since the pre-authorisation studies are typically performed in a relatively small, homogeneous and non-complex group of patients, and for a shorter duration than how the drug is used in clinical practice. This limits the identification of infrequent ADRs or adverse events that take longer to develop or require cumulative exposure to occur. Examples of those PASS are studies that investigate the long-term safety effects of advanced therapy medicinal products (ATMPs), such as gene therapy, somatic-cell therapy, and tissue-engineered drugs [93]. Further, PASS may also be designed to characterise or quantify a specific safety concern or ADR, in terms of severity, risk factors or risk population, and frequency of occurrence. Apart from a limited number of patients exposed to the drug pre-authorisation for a limited duration, such PASS may also be needed as patients with certain comorbidities, worse health status, or other conditions are excluded from pre-authorisation studies. Registries in which pregnant women exposed to the drug are studied or studies in patients with hepatic or renal impairment are examples of such PASS.

A completely different type of PASS are those which are performed to evaluate the effectiveness of risk minimisation measures. Such studies are not intended to provide new insights into the safety profile of a drug but should be able to show whether the measures that are supposed to mitigate the risks of a drug achieve that objective when the drug is used in clinical practice.

While PASS can comprise non-clinical studies, clinical trials, or observational studies, most PASS are observational studies. Data sources for these observational PASS are often existing databases, such as electronic health record databases, insurance or claims databases, or disease or pregnancy registries. These databases may be linked to extend their population coverage or to be able to link the drug of interest, patient characteristics, and outcomes when these data are not collectively present in one database or registry. PASS that are clinical trials are mainly studies designed to investigate the efficacy of a drug but also provide relevant safety information. Notably, not all post-authorisation studies for a drug are considered a PASS since they should be able to meet the aim of PASS as defined in the RMP. In view of the limitations of pre-authorisation studies referred to above, few post-authorisation clinical trials can be considered to add significantly to the knowledge from registrational studies and allow further characterisation of safety concerns. Continuing pivotal clinical trials that are not completed at the time of authorisation of the drug and studies in relevant subpopulations could be PASS, if they are adequate in size, duration, and ability to capture the safety outcome(s) which require further investigation. Non-clinical studies are rarely included as PASS in the RMP since human data is normally preferred. Yet, in specific situations where a mechanism of harm is unclear, but clinical consequences could be significant on theoretical grounds, non-clinical studies may be appropriate PASS as a first step in better understanding the safety concern in question.

3.7 Post-authorisation Efficacy Studies

While pharmacovigilance focuses on adverse reactions and their characterisation and mitigation, the safety profile of a drug is considered in the context of its efficacy. This allows for monitoring of the drug's benefit–risk balance throughout its entire lifecycle. In the same way as important gaps in knowledge of the safety profile may be closed by additional pharmacovigilance activities such as PASS, PAES can be needed to close important gaps in knowledge on the benefits of a drug or to confirm case findings from a single pivotal study. In the EU, imposed PAES, i.e. those that are required by regulators and imposed as a condition of the marketing authorisation, became part of the RMP with the European pharmacovigilance legislation (2012) [78–80]. In 2014, in addition to existing requirements for PAES for specific drugs—such as those granted a Conditional Marketing Authorisation (see Sect. 3.8 below), an Authorisation under Exceptional Circumstances (see Sect. 2.5 above), or ATMPs—other situations that may require a PAES were specified. These situations included investigating clinical outcomes to substantiate already demonstrated efficacy on surrogate endpoints, specific combinations with other drugs, specific subpopulations, long-term efficacy or if the benefit–risk balance is questioned (i.e. real-life use of the drug shows that its efficacy might be significantly worse than previously evaluated) [94].

The design of a PAES will be tailored to a specific drug and the question regarding its efficacy that needs to be answered. To provide reliable estimates of efficacy, randomised studies are the preferred design for PAES such that confounding or bias due to non-comparability between groups is prevented. In certain situations, however, a non-randomised PAES could be an acceptable alternative to a randomised study, for example when randomisation is unethical or unfeasible, or when outcomes are rare or highly predictable. These non-randomised studies then need to be complemented with concurrent comparative data or, if not available, with historical comparative data, to allow for a meaningful interpretation of study results (see Sect. 4.3 below). The role of observational studies in evaluating drug effectiveness is further discussed in Sect. 4 below.

3.8 Expedited Regulatory Pathways

A specific case in which PAES and PASS may be required are the expedited regulatory pathways. Worldwide, several such regulatory pathways for marketing authorisation exist that aim to make promising drugs available to patients earlier. Well-known examples are the EU Conditional Marketing Authorisation and the US Accelerated Approval (see Sect. 2.5 above). Often, earlier authorisation is achieved by accepting less comprehensive clinical data than for standard marketing authorisation, such as a low number of patients studied in the pivotal trial(s), a short duration of follow-up of these patients, the lack of a control to obtain comparative safety and efficacy estimates, or the use of surrogate rather than clinical endpoints [95–97]. An important prerequisite of these regulatory pathways is that comprehensive data are provided post-authorisation, often through additional studies such as PAES and PASS. When these data are ultimately submitted, considered comprehensive and confirm the benefit–risk balance, a standard marketing authorisation can be granted that is not necessarily subject to additional requirements. While PAES and PASS must not be used as a justification for premature granting of marketing authorisation or to compensate for the absence of data on safety or efficacy that are required to demonstrate a positive benefit–risk balance at the time of authorisation, for drugs seeking authorisation via expedited pathways, the results of a PAES or PASS may be more critical.

4 Advanced Pharmacoepidemiological Approaches for Studying Safety and Effectiveness for Drug Regulatory Decision-Making

This section discusses several recent advances in pharmacoepidemiological methods that leverage observational or "real-world" data to generate evidence about drug safety and effectiveness for regulatory decision-making. A detailed discussion on three common observational study designs and the concepts of bias and confounding is presented in Chap. 9.

4.1 Signal Detection

As described earlier in this chapter and elsewhere in this book, spontaneous reporting systems are the cornerstone of post-authorisation drug safety surveillance for signal detection (hypothesis generation). Traditionally, routine electronic health records data and claims data have been used as data sources to enable confirmation and quantification of drug safety signals (hypothesis testing). However, during the past decade, these data sources have been explored as an independent source to improve and refine signal detection. A systematic investigation of the complementarity of spontaneous reporting systems and electronic health record databases for signal detection was conducted by the EU-ADR consortium [98]. This investigation focused on five selected adverse events deemed to be important in pharmacovigilance (bullous eruption, acute myocardial infarction, acute pancreatitis, hip fracture, and upper gastrointestinal bleeding). EudraVigilance identified more signals overall than the EU-ADR databases (41% of signals compared with 32% of signals). Potential explanations for this difference included the worldwide coverage of EudraVigilance compared to the three countries represented in the EU-ADR databases and the fact that EudraVigilance was specifically designed for signal detection. Importantly, whether signals were detected also depended on the nature of the event: acute myocardial infarction and hip fracture were less likely to be detected by EudraVigilance compared to the EU-ADR databases, probably because these events are usually not recognised and reported as ADRs.

Adverse events that are more difficult to attribute to drugs are mostly multifactorial, long-term (delayed) effects, and those with a high background incidence as was confirmed in large drug safety monitoring projects such as the Pharmacoepidemiological Research on Outcomes of Therapeutics by a European ConsorTium (PROTECT) [99], Observational Health Data Sciences and Informatics [100], and the Sentinel Initiative [101]. Electronic health records databases may have added value to detect these adverse events as was demonstrated recently by Kristensen et al. using the Danish National Health registries for screening of the most common cancers in a case–control approach. From a total of 13,577 drug-cancer associations, 274 were associated with high use and a cumulative dose–response pattern. Of these, 65 were classified as not attributable to bias, with 20 established as carcinogens by the International Agency for Research on Cancer. The remaining 45 would require further study to confirm the association [102]. Using multiple data sources may lead to improved signal detection, but development of this approach requires a deeper understanding of the data sources used, additional benchmarks, and further research on methods to generate and synthesise signals [103].

4.2 Multi-database Studies, Common Protocols, and Common Data Models

Traditionally, observational studies have utilised single data sources to assess safety and effectiveness of drugs. During the past decade, it became clear that analysing multiple data sources in parallel offers several advantages such as increased sample size to detect rare adverse events, subgroup effects, and early post-authorisation assessment of safety and effectiveness of drugs during a relatively short time window [104]. Furthermore, the application of a common (study) protocol, with or without a common data model, allows the generation of more consistent results and exploration of sources of heterogeneity of findings across data sources, as further explained below.

Multi-database studies have evolved substantially over the past decade. Initial approaches comprised of implementing a common protocol with details on study design, data specifications, and statistical analyses in parallel and locally in participating data sources [105]. The common protocol approach was used for instance in a multi-database study funded by the EMA to characterise the risk of bleeding associated with direct oral anticoagulants. In this study, four European databases implemented a common protocol and estimates of relative risk of bleeding were pooled across sites. As an extension of this study, the common protocol was also implemented in the Canadian Network for Observational Drug Effect Studies (CNODES) [106] in a collaboration between the EMA and Health Canada. The results of these studies have been used by the EMA's scientific committees PRAC and CHMP to inform healthcare professionals and patients in Europe about the use of direct-acting oral anticoagulants. Their conclusion was that the use of these agents was safe and effective according to current instructions for use. A higher risk of bleeding in patients over 75 years of age prompted the EMA to advise manufacturers to investigate whether a possible change in dosing advice might be beneficial in patients over 75 years of age [107].

Subsequent approaches to multi-database studies developed distributed data networks that used common data models that generally include a set of standardised data files and variables, adopted by all data partners participating within the distributed data network. These also included centrally developed analytical programmes that are distributed to the data partners who then share aggregated results for further meta-analytic pooling of effect estimates [108]. An example of a common protocol—common data model approach was a large investigation on the risk of myocarditis associated with COVID-19 vaccination. The study was funded by the EMA and conducted by the EU PE&PV (Pharmacoepidemiology and Pharmacovigilance) Research Network in collaboration with VAC4EU (Vaccine monitoring Collaboration for Europe). The study used the Conception Common Data Model and used data from five European databases. An increased risk of myocarditis was found, especially when using the Pfizer and Moderna vaccines, and specifically in people younger than 30 years of age who were relatively more often men. These findings have been used by the EMA to educate healthcare workers and the public about the safety of these vaccines [109].

Several regulatory agencies have formalised the distributed data network approach as a tool for drug safety and effectiveness monitoring, including the FDA with the Sentinel Initiative [101], Health Canada with CNODES [106], and most recently the EMA with the Data Analysis and Real World Interrogation Network (DARWIN EU) [110]. Sentinel has delivered more than 400 specific drug safety and exploratory analyses [111]. A recent example of a drug safety analysis investigated the risk of angioedema following sacubitril/valsartan in patients with heart failure using a new-user design matched and stratified on propensity score [112]. CNODES has completed 56 studies so far [113]. A recent drug safety analysis in CNODES evaluated the risk of severe urinary tract infection associated with the use of sodium-glucose transport protein 2 (SGLT2) inhibitors compared to the use of dipeptidyl peptidase-4 (DPP-4) inhibitors. The conclusion was reassuring given the finding of a reduced risk of urinary tract infection for SGLT-2 inhibitors compared to DPP-4 inhibitors [114]. DARWIN EU has recently been launched and the first study results are being generated [115].

4.3 External Control Groups

Another important development for the monitoring of drug safety and efficacy/effectiveness is the use of external control groups (or "external comparators") to contextualise results from long-term uncontrolled extensions of clinical trials and single-arm trials. The authorisation of drugs for rare diseases and novel cancer drugs is often based on single-arm trials [116] because of, for example, ethical restrictions to use a placebo or active comparator arm from the same source population and/or sample size limitations due to a small available population. In such situations, the use of an external control group may become necessary to assess safety or efficacy/effectiveness by providing background rates for outcomes that can be compared with those in the single-arm trial. In contrast to an internal control group that is drawn from the same population, an external control group should be a group of patients that is external to the study, of similar disease severity (at equipoise) but that receives a different treatment [117]. The external control group can consist of patients treated at an earlier time (historical control), or patients treated contemporaneously but in another setting. An important limitation of using an external control group is the lack of randomisation, and therefore the risk of selection and confounding bias [118]. Therefore, the external control group should closely resemble the inclusion and exclusion criteria, and the treatment and healthcare patterns of patients in the single-arm trial to prevent selection bias. When using observational data sources to select external control group patients, it should be considered that not all clinical information that is recorded in the single-arm trial may be recorded in the routine clinical practice that generated the observational data. Furthermore, after selection of an external control group, the distribution of characteristics (especially risk factors for the outcomes of interest) may still be different from the single-arm trial patient population and result in confounding. Traditional epidemiological methods can be applied such as matching (either on key confounding factors or propensity scores), or analytical adjustment such as multivariable regression to control for confounding [119].

4.4 Target Trial Emulation

Finally, an important development during the past decade was the creation of the target trial emulation approach as a framework for causal inference to study drug safety and effectiveness. In the target trial emulation approach, first, the causal question needs to be formulated in a protocol of a hypothetical randomised trial that could provide the answer but for some reason is not feasible. Key components of the causal "estimand" need to be defined (eligibility criteria, treatment strategies, treatment assignment (time zero), the start and end of follow-up, outcomes, causal contrasts) and the statistical analysis plan including approaches to adjust for confounders to emulate random assignment of treatment [120]. The components of the protocol are then explicitly emulated using observational data, for example, from routine clinical practice. In some situations, for instance when there is a lag time before treatment initiation, immortal time bias can be accounted for by "cloning" of patients. This way, patients can be allocated to both arms of the trial that is being emulated, after which further analytical procedures can allow unbiased estimation of the treatment effects [121, 122]. The main advantage of the target trial emulation framework is its transparency and explicit definitions in the different design and analysis elements of drug safety and effectiveness studies, while preventing common sources of bias. Confounding bias remains an issue that still needs to be resolved in non-randomised studies and requires high quality and complete data on confounding factors. Notably, since blinding of outcomes and treatment assignment are not possible for observational data, the target trial that is emulated should be considered a pragmatic study, that is, a study that compares treatment strategies as they are applied in clinical practice [120].

5 Summary and Conclusions

In conclusion, this chapter covered the series of historical events such as drug safety crises that led to the current drug regulatory systems; European and global drug regulatory harmonisation; the current principles of pharmacovigilance and drug regulation and advanced pharmacoepidemiological approaches that contribute to pharmacovigilance and drug regulation, such as new approaches to signal detection, the use of multi-database observational studies, the use of external control groups, and the target trial emulation approach. Looking ahead, important developments can be expected. First, the entire general pharmaceutical legislation of the EU will be revised based on a proposal that was released by the EC in April 2023. The Commission's proposal aims to achieve (1) timely and equitable access to safe, effective, and affordable drugs; (2) an attractive and innovation-friendly environment for research, development, and production of drugs in Europe; (3) reduced administrative burden by speeding up procedures, thereby reducing authorisation times; (4) enhanced availability and security of supply; (5) reduced antimicrobial resistance and the presence of pharmaceuticals in the environment; and (6) more environmentally sustainable drugs [123, 124]. Although these proposals are not expected to change the principles of pharmacovigilance and drug regulation discussed in this chapter, nor how pharmacovigilance is currently being performed as laid down in the GVP guidelines, they may change some of the regulatory procedures that are in place to assess the benefit–risk balance of drugs throughout their lifecycle. Moreover, given the breadth of these legislative proposals and their expected impact on the EU's clinical practice, society, and pharmaceutical market, they will likely also have a global impact on drug development and regulation. Second, even more international collaboration can be expected, both among drug regulators worldwide to facilitate consistent regulatory decision-making based on the same evidence but also with other stakeholders such as health technology assessment organisations that provide recommendations about reimbursement of drugs and with healthcare providers. Eventually, although all these stakeholders have a different role to play in the drug lifecycle, they share the same aim: enabling safe and effective treatments for patients. Increased mutual understanding and, where possible, alignment of the evidence required for each other's decision-making process should facilitate faster patient access to innovative drugs. Third, observational or real-world data will potentially play a greater role in providing evidence of a drug's quality, safety, and effectiveness, while artificial intelligence may make its introduction in supporting pharmacovigilance, for example, in signal detection.

6 Case Studies

6.1 Case Study 1: Valproate

Valproate and its related substances such as valproic acid and valpromide were first authorised in France in 1967 although valproic acid had been used as a solvent already for years.

1. *For which three indications has valproate since been authorised?*

   For treatment of epilepsy and bipolar disorders, and in some countries for prophylaxis of migraine attacks. See for example [125].

After years of use, important ADRs of valproate were discovered that substantially changed how it has been used since.

2. *What ADRs does this refer to?*

   Congenital malformations such as spina bifida and neurodevelopmental disorders such as reduced verbal intelligence quotient (IQ) in children with prenatal exposure to valproate because their mother used valproate during pregnancy. See for example [126].

3. *How often did the EMA advise major regulatory actions to address these ADRs and what were those actions?*

   Major regulatory actions that were incrementally restrictive to the use of valproate during pregnancy were undertaken three times: in 2010, 2014, and 2018.

   (a) In 2009, the Dutch Medicines Evaluation Board requested the CHMP to review the safety and effectiveness of valproate in the treatment of manic episodes of bipolar disorder, the so-called Article 31 referral. In 2010, the CHMP concluded that use of valproate in the treatment of manic episodes should be limited to situations where lithium is contraindicated or not tolerated, and that it should not be used to prevent recurrence of either manic or depressive episodes. Moreover, the CHMP concluded that the use of valproate during pregnancy was associated with a teratogenic risk, including the potential for delayed intellectual development. Therefore, the product information was updated to note that valproate [...] "should not be used during pregnancy and in women of child-bearing potential unless clearly necessary (i.e. in situations where other treatments are ineffective or not tolerated). Women of child-bearing potential have to use effective contraception during treatment". See Ref. [127]. The EC issued a decision in line with the CHMP's conclusions.

   (b) In 2013, the MHRA requested the PRAC to review the safety of valproate, specifically about the risks associated with use in pregnant women and "women of childbearing potential", through an Article 31 referral. In 2014, the PRAC confirmed the risks of congenital malformations and neurodevelopmental disorders and recommended among others that:

   - Valproate "should not be used in female children, women of childbearing potential and pregnant women unless alternative treatments are ineffective or not tolerated" in the existing epilepsy and bipolar disorder indications.
   - Valproate should be contraindicated in the existing migraine indications in case of pregnancy and in "women of childbearing potential who are not using effective methods of contraception".
   - To inform women and healthcare professionals, the product information should be updated with further warnings and precautions, and additional risk minimisation measures such as educational materials and a DHPC were needed.
   - A drug utilisation study was needed to assess the effectiveness of the risk minimisation measures.

   See Ref. [128]. The PRAC's recommendations were endorsed by the Coordination Group for Mutual Recognition and Decentralised Procedures—Human (CMDh) that represents EU member states as overarching regulatory body for marketing authorisations not granted by the EC.

   (c) In 2017, France requested the PRAC to assess the impact of the previously instated risk minimisation measures through an Article 31 referral after French studies suggested that the 2014 measures were not adhered to. In 2018, the PRAC concluded that the risk minimisation measures had not been sufficiently effective to prevent prenatal exposure of children to valproate and recommended among others that:

   - The risk minimisation measures should be strengthened through contraindications for all three indications in women of childbearing potential unless the so-called pregnancy prevention programme was complied with. This included that the patient's potential to become pregnant should be assessed, pregnancy tests should be performed, counselling about the risks and need for contraception should take place and periodic review of treatment should be performed, including the use of a risk acknowledgement form.

- For the treatment of epilepsy, switching to alternative treatments may in some instances not be possible. Therefore, "Every effort should be made to switch to appropriate alternative treatment prior to conception, and before contraception is discontinued. If switching is not possible, the woman should receive further counselling regarding the valproate risks for the unborn child to support her informed decision-making regarding family planning".
- For the treatment of epilepsy, use of valproate during pregnancy is contraindicated unless there is no suitable alternative treatment.
- For the treatment of bipolar disorders and prophylaxis of migraine, use of valproate during pregnancy is contraindicated.
- Educational materials should be updated, among others with a patient card, and a visual reminder of the risks should be added to the outer packaging.
- PASS to assess the effectiveness of the risk minimisation measures should be performed.
- PASS to assess the risks after paternal exposure and the risks to third-generation offspring should be performed.

See Ref. [129]. The PRAC's recommendations were endorsed by the CMDh.

4. *What was the regulatory goal of these actions?*

To prevent that unborn children are exposed to valproate during pregnancy and to better inform women of childbearing potential of the risks of valproate use during pregnancy. Ultimately to ensure that the benefit–risk balance of the use of valproate in the authorised indications remains positive.

5. *What was the impact of PASS?*

The results of multiple PASS are awaited—see also the answer to question 6—and independent scientific studies also continue to be performed and provide insights into the risks associated with valproate treatment. Recently, the impact of the 2018 risk minimisation measures and the revised pregnancy prevention programme on the utilisation and prescribing trends of valproate was studied [130]. There was a small impact of the 2018 measures on valproate use in the studied European countries and regions. The substantial number of concurrent pregnancies with valproate exposure warranted a careful monitoring of implementation of the existing pregnancy prevention programme for valproate in clinical practice in Europe, to see if there is any need for additional measures in the future.

6. *Is more regulatory action needed in the future?*

That cannot be predicted. At the time of writing in October 2023, the PRAC is assessing the final study report for a retrospective observational study to investigate the association between paternal exposure to valproate and the risk of congenital anomalies and neurodevelopmental disorders including autism in offspring. "Initial results of the study may indicate an increased risk of neurodevelopmental disorders in children born to men taking valproate in the 3 months before conception. However, the PRAC has identified important limitations with the data from the study" [131]. Furthermore, in late 2022, the MHRA advised that newly initiated use of valproate should be restricted to patients aged 55 years and older. See Ref. [132].

6.2 Case Study 2: COVID-19 Vaccines

In December 2019, the SARS-CoV-2 virus started the COVID-19 pandemic. Thanks to the development and authorisation of vaccines against COVID-19, many deaths worldwide have been prevented and the course of the pandemic was positively affected [133].

1. *When were the first COVID-19 vaccines authorised?*

   The first COVID-19 vaccines were authorised worldwide in December 2020.

2. *What type of authorisations were initially granted by the EC, FDA, and MHRA?*

   The EC granted a Conditional Marketing Authorisation. The FDA granted an "emergency use authorisation", and the MHRA a batch-specific "temporary authorisation for supply". These latter two are not formal marketing authorisations and can be retracted any time. See for example [134].

3. *What were three important common regulatory elements that sped up the authorisation of COVID-19 vaccines?*

   First, many regulatory authorities performed a so-called rolling review process, in which they continuously assessed available data instead of waiting until the entire data package was available. See for example [135]. Second, regulatory authorities worldwide collaborated intensively, among others through ICMRA, to enable harmonisation of data requirements. Third, initial non-clinical and clinical evidence of safety and efficacy was used to assess whether the benefit–risk balance was positive, while pharmaceutical companies were required to submit data from additional studies post-authorisation. See for example [136, 137], and the explanation of the EU Conditional Marketing Authorisation in Sect. 3.8.

4. *How did regulators prepare for post-authorisation monitoring of the COVID-19 mRNA vaccines?*

   In response to the COVID-19 pandemic, the EMA started with preparing for intensified safety monitoring of COVID-19 vaccines. The EMA and national regulators developed core RMP requirements for COVID-19 vaccines, which included specific guidance on the post-authorisation monitoring of COVID-19 mRNA vaccines. This guidance addressed, among others, signal detection and adverse events of special interest (AESI) to be monitored, the need for observed versus expected (O/E) analyses, summary safety reports (SSRs) to be submitted in addition to regular PSUR reporting and safety surveillance from ongoing clinical trials and in dedicated PASS [138]. The safety monitoring carried out by the EU network throughout the pandemic included near real-time monitoring of AESI. Real-world evidence from observational studies completed the intensified safety monitoring to further characterise emerging safety issues. The EMA contracted in total 11 COVID-19 research projects, one of which was the ACCESS (vACcine Covid-19 monitoring readinESS) project. The ACCESS project provided background rates of AESIs which allowed the analysis of O/E analyses. Furthermore, template protocols were developed for different types of research questions and real-world data sources [139, 140].

5. *What is the current regulatory status of the COVID-19 mRNA vaccines?*

   Full marketing authorisations have been granted for these vaccines throughout 2021 and 2022 when data from additional studies was available.

References

1. World Health Organization. Regulation and Prequalification - Pharmacovigilance. n.d. https://www.who.int/teams/regulation-prequalification/regulation-and-safety/pharmacovigilance. Retrieved 8 Feb 2024.
2. World Health Organization. The importance of pharmacovigilance. 2002.

3. Drews J. Drug discovery: a historical perspective. Science. 2000;287(5460):1960–4. https://doi.org/10.1126/science.287.5460.1960.
4. Dykstra DL. The medical profession and patent and proprietary medicines during the nineteenth century. Bull Hist Med. 1955;29(5):401–19. http://europepmc.org/abstract/MED/13260801.
5. Jones AW. Early drug discovery and the rise of pharmaceutical chemistry. Drug Test Anal. 2011;3(6):337–44. https://doi.org/10.1002/dta.301.
6. Penn RG. The state control of medicines: the first 3000 years. Br J Clin Pharmacol. 1979;8(4):293–305. https://doi.org/10.1111/j.1365-2125.1979.tb04710.x.
7. López-Muñoz F, Ucha-Udabe R, Alamo C. The history of barbiturates a century after their clinical introduction. Neuropsychiatr Dis Treat. 2005;1(4):329–43.
8. Raviña E. The evolution of drug discovery: from traditional medicines to modern drugs. Wiley-VCH; 2011.
9. Jack DB. One hundred years of aspirin. Lancet. 1997;350(9075):437–9. https://doi.org/10.1016/s0140-6736(97)07087-6.
10. Sneader W. Drug discovery: the evolution of modern medicines. John Wiley & Sons; 1985.
11. Bull JP. The historical development of clinical therapeutic trials. J Chronic Dis. 1959;10:218–48. https://doi.org/10.1016/0021-9681(59)90004-9.
12. Dixon WE. Proprietary, patent, and secret remedies. Proc R Soc Med. 1910;3(Ther Pharmacol Sect):82–90. https://www.ncbi.nlm.nih.gov/pubmed/19974854.
13. Journal AMA. "Patent" and secret proprietary medicines. Cal State J Med. 1905;3(10):306.
14. Simmons GH. Proprietary medicines: some general considerations. J Am Med Assoc. 1906;XLVI(18):1333–7. https://doi.org/10.1001/jama.1906.62510450007001c.
15. White Junod S. FDA and clinical drug trials: a short history. 2008.
16. White Junod S. Biologics centennial: 100 years of biologics regulation. 2002.
17. Avorn J. Two centuries of assessing drug risks. N Engl J Med. 2012;367(3):193–7. https://doi.org/10.1056/NEJMp1206652.
18. Cartwright AC, Matthews BR. Pharmaceutical product licensing—requirements for Europe. Ellis Horwood; 1991.
19. Lee PR, Herzstein J. International drug regulation. Annu Rev Public Health. 1986;7:217–35. https://doi.org/10.1146/annurev.pu.07.050186.001245.
20. Mann RD. From mithridatium to modern medicine: the management of drug safety. J R Soc Med. 1988;81(12):725–8. https://doi.org/10.1177/014107688808101216.
21. Paine MF. Therapeutic disasters that hastened safety testing of new drugs. Clin Pharmacol Ther. 2017;101(4):430–4. https://doi.org/10.1002/cpt.613.
22. Vereniging voor Gezondheidsrecht. Geneesmiddelen en recht—preadvies 2006. Sdu Uitgevers; 2006.
23. Williams KJ. The introduction of 'chemotherapy' using arsphenamine—the first magic bullet. J R Soc Med. 2009;102(8):343–8. https://doi.org/10.1258/jrsm.2009.09k036.
24. Toth B. Why the MRC therapeutic trials committee did not introduce controlled clinical trials. J R Soc Med. 2015;108(12):499–511. https://doi.org/10.1177/0141076815618891.
25. Therapeutic Substances Act, 1925. Draft rules and orders. Lancet. 1927;209(5408):895–6. https://doi.org/10.1016/S0140-6736(00)75675-3.
26. Dukes MNG. De toelating van geneesmiddelen in Nederland—pré-advies uitgebracht ten behoeve van de jaarvergadering van de vereniging voor gezondheidsrecht op 15 mei 1981. 1981.
27. Hobæk B, Lie AK. Less is more: Norwegian drug regulation, antibiotic policy, and the "need clause". Milbank Q. 2019;97(3):762–95. https://doi.org/10.1111/1468-0009.12405.
28. Weintraub M. The French drug approval process. J Clin Pharmacol. 1982;22(5–6):213–22. https://doi.org/10.1002/j.1552-4604.1982.tb02664.x.
29. Emanuel M, Rawlins M, Duff G, Breckenridge A. Thalidomide and its sequelae. Lancet. 2012;380(9844):781–3. https://doi.org/10.1016/S0140-6736(12)60468-1.
30. Lenz W. Kindliche Missbildungen nach Medikament-Einnahme während der Gravidität? Dtsch Med Wochenschr. 1961;86:2555.
31. McBride WG. Thalidomide and congenital abnormalities. Lancet. 1961;2:1358.
32. Kinch MS, Kinch GA, Griesenauer RH. Lost medicines: a longer view of the pharmaceutical industry with the potential to reinvigorate discovery. Drug Discov Today. 2019;24(2):382–9. https://doi.org/10.1016/j.drudis.2018.09.006.
33. Stricker BH, Psaty BM. Detection, verification, and quantification of adverse drug reactions. BMJ. 2004;329(7456):44–7. https://doi.org/10.1136/bmj.329.7456.44.
34. Vandenbroucke JP. Observational research, randomised trials, and two views of medical science. PLoS Med. 2008;5(3):e67. https://doi.org/10.1371/journal.pmed.0050067.
35. Goodrich WW. FDA's regulations under the Kefauver–Harris drug amendments of 1962. Food Drug Cosmetic Law J. 1963;18(10):561–9. http://www.jstor.org/stable/26655914.
36. Omar MA, Wilson JP. FDA adverse event reports on statin-associated rhabdomyolysis. Ann Pharmacother. 2002;36(2):288–95. https://doi.org/10.1345/aph.1A289.
37. U.S. Food and Drug Administration. A brief history of the center for drug evaluation and research. 2018. https://www.fda.gov/about-fda/fda-history-exhibits/brief-history-center-drug-evaluation-and-research. Retrieved 22 Oct 2023.

38. Inman B (obituary). BMJ. 2005;331(7530):1477. https://doi.org/10.1136/bmj.331.7530.1477.
39. Committee on Safety of Drugs. Report for 1969 and 1970. 1971.
40. World Health Organization. International drug monitoring: the role of national centres—report of a WHO meeting. Technical report series, issue. 1972.
41. World Health Assembly. Sixteenth World Health Assembly—part I: resolutions and decisions: annexes. 1963.
42. Uppsala Monitoring Centre. Members of the WHO programme for international drug monitoring. 25 Jan 2023. https://who-umc.org/about-the-who-programme-for-international-drug-monitoring/member-countries/. Retrieved 11 Jun 2023.
43. World Health Organization. Pharmacovigilance internationale—rôle de l'hôpital. 1969.
44. European Union. History of the EU. n.d. https://european-union.europa.eu/principles-countries-history/history-eu_en. Retrieved 11 Jun 2023.
45. Council of the European Economic Community. Council Directive 65/65/EEC of 26 January 1965 on the approximation of provisions laid down by law, regulation or administrative action relating to proprietary medicinal products. OJ L. 1965;22:369–73.
46. Council of the European Communities. Council Directive 75/318/EEC of 20 May 1975 on the approximation of the laws of member states relating to analytical, pharmaco-toxicological and clinical standards and protocols in respect of the testing of proprietary medicinal products. OJ L. 1975;147:1–12.
47. Council of the European Communities. Second Council Directive 75/319/EEC of 20 May 1975 on the approximation of provisions laid down by law, regulation or administrative action relating to proprietary medicinal products. OJ L. 1975;147:13–22.
48. Council of the European Communities. Council Directive 83/570/EEC of 26 October 1983 amending Directives 65/65/EEC, 75/318/EEC and 75/319/EEC on the approximation of provisions laid down by law, regulation or administrative action relating to proprietary medicinal products. OJ L. 1983;332:1–10.
49. Council of the European Communities. Council Directive 87/18/EEC of 18 December 1986 on the harmonization of laws, regulations and administrative provisions relating to the application of the principles of good laboratory practice and the verification of their applications for tests on chemical substances. OJ L. 1987;15:29–30.
50. Council of the European Communities. Council Directive 87/21/EEC of 22 December 1986 amending Directive 65/65/EEC on the approximation of provisions laid down by law, regulation or administrative action relating to proprietary medicinal products. OJ L. 1987;15:36–7.
51. Council of the European Communities. Council Directive 87/22/EEC of 22 December 1986 on the approximation of national measures relating to the placing on the market of high-technology medicinal products, particularly those derived from biotechnology. OJ L. 1987;15:38–41.
52. Council of the European Communities. Council Directive 88/320/EEC of 9 June 1988 on the inspection and verification of good laboratory practice (GLP). OJ L. 1988;145:35–7.
53. Council of the European Communities. Council Directive 89/341/EEC of 3 May 1989 amending Directives 65/65/EEC, 75/318/EEC and 75/319/EEC on the approximation of provisions laid down by law, regulation or administrative action relating to proprietary medicinal products. OJ L. 1989;142:11–3.
54. European Commission. Commission Directive 91/507/EEC of 19 July 1991 modifying the Annex to Council Directive 75/318/EEC on the approximation of the laws of member states relating to analytical, pharmacotoxicological and clinical standards and protocols in respect of the testing of medicinal products. OJ L. 1991;270:32–52.
55. Council of the European Communities. Council Directive 93/39/EEC of 14 June 1993 amending Directives 65/65/EEC, 75/318/EEC and 75/319/EEC in respect of medicinal products. OJ L. 1993;214:22–30.
56. Council of the European Communities. Council Regulation (EEC) No 2309/93 of 22 July 1993 laying down Community procedures for the authorization and supervision of medicinal products for human and veterinary use and establishing a European Agency for the Evaluation of Medicinal Products. OJ L. 1993;214:1–21.
57. European Commission. Commission Regulation (EC) No 540/95 of 10 March 1995 laying down the arrangements for reporting suspected unexpected adverse reactions which are not serious, whether arising in the Community or in a third country, to medicinal products for human or veterinary use authorized in accordance with the provisions of Council Regulation (EEC) No 2309/93. OJ L. 1995;55:5–6.
58. Committee for Proprietary Medicinal Products. Note for guidance: summary of the product characteristics (III/9163/89). 1989.
59. Salmon P. The revised SmPC guideline. Presentation at DIA regulatory forum. 2010.
60. Council of the European Communities. Council Directive 92/28/EEC of 31 March 1992 on the advertising of medicinal products for human use. OJ L. 1992;113:13–8.
61. Commission of the European Communities. Report from the commission to the council on the activities of the Committee for Proprietary Medicinal Products (COM(91) 39 final). 1991.
62. European Parliament & Council of the European Union. Regulation (EC) No 726/2004 of the European Parliament and of the Council of 31 March 2004 laying down Community procedures for the authorisation and supervision of medicinal products for human and veterinary use and establishing a European Medicines Agency. OJ L. 2004;136:1–33.

63. Greenberg MD. AIDS, experimental drug approval, and the FDA new drug screening process. N Y Univ J Legis Public Policy. 2000;3:295–350.
64. International Council for Harmonisation of Technical Requirements for Pharmaceuticals for Human Use. History. n.d. https://www.ich.org/page/history. Retrieved 11 Jun 2023.
65. International Coalition of Medicines Regulatory Authorities. History of ICMRA. n.d. https://www.icmra.info/drupal/en/aboutus/history. Retrieved 24 Oct 2023.
66. European Medicines Agency. EMA's final opinion confirms restrictions on use of linear gadolinium agents in body scans (EMA/625317/2017). 2017.
67. European Medicines Agency. EMA review of Zinbryta confirms medicine's risks outweigh its benefits (EMA/286850/2018). 2018.
68. European Medicines Agency. Disabling and potentially permanent side effects lead to suspension or restrictions of quinolone and fluoroquinolone antibiotics (EMA/175398/2019). 2019.
69. European Medicines Agency. Risks of Picato for actinic keratosis outweigh benefits (EMA/368170/2020/Corr.1). 2020.
70. Lane S, Lynn E, Shakir S. Investigation assessing the publicly available evidence supporting postmarketing withdrawals, revocations and suspensions of marketing authorisations in the EU since 2012. BMJ Open. 2018;8(1):e019759. https://doi.org/10.1136/bmjopen-2017-019759.
71. McNaughton R, Huet G, Shakir S. An investigation into drug products withdrawn from the EU market between 2002 and 2011 for safety reasons and the evidence used to support the decision-making. BMJ Open. 2014;4(1):e004221. https://doi.org/10.1136/bmjopen-2013-004221.
72. Onakpoya IJ, Heneghan CJ, Aronson JK. Post-marketing withdrawal of 462 medicinal products because of adverse drug reactions: a systematic review of the world literature. BMC Med. 2016;14:10. https://doi.org/10.1186/s12916-016-0553-2.
73. World Health Organization. Restrictions in use and availability of pharmaceuticals, 2010–2018. 2020.
74. Tsintis P, La Mache E. CIOMS and ICH initiatives in pharmacovigilance and risk management: overview and implications. Drug Saf. 2004;27(8):509–17. https://doi.org/10.2165/00002018-200427080-00004.
75. European Medicines Agency. EudraVigilance. n.d. https://www.ema.europa.eu/en/human-regulatory/research-development/pharmacovigilance/eudravigilance. Retrieved 18 Jun 2023.
76. European Medicines Agency. CHMP Guideline on risk management systems for medicinal products for human use (EMEA/CHMP/96268/2005). 2005.
77. European Parliament & Council of the European Union. Directive 2004/27/EC of the European Parliament and of the Council of 31 March 2004 amending Directive 2001/83/EC on the Community code relating to medicinal products for human use. OJ L. 2004;136:34–57.
78. European Parliament & Council of the European Union. Regulation (EU) No 1235/2010 of the European Parliament and of the Council of 15 December 2010 amending, as regards pharmacovigilance of medicinal products for human use, Regulation (EC) No 726/2004 laying down Community procedures for the authorisation and supervision of medicinal products for human and veterinary use and establishing a European Medicines Agency, and Regulation (EC) No 1394/2007 on advanced therapy medicinal products. OJ L. 2010;348:1–16.
79. European Commission. Commission Implementing Regulation (EU) No 520/2012 of 19 June 2012 on the performance of pharmacovigilance activities provided for in Regulation (EC) No 726/2004 of the European Parliament and of the Council and Directive 2001/83/EC of the European Parliament and of the Council. OJ L. 2012;159:5–25.
80. European Parliament & Council of the European Union. Directive 2010/84/EU of the European Parliament and of the Council of 15 December 2010 amending, as regards pharmacovigilance, Directive 2001/83/EC on the Community code relating to medicinal products for human use. OJ L. 2010;348:74–99.
81. European Medicines Agency. Good pharmacovigilance practices. n.d. https://www.ema.europa.eu/en/human-regulatory/post-authorisation/pharmacovigilance/good-pharmacovigilance-practices. Retrieved 18 Jun 2023.
82. European Medicines Agency & Heads of Medicines Agencies. Guideline on good pharmacovigilance practices (GVP) Annex I—Definitions (Rev 4) (EMA/876333/2011 Rev 4). 2017.
83. European Medicines Agency & Heads of Medicines Agencies. Guideline on good pharmacovigilance practices (GVP) Module V—Risk management systems (Rev 2) (EMA/838713/2011 Rev 2). 2017.
84. International Council for Harmonisation of Technical Requirements for Pharmaceuticals for Human Use. E2E guideline: pharmacovigilance planning. 2004.
85. Psaty BM, Meslin EM, Breckenridge A. A lifecycle approach to the evaluation of FDA approval methods and regulatory actions: opportunities provided by a new IOM report. JAMA. 2012;307(23):2491–2. https://doi.org/10.1001/jama.2012.5545.
86. Health Canada. Guidance document—submission of risk management plans and follow-up commitments. 2015.
87. Therapeutic Goods Administration. Risk management plans for medicines and biologicals—Australian requirements and recommendations (version 3.3). 2019.
88. Buoninfante A, Andeweg A, Baker AT, Borad M, Crawford N, Dogne JM, Garcia-Azorin D,

Greinacher A, Helfand R, Hviid A, Kochanek S, Lopez-Fauqued M, Nazy I, Padmanabhan A, Pavord S, Prieto-Alhambra D, Tran H, Wandel Liminga U, Cavaleri M. Understanding thrombosis with thrombocytopenia syndrome after COVID-19 vaccination. NPJ Vaccines. 2022;7(1):141. https://doi.org/10.1038/s41541-022-00569-8.
89. European Medicines Agency. 2022 Annual report on EudraVigilance for the European Parliament, the Council and the Commission (EMA/900566/2022). 2023.
90. Bate A, Evans SJ. Quantitative signal detection using spontaneous ADR reporting. Pharmacoepidemiol Drug Saf. 2009;18(6):427–36. https://doi.org/10.1002/pds.1742.
91. International Council for Harmonisation of Technical Requirements for Pharmaceuticals for Human Use. E2C(R2) guideline: periodic benefit-risk evaluation report. 2012.
92. European Parliament & Council of the European Union. Directive 2001/83/EC of the European Parliament and of the Council of 6 November 2001 on the Community code relating to medicinal products for human use. OJ L. 2001;311:67–128.
93. European Medicines Agency. Draft guideline on safety and efficacy follow-up and risk management of advanced therapy medicinal products (EMEA/149995/2008 rev.1). 2018.
94. European Commission. Commission Delegated Regulation (EU) No 357/2014 of 3 February 2014 supplementing Directive 2001/83/EC of the European Parliament and of the Council and Regulation (EC) No 726/2004 of the European Parliament and of the Council as regards situations in which post-authorisation efficacy studies may be required. OJ L. 2014;107:1–4.
95. Bloem LT, Schelhaas J, Lopez-Anglada L, Herberts C, van Hennik PB, Tenhunen O. European conditional marketing authorization in a rapidly evolving treatment landscape: a comprehensive study of anticancer medicinal products in 2006-2020. Clin Pharmacol Ther. 2023;114:148. https://doi.org/10.1002/cpt.2906.
96. European Medicines Agency. CHMP guideline on the scientific application and the practical arrangements necessary to implement Commission Regulation (EC) No 507/2006 on the conditional marketing authorisation for medicinal products for human use falling within the scope of Regulation (EC) No 726/2004 (EMA/CHMP/509951/2006, Rev. 1). 2016.
97. Naci H, Smalley KR, Kesselheim AS. Characteristics of preapproval and postapproval studies for drugs granted accelerated approval by the US Food and Drug Administration. JAMA. 2017;318(7):626–36. https://doi.org/10.1001/jama.2017.9415.
98. Pacurariu AC, Straus SM, Trifiro G, Schuemie MJ, Gini R, Herings R, Mazzaglia G, Picelli G, Scotti L, Pedersen L, Arlett P, van der Lei J, Sturkenboom MC, Coloma PM. Useful interplay between spontaneous ADR reports and electronic healthcare records in signal detection. Drug Saf. 2015;38(12):1201–10. https://doi.org/10.1007/s40264-015-0341-5.
99. Innovative Medicines Initiative. PROTECT—The pharmacoepidemiological research on outcomes of therapeutics by a European Consortium. n.d. https://www.imi.europa.eu/projects-results/project-factsheets/protect. Retrieved 13 Jun 2023.
100. OHDSI. OHDSI—observational health data sciences and informatics. n.d. https://www.ohdsi.org/. Retrieved 13 Jun 2023.
101. U.S. Food and Drug Administration. The Sentinel Initiative. n.d. https://www.sentinelinitiative.org/. Retrieved 13 Jun 2023.
102. Kristensen KB, Friis S, Lund LC, Hallas J, Cardwell CR, Andreassen BK, Habel LA, Pottegard A. Identification of drug-cancer associations: a Nationwide screening study. Cancer Res Commun. 2022;2(6):552–60. https://doi.org/10.1158/2767-9764.CRC-22-0026.
103. Harpaz R, DuMouchel W, Schuemie M, Bodenreider O, Friedman C, Horvitz E, Ripple A, Sorbello A, White RW, Winnenburg R, Shah NH. Toward multimodal signal detection of adverse drug reactions. J Biomed Inform. 2017;76:41–9. https://doi.org/10.1016/j.jbi.2017.10.013.
104. Toh S, Pratt N, Klungel OH, Gagne JJ, Platt RW. Distributed networks of databases analyzed using common protocols and/or common data models. In: Strom BL, Kimmel SE, Hennessy S, editors. Pharmacoepidemiology. 6th ed. Wiley-Blackwell; 2019. p. 617–38. https://doi.org/10.1002/9781119413431.ch25.
105. Klungel OH, Kurz X, De Groot MCH, Schlienger RG, Tcherny-Lessenot S, Grimaldi L, Ibáñez L, Groenwold RHH, Reynolds RF. Multi-centre, multi-database studies with common protocols: lessons learnt from the IMI PROTECT project. Pharmacoepidemiol Drug Saf. 2016;25:156–65. https://doi.org/10.1002/pds.3968.
106. CNODES. CNODES—The Canadian Network for observational drug effect studies. n.d. https://www.cnodes.ca/. Retrieved 13 Jun 2023
107. European Medicines Agency. No change is needed in use of direct oral anticoagulants following EMA-funded study (EMA/94424/2020). 2020. https://www.ema.europa.eu/documents/press-release/no-change-needed-use-direct-oral-anticoagulants-following-ema-funded-study_en.pdf.
108. Gini R, Sturkenboom MCJ, Sultana J, Cave A, Landi A, Pacurariu A, Roberto G, Schink T, Candore G, Slattery J, Trifirò G. Different strategies to execute multi-database studies for medicines surveillance in real-world setting: a reflection on the European model. Clin Pharmacol Ther. 2020;108(2):228–35. https://doi.org/10.1002/cpt.1833.
109. Bots SH, Riera-Arnau J, Belitser SV, Messina D, Aragon M, Alsina E, Douglas IJ, Duran CE, Garcia-Poza P, Gini R, Herings RMC, Huerta C, Sisay MM,

Martin-Perez M, Martin I, Overbeek JA, Paoletti O, Palleja-Millan M, Schultze A, et al. Myocarditis and pericarditis associated with SARS-CoV-2 vaccines: a population-based descriptive cohort and a nested self-controlled risk interval study using electronic health care data from four European countries. Front Pharmacol. 2022;13:1038043. https://doi.org/10.3389/fphar.2022.1038043.
110. DARWIN EU. DARWIN EU—The data analysis and real world interrogation network. n.d. https://www.darwin-eu.org/. Retrieved 13 Jun 2023.
111. U.S. Food and Drug Administration. The Sentinel Initiative—Individual drug analyses. n.d. https://www.sentinelinitiative.org/studies/drugs/individual-drug-analyses#undefined. Retrieved 13 Jun 2023.
112. Eworuke E, Welch EC, Haug N, Horgan C, Lee HS, Zhao Y, Huang TY. Comparative risk of angioedema with sacubitril-valsartan vs renin-angiotensin-aldosterone inhibitors. J Am Coll Cardiol. 2023;81(4):321–31. https://doi.org/10.1016/j.jacc.2022.10.033.
113. CNODES. CNODES—Projects. n.d. https://www.cnodes.ca/projects/. Retrieved 13 Jun 2023.
114. Fisher A, Fralick M, Filion KB, Dell'Aniello S, Douros A, Tremblay É, Shah BR, Ronksley PE, Alessi-Severini S, Hu N, Bugden SC, Ernst P, Lix LM. Sodium-glucose co-transporter-2 inhibitors and the risk of urosepsis: a multi-site, prevalent new-user cohort study. Diabetes Obes Metab. 2020;22(9):1648–58. https://doi.org/10.1111/dom.14082.
115. DARWIN EU. DARWIN EU—Studies. n.d. https://www.darwin-eu.org/index.php/studies. Retrieved 13 Jun 2023.
116. Schelhaas J, Mantel-Teeuwisse AK, Hoekman J, Van Hennik PB, Herberts CA, Bloem LT. Unpublished data. 2023.
117. Seeger JD, Davis KJ, Iannacone MR, Zhou W, Dreyer N, Winterstein AG, Santanello N, Gertz B, Berlin JA. Methods for external control groups for single arm trials or long-term uncontrolled extensions to randomized clinical trials. Pharmacoepidemiol Drug Saf. 2020;29(11):1382–92. https://doi.org/10.1002/pds.5141.
118. Burcu M, Dreyer NA, Franklin JM, Blum MD, Critchlow CW, Perfetto EM, Zhou W. Real-world evidence to support regulatory decision-making for medicines: considerations for external control arms. Pharmacoepidemiol Drug Saf. 2020;29(10):1228–35. https://doi.org/10.1002/pds.4975.
119. Hogervorst MA, Soman KV, Gardarsdottir H, Goettsch WG, Bloem LT. Unpublished data. 2023.
120. Hernan MA, Robins JM. Using big data to emulate a target trial when a randomized trial is not available. Am J Epidemiol. 2016;183(8):758–64. https://doi.org/10.1093/aje/kwv254.
121. Hernan MA, Sauer BC, Hernandez-Diaz S, Platt R, Shrier I. Specifying a target trial prevents immortal time bias and other self-inflicted injuries in observational analyses. J Clin Epidemiol. 2016;79:70–5. https://doi.org/10.1016/j.jclinepi.2016.04.014.
122. Maringe C, Benitez Majano S, Exarchakou A, Smith M, Rachet B, Belot A, Leyrat C. Reflection on modern methods: trial emulation in the presence of immortal-time bias. Assessing the benefit of major surgery for elderly lung cancer patients using observational data. Int J Epidemiol. 2020;49(5):1719–29. https://doi.org/10.1093/ije/dyaa057.
123. European Commission. Proposal for a Directive of the European Parliament and of the Council on the Union code relating to medicinal products for human use, and repealing Directive 2001/83/EC and Directive 2009/35/EC—COM(2023) 192 final. 2023.
124. European Commission. Proposal for a Regulation of the European Parliament and of the Council laying down Union procedures for the authorisation and supervision of medicinal products for human use and establishing rules governing the European Medicines Agency, amending Regulation (EC) No 1394/2007 and Regulation (EU) No 536/2014 and repealing Regulation (EC) No 726/2004, Regulation (EC) No 141/2000 and Regulation (EC) No 1901/2006—COM(2023) 193 final. 2023.
125. Tomson T, Battino D, Perucca E. The remarkable story of valproic acid. Lancet Neurol. 2016;15(2):141. https://doi.org/10.1016/S1474-4422(15)00398-1.
126. Tomson T, Battino D, Perucca E. Valproic acid after five decades of use in epilepsy: time to reconsider the indications of a time-honoured drug. Lancet Neurol. 2016;15(2):210–8. https://doi.org/10.1016/S1474-4422(15)00314-2.
127. European Medicines Agency. Assessment report: valproic acid/valproate containing medicinal products—referral under Article 31 of Directive 2001/83/EC (EMA/568844/2019). 2010.
128. European Medicines Agency. Assessment report: substances related to valproate—procedure under Article 31 of Directive 2001/83/EC resulting from pharmacovigilance data (EMA/686022/2014). 2014.
129. European Medicines Agency. Assessment report: Medicinal products containing substances related to valproate—referral under Article 31 of Directive 2001/83/EC (EMA/198940/2018). 2018.
130. Abtahi S, Pajouheshnia R, Duran CE, Riera-Arnau J, Gamba M, Alsina E, Hoxhaj V, Andersen M, Bartolini C, Kristiansen SB, Brown J, Hallgreen CE, Garcia-Poza P, Gardarsdottir H, Gini R, Girardi A, Holthuis E, Huerta C, Ibanez L, et al. Impact of 2018 EU Risk Minimisation Measures and Revised Pregnancy Prevention Programme on utilisation and prescribing trends of medicinal products containing valproate: an interrupted time series study. Drug Saf. 2023;46(7):689–702. https://doi.org/10.1007/s40264-023-01314-3.

131. European Medicines Agency. EMA review of data on paternal exposure to valproate—press release 16 Aug 2023. 2023. https://www.ema.europa.eu/en/news/ema-review-data-paternal-exposure-valproate.
132. Medicines and Healthcare products Regulatory Agency. Valproate: reminder of current pregnancy prevention programme requirements; information on new safety measures to be introduced in the coming months. 2022. https://www.gov.uk/drug-safety-update/valproate-reminder-of-current-pregnancy-prevention-programme-requirements-information-on-new-safety-measures-to-be-introduced-in-the-coming-months. Retrieved 22 Oct 2023.
133. Watson OJ, Barnsley G, Toor J, Hogan AB, Winskill P, Ghani AC. Global impact of the first year of COVID-19 vaccination: a mathematical modelling study. Lancet Infect Dis. 2022;22(9):1293–302. https://doi.org/10.1016/S1473-3099(22)00320-6.
134. Mahase E. Vaccinating the UK: how the covid vaccine was approved, and other questions answered. BMJ. 2020;371:m4759. https://doi.org/10.1136/bmj.m4759.
135. Marinus R, Mofid S, Mpandzou M, Kuhler TC. Rolling reviews during COVID-19: the European Union experience in a global context. Clin Ther. 2022;44(3):352–63. https://doi.org/10.1016/j.clinthera.2022.01.001.
136. Cavaleri M, Enzmann H, Straus S, Cooke E. The European medicines Agency's EU conditional marketing authorisations for COVID-19 vaccines. Lancet. 2021;397(10272):355–7. https://doi.org/10.1016/S0140-6736(21)00085-4.
137. Cavaleri M, Sweeney F, Gonzalez-Quevedo R, Carr M. Shaping EU medicines regulation in the post COVID-19 era. Lancet Reg Health Eur. 2021;9:100192. https://doi.org/10.1016/j.lanepe.2021.100192.
138. European Medicines Agency. Consideration on core requirements for RMPs of COVID19 vaccines core—RMP19 guidance v3.1 (EMA/PRAC/709308/2022). 2022.
139. European Medicines Agency. Report on pharmacovigilance tasks from EU Member States and the European Medicines Agency (EMA) 2019–2022 (EMA/142695/2023). 2023.
140. Willame C, Dodd C, Duran CE, Elbers R, Gini R, Bartolini C, Paoletti O, Wang L, Ehrenstein V, Kahlert J, Haug U, Schink T, Diez-Domingo J, Mira-Iglesias A, Carreras JJ, Vergara-Hernandez C, Giaquinto C, Barbieri E, Stona L, et al. Background rates of 41 adverse events of special interest for COVID-19 vaccines in 10 European healthcare databases—an ACCESS cohort study. Vaccine. 2023;41(1):251–62. https://doi.org/10.1016/j.vaccine.2022.11.031.

Further Reading

Andrews EB, Moore N, editors. Mann's pharmacovigilance. 3rd ed. Wiley; 2014.

McBride L, Schmitt S, editors. Fundamentals of pharmaceutical and biologics regulations: a global perspective. RAPS; 2023.

Strom BL, Kimmel SE, Hennessy S, editors. Pharmacoepidemiology. 6th ed. Wiley; 2019.

Clinical Trials Safety Data

7

Pipasha Biswas, Nilima Justice, and Himal Biswas

Abstract

Patient safety monitoring is a critical component in the clinical development process. In the last few decades, the regulatory landscape has changed for safety data monitoring in clinical trials. The guidelines issued by regulatory authorities specifically for the collection of safety data during clinical trials, documentation, and reporting of serious adverse events have made a significant impact to ensure the safety of clinical trial subjects. The main objective of collecting and reporting safety data from clinical trials is early detection of important safety signals to protect subjects, provide information about new risks, assess the potential risk to future patients, and develop safety profile and product label of the drug contributing to its benefit–risk assessment throughout the life cycle of the product in clinical development.

Keywords

Clinical trials · Data collection · Safety data reporting · Worldwide regulations · Data Safety Monitoring Boards · Data reconciliation · Data integrity · Development Safety Update Report · Integrated Safety Summary · Signal detection

Learning Objectives

- Understand the importance of clinical trials safety data collection, cleaning, and managing safety data arising from patients treated with the drug in clinical development in compliance with worldwide regulatory standards.
- Appraise the significance of clinical trials safety data for discovering new treatments for diseases.
- Appreciate the importance of clinical trials safety data analysis in research towards early detection of adverse events arising from the drugs in development, and associated risk mitigation and minimisation for the patients.
- Contemplate worldwide clinical trial safety data management regulations from different regulatory authorities to apply the knowledge in day-to-day activities whilst handling data originating from clinical trials.

P. Biswas (✉)
Pharmacovigilance & RWE, Symogen Limited, Marlow, UK
e-mail: pippa.biswas@symogen.com

N. Justice
R&I, V&I, AstraZeneca, Pipersville, PA, USA

H. Biswas
FY1, Cardiff University, Cardiff, Wales, UK

J. Jose et al. (eds.), *Principles and Practice of Pharmacovigilance and Drug Safety*,
https://doi.org/10.1007/978-3-031-51089-2_7

Key Points

- The goal of safety monitoring in clinical trials is to identify, evaluate, minimise, and appropriately manage risks.
- Monitoring patient safety during clinical trials is a critical component throughout the drug development life cycle that must be adhered to as per different regulations worldwide to protect patients.
- Clinical trials safety data is important for discovering new treatments for diseases, as well as new ways to detect and reduce the chance of developing any adverse effects to the drug and protecting the patients.

1 Introduction

Monitoring patient safety is an integral and important part in the life cycle of drug development. One of the main objectives of drug development process is to collect safety data from various phases of clinical trials, early detection of important safety signals, and to evolve medically relevant safety label information for the product under development. This is important for protecting patients from risks and developing the safety profile of the drug contributing to its benefit–risk assessment. Safety data collected during clinical trials has a direct impact on the safety and clinical care of patients enrolled in the trials.

The regulatory landscape for safety monitoring of healthcare products in clinical trials changed significantly in March 2006, after the first-in-human (FIH) study with TGN1412 (a CD28 superagonist mAb), resulted in life-threatening, Serious Adverse Events (SAEs) known as Cytokine Release Syndrome (CRS) in the United Kingdom (UK). This tragic episode resulted in several recommendations to improve the safety of initial human clinical studies with drugs in clinical development. This event initiated a new era, with several changes and recommendations put forth by the Medicines and Healthcare products Regulatory Agency (MHRA) in the UK for handling of patient safety data generated from products in clinical development and reporting of serious adverse events (SAEs) have since evolved significantly to help ensure the safety of subjects and patients involved in clinical trials [1].

This chapter provides a brief summary of the tragic events of TGN1412 incident that led to an overhaul of Phase 1 trials on the collection, documentation, and reporting of adverse events (AEs), worldwide regulations of clinical trials safety data collection and reporting, the importance of Drug Safety Monitoring Board (DSMB)/Data Monitoring Committee (DMC), reconciliation of safety data on an ongoing basis, and clinical trials safety data integrity that is very important in the context of drug development and protection of patients.

2 The Events of TGN1412 Incident: Learning from the Past

After a drug is considered safe and efficacious in pre-clinical studies, it is tested in healthy human volunteers for first-in-human (FIH) trials. In March 2006, a phase I clinical study was initiated for a CD28 "superagonist" antibody TGN1412—a new class of monoclonal antibody (mAb) with a stimulatory mode of action on a subset of T cells known as regulatory T cells. TGN1412 binds to CD28 and activates T cells without the need for T cell receptor (TCR) pre-activation, resulting in polyclonal T cell expansion, activation, and concentration-dependent IL-2 production, and TGN1412 was termed a "superagonist". The main aim was to develop TGN1412 as a treatment for B cell chronic lymphocytic leukaemia and for autoimmune diseases, such as rheumatoid arthritis.

1. Phase 1 clinical trial with this antibody was initiated on 13 March 2006 in six human volunteers. Within a span of 30 min, all the six volunteers had been administered TGN1412, while two volunteers were administered a placebo. However, within 90 min of the first infused dose, those who had received TGN1412 had a systemic inflammatory

response, characterised by a rapid induction of proinflammatory cytokines and accompanied by headache, myalgia, nausea, diarrhoea, erythema, vasodilatation, and hypotension. Further 12 and 16 h post infusion, all the six volunteers who had received TGN1412 became critically ill, with pulmonary infiltrates and lung injury, renal failure, and disseminated intravascular coagulation. There was severe and unexpected depletion of lymphocytes and monocytes which occurred within 8 h, reaching a nadir at 24 h. All six volunteers were transferred to an intensive care unit, where they received intensive cardiopulmonary support, including dialysis, high-dose methylprednisolone, and an anti-interleukin-2 receptor antagonist antibody. Prolonged cardiovascular shock and acute respiratory distress syndrome developed in two of six patients, who required intensive organ support for eight and 16 days. It was concluded that TGN1412 had caused a "cytokine storm". The patients later described huge swelling of their body, resembling an elephant and subsequently termed as "The Elephant Man". All six volunteers survived, but the long-term prognosis for these subjects was dismal with one of the volunteers since having to amputate his toes and the tips of several fingers [2].

The MHRA reacted rapidly, immediately suspending the Clinical Trial Authorisation (CTA) and confirming that TGN1412 was not in use in other trials anywhere in the world. Additionally, MHRA also alerted international pharmaceutical regulatory authorities worldwide of the events in case any similar product of this class was in use.

A detailed investigation by the MHRA identified and evaluated potential causes of the adverse reactions. It was concluded that an unpredicted biological reaction of the mAb in humans was likely the cause of serious adverse reactions observed in the trial participants, but not during the pre-clinical toxicity studies conducted on animals.

This incident evoked changes in how human trials are approved by the regulatory authorities and the way clinical trials are conducted. The Expert Scientific Group [3] report found that pre-clinical studies performed with TGN1412 failed to consider what constituted a safe dose for use in humans. In addition, it made 22 recommendations for improving the safety for Phase I trials of higher risk medicines described below [3]:

- Changes in calculations determining the starting point for drug dosing.
- Early discussion between regulators and sponsors with more scrutiny applied to novel agents and access to independent, specialist opinion.
- Sequential clinical testing—one person at a time—rather than simultaneous, with an appropriate period of monitoring for sudden ill effects.
- Careful consideration of the route and rate of administration—i.e. drugs should be administered via slow infusion rather than an injection.

Following this event, the MHRA tightened the UK clinical trial regulations. New guidelines were put in place for trials of certain categories of drugs not yet tested in humans [4].

The guidelines ranged from dosing protocols, timelines for reporting of safety data including AEs and training investigators.

3 Common Terminologies Used in Clinical Trials Safety Data Reporting

This section describes common terminologies and definitions that are used for clinical trial safety data reporting, which is necessary to understand while processing and reporting clinical trials safety data. The definitions, with input from the World Health Organization (WHO) Collaborating Centre, have been accepted for monitoring of AEs arising from drugs in clinical development [5].

3.1 Adverse Event

Any untoward medical occurrence in a patient or clinical investigation subject administered a pharmaceutical product and which does not necessarily have to have a causal relationship with this treatment.

An adverse event (AE) can be any unfavourable and unintended sign (including an abnormal laboratory finding, for example), symptom, or disease temporally associated with the use of a medicinal product, whether or not considered related to the medicinal product.

3.2 Adverse Drug Reaction

In the pre-approval clinical experience with a new medicinal product or its new usages, particularly as the therapeutic dose(s) may not be established:

All noxious and unintended responses to a medicinal product related to any dose should be considered adverse drug reactions.

The phrase "responses to a medicinal product" means that a causal relationship between a medicinal product and an adverse event is a reasonable possibility, i.e. the relationship cannot be ruled out.

Thus, simply an Adverse Drug Reaction (ADR) is defined as "any noxious and unintended response at doses normally used or tested in humans (in cases of approved pharmaceutical products); a noxious and unintended response at any dose(s) (in cases of new unregistered pharmaceutical products); an untoward medical occurrence seemingly caused by overdosing, abuse/dependence, and interactions with other medicinal products (in clinical trials)".

3.3 Unexpected Adverse Drug Reaction

*An adverse reaction, the nature or severity of which is not consistent with the applicable product information (*e.g. *Investigator's Brochure for an unapproved investigational medicinal product).*

3.4 Expectedness of Adverse Drug Reaction

The purpose of expedited reporting is to make regulators, investigators, and other appropriate people aware of new, important information on serious reactions. Therefore, such reporting generally involves events previously unobserved or undocumented, so a guideline is needed to define an event as "unexpected" or "expected" (from the perspective of previously observed, not on the basis of what might be anticipated from the pharmacological properties of a medicinal product). As stated in the definition, *an "unexpected" adverse reaction is one, the nature or severity of which is not consistent with information in the relevant source document(s).* A few examples are as follows:

- Acute renal failure assessed as an ADR with a subsequent new event of interstitial nephritis.
- Hepatitis with a first report of fulminant hepatitis.
- Cerebral thromboembolism can be assessed as unexpected if only cerebral vascular accident is listed in the investigator brochure (IB).

3.5 Serious Adverse Event (SAE) or Serious Adverse Drug Reaction (SADR)

An adverse event (AE) or adverse drug reaction (ADR) is associated with death, inpatient hospitalisation (in case the study was being conducted on outpatients), prolongation of hospitalisation (in case the study was being conducted on inpatients), persistent or significant disability or incapacity, a congenital anomaly or birth defect, or otherwise life-threatening.

Therefore, the criteria(s) for serious adverse events are as follows:

- Results in death
- Is life-threatening, NOTE: The term "life-threatening" in the definition of "serious" refers to an event in which the patient was at risk of death at the time of the event; it does

not refer to an event which hypothetically might have caused death if it were more severe

- Requires inpatient hospitalisation or prolongation of existing hospitalisation
- Results in persistent or significant disability/incapacity or
- Is a congenital anomaly/birth defect

Medical and scientific judgement should be exercised in deciding whether expedited reporting is appropriate in other situations, such as important medical events that may not be immediately life-threatening or result in death or hospitalisation, but may jeopardise the patient or require intervention to prevent one of the other outcomes listed above. These should also, usually, be considered serious.

3.6 Suspected Unexpected Serious Adverse Reaction (SUSAR)

This term is used to refer to an AE that occurs in a clinical trial subject, which is assessed by the sponsor and/or study investigator as being unexpected, serious, and as having a reasonable possibility of a causal relationship with the study drug. Any AE that would have led to one of the consequences that fulfil serious criteria but did not, owing to timely medical intervention, may also be deemed a Suspected Unexpected Serious Adverse Reaction (SUSAR).

4 Current Regulations Governing Clinical Trials Safety Data in Europe, North America, and Asia

Over the last few decades, the regulatory landscape for safety monitoring of medicinal products has rapidly changed and several regulations have been updated on a regular basis. Regulatory guidelines, issued by regulatory authorities worldwide to guarantee documentation and reporting of serious events, have evolved to ensure that the safety of clinical trial subjects is of utmost importance. This section briefly describes the various worldwide regulations for safety data monitoring and reporting for medicinal products during the entire life cycle of clinical development.

4.1 European Union Clinical Trials Regulation

Since 2004, the European Union Clinical Trial Directive 2001/20/EC (EU-CTD) [6] has governed the conduct of clinical trials in the European Union (EU). However, after the implementation of the EU-CTD, it created multiple challenges, where each EU member state had to implement its legal requirements through national legislation. There were several issues with the assessment process for multinational clinical trial applications, as well as a complex data submission framework. Furthermore, the public had limited access to clinical trial applications and results in the EU. In view of these issues, it was decided the EU-CTD be replaced with the new European Union Clinical Trials Regulation (EU-CTR).

As of 31 January 2022, the new EU-CTR designed to simplify and harmonise clinical trials in the EU began to replace EU-CTD, and the new regulation repealed the Clinical Trials Directive (EC) No. 2001/20/EC and national implementing legislation in the EU Member States, which regulated clinical trials in the EU.

4.2 Aims and Benefits of EU Clinical Trials Regulation

The main aims and benefits of the EU-CTR are illustrated below:

- Harmonise the processes for assessment and supervision of clinical trials throughout the EU.
- The evaluation, authorisation, and supervision of clinical trials are the responsibilities of EU Member States and European Economic Area (EEA) countries.

The new regulation will enable sponsors to submit one online application via a single online platform known as the Clinical Trials Information System (CTIS), which is a centralised electronic database for approval to run a clinical trial in several European countries, making it more efficient to carry out multinational trials. The regulation makes it more efficient for EU Member States to evaluate and authorise applications together, via the CTIS. The CTIS will be used for safety reporting, modifications, notifications, corrective measures, results summaries, and other information.

Other key benefits of the current regulation include:

- Improving information sharing and collective decision-making on clinical trials
- Increasing transparency of information on clinical trials
- Ensuring high standards of safety for all participants in EU clinical trials

Additionally, the new regulation has simplified safety data reporting, where a single safety report can be submitted for clinical trials involving more than one Investigational Medicinal Product (IMP), and all unexpected AEs which affect the clinical trial's benefit–risk balance must be reported within 15 days. Additionally, all safety assessments will be governed by separate legislation created by the European Commission. The European Commission is developing supplementary legislation to describe how member states will interact to assess safety reports. Finally, under EU-CTD multiple safety submissions to national competent authorities and ethics committes are permitted, whereas EU-CTR requires all safety reporting via EudraVigilance.

4.3 New Timelines of the EU-CTR

There is a 3-year transition period which started on 31 January 2022:

- 31 January 2022 to 31 January 2023: sponsors may submit clinical trials under the legal framework of EU-CTD or EU-CTR.
- Starting 31 January 2023: all clinical trial applications are subject to EU-CTR. However, trials approved under EU-CTD before 31 January 2023 can continue to be regulated under EU-CTD until 31 January 2025.

Since 31 January 2025, all clinical trials must be regulated under EU-CTR, and sponsors have a maximum of 12 calendar days to respond to application queries or requests for information (RFI) under EU-CTR, otherwise, applications will lapse by default. While authorisations will not expire under EU-CTD, it will, however, expire if no patient is recruited within 2 years under EU-CTR. Similarly, EU-CTR mandates reporting serious breaches within 7 days and archiving the Trial Master File (TMF) after 25 years where EU-CTD sets no timelines for either.

4.4 Medicines and Healthcare Products Regulatory Agency, United Kingdom

As of 1 January 2022, the combined review service formerly known as Combined Ways of Working [7] will now be the way forward for all new Clinical Trials of Investigational Medicinal Products (CTIMPs) where applications are prepared, submitted, and reviewed [5]. Combined review will therefore offer a single application route and co-ordinated review leading to a single UK decision for CTIMPs.

4.4.1 Suspected Unexpected Serious Adverse Reactions

The sponsor of a clinical trial or any other person to whom the sponsor has delegated this responsibility must report all suspected unexpected serious adverse reactions (SUSARs) which occur during the trial to the MHRA.

Fatal or life-threatening SUSARs must be reported as soon as possible, no later than 7 days after the first aware date of the event. Additional relevant information must be sent within 8 days of the initial report.

Non-fatal or non-life-threatening SUSARs must be reported as soon as possible, no later than 15 days after the first aware date of the reaction.

The sponsor of a "trial performed in the United Kingdom" (UK trial) must report the following UK-relevant SUSARs to the MHRA:

- All SUSARs occurring in that trial in UK sites
- All SUSARs occurring in that trial in sites outside the UK
- All SUSARs originating in a non-UK trial of the same medicinal product if the trial is run by the same sponsor of the trial running in the UK
- All SUSARs originating in a non-UK trial of the same medicinal product if the sponsor of the trial outside the UK is either part of the same mother company or develops the medicinal product jointly, on the basis of a formal agreement, with the sponsor of the UK trial

A SUSAR can be reported to the MHRA in one of the following ways:

- Using the eSUSAR website, by registering the details before using the eSUSAR website and completing the eSUSAR registration form and email it to esusar@mhra.gov.uk.
- Using ICSR Submissions, the ICSR Submissions route is used to submit single reports.
- Using the MHRA Gateway, the Gateway route is used to submit bulk reports.

If applicable, dual reports UK-relevant SUSARs can be submitted to the European Medicine Agency's (EMA) EudraVigilance Clinical Trial Module (EVCTM), as well as to other national competent authorities, using the European submission routes.

4.4.2 Development Safety Update Reports

Development Safety Update Reports (DSURs) should consider all new available safety information received during the reporting period. The DSUR should include the following:

- An analysis of the subjects' safety in the concerned clinical trial(s) with an appraisal of its ongoing risk/benefit
- A line listing of all suspected serious adverse reactions (including all SUSARs) that occurred in the trial(s), including all SUSARs from third countries
- An aggregate summary tabulation of SUSARs that occurred in the concerned trial(s)

A DSUR should be submitted to the MHRA by using Submissions via the Human Medicines Tile. However, it should be noted that if at least one of the trials covered by the DSUR has gone through the combined review process, then the report should be submitted via the Integrated Research Application System.

4.4.3 Shortened DSUR Available for Notification Scheme Approved Trials

This is suitable for:

- Individual trials authorised under the Notification Scheme which are not part of a multi-study development programme.
- Phase 4 national (UK only) trials of licenced products that commanded a low fee from the MHRA and where all participants have completed treatment and are only in follow-up.

As an alternative to producing a full DSUR for these trials, the Health Research Authority Annual Progress Report is usually used.

4.5 North America: USA and Canada

4.5.1 United States-Food and Drug Administration

FDA released a draft guidance on 29 September 2021, with the focus on clinical investigators role and responsibility rather than the sponsors [8]. The FDA cited that the current guidance from 2009 and 2012 on safety reporting should continue to be followed until the new document is finalised.

As per the FDA, "Most of the information about the safety of a drug prior to marketing comes from clinical trials", hence, "Adverse event reports from investigators are therefore critically important, given that it is the investigators who observe subjects' responses to an investigational drug [8]".

The new draft was published to separate sponsor responsibility and for clinical investigators. It defines for the clinical investigators, how to identify safety information that raises an "unanticipated problem involving risk to human subjects or others" for investigational drugs or "unanticipated adverse device effects" and how this information should be reported.

This applies to investigational new drug (IND) application studies and investigational device exemption (IDE) studies.

IND Studies

The reporting requirement for clinical investigators is that they must report SAEs to the trial sponsor immediately after identifying the SAE, no longer than one calendar day, regardless of:

- Relatedness of the event to the drug and/or
- Listedness in the safety surveillance plan or the IB as an anticipated event

There can be an exception to this reporting requirement regarding a study endpoint SAE and should be outlined in the study protocol. However, the endpoint SAE has to be reported if it is assessed as having causal relationship that the event was caused by the drug.

FDA requires an identifiable subject, a suspect drug, a reporter, if it is not the clinical investigator, and a description of the event for a case to be valid. The report should include a causality assessment from the clinical investigator of whether there is a "reasonable possibility" that the drug caused the AE, and it is the sponsor's responsibility to determine expectedness.

"FDA interprets reasonable possibility to mean there is evidence to suggest a causal relationship between the drug and the adverse event", the FDA noted in its guidance to investigators. "Factors that should be considered when making a causality assessment include, but are not limited to, temporal relationship of the event to drug administration; biologic plausibility, based on the mechanism of action of the drug or similar drugs in the same class; nonclinical evidence; and dechallenge-re-challenge information".

The investigators are required to report all serious and expected events to the Institutional Review Board (IRB), collect all non-serious AEs, and review all IND safety reports, including safety information from IND-exempt bioavailability/bioequivalence studies received prior to submitting the reports to the IRB unless it is communicated that the sponsor has sent the information to the IRB. The investigators must also report to the IRBs, medication errors, breach of privacy or confidentiality, and untimely destruction of study records, as these are considered unanticipated problems related to study procedures.

IDE Studies

For IDE studies, investigators must report unanticipated adverse device effects (UADEs) to both the trial sponsors and the IRBs as soon as possible, no later than 10 working days after the investigator discovers the effect.

In the guidance, the FDA writes "What qualifies as a UADE is expected to vary depending on the specific device and the way the device is used within the study". "Therefore, sponsors are required to include risk information in the investigational plan, which may help investigators identify and assess potential UADEs".

As per the draft guidance, clinical investigators are also responsible for providing updates on adverse device effects at regular intervals to sponsors, monitors, and IRBs.

4.5.2 Health Canada

Biological Drugs, Pharmaceutical Drugs, and Radiopharmaceuticals

All trial sponsors, or applicants, must report any serious and unexpected ADR that occurred inside and outside Canada to Health Canada, while the drug (including biological drugs) is in clinical trials in Canada [9].

For clinical trials in Canada, only ADRs that are both serious and unexpected are reported in an expedited manner to Health Canada, regardless of whether the ADR occurred inside or outside of Canada. Expedited reporting of serious and expected cases is not required as well as serious events from clinical investigations that are considered unrelated to the study product, whether the event is expected.

IND Annual Reports for Both FDA and Health Canada

The sponsors have to provide IND annual reports within 60 days of the anniversary date that the application went into effect, and Form 1571 is expected to be sent along with each annual report submission [10].

The FDA will accept DSURs in lieu of IND Annual Reports (76 Federal Register 52667 (23 Aug 2011) provided all the requirements of the US Annual Report are provided in the region-specific appendices of the DSUR.

4.6 Asia: Japan, China, and India

4.6.1 Japan

In Japan, sections 80-2-6 and 66-7 of the Pharmaceutical Affairs Law includes information on the AE and ADR reporting occurring during clinical trials [11]. This section of the law describes reporting to the Ministry of Health, Labour, and Welfare (MHLW). However, in practice, AE and ADR reports are submitted to the Pharmaceuticals and Medical Devices Agency (PMDA).

Japanese regulation on Good Clinical Practice (GCP) [12] requires sponsors to report AEs and ADRs "immediately" to investigators and to the heads of institutions involved in the clinical trial. There are, however, several differences in reporting of safety data between The International Council for Harmonisation of Technical Requirements for Pharmaceuticals for Human Use (ICH) E2A, US, and EU regulations with that of the Japanese regulations as detailed below.

Differences Between ICH E2A, US, and EU Regulations with the Japanese Regulations

Determination of Serious AE

Per ICH E2A, US, and EU regulations, all hospitalisations are considered "serious". However, in Japan, only hospitalisations or extension of hospitalisation "for treatment" qualify as serious, Section 66-7 of the Pharmaceutical Affairs Law [11]. In practice, however, this situation can be difficult to determine if hospitalisation is "for treatment" and counts as serious under Japanese regulations.

Another additional difference in the definition of "serious" is that where the ICH, EU, and US regulations use the phrase "persistent or significant disability/incapacity", the Japanese regulation uses a term equivalent to "disability".

"Expectedness" of a New Event in Japan

In both the USA and Europe, an AE is considered unexpected if its severity or nature are inconsistent with what is written in the IB, and all subsequent reports of a previously reported event continue to be unexpected until the IB has been updated to include it. However, in Japan, once an event has been distributed to investigators as a SUSAR, it is considered "expected".

Expected Life-Threatening and Death SUSARs

The USA, EU, and Japan all require 7-day reporting to regulators of unexpected life-threatening and death SUSARs, although none of these territories specifies a 7-day timeline for reporting to investigators. In all three regions, unexpected serious reactions, which are serious by any of the other criteria, are to be reported to regulators within a 15-day timeline. It should be noted, however, that in Japan, unlike the USA and EU, expected life-threatening and death SUSARs qualify as 15-day reports to the PMDA and must also be reported to investigators as well.

Reporting Timelines

Only US regulations give a clear, 15-day timeline for reporting SUSARs to clinical investigators. The EU Clinical Trials Directive [6] states that "The Sponsor shall also inform all investigators, but gives no timeline on reporting to investigators, except that reporting should be prompt". Similarly, the Japanese regulations indicate that reporting should not be delayed but does not specify reporting timelines.

Format of Report

Both the US and Japanese regulations indicate that individual reports of SUSARs should be provided to investigators in the same format they are provided to the regulatory authorities. However, the EU Guidance states that line listings accompanied by a summary is an appropriate format for informing investigators.

Reporting to Ethics Committee and Institutional Review Boards

EU regulations give the same 7 and 15-day timelines for reporting to regulators as to ECs and clearly state the sponsor is responsible for reporting to Ethics Committee (EC). Japanese regulations also have the responsibility for reporting to the IRB on the sponsor, but US regulations give investigators the responsibility for reporting to the IRB.

4.6.2 China

Clinical Trials Safety Data Reporting

In China, the Clinical Trials Management Office [13] is responsible for the reception, analysis, and evaluation of SUSARs during clinical trials, as well as DSURs.

China: Expedited Adverse Event Reporting in Clinical Trials

In China, any SAEs that occur during the trial should be reported to the EC in time. Regulations state that if any SAE occurs during the clinical trial, the investigators will be responsible for reporting to the drug regulatory departments of the relevant provinces, autonomous regions, or municipalities directly under the Central Government. The applicant must be notified within 24 h and report to the EC in time.

If there are large numbers of unexpected adverse reaction or SAEs, the China Food and Drug Administration (CFDA) may order to change the protocol, suspend, or terminate the clinical trial. This is also the case for SAEs unreported within the specified timeline [SFDA Order No. 28, Chapter III, Article: 42–43] [13].

When conducting an international multi-centre clinical trial in China, if there are observed serious adverse reactions and unexpected adverse reactions associated with the drug in any country, the applicant shall, in accordance with relevant regulations, report to the CFDA in time [SFDA Order No. 28, Chapter III, Article: 44] [13].

4.6.3 India

The Indian Good Clinical Practice (IGCP) guidelines, published in 2001, provided definition of AE and ADR and defined responsibilities of the investigator and sponsor regarding safety reporting during clinical trials. As per this guideline, investigators should promptly report all ADRs and AEs that are serious and/or unexpected to the EC and the sponsor, while the sponsor should expedite reporting of all serious and/or unexpected ADRs to all concerned, including EC and regulatory authorities [14].

In 2005, Schedule Y was amended and came into existence with several updates to the Indian pharmacovigilance [15]. Amended Schedule Y marked the beginning of compulsory and time-bound pharmacovigilance practice in India and specified reporting timelines for SAEs for sponsors and investigators, enlisted data elements required for reporting of SAE, and general reporting structure for such events.

Amended Schedule Y [15] requires "all serious and unexpected AEs" to be reported to the regulators and other investigators, but the trial approval letter issued by the office of Central Drugs Standard Control Organisation (CDSCO) states that, "in case any unexpected serious adverse reaction (SADR) is observed during trial, the same should be immediately communicated" [15]. It should be noted that while both ICH E2A and 21 CFR 312.32 define the term "unexpectedness", neither Schedule Y nor Indian GCP clarifies the criteria of "unexpectedness".

India: Reporting Timelines for Serious Adverse Events

The reporting timelines as per Schedule Y for SAEs are as follows:

- All unexpected serious AEs are to be reported by the investigator within 24 h of the occurrence to regulatory authority and to site EC within 7 working days, while globally the timeline for reporting fatal/life-threatening SUSAR to regulatory agencies is 7 calendar days.

In the event of death or fatality, the site EC will be aware of the event in 7 working days, which in practice may exceed 7 days, considering public holidays/weekends.

Expedited Reporting Requirements and Reporting Requirements for Global Sites

In the amended Schedule Y, there is no mention in the definition and standards for expedited reporting. Thus, as per Schedule Y, any "unexpected and serious" adverse events can be reported to CDSCO and other investigators within 14 calendar days.

There is no requirement to prioritise reporting of events that are suspected of having a causal association, nor is there any provision to differentiate reporting timelines for unexpected deaths or life-threatening events that are suspected to be due to study medication. This contrasts with both ICH E2A and 21 CFR 312.32, which mandate reporting of fatal or life-threatening SUSAR to regulators within 7 calendar days, while other SUSARs can be reported in 15 days time.

There is also no mention of reporting requirements from foreign sites for multinational trials and Schedule Y does not include the term "SUSAR" and does not specify expedited reporting requirements for SUSARs. Since CDSCO does not specify the expedited reporting timeline, the event can be reported to CDSCO anytime within the 14-day timeframe.

Development Safety Update Reports in India

The concept of a DSUR was first introduced by the Council for International Organizations of Medical Sciences (CIOMS) VI working group and taken forward by the CIOMS VII working group.

Both the US FDA and EU Clinical Trial Directive required what is termed as IND Annual Report and Annual Safety Report (ASR), respectively, the content, format, and timings differed between the US and EU reports [16, 17]. CDSCO does not require DSUR for Indian pharmaceutical companies undertaking global trial for a locally developed drug. However, sponsors are required to submit a status report on the clinical trial to the licencing authority at the prescribed periodicity.

4.7 Australia

4.7.1 Clinical Trials Safety Data Reporting in Australia and Therapeutic Goods Administration Notification and Safety Reporting Requirements

In Australia, the Therapeutic Goods Administration (TGA) has set clear regulations and guidelines for clinical safety data reporting.

It is advised that trial sponsors should refer to the *NHMRC Safety Monitoring and Reporting in Clinical Trials Involving Therapeutic Goods (2016) (NHMRC Guidance)* [18], for safety reporting requirements. The National Health and Medical Research Council (NHMRC) guidance addresses the monitoring, collection, and reporting of AEs that occur in clinical trials. This involves therapeutic goods conducted under the Clinical Trials Notification (CTN) or Clinical Trials Exemption (CTX) schemes. The NHMRC

Guidance has aligned with the European Union's Clinical Trial Regulations: Regulation EU No. 536/2014 [6].

According to the NHMRC Guidance, the trial sponsor is responsible for reporting to the TGA. The NHMRC Guidance outlines the trial sponsor's safety reporting responsibilities for CTN and CTX trials. Further information on how the trial sponsor should notify all relevant safety reports for CTN and CTX trials is in the following Tables 7.1 and 7.2.

4.7.2 Safety Reporting Timeframes for CTN and CTX Trials Single Case Events from Australian Sites: Suspected Unexpected Serious Adverse Reactions and Unanticipated Serious Adverse Device Effects

Individual SUSARs and Unanticipated Serious Adverse Device Effects (USADEs) from Australian sites must be reported to the TGA [18], even if initial information is limited (i.e. less than the minimum information required for expedited reporting as outlined in the CPMP/ICH/377/95 Guideline for Clinical Safety Data Management: Definitions and Standards for Expedited Reporting), and these details should still be forwarded to the TGA pending receipt and provision of further data (Tables 7.1 and 7.2) [18].

Other Report Types

Annual Safety Report

Summary of all new available safety information relevant to a trial that is received over a 12-month period (the Executive Summary of safety information produced for international regulators, such as the DSUR may serve as the Annual Safety Report). The reporting timelines for annual safety report and single AEs is represented in Table 7.3 [18].

Table 7.1 Suspected Unexpected Serious Adverse Reactions and Unanticipated Serious Adverse Device Effects

Type of event	Type of good	Report format	Timeline
Suspected Unexpected Serious Adverse Reactions (SUSARs) from Australian sites only	Medicines and biologicals	The new Electronic Data Interchange (EDI) functionality allows sponsors to submit adverse event reports directly from their system to Therapeutic Goods Administration OR Adverse event reports can be submitted using the new online reporting form. This can be accessed from the reporting problems page—https://www.tga.gov.au/safety/reporting-problems OR Blue Card or CIOMS form emailed to adr.reports@health.gov.au	For fatal or life-threatening Australian SUSARs, immediately, no later than 7 calendar days after being made aware of the case, with any follow-up information within another 8 calendar days For all other Australian SUSARs, no later than 15 calendar days after being made aware of the case
Unanticipated Serious Adverse Device Effects (USADEs) from Australia	Medical devices	Medical device incident reporting system OR Users medical device incident report form emailed to iris@health.gov.au	For fatal or life-threatening Australian USADEs, immediately, no later than 7 calendar days after being made aware of the case, with any follow-up information within a further 8 calendar days For all other Australian USADEs, no later than 15 calendar days after being made aware

Table 7.2 Significant Safety Issues and Urgent Safety Measures reporting timelines for Australia: significant safety issues[a] and overseas regulatory action

Type of event	Type of good	Report format	Timeline
Significant safety issues (SSIs) requiring implementation of urgent safety measure (USMs)	All therapeutic goods	In writing to the pharmacovigilance and special access branch via email to clinical. trials@health.gov.au	Within 24 h (where possible) and in any case, no later than 72 h of the measure being taken
Action with respect to safety that has been taken by another country's regulatory agency (relevant to an ongoing clinical trial in Australia)	All therapeutic goods	In writing to the pharmacovigilance and special access branch via email to clinical. trials@health.gov.au	Without undue delay, no later than 72 h of the trial sponsor becoming aware of the action
All other SSIs: Notification of an amendment[b] Temporary halt of a trial for safety reasons Early termination of a trial for safety reasons	All therapeutic goods	In writing to the pharmacovigilance and special access branch via email to clinical. trials@health.gov.au	Without undue delay, no later than 15 calendar days of the trial sponsor becoming aware of the issue or temporary halt or early termination

Note: A Suspected Unexpected Serious Adverse Reaction or Unanticipated Serious Adverse Device Effect may also meet the definition of an SSI

[a] SSIs that arise from analysis of overseas reports (relating to a clinical trial in Australia) should be reported to the TGA as per the timeframes above

[b] Therapeutic Goods Administration should receive notification that an SSI has occurred but the amendment revising trial documentation should be submitted to the Human Research Ethics Committee only

Table 7.3 Annual safety report and single adverse events reporting timelines for Australia

Type of event	Type of good	Report format	Timeline
Other single case AEs	All therapeutic goods	Up-to-date tabulations or line listings	On TGA's request
Annual safety reports	All therapeutic goods	Development safety update reports or other annual safety reports	On TGA's request

5 Collection and Management of Safety Data Arising from Clinical Trials

Regulatory authorities worldwide critically review whether a drug is safe for its intended use during the safety review of a New Drug Application (NDA). They assess safety and determine the significance of the AEs, including their impact on the approvability of the drug. Finally, regulatory authorities determine the safety issues to be included in the product labelling should the drug be approved and decide whether additional safety studies are needed [19].

Data collected during clinical trials serve as an important source of safety information that generates evidence for regulators, sponsors, physicians, and patients. Data collection methods used during the conduct of clinical trials are important part of the process of safety monitoring to investigators, sponsors, regulators, and patients. In the pre-approval setting, comprehensive safety data collection is required to understand the frequency, severity, seriousness, and dose–response of AEs, including potential differences across subsets, e.g. demographic, concomitant illnesses, and/or concomitant therapy. Hence, when a clinical trial is being designed, it is important to plan how and what type of safety data will be collected and captured during the trial.

5.1 Types of Data Collection Methods in Clinical Trials

Safety data from clinical trials are usually generated and collected by the following:

- Study investigator
- Study sponsor
- Directly by patients called patient-reported outcomes (PROs)

Throughout the clinical development process of the medicinal product, safety data are collected through various ways.

5.1.1 Traditional Data Collection

- On paper such as Case Report Forms (CRFs), patient diaries, or questionnaires

Paper CRFs are common and usually designed for collection from handwritten information. This method of data collection is cheap and allows for creation of direct copies and faxing; however, there are several disadvantages such as storage issues for large volume of paper, space, and correction limitations of the form itself and scope of mistakes and errors while transferring information from paper to electronic database.

5.1.2 Electronic Data Collection

- Electronic CRFs (eCRFs)
- Through dedicated Apps—mobile phones or tablets to collect data directly from patients through patient-reported outcomes (ePROs)
- Direct Data Capture (DDC)—here data is directly generated by electronic devices and entered directly into the database, for example, laboratory data, ECG data, central image reading data, i.e. MRI results, electronic patient questionnaires, or patient diaries

eCRFs are a very popular method of data collection, but they are more complicated to produce and have to adhere to strict data regulations. In this method of data collection, the computer programmes and software should be validated, and every correction that is made to the data entered must be traceable and only authorised persons have access to the programme.

Regulatory requirements that eCRFs must conform to are as follows:

- In Europe: ICH GCP E-6, Section 5.5.3 [20]
- In the USA: FDA—21CFR Part 11 and Guidance for Industry—Computerised Systems used in Clinical Trials [21]

If data collection is through eCRFs, validation of electronic systems is mandatory. The system must have an audit trail; any change made should be electronically recorded and traceable; be protected against unauthorised access; and data should be backed up regularly on a different server or computer that can be accessed for the lifetime of the product.

5.1.3 Patient Reported Outcomes (PROs) and Electronic Captured PROs (ePROs)

In this method of data collection, data is directly provided by patients, which includes all types of questionnaires and diaries that are recorded on paper or via electronic systems. Typically, electronic data are either in the form of a daily diary at the patient's home or quality of life (QoL) questionnaires administered during site visits.

5.2 Available Safety Data Sources from Premarketing Clinical Trials

Throughout the drug development process, safety data is continuously evaluated at all stages of drug development. The safety profile of an investigational drug is determined from the analysis of safety information obtained from both non-clinical and clinical studies.

The clinical phase of development involves the following:

- Phase 0 usually only involves a small number of subjects and very small dose of a drug, and the aim is to find out whether the drug reaches the cells.

- Phase I studies determine safety and dosing in healthy volunteers (patients in oncology studies).
- Phase II studies determine efficacy and safety in patients with the disease or condition.
- Phase III studies determine safety and efficacy in sufficiently large number of patients with the disease or condition.

The safety information collected from clinical trials during the drug development process include AEs, laboratory measurements, vital signs, clinical investigations such as ECGs, X-ray, MRI, and CT scan and other tests relevant to the indication being studied. Randomised controlled trials are the gold standard of scientific testing for new drugs, and this is based on the premarketing safety data.

AEs are normally collected according to the following domains:

- Seriousness
- Expectedness of the event
- Relatedness
- Intensity or severity
- Incidence
- Duration
- Latency
- Time to resolution

The relationship between drug exposure and AEs is also assessed through causality assessment using several algorithms. However, there are several limitations from the premarketing safety database based on clinical trials for several reasons.

5.3 What Data Should Be Reported?

5.3.1 Single Cases of Serious, Unexpected ADRs

All ADRs that are both serious and unexpected are subject to expedited reporting. This applies to reports from spontaneous sources and also from any type of clinical or epidemiological investigation, independent of design or purpose. It also applies to cases not reported directly to a sponsor or manufacturer (e.g., those found in regulatory authority-generated ADR registries or in publications). Expedited reporting is inappropriate for serious events from clinical investigations that are considered not related to study product, whether the event is expected or not. Similarly, non-serious adverse reactions, whether expected or not, are usually not subject to expedited reporting. Information obtained by a sponsor or manufacturer on serious, unexpected reports from any source should be submitted on an expedited basis to appropriate regulatory authorities if the minimum criteria for expedited reporting are met.

5.4 Baseline Data Collection

Baseline data are needed to ensure that subjects meet inclusion and exclusion criteria for study enrolment and are important in safety assessment. For example, particular SAEs may occur more frequently in subgroups defined based on ICH E19 Guideline demographics, baseline disease characteristics, coexisting illnesses, or concomitant therapies; analyses of such information can be important in considering the benefit–risk profile of the drug. Use of a selective safety data collection approach does not change considerations for baseline data collection.

5.5 Blinded Data in Clinical Trials

A "blind" study is a clinical trial in which the subject or the investigator (or both) are unaware of which trial product/drug the subject is taking [22]. In a clinical trial, blinding is necessary to prevent observer bias.

When the term "double blind" is mentioned, it usually refers to keeping the study participants, those involved with the trial management, and those collecting/analysing clinical data unaware of the assigned treatment to prevent influence. Different parties that are involved in a clinical trial are possible sources of bias and therefore should be blinded to ensure trial objectivity, including:

- The patient being treated
- The clinical staff administering the treatment
- The physician assessing the treatment
- The team interpreting the results

There are different types of blinded studies and these include the following:

- Single-blind studies are those where the subjects in the trial are unaware of which treatment group they are in, but the sponsor team knows about it.
- Double-blind studies are those where both the sponsor team and subjects do not know which subject is assigned to which treatment group.
- Triple-blind studies are those that further extend the blinding to the data analysts, so the subjects, clinicians/data collectors, and outcome adjudicators/data analysts are all unaware of the treatment the participant has received.

5.5.1 Unblinding of Clinical Trial Data

Unblinding in a clinical trial refers to as code-break, and the process by which the treatment or allocation details are made available either purposefully (i.e. according to the code-break procedures) or accidently.

The main aim and purpose of unblinding are as follows:

- Unblinding a subject in an emergency situation
- Unblinding data for the purpose of notification to Drug safety monitoring board/Drug monitoring committee
- Manage accidental unblinding
- Unblinding at the end of the trial

Blinding in clinical trials is a vital procedure that needs to be handled with attention and confidentiality to prevent any form of bias. Blinded data is an important piece of information, and the unblinding process should be mentioned clearly in the clinical study report (CSR) in detail at the end of the study and to the regulatory authorities.

6 Drug Safety Monitoring Board (DSMB)/Drug Monitoring Committee (DMC)

A Drug Safety Monitoring Board (DSMB) or Data Monitoring Committee (DMC) is an independent committee consisting of a group of three to seven expert members who are independent from the entity conducting clinical trial [23, 24]. The main activity of the DSMB/DMC is to protect patient safety. The DSMB/DMC serves as an advisory body, responsible for the oversight of the activities related to the clinical trial and more specifically, the monitoring of safety and conduct to ensure patient safety, adherence to the clinical protocol, overall performance of the study, including study officer, coordinating centre, clinical sites, and integrity of the data being collected. The committee also ensures that safety monitoring is carried out while maintaining the blinding of the trial so that the trial remains valid.

The composition of the DSMB/DMC consists of at least one independent statistician and clinicians who have sufficient knowledge about the disease indication and major suspected safety effects, as well as ethicists or representatives from patient advocacy group, especially for trials involving vulnerable populations.

DSMB/DMC is indicated by the clinical and safety departments in the following situations:

- If the trial is intended to provide definitive information about effectiveness and/or safety of a medical intervention.
- If there are prior data to suggest that the intervention being studied has the potential to induce potentially unacceptable toxicity.
- If the trial is evaluating mortality or another major endpoint, such that inferiority of one treatment arm has safety as well as effectiveness implications.
- If there are questions of ethical importance for the trial to stop early, if the primary question addressed has been definitively answered, even if secondary questions or complete safety information were not yet fully addressed.

It is generally expected by the clinical and safety department that a DSMB/DMC will be needed in the following situations:

- All Phase III studies require a DSMB, with the exception of low-risk behavioural and nutritional studies.
- Multi-centre randomised Phase II clinical trials require a DSMB, with the exception of low-risk behavioural and nutritional studies.
- Phase II studies which are "high risk" require a DSMB. In this context, high risk is usually referred to trials or interventions that are associated with substantial adverse effects that are usually serious and could result in serious morbidity or death.
- For some studies involving particularly vulnerable study participants (e.g. children or persons with impaired ability to consent), it may be beneficial to utilise a DSMB as an additional measure of subject protection.

A DSMB/DMC is not generally needed in the following situations:

- Single-centre open-label Phase I and II clinical trials generally do not need a DSMB since the local investigator will have access to all data.
- A multi-centre, high-risk Phase I clinical trial should not require a DSMB if there are very clear rules for stopping the trial. For example, a DSMB is generally not required for a classic open-label dose escalation trial with clear and objective criteria for halting the dose escalation when unacceptable side effects are observed.
- A DSMB may not be feasible for clinical trials that are expected to accrue too quickly to allow for a DSMB to be constituted and complete data and safety monitoring.

The role of DSMBs/DMCs is of importance for both industry-sponsored and investigator-initiated trials due to the increasing number of industry-sponsored trials with mortality and major morbidity endpoints.

7 Types of Safety Data That Should Generally Be Collected Under All Circumstances

For detailed analysis of the event that is received, the following types of events/data, comprehensive details should generally be provided to allow adequate assessment of the event/data, e.g. history, associated AEs, relevant underlying disease of the patient, laboratory values, concomitant medications, vital signs, and/or follow-up outcome. The following information detailed below are also required for complete assessment of products in clinical development [19].

1. Deaths
2. SAEs
3. Significant AEs that led to an intervention, including withdrawal or dose reduction of IMP or addition of concomitant therapy
4. Marked laboratory abnormalities (other than those meeting the definition of serious)
5. Overdose
6. Pregnancies
7. AEs of special interest (if defined). These AEs may warrant collection of additional information across the entire study population to better characterise these events (e.g. particular laboratory parameters, vital signs, risk factors, concomitant therapies, and/or concomitant illnesses). For example, if gastrointestinal haemorrhage was an AE of special interest, one might want to proactively collect concomitant antithrombotic therapy across the entire study population
8. Laboratory data, vital signs, electrocardiograms of special interest (if defined)

Sponsors should be aware that the following types of data are generally not appropriate for selective safety data collection and should always be collected:

- Data on all SAEs
- Data on non-SAEs that lead to dose modification, drug discontinuation, or withdrawal from the trial

- Data on unscheduled study visits, hospitalisations, and accidental injuries because these events may reflect SAEs of the drug
- In an oncology setting, data from all Grade 3 and Grade 4 AEs, as well as Grade 2 AEs that affect vital organs (e.g. heart, liver)
- Pregnancy data

7.1 Selective Safety Data Collection Considerations

Selective safety data collection is considered for studies using lower doses and/or shorter durations than in previous studies. Selective safety data collection would generally not be acceptable if higher doses and/or longer treatment durations than previously studied are planned.

When sponsors choose to implement selective safety data collection for a clinical study, a scientific justification should be provided. Factors that contribute to a determination that selective safety data collection would be appropriate include the following:

- The medicinal product has received marketing authorisation from a regulatory authority for the indication under investigation.
- Availability of post-approval safety data and findings.
- The dose, dosing regimen, dosage form, route of administration and treatment duration used in the previously conducted studies are comparable to the planned use of the drug in the proposed study.
- The patient population from previously conducted studies is representative of subjects in the planned study regarding demographic characteristics, underlying medical conditions, concomitant drugs, and other important factors (e.g. Cytochrome P450 enzymes (CYP) metaboliser status).
- Exposure in previously conducted (or ongoing, if applicable) studies that contribute to the overall safety database, i.e. number exposure to drug, treatment duration
- Consistency of the safety profile across previous studies.
- Characteristics of previous studies, e.g. study design, study conduct, adequacy of safety monitoring/safety data collection, availability of protocols, statistical analysis plan, and/or access to data.
- Knowledge of the mechanism of action of the medicinal product under study.
- Knowledge of the safety profile of approved drugs in the same pharmacologic class.

In the pre-approval setting, selective safety data collection may be justifiable if sufficient safety data are available from completed studies. Furthermore, when sufficient safety data becomes available from one or more ongoing late-stage study(ies), selective safety data collection may be appropriate for a concurrently conducted study-initiated pre-approval.

7.1.1 Examples Where Selective Safety Data Collection May Be Considered

Selective safety data collection may be appropriate in studies used to evaluate some of the following objectives. These are not the only circumstances where selective safety data collection may be appropriate.

- New indications of approved drugs
- To study additional endpoints, e.g. patient-reported outcome for symptomatic improvement, quality of life, and/or outcome studies (e.g. mortality, morbidity, and/or specific safety issues)
- To study comparative effectiveness/efficacy
- Demonstration of superiority when non-inferiority has been demonstrated
- Characterisation of AEs of special interest
- Fulfilment of post-approval requirements, post-authorisation safety studies based on data collection from registries or electronic health records
- Late-stage premarketing outcome study in a large population

7.2 Types of Safety Data Where It May Be Appropriate to Limit or Stop Collection

- Non-SAEs
- Routine laboratory tests
- Information on concomitant medications
- Physical examinations (including vital signs)
- Electrocardiograms

7.3 Collection of Safety Data for Clinical Trials in Rare Diseases

For drug development studies for rare disease indications, complete safety data should be collected because these trials generally have limited patient populations and are unlikely to meet the recommendations for selective safety data collection. For these types of safety data, it is generally important to collect information on all occurrences to better understand the following:

- Causality
- Incidence
- Severity of AEs
- Populations that are at risk
- Dose–response
- Other factors that contribute to our understanding of the nature of the event and who is at risk

8 Safety Data Output(s) Originating from Clinical Trials

8.1 Integrated Safety Summary

At the end of a clinical development programme for a medicinal product, sponsors are required to summarise the safety information from all clinical trials for submission to the regulatory authorities along with the marketing registration application. Detailed analyses of integrated data of multiple studies from several treatment arms of a clinical development programme are required to identify safety signals that may not be detected in individual trials. Integrated Safety Summary (ISS) is required for regulatory submission in applications submitted to the FDA and other regulatory authorities in accordance with the regulations for New Drug Applications (NDA) submissions (21 CFR 314.50(d)(5)(v) and 21 CFR 314.50(d)(5)(vi)(a), respectively) [25]. The Clinical Trial Directive (CTD)/electronic CTD (eCTD) Module 2 contains several clinical sections that include the summaries of ISS.

ISS is defined as a section of the NDA that provides comprehensive safety data information collected throughout the drug development process. ISS is the most important safety data output from all the clinical trials from various treatment arms in the drug development process and a team consisting of regulatory affairs, pharmacovigilance safety physicians and scientists, biostatisticians, data managers, and medical writers are involved in writing the report. The ultimate goal of the ISS is to characterise the overall safety profile of the drug and to identify risks that should be included on the Reference Safety Information (RSI) or the product label. The ISS-related sections with corresponding regulations are reported in Table 7.4 [25].

The aim of the ISS is to provide an overall analysis and summary of the safety data arising from the various treatment arms of the clinical development programme. The following are the key elements in an ISS, as detailed below:

- A summary of the safety profiles from all clinical studies and assessment of summaries and statistical analysis of safety data collected from various clinical studies (can include Phase I studies in healthy volunteers; normally presented separately from study patients).
- AEs
  - Overall analysis of AEs including event rates, deaths, adverse dropouts, and other potentially serious events.

Table 7.4 Integrated safety summary-related sections with corresponding regulations

CTD section	US Regulation	Comment
2.5 Clinical Overview 2.5.5 Overview of Safety	N/A	Not a US requirement, but recommended by ICH M4E
2.7 Clinical Summary 2.7.4 Summary of Clinical Safety	21 CFR 314.50(c)(2)(viii)	US requirement for a clinical summary
5.3 Clinical Study Reports 5.3.5.3 Reports of Analyses of Data from More than One Study (Including Any Formal Integrated Analyses, Meta Analyses, and Bridging Analyses)	21CFR 314.50(d)(5)(vi)	Integrated summary of safety

- Evaluation of AE effects in various subgroups of the variable patient base including impact of concomitant medications' safety and efficacy.
- Analysis of adverse effects relating to dose–response information—this includes any evidence of dose–response variations relating to age, sex, or any other subpopulations
  - Drug–drug, drug–demographic, and drug–disease interactions
  - Any other pharmacologic properties—including effects on liver, kidneys, etc.
  - Long-term adverse effects and withdrawal effects
- The extent of exposure—the number of patients exposed (by gender and other demographic subgroups) and number exposed to various doses for defined durations.
- Demographic and other characteristics of study population—age, gender, race, body weight, primary and secondary outcomes, and other relevant prognostic variables.
- Laboratory assessments.
- Summary of animal data important to human safety.

In an ISS, for analysis of the AEs, it must clearly define the treatment-emergent adverse events (TEAE) consistently across studies. It is important to specify the analysis rules used to identify TEAE. Also, the analysis rules for assigning AEs in crossover studies (e.g. an AE that occurs during washout between treatment periods 1 and 2) should be specified and stay as consistent as possible with individual study analyses. Finally, it is necessary to clearly specify all analysis rules in the ISS, statistical analysis plan, so regulatory agencies can provide input on the proposed approach ahead of time.

9 Aggregate Safety Data in Clinical Development and Timelines for Submissions to Regulatory Authorities

9.1 Development Safety Update Report

A Development Safety Update Report (DSUR) is a premarketing aggregate periodic report that covers safety information of drugs, biological, vaccines, and combination products under development (including marketed drugs that are under further study) among the ICH regions [26].

DSURs are internationally harmonised, safety documents which became mandatory in EU member states in September 2011. It covers the safety summary of medicinal products during their development or clinical trial phase.

The DSUR format replaced the previous EU Annual Safety Report (EU-ASR) and the United States IND Annual Report and is based heavily on the Periodic Safety Update Report (PSUR) format that is used for post-marketing products.

The main objective of a DSUR is to present a comprehensive annual review and evaluation of pertinent safety information collected during the reporting period related to a drug under investigation, whether or not it is marketed, by:

- Examining whether the information obtained by the sponsor during the reporting period is in accord with previous knowledge of the investigational drug's safety.

- Describing new safety issues that could have an impact on the protection of clinical trial subjects.
- Summarising the current understanding and management of identified and potential risks.
- Providing an update on the status of the clinical investigation/development programme and study results.

A DSUR should be concise and provide information to assure regulators that sponsors are adequately monitoring and evaluating the evolving safety profile of the investigational drug. All safety issues obtained during the reporting period should be discussed in the DSUR; however, it should not be used to provide the initial notification of significant new safety information or provide how new safety issues are detected.

9.1.1 DSUR Reporting and Submission Timelines

Sponsors are required to submit a DSUR within 1 year of the Development International Birth Date (DIBD)—the date of first authorisation of a clinical trial in any country worldwide and provide annual DSUR submissions until all open clinical studies have ended (the final clinical study is completed, and its study report has been submitted). Thus, the DIBD is used to determine the start of the annual reporting period for the DSUR. The data lock point of the DSUR is the last day of the 1-year reporting period. The start of the annual period for the DSUR is the month and date of the DIBD. The DSUR is submitted to all applicable regulatory competent authorities in countries where the trial is being conducted and approving Research Ethics Committes (RECs) no later than 60 calendar days after the DSUR data lock point. A DSUR must be submitted during every 12-month reporting period until the End of Trial Notification has been submitted to the competent authority of the member state where the trial is being conducted.

9.1.2 Reference Safety Information Used for DSUR

From start of the reporting period, the IB serves as the Reference Safety Information (RSI) to determine whether the information received during the reporting period remains consistent with previous knowledge of the safety profile of the investigational drug. Section 7.1 of the DSUR should clearly indicate the version number and date of the IB used for this purpose. The IB is a compilation of the clinical and non-clinical data on the investigational drug that are relevant to the study of the drug in human subjects. When an IB is not required by national or regional laws or regulations, the applicable national or regional product label serves as the RSI. Usually, a single document should serve as the RSI, but in certain circumstances, it might be appropriate to use more than one reference document to support the DSUR (e.g. for a DSUR providing information on an investigational drug used in combination and as monotherapy) [26].

If the IB has been revised during the reporting period and not previously submitted to the relevant regulatory authority, the sponsor should provide a copy of the current version of the IB as an attachment to the DSUR. If the IB or Summary of Product Characteristics (SmPC) has been revised during the reporting period, the sponsor should provide a copy of the current version of the IB or SmPC as an attachment to the DSUR, listing any significant safety-related changes in the relevant section of the DSUR. Despite the change in the RSI, the RSI in effect at the start of the reporting period serves as the RSI during the reporting period.

10 Signal Detection and Data Management in Clinical Trials

Signal detection and data management is an important activity that takes place continuously throughout the entire life cycle of the drug development process, where related and not related AEs to drugs are anticipated during drug development programmes. An increase of AEs associated with a product's use compared with the expected rate is referred to as a safety signal. Signals are detected at any time during the lifespan of a drug, from the pre-clinical phase through the post-marketing phase.

An important factor in signal detection for a medicinal product during the premarketing period is the availability of denominator data and the ability to compare AE incidence rates between two or more selected populations. This is possible due to structured data collection under strictly controlled conditions in accordance with GCP. The blinding of investigators and study subjects to therapy assignment in randomised controlled studies also helps reduce bias in ascertaining AEs. This contrasts with spontaneous reporting systems during post-marketing period, which rely on spontaneous reports where the quality of data received are not complete. A detailed discussion of evaluating safety from clinical trials, and identification of emerging safety signals, is included in the report of CIOMS Working Group VI (Management of Safety Information from Clinical Trials) [27].

There are several methodologies for detecting signals in clinical trials. These include quantitative signal detection, which is most useful on large pivotal studies or pooled studies, and qualitative methods, which remain the basis of signal detection in early stages. Signal detection methods are ranked according to their performance with regard to positive predictive value (PPV), specificity, and sensitivity [28]. The EMA has published scientific guidance on routine signal detection methods in EudraVigilance for use by the agency, national competent authorities, and Marketing Authorisation Holders (MAHs).

CIOMS VI includes the following key sources of new safety information:

1. Evaluation of serious individual case safety reports.
2. Periodic aggregate assessment of available clinical safety data (including clinical AEs and laboratory parameters) without regard to seriousness or causality.
3. Evaluation of unblinded studies including individual study results and pooled analyses where appropriate.

While randomised clinical trial data are generally thought to accrue from the pre-approval period, there is often a substantial body of randomised clinical trial safety data that accumulates after approval. The data from both pre- and post-approval randomised clinical trials can be pooled in a cumulative meta-analysis to understand the previously unrecognised ADRs that the pre-approval human safety database was unable to detect because of insufficient sample size due to the lack of adequate statistical power.

11 Clinical Trials Safety Data Reconciliation

As already discussed, SAE information is continuously collected throughout the life cycle of the clinical trials. Usually, SAEs are captured in two different databases—a clinical database that includes the AE information recorded in the CRFs and a safety database that contains information collected on the SAE form and their respective follow-ups. It is a challenge to continuously match these two databases, making sure that the information pertaining to the SAEs collected during the clinical trial, particularly at the time of study database lock, does not impact the data quality, operations performance, and compliance. The parallel processing of SAEs in two different databases may create discrepancies that need to be clarified and reconciled before the clinical database is locked.

Reconciliation is therefore defined as a process of comparing key safety data variables between the drug or device safety SAE database and the clinical database in order to identify any discrepancy, determine whether a discrepancy is acceptable or not and, if acceptable, document the discrepancy [29]. It is an iterative process and an important activity that occurs regularly throughout and during the entire study. The timeline for reconciliation is determined by the frequency of data receipt, scheduling of safety updates, and timing of interim and final reports. The objective is to reconcile all discrepancies before final clinical database lock to submit validated data to regulatory authorities.

The SAE reconciliation process is undertaken on a periodic basis, where data is reviewed in the clinical database and compared with the corresponding records in the safety database. Several departments are involved in this activity, including drug safety and clinical research departments, but also data management and clinical operations. During the reconciliation process, verbatim descriptions, coding terms, treatment and event onset/resolution dates, causality assessment, seriousness criteria, SAE outcome, and other information that is found to be different are first matched and then corrected. Based on each company's standards and processes, the discrepancies are resolved and corrected in either dataset before the clinical database lock at the end of the trial. Therefore, a mismatch between the safety database and clinical database is identified during the reconciliation process. A discrepancy can be for example:

- SAE present in one database but missing in the other one
- Inconsistent SAE associated data between the databases
- Mismatched SAE preferred term

Once the discrepancies are identified, actions are then taken to address the discrepancies, and the status relevant to the action taken are recorded in the SAE manual or electronic reconciliation tool. The SAE data listing is generally in Excel format and is used to review and document all the discrepancies found during SAE data reconciliation.

After the database has been corrected and updated, the evidence of SAE reconciliation and the resulting outcome is documented and filed in the Trial Master File (TMF) for future inspection by health authorities.

12 Clinical Trial Safety Data Integrity

As clinical trial methodologies and new technologies are deployed, data integrity, and the safety of clinical trial participants remain at the forefront of regulatory oversight. Officials from the US FDA and the UK MHRA have written an article published in *Clinical Pharmacology & Therapeutics* [30], on this topic.

Data integrity as defined by the WHO "is the degree to which data are complete, consistent, accurate, trustworthy and reliable". The data in good practice environments is collected and maintained in a secure manner, so that they are attributable, legible, contemporaneously recorded, original (or a true copy), and accurate.

In the USA, the FDA uses the ALCOA acronym [31] to define expectations with respect to data integrity as stated below:

- Accurate: Recorded data should be correct, complete, valid, reliable, and free from errors.
- Legible: The record that is created, especially paper-based records should be legible, should be permanent, and not erasable so that they are reliable throughout the data life cycle.
- Contemporaneous: The evidence of actions, events, or decisions should be recorded as it is generated.
- Original: The record should be a true copy, and the data is to be used or presented as it was created.
- Attributable: The evidence or every piece of data entered into the record must be capable of being traced back to the person collecting the data.

12.1 Ensuring and Monitoring Data Integrity in Clinical Trials

To ensure that the data that is collected is fit for purpose, data is monitored by keeping a close eye on the following areas:

- Source data verification (SDV)
- Validation of computer systems supporting data collection, data processing, data reporting, etc.
- Data access and control
- Training of personnel involved in data collection, data processors, analysts, site staff, and report writers
- Data monitoring: onsite, centralised, and risk-based monitoring
- Clinical trial quality assurance and quality control: ensuring vendors and Contract Research Organisations (CROs) have efficient quality management system in place with Standard Operating Procedures (SOPs) and controlled records

As clinical trials become more complex and multinational, involving multiple sites vendor protecting the data becomes immensely critical. Collection of accurate clinical trial data is essential for compliance with good clinical practice (ICH GCP E6 R2), regulatory compliance (FDA-21 CFR part 11, EMA, etc.), and clinical research ethical principles [31]. Worldwide regulatory authorities, especially the FDA and EMA, are particularly interested in ensuring data integrity in clinical trials to maintain their ability to not only accurately evaluate safety and efficacy of the medical product that is in clinical development but also protect the patient and the public, as a lack of acceptable data integrity practices in clinical research can lead to serious regulatory and financial consequences.

In October 2018, FDA and MHRA held their first joint GCP workshop to discuss data integrity in clinic trials. Several examples were cited by the FDA and MHRA on data integrity issues, including data integrity issues in some of the largest biopharma companies. A joint article written by the FDA and MHRA cited several concerns with audit trails, blinding, and data management in addition to sponsor oversight of electronic systems and electronic health records used at sites, electronic source data, protocol deviations and management of these deviations, and novel clinical trial designs and the challenges in ensuring the quality and reliability of study data [30].

13 Summary and Conclusions

Patient safety monitoring is a critical component of the drug development process. The main objective of collecting safety data from clinical trials is the early detection of important safety signals to protect subjects in clinical trials and provide information about new risks, assess the potential risk to future patients, and develop safety profile/product label of the drug contributing to its benefit–risk assessment.

Safety data, obtained from ongoing clinical trials, has a direct effect on the safety and clinical care of research subjects enrolled in these trials. The ultimate goal of safety signal detection in clinical trials is to translate clinically significant safety information to the product label under development and protect research subjects from experiencing ADRs. The last few decades have changed the regulatory landscape of safety data monitoring in clinical trials and the guidelines issued by regulatory authorities specifically for the collection of appropriate safety data during clinical trials, documentation and reporting of serious events have made a significant impact to ensure the safety of clinical trial subjects. With the advent of new technology and artificial intelligence, it remains to be seen if there can be a harmonised and structured way of data collection and analysis worldwide that would be acceptable to the regulatory authorities that would help detect early safety signals from the enhanced safety data, thus protecting the trial subjects and patients from serious risks.

14 Case Studies

Clinical trial AEs referred to as safety data are required to be collected in all clinical trials. The data collected consists of non-SAEs and SAEs and are collected separately as two separate data sets. One dataset collected by the data management team consists of both non-SAEs and SAEs, while the safety database managed by the pharmacovigilance/drug safety team comprises of SAEs only. The safety analysis is conducted using only the AE dataset from the data management which has all safety events reported in the clinical trial.

14.1 Case Study 1: Clinical Trial Data Review for Risk of Respiratory Adverse Events for Treatment of Hepatorenal Syndrome

A pharmaceutical company evaluates clinical trial data for the treatment of Hepatorenal Syndrome to determine why a drug was linked to a high number of respiratory AEs.

Literature search for articles on the active moiety were conducted as the product was marketed in countries outside of the USA as well of the EudraVigilance database for AEs reported in the post-marketing arena. A dataset was created for all respiratory-reported AEs by standardising the MedDRA coding with the AEs reported in the clinical trials in the respiratory system organ classification (SOC). A combined dataset of all unique safety events (whether reported in the post-marketed or clinical trial dataset) was created and safety analyses re-performed. To evaluate if these were true ADRs, all data from time to onset of the AE, to start and stop date of the AEs, concomitant medications, medical history had to be determined to assess if the injury was causally related to the drug.

In-depth analysis of the post-marketing data showed that there was an increase in the respiratory disorders in patients with decompensated cirrhosis and the clinical safety data showed that the subjects that experienced respiratory failure had a history of cardiorespiratory, recent upper GI haemorrhage, or increasing hepatic encephalopathy, and it was advised that the drug should be used with caution in these patients.

1. *What are the major lessons learnt from the above case study?*

   Pharmacovigilance personnel need to gather literature articles and ICSRs for health authority databases for a marketed product used for other indications and determine if the product is being used off-label and if yes, is it the indication of interest. This needs to be performed earlier on in the clinical trial.

2. *What significant data was obtained from in-depth analysis of post-marketing and clinical safety data and what safety measure was taken with the obtained data?*

   Post-marketing data demonstrated an increase in respiratory disorders in patients with decompensated cirrhosis. Clinical trial data identified history of cardiorespiratory disorders, recent GI haemorrhage, or increasing hepatic encephalopathy as the potential predisposing factors for the development of respiratory disorders as an adverse effect in the patients on the drug in question.

14.2 Case Study 2: Clinical Trial Data Review for Risk of Lung Cancer with Inhaled Insulin

A small pharmaceutical company evaluating an inhaled drug/device combination product consisting of Technosphere insulin powder (known as TI), the inhaler, and the cartridges containing TI. TI consists of recombinant human insulin and fumaryl diketopiperazine (FDKP an inert excipient). The insulin powder particles are adsorbed onto uniform-sized (approximately 2 μm) carrier Technosphere particles that contain mostly crystallised FDKP and when inhaled, the Technosphere particles carry the insulin into the alveoli where the particles dissolve. The insulin and the FDPK are rapidly absorbed across the alveolar walls independently of each other, leading to insulin uptake into the blood stream faster than that of any other approved insulin.

The risk of lung cancer was raised as a safety concern to the use of inhaled insulin. In the registration trials, two heavy smokers developed lung cancer—one while in a controlled comparative clinical trial and one while in an extension. Pharmacoepidemiology was the safety tool used to compare the frequency risks in the general patient population with lung malignancies to the patient population in the clinical trials. The results showed that incidence of lung cancer (0.8 cases per 1000 patient-years) was felt by the company to be within the range of lung cancer observed in the general population (approximately 0.23–1.22 cases per 1000 patient-years, according to the American Lung Association).

1. *What are the major lessons learnt from the above-mentioned case?*

   The incidence rate of the AE of interest in the clinical trial vs. incidence rate of the AE of interest in the general patient population needs to be determined proactively to mitigate any risks seen in the trial. If there is an imbalance where the risk is associated with the drug, the pharmacovigilance team can then proactively mitigate the risk by putting a strategy in place for a successful filing.

References

1. Medicine and Healthcare products Regulatory Agency. NIBSC. TGN1412 – learning from a clinical trials disaster. https://www.nibsc.org/about_us/world-wide_impact/tgn1412.aspx.
2. Gibb F. Victim Ryan Wilson in "elephant man" drug trial to get £2m. The Times, London. 2008.
3. Expert Group on Phase One Clinical Trials. Final report. 2006. https://webarchive.nationalarchives.gov.uk/ukgwa/+/dh.gov.uk/en/publicationsandstatistics/publications/publicationspolicyandguidance/dh_063117.
4. Medicines and Healthcare Products Regulatory Agency (MHRA). Clinical trial suspension: latest findings, 5 Apr 2006. https://www.ema.europa.eu/en/news/first-man-clinical-trials-guideline-released-public-consultation. http://www.mhra.gov.uk/NewsCentre/Pressreleases/CON2023515.
5. WHO International Drug Monitoring Centre (Uppsala, Sweden), Edwards IR, et al. Harmonisation in pharmacovigilance. Drug Saf. 1994;10(2):93–102.
6. Regulation (EU) No. 536/2014 of the European Parliament and of the council of 16 April 2014 on clinical trials on medicinal products for human use, and repealing Directive 2001/20/EC.
7. Medicines and Healthcare products Regulatory Agency. Clinical trials for medicines: apply for authorisation in the UK. 2014. https://www.gov.uk/guidance/clinical-trials-for-medicines-apply-for-authorisation-in-the-uk.
8. Center for Drug Evaluation and Research (CDER). Investigator responsibilities–safety reporting for investigational drugs and devices. 2021. https://www.fda.gov/regulatory-information/search-fda-guidance-documents/investigator-responsibilities-safety-reporting-investigational-drugs-and-devices.
9. Government of Canada. Adverse drug reactions (ADR) reporting. https://www.canada.ca/en/health-canada/services/drugs-health-products/drug-products/applications-submissions/guidance-documents/clinical-trials/post-authorization-requirements.html#adr.
10. U.S. Department of Health and Human Services. Guidance for industry and investigators safety reporting requirements for INDs and BA/BE studies. 2012. https://www.fda.gov/files/drugs/published/Safety-Reporting-Requirements-for-INDs-%28Investigational-New-Drug-Applications%29-and-BA-BE-%28Bioavailability-Bioequivalence%29-Studies.pdf.
11. Pharmaceutical Regulations in Japan. Pharmaceutical Laws and Regulations (Chapter 12). 2020. https://www.jpma.or.jp/english/about/parj/eki4g6000000784o-att/2020e_ch02.pdf.
12. Ministerial Ordinance on Good clinical practice for drugs. https://www.pmda.go.jp/files/000152996.pdf.
13. Song H, Pei X, Liu Z, Shen C, Liu Y, Zhou L, Sun F, Xiao X, Sun J. Pharmacovigilance in China: Evolution and future challenges. Br J Clin Pharmacol. 2023;89:510–22.
14. Central Drugs Standard Control Organisation. Good clinical practices for clinical research in India. 2001. Available from: http://cdsco.nic.in/html/GCP.htm.
15. Central Drugs Standard Control Organisation. Schedule Y (Amended version). 2005. Available from: http://cdsco.nic.in/html/GCP1.html.
16. International conference on harmonization of technical requirements for registration of pharmaceuticals for human use. Development safety update report E2F. 2010. Available from: http://www.ich.org/LOB/media/MEDIA4727.pdf.
17. European Commission. Detailed guidance on the collection, verification and presentation of adverse reaction reports arising from clinical trials on medicinal products for human use. 2006. Available from: http://ec.europa.eu/health/files/eudralex/vol-10/21_susar_rev2_2006_04_11_en.pdf.
18. National Health and Medical Research Council. Guidance: safety monitoring and reporting in clinical trials involving therapeutic goods. 2016. https://www.nhmrc.gov.au/sites/default/files/images/NHMRC-guidance-safety-monitoring-and-reporting.pdf.
19. European Medicines Agency. ICH guideline E19 on a selective approach to safety data collection in specific late-stage pre-approval or post-approval clinical trials. 2022. https://www.ema.europa.eu/en/ich-guideline-e19-optimisation-safety-data-collection-step-2b.
20. European Medicines Agency. Clinical safety data management: definitions and standards for expedited reporting. 1995. https://www.ema.europa.eu/en/documents/scientific-guideline/international-conference-harmonisation-technical-requirements-registration-pharmaceuticals-human-use_en-15.pdf.
21. U.S. Department of Health and Human Services. Guidance for industry: computerized systems used in clinical investigations. 2007. https://www.fda.gov/files/drugs/published/Guidance-for-Industry%2D%2DComputerized-Systems-Used-in-Clinical-Investigations.pdf.
22. Monaghan TF, Agudelo CW, Rahman SN, Wein AJ, Lazar JM, Everaert K, Dmochowski RR. Blinding in clinical trials: seeing the big picture. Medicina. 2021;57:647. https://doi.org/10.3390/medicina57070647.
23. National Institute on Deafness and Other Communication Disorders (NIDCD). NIDCD guidelines for data and safety monitoring of clinical trials. https://www.nidcd.nih.gov/research/clinical-studies/nidcd-guidelines-data-and-safety-monitoring-clinical-trials.
24. Ellenberg SS, Fleming TR, DeMets DL. Data monitoring committees in clinical trials: a practical perspective. Chichester: John Wiley; 2002. Also, see Ellenberg, S.S. Independent data monitoring com-

mittees: rationale, operations and controversies. Stat Med. 20:2573–2583, 2001.
25. Center for Drug Evaluation and Research. Integrated summaries of effectiveness and safety: location within the common technical document. 2009. https://www.fda.gov/regulatory-information/search-fda-guidance-documents/integrated-summaries-effectiveness-and-safety-location-within-common-technical-document.
26. European Medicines Agency. ICH guideline E2F on development safety update report. 2011. https://www.ema.europa.eu/en/documents/scientific-guideline/international-conference-harmonisation-technical-requirements-registration-pharmaceuticals-human-use_en-26.pdf.
27. Council for International Organizations of Medical Sciences. Management of safety information from clinical trials—report of CIOMS working group VI. 2005. https://cioms.ch/wp-content/uploads/2017/01/Mgment_Safety_Info.pdf.
28. Spontaneous reporting systems and pharmacovigilance. WHO programme perspective. imi-protect.eu.
29. Burnstead B, Furlan G. Unifying drug safety and clinical databases. Curr Drug Saf. 2013;8(1):56–62. https://doi.org/10.2174/15748863113080l0008.
30. Khin NA, Francis G, Mulinde J, Grandinetti C, Skeete R, Yu B, Ayalew K, Cho S-J, Fisher A, Kleppinger C, Ayala R, Bonapace C, Dasgupta A, Kronstein PD, Vinter S. Data integrity in global clinical trials: discussions from Joint US Food and Drug Administration and UK Medicines and Healthcare Products Regulatory Agency Good Clinical Practice Workshop. Clin Pharmacol Ther. 2020;108(5):949–63.
31. U.S. Department of Health and Human Services. Data integrity and compliance with CGMP guidance for industry. 2016. https://www.fda.gov/files/drugs/published/Data-Integrity-and-Compliance-With-Current-Good-Manufacturing-Practice-Guidance-for-Industry.pdf.

8 Causality Assessment in Pharmacovigilance

Madhan Ramesh and Anand Harugeri

Abstract

Causality assessment is an essential component of, and routine procedure in, any pharmacovigilance system. Establishing a causal relationship between the suspected drug and the adverse event is a complex process and should consider both patient- and medication-related factors. There are three broad approaches, or categories, of causality assessment adopted for establishing causation in pharmacovigilance. The methods adopted to assess the causal relationship generally consider a few criteria in common. There are multiple criteria or algorithms available for establishing a causal relationship in cases of adverse events. The causality assessment tools help clinicians in identifying the culprit drugs. Establishing a causal relationship is important to incorporate the individual case safety reports in benefit–harm analysis, identification of new adverse drug reactions, and regulatory decision-making process. Causality assessment is a continuous process and has wider applications across various fields including academic research, clinical practice, sponsored clinical research, and regulatory activity. Therefore, knowledge of its applications, and associated challenges, is important in enabling stakeholders to play their role at all levels to improve patient safety.

Keywords

Causality assessment · Causality assessment algorithms · Pharmacovigilance · Adverse drug reactions · Adverse events · Artificial intelligence

Learning Objectives

- Understand the importance and basic principles of causality assessment.
- Describe the categories of causality assessment.
- Apply various methods of causality assessment.
- Understand the clinical, industry, and regulatory perspectives of causality assessment.
- Appreciate the applications of causality assessment.

M. Ramesh (✉)
Department of Pharmacy Practice, JSS College of Pharmacy, JSS Academy of Higher Education & Research, Mysuru, Karnataka, India
e-mail: mramesh@jssuni.edu.in

A. Harugeri
PV Projects Leadership and Strategic Solutions, Lifecycle Safety, IQVIA RDS Inc., Durham, NC, USA

J. Jose et al. (eds.), *Principles and Practice of Pharmacovigilance and Drug Safety*,
https://doi.org/10.1007/978-3-031-51089-2_8

Key Points

- Causality assessment is one of the essential elements and challenging aspects of pharmacovigilance.
- Causality in pharmacovigilance should be viewed considering both patient-related and medication-related factors.
- WHO probability scale and Naranjo's algorithm are widely accepted and used across the globe.
- Pharmaceutical industry uses structured causality assessment methods for individual case safety reports to facilitate case processing.
- Causality assessment is important for inclusion of reports into benefit–harm analysis, identification of new adverse drug reactions, and regulatory decision-making process.
- Although causal association is established, there exists some degree of uncertainty.
- There is a need to develop a high-quality assessment tool which can meticulously, accurately, and consistently establish suitable diagnostic criteria for adverse drug reactions with universal acceptance.

1 Introduction

Adverse drug reactions (ADRs) are inevitable in clinical practice and if unrecognised and not adequately managed may cause prolonged harm, additional medical costs, and hospitalisation or prolongation of hospitalisation. As ADRs can mimic naturally occurring disease process, it is often difficult to distinguish them from the patient's disease condition. Nevertheless, early detection of ADRs is important in their management and to minimise the human sufferings. Epidemiological studies have reported that ADRs are an important cause of morbidity, hospital admission, and even death [1–4]. Establishing a relationship likelihood (causal association) for case reports of suspected ADRs is important for decision-making at a regulatory and clinical level. Although the term 'adverse event' (AE) and 'adverse drug reaction' are often used interchangeably in clinical practice, the term adverse event refers to reported safety information, mainly in clinical trials, where the causality may or may not exist. If causality is established, then these events are termed as an ADR. Causality assessment is an essential component and routine procedure in pharmacovigilance system. Causality assessment is a standardised method for establishing the causal relationship between suspect drug and observed adverse event. It contributes to the assessment of pharmacovigilance signals, better knowledge of benefit–harm profiles of medicines, and regulatory decision-making process. In clinical settings, it is useful in understanding the possible causal relationship between the drug and the event and accordingly deciding the future course of action. Recognising ADRs at their early stage of manifestations and establishing a likelihood relationship between the drug and the adverse event in order help ensure early and proactive management to avoid further, or more serious, adverse consequences [5, 6].

2 Importance of Causality Assessment

Causality assessment aims to reduce data ambiguity and plays a role in data exchange and preventing erroneous conclusions. This is especially of significance when reports are submitted to a pharmacovigilance system since it aids in the regulatory decision-making process. Use of standardised causality assessment system in clinical practice may also reduce the ambiguity in the process of evaluation of ADRs. Furthermore, causality assessment contributes to the efficient evaluation of the benefit–harm profile of the drug and serves as an essential part of evaluating ADR reports in early warning systems and for regulatory reporting purposes [7]. In regular clinical practice, it is an important element to understand the possible causal relationship between the observed adverse event and the suspected drug/s. Causality assessment of ADRs supports prevention and management of ADRs, aids in differential diagnosis, helps manage patient's drug therapy including dosage adjustments, and helps to identify interacting drugs [8].

3 Stages of Data Assessment

In assessing the causality, there are two important issues that need to be addressed. First, is there a convincing relationship between the drug and the event? And second, did the drug cause the event? During clinical research, as well as from the perspective of industry or regulatory agencies during regular use of drugs, the assessment of reported adverse event can happen in two stages. The first stage is the assessment of the individual case safety report (ICSR) that is usually carried out soon after the event is reported and is assessed on case-to-case basis, whereas the second stage is the interpretation of aggregated data and is adopted during the benefit–harm analysis and signal detection process [7]. This kind of assessment is an integral part of the work of regulatory authorities and marketing authorisation holders and helps in identifying new ADRs, therefore in getting a better knowledge of medicines' safety profile. For a healthcare professional facing an individual patient with an adverse event, it can be difficult to make a proper assessment of causality. However, it is important to try to confirm the suspicion of causality, as it could be crucial for patient management to withdraw a suspected medicine/adjust the dose and start an appropriate treatment in a timely manner.

4 Basic Criteria/Principles of Causality Assessment

In clinical practice, the methods adopted to assess the causal relationship generally consider few criteria in common [9–11]. These include the following.

4.1 Complete Knowledge of Clinical Event

The knowledge of reported adverse event should encompass complete description of event rather limiting to the specifics of nature of event.

4.2 Patient's Medical and Medication History

The patient medical history should include chief complaints, history of present illness, review of systems, relevant past medication and vaccination history, as well as family, social, and allergy history. Medication history should encompass the complete dosing regimen details of all current and recently prescribed medications, any over-the-counter (OTC) medications including herbal or alternative medicines, and details on adherence to therapy.

4.3 Temporal Relationship (Time to Onset)

The *temporal relationship* is the *time gap* between the administration of the suspect drug (start date and duration of therapy) and the occurrence of the adverse event (date of onset of event/initial symptoms observed).

4.4 Biological Plausibility and Possible Alternative Causes

Biological plausibility is considered as an important criterion, and it should be explicable biologically based on the available facts. The possible contributing factors that could as well be attributed to an adverse event include (i) medical condition—underlying concurrent medical conditions of patient (e.g. diabetes, asthma, etc.) or past medical history and prior/ongoing surgical procedures; (ii) other concurrent/concomitant medication use and past medication history; (iii) social history such as alcohol use, smoking, diet, etc.; and (iv) predisposing factors such as age and intercurrent diseases (hepatic and renal impairment).

4.5 Dechallenge

Dechallenge refers to the withdrawal/cessation or reduction in dose of the suspected drug. If there is a complete or partial resolution of adverse event following withdrawal/cessation or reduction in the dose (in the case of type A reaction) of the suspected drug, it is called as positive dechallenge. On the other hand, if there is no change in the outcome of an event and continued to exist in the same intensity or worsened further despite the cessation of the suspected drug, it is called as negative dechallenge. Outcome of dechallenge could be influenced by corrective treatment for the adverse event in addition to the dechallenge. Hence, this potential influence needs to be considered while deciding positive dechallenge.

4.6 Rechallenge

Rechallenge is the reintroduction of the suspected drug in a similar manner to the previous exposure and is applicable in the positive dechallenge scenario. The re-occurrence of similar adverse event following the reintroduction of suspected drug refers to positive rechallenge while failure to recur even after the reintroduction of suspected drug is referred to as negative rechallenge. Well-proved positive rechallenge is one of the strongest associations for causal relationship between the event and the medicine. In real practice, only very less often a rechallenge is done specifically to establish causality, due to ethical issues and concerns of causing harm in the patient, especially in the case of type B ADRs. Rechallenge is done in specific circumstances (like when there are no suitable safe and effective treatment alternatives available) depending on various factors including nature and severity of initial presentation of the adverse event, under strict medical supervision and appropriate monitoring.

5 Approaches or Categories of Causality Assessment

There are three broad approaches or categories of causality assessment adopted for establishing causation in pharmacovigilance. They include:

- Expert/clinical judgement or global introspection method
- Algorithms or standardised assessment method
- Probabilistic or Bayesian method

5.1 Expert/Clinical Judgement or Global Introspection Method

In this approach, the causation of the adverse drug reaction is established based on the clinical judgement of the expert or panel of experts using no standardised tool to arrive at conclusions in assigning the causality category. Instead, an individual assesses the causation based on previous knowledge and clinical experience in the field of pharmacovigilance. The expert(s)/clinician(s) analyses all the available data on the reported adverse event, following which an opinion is formulated on causality category based on the likelihood involvement of suspected drug in causing the adverse event [6, 12].

The expert(s)/clinician(s) would carefully evaluate each case to determine if the adverse event was likely caused by the drug or occurred due to other reasons. However, there are greater chances of inter-individual variability as there may be information bias between different experts. Causality assessment using this method is highly subjective and is based on the individual assessor's judgement and influenced by several other factors such as depth of clinical knowledge, evidence, extent of available information, and expertise and/or experience of the assessor. Therefore, one assessor's 'probable' may be another assessor's 'possible' for the given case causality assessment [6]. Other important considerations such as pharmacologic plausibility, dose–response, and timing may or may not be included. These assessments done by experts are generally expressed in terms of a qualitative probability scale such as 'definite', 'probable', 'possible', 'doubtful', or 'unrelated' [9, 12–15]. World Health Organization—Uppsala Monitoring Centre (WHO-UMC) causality assessment method is a widely used global introspection method to assess the causality of individual case safety reports required for the submission to pharmacovigilance systems worldwide [16]. There is some degree of ambiguity as to whether WHO-UMC causality assessment method should be considered as global introspection or as an algorithm. More ideally, it could be considered as a global introspection method as in the assessment using this scale, the assessor considers factors that might contribute to a causal link between one or more drugs and an observed ADR, weighs their importance, and decides the probability of drug causation, but no specific checklist or algorithm is given. It could be considered as a global introspection method, used for causality assessment, based on expert judgement, though delimited by specific criteria.

5.1.1 Advantages

The major advantage of global introspection method is its pivotal role in the identification and rating of potential ADRs over the years. There is also widespread support for continuing to value expert clinical judgement [17–20].

5.1.2 Limitations

The main drawback of global introspection is that clinical judgement is characterised by inter- and intra-rater dissimilarity, ambiguity, lack of reproducibility, and discernible prejudice [21–23].

5.2 Algorithms

Algorithms are problem-specific flow chart or sets of specific questions with associated scores that provide step-by-step guidance on how to arrive at conclusions on causality of the reported adverse event. These algorithms give a structured and standardised method of assessment in a systematic approach in identifying the adverse drug reaction or temporal sequence, previous drug/adverse reaction history, dechallenge, and rechallenge [24–26].

Most algorithms are in the form of a questionnaire that allows the user to gather adequate information and also assess the causal relationship between the drug and the suspected reaction. In algorithms-based approach, as causation is established using a well-structured, standardised, and validated scale, the chance of difference of opinion between two assessors (inter-individual variability) is greatly minimised. Naranjo's [27] scale is widely accepted and used worldwide in case causality assessment by personnel in clinical practice, pharmacovigilance, and researchers. A number of other algorithms have been published including the Karch and Lasagna algorithm [21], the Jones algorithm [28], the Yale algorithm [29], and the Begaud algorithm [30]. None of the existing algorithms are unanimously acknowledged as a recognised tool or a gold standard method as the evaluation of the same ADR reports by using different algorithms demonstrated significant variations in the results [11, 27, 31].

5.2.1 Advantages

Algorithmic methods are widely used for their simplistic and comprehensive approach, which creates a logical approach to causality assessment and scientific validity. These methods have poor sensitivity, but good specificity, and provide better reproducibility between assessors as they eliminate or at least reduce inter- and intra-rater disagreement [17, 18, 31, 32].

5.2.2 Limitations

Algorithmic methods do not provide certainty of case diagnosis. Also, they fail to ascertain the causality consistently due to a lack of regard to the confounding variables. Moreover, their inability to verify and invalidate the causality and to provide precise quantitative measurement of the probability of a causal relationship are the major drawbacks [18, 32].

5.3 Probabilistic or Bayesian Approaches

Probabilistic, or Bayesian, approaches involve the use of a statistical approach to assess the causal relationship between the drug and the outcome. It involves the use of specific findings in a case to transform the prior estimate of probability into a posterior estimate of probability of drug causation. The prior probability is calculated from epidemiological information, and the posterior probability combines this background information with the evidence in the individual case to provide an estimate of causation [6, 9, 19, 32]. Examples are the Australian method [33], the Bayesian Adverse Reactions Diagnostic Instrument (BARDI), and MacBARDI [24, 34].

5.3.1 Advantage

The probabilistic/Bayesian methods are trustworthy in assessing the ADRs in routine practice or automated evaluation of suspected case reports as they are highly sensitive, and have positive predictive value, and provide an outcome as probabilities [35].

5.3.2 Limitations

The major drawbacks of probabilistic/Bayesian methods are poor specificity and the fact that they are complex in practical approach as they require specifically calculated information data, such as specific ADR incidence, to reproduce the likelihood distribution [35].

6 Methods of Causality Assessment

Different methods ranging from simple questionnaires to comprehensive algorithms are available to determine the causal relationship between a suspected drug and adverse event. However, it is essential/desirable that the causality of a reported event is objectively assessed using a well-structured, standardised, and validated scale so as to ensure that the assessment is reliable and reproducible. Despite many systems being developed for a structured and harmonised assessment of causality, none of these systems have been shown to produce a reliable and quantitative estimation of likelihood relationship. Nevertheless, in clinical practice, the WHO probability scale and Naranjo's algorithm are widely used as they offer convenience of ease of use and are less time-consuming owing to their simple methodology. The following are the common methods adopted for establishing causation in pharmacovigilance [36].

6.1 WHO-UMC Causality Assessment Scale

The WHO-UMC causality assessment scale is a practical tool for the assessment of case reports. It basically considers the clinical-pharmacological aspects of the case history and the quality of the documentation of the observation. This scale establishes the causal relationship between suspected drug and observed event under any of the six categories and guides the assessor in the selection of one category over another [16]. The various causality categories of WHO-UMC causality assessment scale are listed in Table 8.1.

Table 8.1 WHO-UMC causality categories

Causality category	Criteria
Certain	• Event or laboratory test abnormality, with plausible time relationship to drug intake • Cannot be explained by disease or other drugs • Response to withdrawal plausible (pharmacologically, pathologically) • Event definitive pharmacologically or phenomenologically (*i.e. an objective and specific medical disorder or a recognised pharmacological phenomenon*) • Rechallenge satisfactory, if necessary
Probable/likely	• Event or laboratory test abnormality, with reasonable time relationship to drug intake • Unlikely to be attributed to disease or other drugs • Response to withdrawal clinically reasonable • Rechallenge not required

Table 8.1 (continued)

Causality category	Criteria
Possible	• Event or laboratory test abnormality, with reasonable time relationship to drug intake • Could also be explained by disease or other drugs • Information on drug withdrawal may be lacking or unclear
Unlikely	• Event or laboratory test abnormality, with a time to drug intake that makes a relationship improbable (but not impossible) • Disease or other drugs provide plausible explanations
Conditional/ unclassified	• Event or laboratory test abnormality • More data for proper assessment needed • Additional data under examination
Unassessable/ unclassifiable	• Report suggesting an adverse reaction • Cannot be judged because information is insufficient or contradictory • Data cannot be supplemented or verified

6.2 Naranjo's Algorithm [27]

Naranjo's ADR probability scale is a simple questionnaire used to assess the causality of ADRs in a variety of clinical situations. It consists of ten questions, and the answer to each of the questions could be positive (yes), negative (no), or unknown or inapplicable (do not know). Each of the questions is assigned with score ranging from −1 to +2, and based on the total score, the causality of reported adverse event is categorised into any of the four categories as 'Definite' (≥9), 'Probable' (5–8), 'Possible' (1–4), and 'Doubtful' (≥0) (Table 8.2). Simplicity and wider applicability are the advantages of this ADR probability scale and is reliable and valid in assessing the adverse drug-related events, while some minor modifications may be required in special circumstances.

Table 8.2 Naranjo's algorithm

Sl. No.	Criteria	Yes	No	Do not know
1	Are there previous conclusive reports on this reaction?	+1	0	0
2	Did the adverse event appear after the suspected drug was administered?	+2	−1	0
3	Did the adverse reaction improve when the drug was discontinued or a specific antagonist was administered?	+1	0	0
4	Did the adverse reaction reappear when the drug was readministered?	+2	−1	0
5	Are there alternative causes (other than the drug) that could on their own have caused the reaction?	−1	+2	0
6	Did the reaction reappear when a placebo was given?	−1	+1	0
7	Was the drug detected in the blood (or other fluids) in concentrations known to be toxic?	+1	0	0
8	Was the reaction more severe when the dose was increased, or less severe when the dose was decreased?	+1	0	0
9	Did the patient have a similar reaction to the same or similar drugs in any previous exposure?	+1	0	0
10	Was the adverse event confirmed by any objective evidence?	+1	0	0

7 Various Perspectives

7.1 Clinical Practice Perspective

Understanding and assessing the causal relationship between the observed adverse event and the suspected drug/s will greatly influence the determination of the possibility of the drug causing the observed event and future course of action including prescribing decisions. Clinicians should always consider ADRs as a differential diagnosis. When all the other alternative explanations for observed AE fail, the cause suspicion will fall on the drug. However, in many cases a decisive causal relationship may not always be practically possible, and a level of uncertainty will exist.

Identifying the culprit drug(s) can be lifesaving or helpful in preventing the further drug-related harm. Assessing causality is of importance as it directly influences decision-making by a clinician on future course of action which could be either to continue or to withdraw the likely drugs, need for any dose adjustment of the likely drugs, and need for any specific/non-specific treatment for the ADR. A causality assessment should be performed based on patient's detailed clinical history, examination to look for temporal correlation between suspected drug and drug reaction, biological plausibility, and outcomes of dechallenge and rechallenge, if carried out. At times, these assessments are highly subjective in nature and are mainly based on clinical knowledge and experience of an individual clinician. Identifying the culprit drug could be challenging at many times when multiple drugs are suspected to be responsible for causing a drug reaction. The situation becomes further challenging when the underlying disease is capable of producing the same manifestation as caused by the drug. To a good extent, the principles and methods of causality assessment or causality assessment tools help clinicians to identify the culprit drugs. Though none of the multiple criteria or algorithms available is specific or complete, the causality assessment system proposed by the WHO-UMC and the Naranjo probability scale are the generally accepted and most widely used methods in clinical practice as they offer a simple methodology and they are time tested.

Formalised causality assessment offers some objectivity and reduced inter-individual variations. Causality assessment tools can be used in clinical practice, but an awareness of their potential limitations is required. A few of the difficulties in causality assessment noticed in clinical practice are incomplete information about the suspected ADR, polypharmacy, variable clinical responses, poor understanding of biological plausibility, other alternative causes, and lack of healthcare professional training. Establishing causality in patients with polypharmacy is difficult as dechallenge–rechallenge analysis may not be possible or ethical for every individual drug. It should be borne in mind that clinical judgement obviously is helpful in identifying the relationship likelihood in actual clinical practice and there is no substitute for clinical observations and experience of the healthcare professionals when it comes to identifying the cause of an adverse event.

In addition to its benefits in determining the relationship likelihood between the event and the drug/s and subsequent course of action, causality assessment is beneficial for other reasons as well. If case reports/case series based on drug reactions are being submitted for publication, completion of causality assessment is an expectation. When completing in-house documentation of ADR reports in a healthcare institution, causality assessment of the reported ADRs is useful to quantify the type of ADRs based on causality as well as for routine dissemination of the evaluated ADR data. From the patient perspective, data on the causality assessment will be helpful when communicating the details of the observed ADR to the individual patient. Additionally, causality assessment will be helpful in deciding the need of providing an alert card for the patient regarding the specific ADR, as well as documenting the ADR details in the patient medical records to caution future prescribing. The relevance of causality assessment in clinical practice signifies the importance of training healthcare professionals on the concept, basis, and process of causality assessment [11, 16, 37].

7.2 Industry Perspective

Reporting of safety information by the pharmaceutical companies for their proprietary molecules is mandated by most of the regulatory authorities worldwide. The major focus of regulators is to scrutinise the products in clinical development and post-marketed products to ensure medications with a favourable benefit–harm ratio are available in the market. This requires clinical trial sponsors and marketing authorisation holders to continuously evaluate their products for potential adverse events, ensuring the benefits outweigh its harms. Therefore, pharmaceutical companies must have a robust pharmacovigilance system in place to closely monitor the adverse events associated with their products both as a regulatory requirement and product liability. Many multinational pharmaceutical companies have adopted a structured way of capturing ADRs and their subsequent causality assessment, in comparison to the relatively less developed systems in academic research and general healthcare provision. However, establishment of confirmed causal relationship between the drug and the adverse event is a challenge and carries utmost importance in the continuing scenario of emerging drug safety concerns. Initially, investigators/sponsors were conservative in their interpretation of 'reasonable possibility' of association between the drug and the adverse event. The spontaneous reports are considered by pharma companies as reports with implied causality by reporter.

Solicited reports are classified as study reports and therefore should have an appropriate causality assessment by a healthcare professional or pharmaceutical company (International Council for Harmonisation [ICH] E2D, 2003). A method of causality assessment is recommended to be applied for assessing the causal role of medicinal products in the solicited adverse events. Spontaneous reports are considered suspected adverse reactions, since they convey the suspicions of the primary sources, unless the reporters specifically state that they believe the events to be unrelated or causal relationship can be excluded [38]. Comments from the primary source regarding causality assessment are reported by pharmaceutical companies to regulatory authorities as 'Reporter's comments' (ICH-E2B (R2) B.5.2). Change in the causality assessment in the follow-up reports of ADRs is considered as significant new information. In pharmaceutical industry, structured causality assessment methods for individual cases have been used primarily to facilitate case processing rather than to reach definitive conclusions. Events are considered 'related' or 'not related' for the purpose of case processing and regulatory reporting. Pharma companies' designation of relatedness for regulatory reporting purposes is independent of the investigator's/report's assessment. Despite follow-up attempts, usually complete information required for comprehensive causality assessment is barely received by pharma companies particularly from unsolicited sources.

To date, there are no internationally agreed-upon standards or criteria by pharma companies for assessing causality in ICSR. Nature of the event, consistency with the known drug profile, physiological plausibility, temporal association, availability of sufficient and consistent information, specific laboratory investigations, more probable/likely alternative reasons, confounding medical conditions/medications, and dechallenge/rechallenge results are the criteria typically considered by the pharma companies for causality assessment. Definitive decisions about causality (leading to risk management plan/label changes, etc.) usually incorporate evidence from various sources. However, no single 'one size fits all' approach exists as sometimes individual case reports provide compelling evidence of causality [37–40].

7.3 Regulatory Perspective

Causality assessment is necessary for adverse events reported in clinical trials. Most of the clinical trial protocols require investigator's causality assessment for both serious and non-serious adverse events. The investigator's assessment of causality is not required for non-serious adverse events by the regulations, except some circumstances like non-serious adverse events of special interest. Serious adverse events (SAEs) that are either expected or unexpected and related to the suspected drug qualify for expedited reporting to regulatory authorities. Causality assessment is well described in the International Council for Harmonisation (ICH) E2A Guideline and the report of Council for International Organizations of Medical Sciences (CIOMS) working group VI. The adverse events do not imply any judgement about causality. Suspected adverse reaction suggests a causal association. ADRs imply 'reasonable possibility' that there is evidence to suggest a causal relationship between the drug and the adverse event as judged by either the reporter or the sponsor. The United States Food and Drug Administration (US FDA) considers causality assessment as sponsor's responsibility to decide expedited reporting needs as they are better positioned for assessment than the individual clinical trial investigators. However, for all serious adverse events reported to the sponsor, as per 21 Code of Federal Regulations 312.64, clinical trial investigators are required to provide a causality assessment. In general, 'reasonable possibility' conveys that there are evidence or opinions to suggest a causal relationship even if the relationship is unknown or unstated.

Causal association between the drug and the adverse event in clinical trials is supported by evidences like uncommon event and known to occur with drug exposure, one or more uncommon events in the population exposed, and higher frequency of occurrence in treatment group than control group. The sponsor decides the causality assessment scale to be used by investigators. Many sponsors usually demand 'Yes/No' answer to the question 'Was there a reasonable possibility that the drug caused the adverse event?' for the causality assessment as CIOMS VI Working Group recommends using a simple binary decision for causality assessment. Although many sponsors use home-grown causality assessment methods, the 'Introspection' is the sponsors' causality assessment method of choice. ADRs associated with marketed drugs (unsolicited reports) usually considered to imply causality for reporting purposes to regulatory authorities. For the purposes of safety reporting to regulatory authorities, solicited reports associated with marketed products are classified as study reports and therefore should have an appropriate causality assessment by a healthcare professional or a Marketing Authorisation Holder (MAH). Currently, there are no standard international causality assessment methods and nomenclature to describe the attributability between drug exposure and adverse event; hence, terms like certainly, definitely, likely, probably, possibly, or likely related or not related are in use [40–42].

8 Application of Artificial Intelligence and Machine Learning in Causality Assessment

With the increasing number of reports, it has become ever more necessary to implement computer-based approaches to support the efforts of human expert causality assessment of ADRs. An automated solution for causality assessment is yet to be found as the assessment workflow is not fully standardised to a level required for computation [43]. The US FDA requires pharmaceutical companies to have procedures for receipt, assessment, and reporting of post-marketing adverse drug experiences [44]. Efforts to standardise the workflow for purposes of computation need expert judgement and flexibility. Artificial intelligence (AI) approaches expected to be applied for causality assessment need the understanding of both the individual tasks and how they are further assembled into a cognitive framework for causality assessment. Causality assessment by human expert processes involves use of information that is both internal and external to the case report. Drug exposure, ADR outcome, temporality, and alternative explanations are some of the important elements that need to be considered by cognitive framework for causality assessment [45].

The MOdified NARanjo Causality Scale for ICSRs (MONARCSi) is an early effort in developing machine-based learning tool for causality assessment. The MONARCSi approach uses matrix and weights determined by aggregating the importance of presence or absence of a specific drug-event feature. The final scores obtained for a specific drug–event pair are then logistically transformed to estimate the probability or confidence level in the 'relatedness' or 'unrelatedness' for drug–event causality. Based on this logistic probability level, the model then assigns causality as related or unrelated [46]. DeepCausality provided an AI-powered promising solution for causality assessment from free text by integrating transformers, named entity recognition, and Do-calculus into a unified framework to empirically estimate the causal factors for suspected endpoints embedded in the free text [47].

Identification of low-value reports is important in applying AI to causality assessment of ICSRs, since computerised algorithms can achieve better causality assessment results (in cases containing enough information) to make an informed causality assessment. This can be achieved by training the algorithm on reports classified as either 'assessable' or 'unassessable' [43]. Machine learning capabilities have been explored to predict ICSRs that are most useful for causality assessment. Natural language processing extraction and visualisation of clinical data have been used to support case series analyses for causality assessment [48].

It is believed that pharmacovigilance was lagging in adopting machine learning–causal assessment integrated models [49]. AI may become increasingly important for improving the efficiency and scientific value of ICSRs including reducing the inconsistencies in assessment processes and improving overall decision-making [45]. Using AI-powered language models to conduct causal inference, similar to human experts, is still at the infant stage. AI for causality assessment will have to be aligned with the emerging best practices for the field to reach a state of maturity, as causality assessment still remains a challenge [50]. Regulatory authorities have not yet endorsed any specific approach for applying AI to ADR case processing and evaluation. Research on enhancing data quality and data representation will be an important step in successful implementation of AI in causality assessment. The likelihood of AI systems that will reach a level of full automation performance in the near term has been assessed as low [45]. However, incorporating causal inference paradigms to address currently prominent machine learning issues in causality assessment could be a new future. Learning from AI applications in the aviation industry, it may be that AI supporting, rather than supplanting, human expertise in causality assessment be beneficial.

9 Applications of Causality Assessment

Continuous specification of the safety profile of a drug product is an essential component throughout its life cycle, from the drug discovery, to post-marketing and until the drug is out of the market. Thus, the need for causality assessment continues and has wider applications across various fields including academic research, clinical practice, sponsored clinical research, national pharmacovigilance programmes, and regulatory decision-making. It is an integral part of clinical management as early detection of adverse event and identification of culprit drug can aid healthcare professionals to make therapeutic decisions to improve patient safety. Causality assessment is legally required by health authorities including US FDA, European Medicines Agency, and other health authorities for expediting reporting of all serious adverse events (SAEs). Furthermore, causality assessment is needed to determine whether the adverse event should be considered in the signal detection process, benefit–harm determination, and whether it should be listed in the reference safety information (Investigator Brochure, Company Core Safety Datasheet) and label (including Package Inserts and the Summary of Product Characteristics). Also, as an essential component of pharmacovigilance contributing to better patient care, establishing causation of the reported event is important prior to dissemination of safety information amongst healthcare professionals, investigators, patients, and other stakeholders [7, 42].

10 Challenges in Causality Assessment

Causality in pharmacovigilance is a complex process and should be viewed considering both patient-related and medication-related factors. It is often highly subjective based upon clinician's judgement that is influenced by several factors including the assessor's knowledge of the event, experience, availability of time, and amount of information. These factors lead to higher chances of inter- and intra-individual variability in assigning causality. ADRs also frequently mimic disease symptoms with no distinct characteristic features that can differentiate the iatrogenic cause from disease process. Eliminating all possible alternative causes is often key to assigning causality. However, in a routine clinical practice, this can be a challenge and may not also be possible considering the time and economic constraints within healthcare systems. Also, many of the symptoms attributed to ADRs occur in healthy individuals taking no medications. For example, headache can occur in any individual due to various reasons, making it more difficult to attribute to a medication. In addition, incomplete information of ADR, polypharmacy, variable clinical responses, poor understanding of biological plausibility, and lack of training among assessors pose additional challenges in causality assessment [6, 7, 9].

What causality assessment aids in:[7]

- Decreasing the disagreement between assessors
- Classifying uncertainty
- Marking individual case reports
- Improving scientific basis of evaluation

What causality assessment lacks:

- Giving accurate quantitative measurements of the causation
- Distinguishing between valid and invalid cases
- Confirming the relationship between drug and event
- Quantification of the contribution of the drug in the development of the adverse event
- Changing uncertainty to certainty

11 Summary and Conclusions

Causality assessment is an essential and challenging aspect of pharmacovigilance. It is important in clinical practice to identify the culprit drugs as the safety of the patients is paramount. Using causality assessment tools may help clinicians in identifying the culprit drugs, understanding the probability that the suspected drug has caused the event observed, and determining future course of action including informed future prescribing. There are multiple criteria or algorithms available for establishing a causal relationship in case of suspected ADR. However, a standardised causality assessment method that offers reliable and reproducible measures of the relationship likelihood in suspected cases of ADR seems to be unfeasible, since no single method has achieved this to date, with no single method universally accepted. Differences in ADR causality assessment methods, and the unavoidable subjectivity of judgements, will likely impact reproducibility for most published methods. Therefore, there is a need to develop a high-quality causality assessment tool that can establish a suitable diagnostic criterion for ADRs, with universal acceptance.

12 Case Studies

12.1 Case Study 1: Causality Assessment Using WHO-UMC Causality Assessment Scale

Mr. K is a 38-year-old man, weighing 50 kg, private employer, and married. He was diagnosed with pulmonary tuberculosis (TB) 20 days ago at a tertiary care hospital. His lab investigations at the time of diagnosis were as follows. Sputum Acid Fast Bacillus (AFB): Positive (2 samples); Haemoglobin (Hb): 8.5 g%; WBC: 3800 cells/mm^3; platelets: 2,10,000 cells/mm^3; liver tests: aspartate aminotransferase (AST): 45 IU/L (0–40 IU/L); alanine aminotransferase (ALT): 40 IU/L (0–40 IU/L); alkaline phosphatase (ALP]: 160 IU/L (150–280 IU/L); albumin: 3.5 mg/dL (3–5 mg/dL); chest X ray: indicative of tuberculosis, presence of granuloma. Mr. K is a non-smoker and non-alcoholic. Diet: Mixed type. Clinician referred Mr. K to Directly Observed Therapy (DOT) centre where he was put on treatment with a combination of Tab. Isoniazid 300 mg + rifampicin 450 mg + pyrazinamide 1500 mg + ethambutol 375 mg PO once daily in empty stomach, Tab. Pyridoxine 40 mg PO once daily. Other medications include Tab. Paracetamol 650 mg PO 1-1-1 for 2 weeks to ameliorate fever and malaise, Tab. Pantoprazole 40 mg PO 1-0-0 (1 h before anti-TB drugs), protein powder 2 teaspoon in milk twice daily. Mr. K was asked to follow as per given schedule at DOT centre.

Later, 14 days after treatment, Mr. K visited hospital again with complaints of abdominal pain, yellowish discolouration of eyes and skin. Treating doctor examined the patient and ordered for liver tests. The liver function tests results were as follows. AST: 140 IU/L (baseline: 45 IU/L); ALT: 160 IU/L (baseline: 40 IU/L); ALP: 400 IU/L (baseline: 160 IU/L). Considering the elevated liver enzymes and symptoms in the patient, clinician suggested to hold anti-TB drugs temporarily.

Task: *Interpret the available information and perform the causality assessment using WHO probability scale.*

1. *Can elevated liver enzymes (hepatotoxicity) in this case be reported as an adverse event?*

   The elevated liver enzymes (hepatotoxicity) could be reported as an adverse event as it manifested in Mr. K while the patient was on medications.

2. *Is the adverse event attributable to any single agent?*

   No. As Mr. K was receiving anti-tubercular medications as combination therapy and multiple antitubercular agents are reported to cause the same reaction, at this stage, the adverse event cannot be attributable to a single agent.

3. *Is the data complete/adequate/inadequate to assess this reaction?*

   At this stage, the data appears to be neither complete nor inadequate. As the basic information on patient's medical history, event, and all medications are available for the assessment, it is considered as adequate, but additional information is warranted for complete case causality assessment.

4. *What is the causality category of the adverse reaction?*

   As assessed using the WHO probability scale, with the current available information, the causality category of the reported adverse reaction (hepatotoxicity) is categorised as *possible* as this case fulfil three criteria that are required for the event to be categorised under the said causality category. In this case, the causality could not be categorised as either certain or probable due to non-availability of information on the rechallenge and the outcome of dechallenge.

What happened next?

During the same hospital visit, clinician provided supportive care for 4 days to the patient and asked Mr. K to wait for treatment till liver enzymes are normal. After a week, Mr. K's liver enzymes were observed to be normal. Clinician wanted to identify the offending drug and hence suggested for rechallenge with anti-tubercular drugs.

5. *Will the causality category change at this stage of assessment?*

   Now, the causality category is expected to change with the available additional information on outcome of dechallenge. As Mr. K's elevated liver enzymes are normal after the cessation of suspected drugs, there is a positive dechallenge, and thus the causality category could now be assigned as *probable*.

6. *Can rechallenge be conducted in this case and why?*

   In this case, as Mr. K must be treated for his tuberculosis as otherwise it may lead to unnecessary complications leading even to death. Rechallenge is important to identify the culprit drug in causing the hepatotoxicity so that the treatment can be reinitiated with anti-tubercular agents along with secondary medications—avoiding the culprit drug.

7. *If we perform rechallenge, will there be a change in the causality category?*

   Further change in the causality category depends on the outcome of rechallenge. If there is a positive rechallenge, the causality would change from *probable* to *certain* or else the causality remains as *probable*.

What happened next?

A day after liver enzymes became normal, Mr. K was re-administered with rifampicin for 7 days. Post 7 days of treatment, liver tests were performed, and it was observed to be normal. Later, Isoniazid was added to the patient's regimen, and after three days, liver enzymes were elevated.

8. *What is the status of dechallenge/rechallenge in Mr. K's case?*

   At this stage, both dechallenge and rechallenge were performed, and the outcome of them was positive as there was recovery from the adverse reaction following cessation of suspected drugs (positive dechallenge) and also there was recurrence of same event (elevation of liver enzymes) after the rechallenge with the anti-tubercular agents.

9. *Can the adverse event be attributed to any single agent?*

   At this stage, as Mr. K developed the similar event (elevated liver enzymes) following re-administration of isoniazid, the event now is more likely to be attributable to single agent (isoniazid). The involvement of rifampicin in causing the hepatotoxicity could be ruled out as Mr. K did not experience a similar event following the re-administration of rifampicin for 7 days. However, in similar line, the possibilities of the likelihood involvement of other agents should also be ruled out prior to arriving any conclusion. Though paracetamol may not be the culprit drug considering the dose that was used and there are more likely drugs, the contribution of paracetamol in increasing the risk of hepatotoxicity associated with anti-tubercular agents as well needs to be considered.

10. *Will causality category of the reaction change now?*

    Yes. In Mr. K's case, the likelihood involvement of isoniazid causing hepatotoxicity is *certain* as it currently fulfils all the required criteria for the said causality category as per the WHO probability scale.

12.2 Case Study 2: Causality Assessment Using Naranjo's Algorithm

A 50-year-old Asian male weighing 60 kg was admitted to the hospital with fever, loose stools, cough, breathlessness, and upper abdomen tenderness over the preceding week. Three years ago, he was diagnosed to have had human immunodeficiency virus (HIV) infection with pulmonary tuberculosis. Following the completion of 6-month treatment for his tuberculosis, he was initiated on anti-retroviral treatment with zidovudine 300 mg BD, lamivudine 150 mg BD, and nevirapine 200 mg BD. Also, he was on prophylaxis for *pneumocystis carinii pneumonia* (PCP) with co-trimoxazole 80 mg OD since 2 years. At the time of initiating the anti-retroviral treatment, his CD4+ count was 290 cells/mm^3. After 18 months, his antiretroviral therapy was changed to nevirapine 200 mg BD, lamivudine 150 mg BD, and stavudine 30 mg BD as he has had anaemia (Hb 10 g/dL). He was prescribed multivitamins for anaemia. After 2 months of treatment with nevirapine, lamivudine, and stavudine, patient's Hb was 13.5 g/dL.

After 6 months of treatment with nevirapine, lamivudine, and stavudine, he was hospitalised with the complaints of nausea, vomiting, anorexia, and pain in epigastric region. His serum amylase and lipase levels were 211 U/L (normal reference range—up to 100 U/L) and 1267 U/L (normal reference range—114 to 286 U/L), respectively. He was diagnosed to have had pancreatitis. Stavudine was discontinued, and he was treated symptomatically, and subsequently he was discharged after 7 days of hospitalisation. At the time of discharge, serum amylase and lipase levels were 195 U/L and 1021 U/L, respectively. After 8 weeks of discharge from the hospital, the amylase and lipase levels decreased to 140 U/L and 440 U/L, respectively. After 20 weeks of discharge from the hospital, considering his CD4+ count (23 cells/mm^3), he was initiated on the antiretroviral treatment with emtricitabine 200 mg OD, tenofovir 300 mg OD, and the fixed dose combination of lopinavir–ritonavir (200 mg + 50 mg) BD.

1. *What are the suspected adverse reactions in this patient?*

   Anaemia and pancreatitis are adverse events identified in this patient. It is essential to note that both these conditions were not present in the patient prior to starting the drug therapy and manifested only after 18 and 6 months of treatment with the suspected drugs, respectively. It is also important to note that certain ADRs may take longer duration to manifest, while others may occur within a few minutes to days.
2. *Which are the suspected drugs associated with the adverse reactions?*

   Zidovudine and stavudine were implicated for anaemia and pancreatitis, respectively. It is important to narrow down, considering various factors, to the single causative agent when two or more drugs are known to cause the similar ADRs. For example, co-trimoxazole is also known to cause pancreatitis but rarely, and also it is reported to cause pancreatitis at high doses. In this case, patient was receiving the co-trimoxazole at lower prophylaxis dose for over 18 months and before initiating stavudine. Hence, the likely association of co-trimoxazole causing pancreatitis is weak.
3. *Assess the causality of the suspected adverse reactions using Naranjo's algorithm.*

   Upon the assessment using Naranjo's algorithm, the causality category of both zidovudine-induced anaemia and stavudine-induced pancreatitis is found to be *probable* owing to the facts that there is a reasonable time relationship to drug intake and event or laboratory test abnormality, and furthermore, these reactions are unlikely to be attributed to disease, and the response to withdrawal of the suspected drugs has been clinically reasonable.
4. *What are other learning points in this case?*

   A safe drug does not mean it is devoid of risk. Clinicians and patients always need to take an informed decision considering the benefit–harm ratio of suspected medications.

   When a patient develops more than one adverse reaction, the process of estimating the causal association needs to be carried out separately for each of the reported ADRs considering all other possible drug-related and patient-related causes.

References

1. Lazarou J, Pomeranz BH, Corey PN. Incidence of adverse drug reactions in hospitalized patients: a meta-analysis of prospective studies. JAMA. 1998;279(15):1200–5. https://doi.org/10.1001/jama.279.15.1200.
2. Malhotra SJ. Drug-related visits to the medical emergency department: a prospective study from India. Int J Clin Pharmacol Ther. 2001;39(1):12–8.
3. Patel KJ, Kedia MS, Bajpai D, Mehta SS, Kshirsagar NA, Gogtay NJ. Evaluation of the prevalence and economic burden of adverse drug reactions presenting to the medical emergency department of a tertiary referral centre: a prospective study. BMC Clin Pharmacol. 2007;7:8. https://doi.org/10.1186/1472-6904-7-8.
4. Pirmohamed M, James S, Meakin S, Green C, Scott AK, Walley TJ, Farrar K, Park BK, Breckenridge AM. Adverse drug reactions as cause of admission to hospital: prospective analysis of 18 820 patients. BMJ (Clin Res Ed). 2004;329(7456):15–9. https://doi.org/10.1136/bmj.329.7456.15.
5. Khan LM, Al-Harthi SE, Osman AMM, Sattar MAAA, Ali AS. Dilemmas of the causality assessment tools in the diagnosis of adverse drug reactions. Saudi Pharm J. 2016;24(4):485–93. https://doi.org/10.1016/j.jsps.2015.01.010.
6. Parthasarathi G, Nyfort-Hansen K, Nahata MC, editors. A textbook of clinical pharmacy practice: essential concepts and skills. 2nd ed. Universities Press (India) Private Limited; 2012.
7. Meyboom RHB, Hekster YA, Egberts AC, Gribnau FWI, Edwards R. Causal or casual? The role of causality assessment in pharmacovigilance. Drug Saf. 1997;17(6):374–89. https://doi.org/10.2165/00002018-199717060-00004.
8. Horn JR, Hansten PD, Chan LN. Proposal for a new tool to evaluate drug interaction cases. Ann Pharmacother. 2007;41(4):674–80. https://doi.org/10.1345/aph.1H423.

9. Agbabiaka TB, Savović JS, Ernst E. Methods for causality assessment of adverse drug reactions a systematic review. Drug Saf. 2008;31(1):21–37.
10. Fedak KM, Bernal A, Capshaw ZA, Gross S. Applying the Bradford Hill criteria in the 21st century: how data integration has changed causal inference in molecular epidemiology. Emerg Themes Epidemiol. 2015;12(1):14. https://link.springer.com/article/10.1186/s12982-015-0037-4.
11. Pande S. Causality or Relatedness assessment in adverse drug reaction and its relevance in dermatology. Indian J Dermatol. 2018;63(1):18–21. https://journals.lww.com/ijd/fulltext/2018/63010/causality_or_relatedness_assessment_in_adverse.4.aspx.
12. Mannino RE. Causality assessment of adverse drug reactions using decision support and informatics tools. Pharmacoepidemiol Drug Saf. 1992;1(5):235–49.
13. Teschke R, Eickhoff A, Wolff A, Frenzel C, Schulze J. Herbal hepatotoxicity and WHO global introspection method. Ann Hepatol. 2013;12(1):11–21. PMID: 23293189.
14. Behera SK, Das S, Xavier AS, Velupula S, Sandhiya S. Comparison of different methods for causality assessment of adverse drug reactions. Int J Clin Pharm. 2018;40(4):903–10. https://doi.org/10.1007/s11096-018-0694-9. Epub 2018 Jul 26. PMID: 30051231.
15. Rezende de Menezes R, Graciano Silva MDD, Pinho Ribeiro AL, Martins Pinto Filho M, Martinho GH, Carvalho Ferreira LE, Parreiras Martins MA. Causality assessment of adverse drug reactions by applying a global introspection method in a high complexity hospital. Explor Res Clin Soc Pharm. 2021;3:100064. https://doi.org/10.1016/j.rcsop.2021.100064. PMID: 35480605; PMCID: PMC9032013.
16. World Health Organization (WHO), Uppsala Monitoring Centre. The use of the WHO-UMC system for standardised case causality assessment. Retrieved August 23, 2022, from http://www.who-umc.org/graphics/4409.pdf
17. Arimone Y, Bégaud B, Miremont-Salamé G, Fourrier-Réglat A, Moore N, Molimard M, Haramburu F. Agreement of expert judgment in causality assessment of adverse drug reactions. Eur J Clin Pharmacol. 2005;61(3):169–73. https://doi.org/10.1007/s00228-004-0869-2.
18. Arimone Y, Miremont-Salamé G, Haramburu F, Molimard M, Moore N, Fourrier-Réglat A, Bégaud B. Inter-expert agreement of seven criteria in causality assessment of adverse drug reactions. Br J Clin Pharmacol. 2007;64(4):482–8. https://doi.org/10.1111/j.1365-2125.2007.02937.x.
19. Théophile H, Arimone Y, Miremont-Salamé G, Moore N, Fourrier-Réglat A, Haramburu F, Bégaud B. Comparison of three methods (consensual expert judgement, algorithmic and probabilistic approaches) of causality assessment of adverse drug reactions an assessment using reports made to a French pharmacovigilance centre. Drug Saf. 2010;33(11):1045–54. https://doi.org/10.2165/11537780-000000000-00000.
20. Pillans PI. Clinical perspectives in drug safety and adverse drug reactions. Expert Rev Clin Pharmacol. 2008;1(5):695–705. https://doi.org/10.1586/17512433.1.5.695.
21. Karch FE, Lasagna L. Toward the operational identification of adverse drug reactions. Clin Pharmacol Ther. 1977;21(3):247–54.
22. Koh Y, Yap CW, Li SC. A quantitative approach of using genetic algorithm in designing a probability scoring system of an adverse drug reaction assessment system. Int J Med Inform. 2008;77(6):421–30. https://doi.org/10.1016/j.ijmedinf.2007.08.010.
23. Kramer MS, Leventhal JM, Hutchinson TA, Feinstein AR. An algorithm for the operational assessment of adverse drug reactions I. Background, description, and instructions for use. JAMA. 1979;242(7):623–32.
24. Lanctot KL, Naranjo CA. Computer-assisted evaluation of adverse events using a Bayesian approach. J Clin Pharmacol. 1994;34(2):142–7. https://doi.org/10.1002/j.1552-4604.1994.tb03978.x.
25. Leventhal JM, Hutchinson TA, Kramer MS, Feinstein AR. An algorithm for the operational assessment of adverse drug reactions. III. Results of tests among clinicians. JAMA. 1979;242(18):1991–4.
26. Venulet J. Recognition and assessment of adverse drug reactions in children. Bratisl Lek Listy. 1991;92(11):540–3.
27. Naranjo CA, Busto U, Sellers EM, Sandor P, Ruiz I, Roberts EA, Janecek E, Domecq C, Greenblatt DJ. A method for estimating the probability of adverse drug reactions. Clin Pharmacol Ther. 1981;30(2): 239–45.
28. Jones JK. Adverse drug reactions in the community health setting; approaches to recognizing, counseling and reporting. Fam Community Health 1982;5(2): 58–67. 12.
29. Kramer MS, Hutchinson TA. The Yale algorithm. Special workshop-clinical. Drug Inf J 1984;18:283–91.
30. Begaud B, Evreux JC, Jouglard J, Lagier G. Imputation of the unexpected or toxic effects of drugs. Actualisation of the methods used in France. Therapie 1985;40:115–8].
31. Théophile H, André M, Miremont-Salamé G, Arimone Y, Bégaud B. Comparison of three methods (an updated logistic probabilistic method, the Naranjo and Liverpool algorithms) for the evaluation of routine pharmacovigilance case reports using consensual expert judgement as reference. Drug Saf. 2013;36(10):1033–44. https://doi.org/10.1007/s40264-013-0083-1.
32. Macedo AF, Marques FB, Ribeiro CF, Teixeira F. Causality assessment of adverse drug reactions: Comparison of the results obtained from published decisional algorithms and from the evaluations of an expert panel. Pharmacoepidemiol Drug Saf. 2005;14(12):885–90. https://doi.org/10.1002/pds.1138.

33. Mashford ML. The Australian method special workshop-regulatory of drug-event assessment. Drug Inform J. 1984;18(3–4):271–3.
34. Lane DA. A Bayesian approach to causality assessment for suspected adverse drug reactions I: conceptual framework. Minneapolis, MN: University of Minnesota; 1986a.
35. Du W, Lehr VT, Lieh-Lai M, Koo W, Ward RM, Rieder MJ, van den Anker JN, Reeves JH, Mathew M, Lulic-Botica M, Aranda JV. An algorithm to detect adverse drug reactions in the neonatal intensive care unit: a new approach. J Clin Pharmacol. 2013;53(1):87–95. https://doi.org/10.1177/0091270011433327.
36. Talbot J, Aronson JK. Stephens' detection and evaluation of adverse drug reactions: principles and practice. 6th ed. John Wiley & Sons; 2012.
37. Naidu RP. Causality assessment: a brief insight into practices in pharmaceutical industry. Perspect Clin Res. 2013;4(4):233. https://doi.org/10.4103/2229-3485.120173.
38. European Medicines Agency. Guideline on good pharmacovigilance practices (GVP); 2014. https://www.ema.europa.eu/en/documents/scientific-guideline/guideline-good-pharmacovigilance-practices-module-vi-management-reporting-adverse-reactions_en-0.pdf
39. Crout JR. Introduction to causality the manufacturer's perspective assessment—who, what and why? Drug Inform J. 1986;20(4):395–7.
40. U.S. Department of Health and Human Services Food and Drug Administration. Guidance for industry and investigators safety reporting requirements for INDs and BA/BE studies; 2012. https://www.fda.gov/files/drugs/published/Safety-Reporting-Requirements-for-INDs-%28Investigational-New-Drug-Applications%29-and-BA-BE-%28Bioavailability-Bioequivalence%29-Studies.pdf
41. CIOMS. Management of safety information from clinical trials. Report of CIOMS Working Group VI; 2005. https://cioms.ch/wp-content/uploads/2017/01/Mgment_Safety_Info.pdf
42. ICH Harmonized Tripartite Guideline. Clinical safety data management: definitions and standards for expedited reporting E2A; 1994. https://database.ich.org/sites/default/files/E2A_Guideline.pdf
43. Kreimeyer K, Dang O, Spiker J, Muñoz M, Rosner G, Ball R, et al. Feature engineering and machine learning for causality assessment in pharmacovigilance: lessons learned from application to the FDA adverse event reporting system (FAERS). Comput Biol Med. 2021;202(135):104517. https://doi.org/10.1016/j.compbiomed.2021.104517.
44. Electronic Code of Federal Regulations. Title 21: food and drugs part 314.80; 2021. https://www.accessdata.fda.gov/scripts/cdrh/cfdocs/cfcfr/cfrsearch.cfm?fr=314.80. Accessed 4 Apr 2023.
45. Ball R, Dal Pan G. "Artificial Intelligence" for pharmacovigilance: ready for prime time? Drug Saf. 2022;45:429–38. https://doi.org/10.1007/s40264-022-01157-4.
46. Comfort S, Dorrell D, Meireis S, Fine J. MOdified NARanjo causality scale for ICSRs (MONARCSi): a decision support tool for safety scientists. Drug Saf. 2018;41:1073–85.
47. Wang X, Xu X, Tong W, Liu Q, Liu Z. DeepCausality: a general AI-powered causal inference framework for free text: a case study of LiverTox. Front Artif Intell. 2022;5:999289. https://doi.org/10.3389/frai.2022.999289.
48. Spiker J, Kreimeyer K, Dang O, Boxwell D, Chan V, Cheng C, et al. Information visualization platform for post-market surveillance decision support. Drug Saf. 2020;43:905–15.
49. Zhao Y, Yu Y, Wang H, Li Y, Deng Y, Jiang G, Luo Y. Machine learning in causal inference: application in pharmacovigilance. Drug Saf. 2022;45(5):459–76. https://doi.org/10.1007/s40264-022-01155-6.
50. Ralph Edwards I. Causality assessment in pharmacovigilance: still a challenge. Drug Saf. 2017;40:365–72. https://doi.org/10.1007/s40264-017-0509-2.

Pharmacoepidemiologic Studies 9

Deborah Layton

Abstract

Over the last 30 years, observational studies applying epidemiological methods to real-world clinical data from electronic medical records, registries and health insurance claims are highly regarded as generating quality real-world evidence that provides complementary information on safety, particularly post-marketing. This chapter will explore why pharmacoepidemiology is an important part of pharmacovigilance and describe some common epidemiological study designs—namely the cross-sectional study design, the cohort study design and case–control study design—which can be used to study safety (and effectiveness) of medicines. Considerations in objectively assessing such methods will be outlined, including potential confounding and bias, supported by case studies that explore the application of three common epidemiological techniques in support of addressing emergent safety issues. Finally, important initiatives are introduced that collectively aim to improve quality, transparency and reproducibility in generating real-world evidence from observational pharmacoepidemiologic studies that is important for regulatory decision-making.

Keywords

Pharmacovigilance · Pharmacoepidemiology · Pharmacoepidemiologic study methods · Post-authorisation safety studies · Measures of risk and of association · Observational study designs · Confounding and bias · Secondary use data sources · Quality, transparency and reproducibility · Real-world evidence

Learning Objectives

At the end of the chapter, the reader will be able to:

- Define pharmacoepidemiology, pharmacovigilance and real-world evidence.
- Explain the need for observational post-authorisation safety studies and where these fit within pharmacovigilance.
- Identify three commonly used observational study designs and the statistics that are used to report results.
- Explain important limitations of observational study designs and how these impact our interpretation of study results.
- Describe some key considerations of using database networks for post-marketing safety studies.
- Describe the need for quality, transparency and reproducibility of real-world evidence.

D. Layton (✉)
PEPI Consultancy Limited, Southampton, UK
e-mail: drdeborahlayton@outlook.com

J. Jose et al. (eds.), *Principles and Practice of Pharmacovigilance and Drug Safety*,
https://doi.org/10.1007/978-3-031-51089-2_9

Key Points

- The Good Pharmacovigilance Guidelines (GvP) reinforce the mandatory requirement for risk management planning and underpin the importance of pharmacoepidemiological observational techniques in supporting regulatory decision-making across the post-marketing lifecycle of a drug.
- Observational methods can enable the timely identification of any significant safety concerns that arise when a medicinal product is used in the real-world 'uncontrolled' setting.
- As the availability of electronic healthcare databases expands, post-authorisation safety studies are being increasingly conducted to provide real-world evidence, often requested by regulatory agencies.
- It is essential that high-quality data are used and that stakeholders not only understand the strengths and limitations of the methods used but can also interpret the results appropriately in order to improve clinical decision-making. This is essential to protect the health and quality of life of patients.

1 Introduction

Whilst there are many examples of harms associated with medicines since the 1900s, some have been significant enough to have remarkable influence on regulating the safety of medicines and public health policy, as described in Chaps. 6 and 13. Randomised controlled trials (RCTs) conducted during drug development have traditionally been regarded as the gold standard for generating evidence on the efficacy of new medicines, with somewhat limited scope for safety. However, over the last 30 years, observational studies applying epidemiological methods to real-world clinical data from electronic medical records, registries and health insurance claims are highly regarded as generating quality real-world evidence (RWE) that provides complementary information on safety, particularly post-marketing. In this chapter, the reader will explore why pharmacoepidemiology is an important part of pharmacovigilance and gain an understanding of common epidemiological study designs—namely the cross-sectional study design, the cohort study design and case–control study design—which can be used to study safety (and effectiveness) of medicines. Concepts and definitions introduced in Chap. 1 will be further applied in these contexts. Considerations in objectively assessing such methods, including confounding and bias, will be outlined. Notably, it is out of scope of this chapter to have a detailed deep dive into technical aspects of epidemiological methods; other solid introductory texts are available for this. Finally, the reader will be introduced to important initiatives that collectively aim to improve quality, transparency and reproducibility in generating real-world evidence from observational pharmacoepidemiologic studies that are important for regulatory decision-making.

2 The Origins of Drug Safety in the UK and EU

Note: Origin of drug regulation globally is discussed in Chap. 6.

Originally thalidomide was introduced in West Germany in 1956 and marketed in 1958 in the United Kingdom as Distaval®. By 1960, doctors became concerned about possible side effects, and in November 1961, investigations at obstetric units in West Germany showed a significant rise in the number of children born with limb deformities. During drug development, animal tests did not include monitoring for congenital effects during use in pregnancy. By the time thalidomide was withdrawn, over 10,000 babies had been born deformed [1]. This appalling human toll led to the establishment of drug regulatory bodies in a concerted effort to ensure adequate testing of drugs before marketing and pharmacovigilance systems to identify drug safety hazards earlier. Pharmacovigilance is defined as the science and activities relating to the detection, assessment, understanding and prevention of adverse effects or any other medicine-related problem [2]. The lesson learnt was that no pharmacologically effective drug is without hazard.

In the UK, the Committee on Safety of Drugs (subsequently the Committee on Safety of Medicines—CSM and now the Commission on Human Medicines—CHM) was formed [3]. This was followed in May 1964 by the launch of a voluntary spontaneous adverse drug reaction (ADR) reporting system called the Yellow Card Scheme. Crucially, the scheme depended (and still does to this day) on the willingness of healthcare professionals to transmit their suspicions of ADRs that they encountered during their regular work [4]. However, it soon became clear that this system was not entirely fit for purpose. In 1976, practolol (a selective beta-blocker) was withdrawn following the development of a serious ADR—oculomucocutaneous syndrome in hundreds of people [5]. Multiple issues were identified—not only misdiagnosis of early symptoms as conjunctivitis (a common condition in the elderly) but also failure of clinicians to submit spontaneous reports and the ability to generate alerts of seemingly common side effects. In 1980, following several proposals for a complementary safety monitoring scheme aimed at generating evidence around common and uncommon side effects (both serious and non-serious), a small pilot study conducted by the University of Southampton paved the way for an improved method for early detection of potential hazards of drugs destined for widespread, long-term use in primary care, not only for new products but also for established medicines. This scheme, endorsed by the CSM in 1983, was called Prescription-Event Monitoring [6]. Its underlying purpose is to extend the safety database of a new drug to at least 10,000 exposed individuals. The scheme run by the Drug Safety Research Unit (DSRU) remains active to the present day and is available to all primary care general practitioners (GPs), with some modification [7].

In 2005, new pharmacovigilance legislation formally integrated the principles of risk management within the drug safety (and effectiveness) landscape [8]. According to the European Medicines Agency [9] 'Medicines in the European Union (EU) are authorised on the basis that their benefits outweigh their risks for the target population. However, not all potential or actual adverse reactions are identified at the time of initial marketing authorisation. The aim of risk management is to address uncertainties in the safety profile at different points in the product lifecycle, and to plan accordingly'.

Guidance on risk management activities to the pharmaceutical industry was available in Volume 9A of the Rules Governing Medicinal Products in the EU [10]. In brief, a risk management plan (RMP) must include *information* on a medicine's safety profile and plans for pharmacovigilance activities designed to gain greater knowledge. The RMP also explains how risks will be minimised in patients and how those efforts will be measured. Every new medicinal product must have comprehensive RMP in place as part of its approval and to retain its approved status. In 2012, a revised set of guidelines for the conduct of pharmacovigilance was developed which replaced those rules, known as the Good Pharmacovigilance Guidelines (GvP) [11]. These reinforced the requirement for risk management planning through extension of components of the RMP and further guidance on pharmacovigilance processes such as inspections, audits and safety communications as well as product- or population-specific considerations such as management of ADRs. The importance of observational studies in supporting regulatory decision-making across the post-marketing lifecycle of a drug was also recognised formally within the updated pharmacovigilance legislation. In terms of studying specific safety concerns, Part III: The Pharmacovigilance Plan describes the inclusion of additional pharmacovigilance activities which includes (but not limited to) non-interventional studies that may be conducted to provide additional characterisation of the (long-term) safety of a medicinal product.

The GVP Module VIII uses the legal definition of a post-authorisation safety study (PASS) as defined in Directive 2001/83/EC (DIR) Art 1(15), namely any study relating to an authorised medicinal product conducted with the aim of identifying, characterising or quantifying a safety hazard, confirming the safety profile of the medicinal product, or of measuring the effectiveness of risk management measures (see Box 9.1 for additional conditions of a non-interventional PASS) [12]. A PASS may be initiated, managed or financed by a Marketing Authorisation Holder (MAH) either voluntary or following an obligation imposed by a competent authority. The most important consideration of that PASS is that they are post-marketing studies intended to study a drug under real-world conditions, where the data reflect such use, outside the context of RCTs. The term real-world evidence' (RWE) has been used for evidence obtained from the analysis of real-world data (RWD) and is often used to support regulatory decision-making (see Sect. 5).

Box 9.1 The Additional Conditions of a Non-interventional PASS [12]

- The medicinal product is prescribed in the usual manner in accordance with the terms of the marketing authorisation.
- The assignment of the patient to a particular therapeutic strategy is not decided in advance by a trial protocol but falls within current practice, and the prescription of the medicine is clearly separated from the decision to include the patient in the study.
- No additional diagnostic or monitoring procedures are applied to the patients, and epidemiological methods are used for the analysis of collected data.

Other types of non-interventional studies also include those that are prospective (where subjects are recruited before outcomes of interest are developed) with de novo primary data collection, provided the conditions set out above are met [12]. However, non-interventional studies with primary data collection may be subject to other pharmacovigilance processes, such as reporting of individual cases of suspected ADRs [13]. Clinical trials may be considered as a PASS, but these are uncommon and will not be discussed here.

A PASS may have several objectives which may include the quantification of risks identified with the RMP as 'potential' or 'identified' within all users (often compared to patients taking another drug), and/or in sub-populations of special interest for which safety information is limited or missing (e.g. pregnant women, elderly or young); risks associated with long-term use; patterns of drug utilisation that add to knowledge on safety and effectiveness of a risk minimisation activity (e.g. such as healthcare professional communications).

3 Epidemiological Techniques for Post-marketing Studies

The ability to characterise the certainty of strength of evidence for a safety concern relies on a robust understanding of scientific methods, including observational epidemiological methods and where that evidence falls short. Pharmacoepidemiology has traditionally been defined concisely as 'An applied science which uses epidemiologic techniques to study drug effects' [14]. The current concise definition endorsed in 2023 by the International Society for Pharmacoepidemiology (ISPE) is 'Pharmacoepidemiology is a scientific discipline that uses epidemiological methods to evaluate the use, benefits and risks of medical products and interventions in human populations' [15]. Accordingly, such studies quantify drug use patterns and adverse drug effects. In this section, it is hoped that the reader will get some appreciation of the varied architecture of the most common observational epidemiological techniques, their application to real-world drug safety questions and the necessary considerations regarding study validity and bias. The GVP Module VIII provides a summary of methods used for PASS. The focus of this section will be restricted to those listed as the following observational study designs: cross-sectional, case–control and cohort studies [12]. As also stated therein, the classification of a PASS is not constrained by the type of study design chosen, but by its aims and objectives. The most up-to-date advances in quantitative methods and innovative concepts are beyond the scope of this section, and the reader should refer to other bespoke texts [16]. However firstly, some fundamental concepts should be outlined.

3.1 Common Terms

Understanding the nomenclature presented in publications can be challenging. For each study design, it is important to know how the results are presented and their interpretation. This section is not intended to be a fully comprehensive overview; the reader should again refer to other texts for that [16].

3.1.1 Measures of Disease Frequency and Association

A measure of disease frequency is the epidemiological term that characterises the occurrence of health outcomes (be it an adverse event, adverse drug reaction or some other health condition in a study population). It is descriptive in nature and is expressed most commonly as risk (incidence), rate and prevalence (Table 9.1). Notably, these measures can be correctly estimated because the population at risk at the start of the study can be defined; however, there are some situations where this is not possible. This situation occurs for case–control studies where the approximation of a measure of frequency is given as the odds (see Sect. 3.2.3 for further details on case–control study design).

Table 9.1 Common measures of disease frequency
These estimates should always be reported with 95% confidence interval

Measure	Definition	Example
Risk	Also known as '*incidence*' This measure defines the probability of an unaffected individual developing a specified health outcome over a given period of time. Risk = numerator (number of new cases with the health outcome)/denominator (total number of individuals at risk at the start of study period)	The incidence of first-time use of oral contraceptive (OC) as recorded in a primary care database among women aged 15–44 years in England in 2022 would be calculated as follows: numerator (number of women with their first ever (OC) prescription)/denominator (number of women in database at the start of 2022) *A risk of 0.1 indicates that 1 in 10 women within that age group will start an OC for the first time*
Rate	This measure defines how quickly the health outcome occurs in the population over time. Rate = numerator (number of new cases with the health outcomes)/denominator (total person-time observed for the individuals during the study where person-time is the sum of time that each at-risk individual contributes to the study	The incidence rate of myocardial infarction (MI) in first-time users of an NSAID in the first month after starting treatment, as recorded in a primary care database would be calculated as follows: numerator (number of patients newly diagnosed with MI)/denominator (the sum of person-time (months) from each individual newly prescribed the NSAID within the first month) *A rate of 1 per 1000 person-months indicates that, on average for every 1000 people given an NSAID and followed for one month, 1 new case of an MI will develop*

(continued)

Table 9.1 (continued)

Measure	Definition	Example
Odds	Used in a case–control study, this measure defines the probability (p) of a health outcome occurring divided by the probability of the health outcome not occurring ($1 - p$)*, in a group defined by a characteristic, e.g. exposure Odds = numerator (number of cases of the health outcome)/denominator (number of subjects who did not have the health outcome) *when p is very small $1 - p$ is close to p, so odds approximates risk	The odds of rhabdomyolysis in patients exposed to a statin for 1 year would be calculated as follows: numerator (number of patients who had the diagnosis)/denominator (number of patients who did not have the diagnosis) *if the probability (p) of rhabdomyolysis is 0.75, then the odds of rhabdomyolysis in this exposed population is* $p/(1 - p) = 0.75/(1 - 0.75) = 3$
Prevalence	This measure defines the proportion of a health outcome at a given period of time, irrespective of new or pre-existing. It indicates how widespread the health outcome is at a given time Prevalence = numerator (number of **all** cases of the health outcome)/denominator (total number of individuals at risk at a particular point in time [termed point prevalence] (or over a given time (study) period [termed period prevalence]	The point prevalence of heart disease as recorded in a primary care database among men aged 18–65 years in England at the start of 2020 would be calculated as follows: numerator (number of men with a diagnosis of heart disease (new or pre-existing)/ denominator (number of men in database at the start of 2020).The point prevalence of 0.25 indicates that 25% of men within that age group were affected by heart disease at the start of 2020. The period prevalence would be the proportion of cases of heart disease during 2020 *A period prevalence of 0.25 indicates that 25% of men within that age group were affected by heart disease in that year.*

When estimating these measures, there is always uncertainty around that estimate because the number is based on a sample of the population under study. The confidence interval (CI) is the range of values that one expects the estimate to fall between a certain percentage of the time if you repeat the study or re-sample the population similarly. The 95% CI is often reported—it is beyond the scope of this chapter to provide details of the statistical foundation of measuring the variability of estimates but suffice to say, based on the normal distribution and that the central value represents truth, it is assumed that one can be confident that the estimate reported lies within the range that spans the true estimate, should the study be repeated many times.

Measures of association quantify the relationship between two variables—for example, between a specific exposure and a health outcome (such as an adverse event or adverse drug reaction), and enable comparisons to be made on health outcomes between study populations, for example, between those with a particular exposure and those without. Common measures of association include the absolute difference or the relative difference (as a ratio) between risks, rates or odds (Table 9.2).

3.1.2 *P*-value

The probability (p)-value is used in medical statistics to allow one to make a decision about whether any differences in the observed effect estimates may have occurred by chance. It indicates the strength of evidence against the hypothesis of no difference (reflected by the relevant null values). The basis of that decision is usually taken to be a fixed value of 0.05. When the p-value is large (and above this threshold of 0.05), investigators often report this as statistically non-significant result and proceed as if they have proved there is no effect—but actually this can also demonstrate a failure to detect a statistically significant one. There is a relationship between p-value and the CI such that the 95% upper and lower bounds do not include the

Table 9.2 Common measures of association
These estimates should always be reported with 95% confidence interval

Measure	Definition	Example
Risk (rate) difference	This measure represents the absolute difference between two groups and represents the excess risk (or rate) attributable to the exposure of interest. The value may be positive indicating higher risk or negative indicating a protective effect. If the value is zero (referred to as 'null' value for a difference), then there is no absolute difference in effect Risk difference* = $\text{Risk}_{\text{exposed}} - \text{Risk}_{\text{unexposed}**}$ Rate Difference = $\text{Rate}_{\text{exposed}} - \text{Rate}_{\text{unexposed}**}$ * may also be referred to as Attributable Risk (AR) **the unexposed group may also be called the reference group if exposed to an alternative treatment	The risk of serious gastrointestinal bleeds in the first year after starting treatment is 0.05% for a COX-2 selective inhibitor (exposure of interest) and 0.1% for another NSAID (reference group). *The risk difference (attributable risk) is −0.05% with a 95% CI (−0.07, −0.02) indicating that since the upper 95% CI bound does not go above zero (i.e. −0.02), the exposure of interest is associated with a protective effect*
Risk (rate) ratio (RR)	The relative difference is defined as a ratio of risk (or rate) in the exposed group to the risk in the unexposed group. The value may be higher than 1 indicating higher risk or lower than indicating a protective effect. If the value is 1 (the null value for a ratio), then there is no difference in effect Risk ratio*** = $\text{Risk}_{\text{exposed}}/\text{Risk}_{\text{unexposed}}$ *** may also be referred to as Relative Risk (RR) Rate ratio = $\text{Rate}_{\text{exposed}}/\text{Rate}_{\text{unexposed}}$	The rate of deep vein thrombosis in first 6 months after starting treatment is 1.15 per 1000 person-years for a COX-2 selective inhibitor (exposure of interest) and 0.69 per 1000 person-years for another NSAID (reference group). *The crude RR is 1.66 and the 95% CI is (1.16, 2.38), indicating that since the 95% CI does not go below 1, the exposure of interest is associated with a higher rate of this adverse event*
Odds ratio (OR)	This is a relative measure, that is, the ratio of the odds of an event in the exposed group to the odds of the same event in the nonexposed group. The OR can range from zero to infinity. OR > 1 indicates exposure increases risk while OR < 1 indicates that exposure is protecting against risk. If the value is 1 then there is no difference in effect Odds ratio = Odds of event in exposed group/Odds of event in unexposed group	For a trial comparing a new anticoagulant to warfarin, the odds of all-cause mortality for the new anticoagulant was 0.4 and for warfarin the odds was 0.8. *The crude OR is 0.5 and the 95% CI is (0.4, 0.6), meaning that since the 95% CI does not go above (1) the odds of death in those exposed to the new anticoagulant is 50% less than those exposed to warfarin*

null value; it is likely that the observation will be significant. The term 5% significance is often used in observational epidemiology. For example, consider the hypothetical statement 'In a cohort study comparing the risk of rhabdomyolysis between statin users and non-statin users within the first 3 months of use, a risk ratio of 4.96 (with a 95%CI of 2.8, 8.7) was reported'. The *p*-value was $p < 0.0001$. This would be considered a statistically significant result at the 5% level of significance. However, a 5% significance level indicates that once in every 20 times a test is undertaken on the same sample, the result is likely to be significant by chance alone. Therefore, there is always the possibility of making the wrong decision, and one should not rely on an absolute *p*-value alone but evaluate this in combination with other information such as clinical significance and the 95% CI.

3.1.3 Bias

As alluded to in the previous section, the variability of any estimate is an inherent part of the data being measured and the measurement process. In statistics, the term 'error' is used to define the difference between a calculated value and the 'true' value. It does not imply a mistake. This error can be divided into two components—random and systematic.

- Random errors: are chance fluctuations in the data through natural variation. It is random, such that the next measurement cannot be predicted from the previous value. Natural variation means that on occasion, measures may be imprecise (reflected by a wide 95% CI), but it still represents the population value.

- Systematic errors: are introduced through inaccuracy in the research methodology which contains some constant 'offset' that can occur reproducibly. Bias is a term used to describe any systematic error in an epidemiological study that results in an incorrect estimate of the association between exposure and risk of disease. Notably the 95% CI may appear to be narrow (indicating a precise measure), but it may still be biased.

Avoidance of random error is influenced by using good quality assurance systems to ensure high internal validity. However, in contrast, the presence of systematic error is hard to avoid and can result in a distortion of the study estimate in any direction. It can lead to an underestimation or overestimation of a measure and cannot be corrected for at the analysis stage. Bias may occur at any stage of a study. The presence of bias cannot be determined internally, and one must look to some sort of external standard. There are many types of bias; however, we will focus on one of the most important for epidemiological studies—selection bias.

Selection bias occurs when the association between exposure and disease is different for those who complete a study compared with those who are in the target population (this phenomenon is call 'depletion of susceptibles'); or where the study members are systematically different through a sampling method, compared to the overall population for which the measure of effect is intended to provide inference about (e.g. Box 9.2).

Box 9.2 Loss to Follow-Up Bias in Medical Research

Suppose in a hypothetical cohort study below, investigators compared the incidence of myocardial infarction (MI) in 10,000 men taking an NSAID and 10,000 men not taking an NSAID for 1 year. MI occurred in 20 subjects taking the NSAID and in 10 subjects not taking the NSAID, so the unbiased risk ratio is (20/10,000)/(10/10,000) = 2.0, with the rate ratio as (20/10,000 person-years (pyrs))/10/10,000 pyrs) = 2.0.

However, suppose there were substantial losses (attrition) to both groups over the period after entering the study (follow-up) for any reason, i.e. 6000 in the exposed group and 4000 in the unexposed group had less than 1 year of follow-up.

This substantially reduces the number of patients in not only the 'denominator' for risk but also the rate. In addition, suppose here was a greater tendency to lose subjects taking the NSAID who subsequently developed MI. Assume there was a loss of 12 diseased subjects in the group taking NSAIDs (leaving 8 subjects), but only 2 subjects with MI in the unexposed group (leaving 8 subjects). In other words, there is a differential loss between the groups and there is also a change in the numerator of cases of MI. This would result in a biased risk ratio of (8/10,000)/8(10,000) = 1.0. Remember the denominator is of persons at risk at the start of the study which is the same as before.

However, assuming those subjects that left contributed an average of 6 months of follow-up time in the year, the denominator would be less, i.e. in the exposed group, 4000 patients contribute 4000 pyrs but 6000 contribute 3000 pyrs giving a sum of 7000 pyrs, whilst in the unexposed group 6000 patients contribute 6000 pyrs and 4000 contribute 2000 pyrs giving a sum of 8000 pyrs, such that the biased rate ratio would be (8/7000 pyrs)/(8/8000pyrs) = 1.14.

So in this scenario, whilst there was substantial attrition in both groups, there was greater loss of diseased patients in the exposed group than the unexposed group.

For a more detailed understanding of selection bias and other different types of bias, the reader is referred to other texts [16, 17].

3.1.4 Confounding

Confounding is another type of systematic error. It is an important concept because if present it can also cause an under- or over-estimate of the association between exposure and an outcome. It occurs when other factors that are independently related to both the disease and primary exposure distort the observed association. The distortion may be large or even change the direction of the association effect. It must be understood that it is rarely only the exposure that is associated with an outcome and other factors may be associated with that outcome independent of the exposure. Therefore, these other factors (called 'confounders') need to be accounted for when evaluating any association. Whilst confounding is a form of bias which can occur in any epidemiological study, it can, unlike most bias, be handled in the analysis of a study. Each potential confounder should be assessed according to (a) whether it is a known risk factor for the outcome of interest and (b) independently associated with the main exposure of interest (and not caused by it). For more details, the reader is referred to other texts [16]. An example of confounding (in the form of channelling) is given in Box 9.3.

Box 9.3 Channelling and Confounding

In RCTs, the process of randomisation ensures that the allocation of treatment is independent of patients' health characteristics and also balances the profile of health characteristics between the two groups. However, pharmacoepidemiological observational studies do not employ randomisation and are thus used in real-world clinical practice data to compare groups of patients taking a drug compared to those who do not. In this situation, it is the patient or their doctors who choose whether or not to use the medicine based on clinical need, so allocation is not random. The indication for treatment will be related to the choice of treatment and could be related to any outcome the patient experiences. This phenomenon therefore introduces a selection bias through preferential prescribing of a drug to subsets of patients who have a different underlying risk to those who are not exposed to the drug. The validity of then comparing safety outcomes between the exposed and unexposed is determined by the extent to which the observed difference in the risk of an event between the comparison groups can be attributed to the drug rather than other factors.

An example of where channelling may have had a profound effect on the interpretation of safety is that of rofecoxib—this being an NSAID associated with a lower risk of gastrointestinal bleeding (through its selective mechanism of action via inhibition of the cyclooxygenase (COX) 2 enzyme). Rofecoxib and similar NSAIDs were commonly known as 'coxibs' and were different to NSAIDs that had been available for many years which did not demonstrate this selective inhibition [18]. That rofecoxib was advocated as a pharmacologically 'cleaner' drug with a reduced risk of gastrointestinal bleeding resulted in the product being prescribed in real-world clinical practice to patients who were considered at high risk of GI bleed [19]. Whilst this advantage was indeed observed, it was noted that coxibs were being prescribed instead of traditional NSAIDs to high comorbidity patients susceptible to other types of adverse health outcomes including those of cardiovascular origin.

Many observational studies were conducted to explore this safety issue, but due to the type of data available, it was often not possible to account for differences in baseline cardiovascular risk between study populations, not only for the prevalence of cardiovascular disease but also for other risk factors associated with cardiovascular disease. Thus, missing or partial information on cardiovascular risk factors is likely to have confounded (distorted) the study findings [20].

3.2 Observational Study Designs

3.2.1 Cross-Sectional Studies

These studies measure the prevalence of health outcomes (e.g. adverse event or adverse drug reaction) and/or a particular determinant of health (e.g. exposure to a drug) at the same point in time [12] (Fig. 9.1). There is no evaluation of what happens to a patient after that point in time (or several fixed points of time) or what happened to the patient before that point, so no temporal sequence between an exposure and health outcome can be established. This in turn means this type of study cannot infer any causal relationship. However, it can offer insights into drug prescribing or disease burden. This type of approach may also be used to examine associations between exposure and outcome at the population level for ecological studies. In terms of applications, this design may be applied for drug utilisation research—an essential part of pharmacoepidemiology as it describes the extent, nature and determinants of drug exposure at the patient level.

How the data are sampled and the response rate to the survey (if applicable) will determine the generalisability of results from a cross-sectional study to the broader population. The optimum situation would be the sampling frame based on the whole population, but for representativeness of the population, responders should also be representative. If performing an active survey rather than using existing data, nonresponse is a problem which has been observed for descriptive safety surveillance studies such as Prescription-Event Monitoring which relies on general practitioners to fill out questionnaires [21].

Case Study 1 (Sect. 7.1) explores the application of a cross-sectional design to address a regulatory issue. Concerns of the persistence and severity of the adverse effects of fluoroquinolones, mainly involving the nervous system, muscles and joints, resulted in the 2018 referral procedure led by the European Medicines Agency (EMA). They advised to stop prescribing fluoroquinolones for infections of mild severity or of a presumed self-limiting course and for prevention

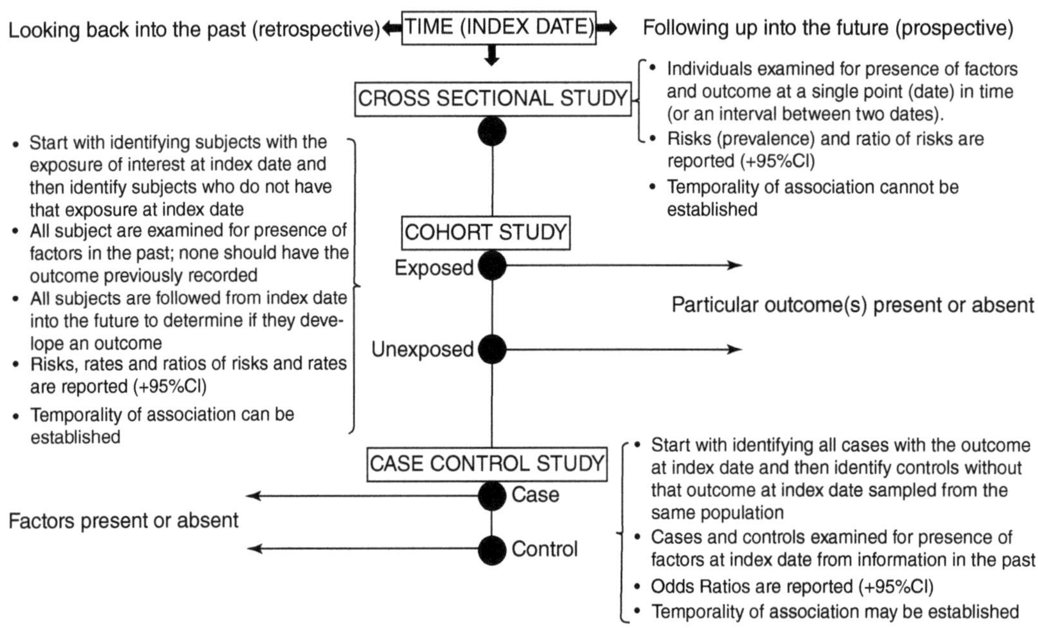

Fig. 9.1 Overview of cross-sectional, cohort and case–control study designs
Adapted from: Dupépé, Esther & Kicielinski, Kimberly & Gordon, Amber & Walters, Beverly. (2019). What is a Case-Control Study? Neurosurgery. 84. 819–826. 10.1093/neuros/nyy590

of infections, plus to restrict prescriptions in cases of milder infections where other treatment options are available and restrict in at-risk populations. The drug utilisation study utilised a cross-sectional approach in the analysis by estimating fluoroquinolone prescribing trends for each month between 2018 and 2019 [22].

3.2.2 Cohort Studies

Cohort studies can be used to estimate the incidence risk and rate of an event after exposure to a medicine (see Sect. 3.1.1). They are particularly suitable for assessing multiple health outcomes following exposure, especially over a long-term period. In particular, cohort studies have the advantage that the temporal relationship between an exposure (e.g. to a medicine) and an outcome (e.g. adverse event or adverse drug reaction) can be established since the selection of the population is based on a particular exposure before the event has occurred, i.e. at the start of follow-up, given that all subjects are free of the outcome (Fig. 9.1). Such a study may also be referred to as a longitudinal study. However, there are several disadvantages in that cohort studies often require large sample sizes and possibly a long study duration especially if the outcomes are rare.

A cohort study may be prospective, which identifies a cohort based on present day and follows a cohort into the future for an outcome, whilst a retrospective study uses historical information tracing the cohort back in time for exposure information knowing the outcome may have already occurred (Fig. 9.1). More often retrospective studies will use data that already exists in data sources such as registries, health insurance claims or primary care clinical practice electronic medical records. In such circumstances, these data are being re-used, and the term 'secondary use of data' is applied to indicate that the data has not been specifically generated for the study.

In designing a cohort study, as with any study, a protocol must be developed, and the following general steps would be used:

- After defining the research aims and objectives, the investigator should identify all of the criteria that would be used to characterise the population at risk, the exposure and the outcomes. This may be through code lists if using secondary data sources.
- Once the general framework of the desired characteristics is defined, the investigator must identify the best source data that are fit for purpose to address the research question (see Sect. 5.3). The source data should be generalisable to the region or country to which the result would apply.
- From that data source, the study subjects at risk of the outcome and who would be treated with the medicine of interest will be identified. The investigator should construct relevant inclusion criteria and minimal inclusion criteria to identify the eligible study population using the characteristics previously defined. Since not all subjects within that data source may be used, the selection of subjects from the data source should ideally be representative of the data source and also the target population to which the results would apply.
- If the study aims to contextualise the risk or rate of the outcome(s) against, e.g. another drug or subjects unexposed to the medicine of interest, two or more groups of subjects (referred to as study cohorts) that differ according to their exposure may be identified. In this scenario, the measure of effect (ratio of risks or rates—see Sect. 3.1.1) can be calculated.
- The study investigator should define the relevant calendar period to capture all data (this defining study start and stop date). In addition, the length of time that each study subject should be observed from first exposure to the medicine (defined as index date) should be defined, including the criteria that outline what to do when a patient can no longer be followed (called censoring). Each group (exposed to a medicine or not) should be followed from index date with sufficient time to observe the occurrence of the outcome(s) of interest, should it occur. For example, if an event only occurs after 6 months, then subjects should be observed for at least 7 months in order for information for that event to be captured, should it occur.
- The study investigator should also define how far back records will be examined to define

clinical characteristics at index date for each cohort (termed 'look back'); often a minimum of 12 months is needed.

- The statistical analysis plan should not only include how the risk and rate (or risk or rate ratio) will be calculated but also how to best account for other characteristics that may be associated with the outcome itself (risk factors) or characteristics that may be associated with both exposure and the outcome (confounders). The study investigator should define appropriate statistical modelling approaches for 'adjusting' for these variables. In this sense, to adjust is to try and balance the groups in terms of particular characteristics so that any effect of a particular characteristic is effectively reduced. Various methods exist, and it is beyond the scope of this chapter to review these [23]. In addition, the study investigator should consider how to test the robustness of any results. This may be through examining model diagnostics and/or conducting sensitivity analyses whereby, for example, definitions of variables or follow-up time may be modified to see if the results change in any way.
- Finally the study investigator should consider all of the possible biases and sources of error that may affect the study conduct and/or results. By identifying as many in advance as possible, steps can be put in place to reduce that risk. However, sometimes risks that occur are beyond the control of the study investigator.

Case Study 2 (Sect. 7.2) explores the application of a cohort study design for contextualisation of safety signals arising from spontaneous reporting data. A particular concern arose regarding thrombotic events, with concurrent thrombocytopenia reported among individuals vaccinated with adenovirus-based vaccines against SARS-CoV-2. As of May 26, 2021, 348 spontaneous reports of major thromboembolic events with thrombocytopenia had been documented following 24 million first doses and 13 million second doses of an adenovirus-based COVID-19 vaccine in the UK. Although fewer concerns have been raised about safety signals for an mRNA-based COVID-19 vaccine, instances of immune thrombocytopenia had also been observed among recipients of this vaccine. In this cohort study, the authors estimated the incidence of thrombosis, thrombocytopenia and thrombosis with thrombocytopenia over the 28 days following a first dose of the an adenovirus-based COVID-19 vaccine and an mRNA-based COVID-19 vaccine and compared these rates with historical, pre-pandemic rates in the general population [24].

3.2.3 Case–Control Study

Case–control studies are particularly useful if investigating whether there is an association between a medicinal product (or several products) and a rare outcome (e.g. a specific rare adverse event), as well as to identify other multiple risk factors for that rare outcome. Advantages of a case–control study include a computational efficiency far superior to the cohort design, the possibility to initiate a study based on a set of cases already identified (e.g. in a hospital); they require fewer subjects and are less expensive to conduct. In contrast to a cohort study (whereby the investigator identifies a subject based on exposure before the event has occurred), in a case–control study, the investigator identifies subjects on the basis of whether they had the event (cases) and looks backwards to examine a range of factors including exposures to medicines that may have contributed to being a case (Fig. 9.1). Thus, case–control studies are usually retrospective. However, in order to make any meaningful interpretation, the distribution of these factors must also be examined for subjects who originate from the same population as cases but do not have the event called (controls). In contrast to cohort studies, case–control studies do not measure incidence because of the sampling method (see below), so only the 'relative' size of a measure of disease frequency can be estimated, namely the odds of a case being exposed to a particular factor (medication) can be compared to the odds of a control being exposed to that same factor and the odds ratio calculated (see Sect. 3.1.1).

In designing a case–control study, whilst some common steps overall should be followed as outlined for the design of a cohort study (protocol, data feasibility and possible bias/sources of error), some different aspects should be considered:

- After defining the research aims and objectives, the investigator should identify all of the criteria that would be used to define the case and any risk factors (including exposures) that need to be investigated.
- From the chosen data source, the study subjects who are cases will be identified. The investigator should construct relevant inclusion criteria and minimal inclusion criteria to identify the eligible case population using the characteristics previously defined.
- An important aspect that the investigator must specify is how the 'control' subjects who are not cases will be sampled from the same source from which the cases originate. Controls should be as comparable as possible (termed 'counterfactual') to the cases with the only exception being that they are not a case. In order to do this, a process of 'matching' is necessary. For each case, the investigator should specify how many controls are desired per case and the factors to match on. Through a random allocation process, a pseudo-case date is created for each control. Generally matching factors are measured at this pseudo-index date and are most often those for which the confounding effect is well known, e.g. age (often ±5 year age bands), sex and calendar time. This creates a set of eligible controls for each case; this group of cases and controls is called a 'risk set'. Although this matching may help to control for some unmeasured confounders making cases and controls more similar, it may also introduce a distribution of that matching factor in the study population that is different to the overall source population which itself can reduce generalisability to other populations. Once a risk set has been created, further refinement of the risk set may be specified, e.g. matching on several other factors using methods such as propensity scores [23]. Up to 10 controls per case can be used.
- As for the cohort study, the study investigator should define the relevant calendar period to capture all data (thus defining study start and stop date). In addition, the length of time that each study subject should be observed historically (the look back period) should be defined up to the date of the matched event date. This should be relevant to the outcome, for example, if an important risk factor could be long-term exposure to a drug, the look back period should be sufficiently long enough to capture such exposure, should it have occurred for both cases and controls. The creation of these risk sets also requires a specific analytical approach called conditional logistic regression modelling which the study investigator should specify, along with other risk factors and confounders that should be adjusted for, excluding the matching factors.

However, there are some important limitations. Because of the way that the study population is assembled, there is risk of differential sampling of cases and controls such that the distribution of exposure categories among controls is not a valid representation of the distribution of exposure in the source population. Furthermore, being retrospective in nature, such studies are subject to recall bias, where knowledge regarding exposure or other risk factors may not be accurately recalled by participants or care providers or recorded in the databases. Another disadvantage is the difficulty to study very rare exposures, as a large sample of cases and controls would be needed to identify exposed groups large enough for the planned statistical analysis.

In order to increase the efficiency of exposure assessment in case–control studies, an alternative approach is a design in which the source population is a cohort. The nested case–control design includes all cases occurring in the cohort and a pre-specified number of controls randomly chosen from the population at risk at each time a case (or other relevant event) occurs [25]. Another study design, a case–cohort study includes all cases and a randomly selected sub-cohort from the population at risk [26]. Advantages of such designs are to allow the conduct of a set of case–control studies from a single cohort and use efficiently electronic healthcare records (EHRs) databases where data on exposures and outcomes are already available.

Case Study 3 (Sect. 7.3) explores the application of a case–control study that has been nested within a cohort study for purposes of further exploring a safety signal (termed signal strengthening).

Selective serotonin re-uptake inhibitors (SSRI) are associated with an increased risk of bleeding, most notably upper gastrointestinal bleeding [27]. Results from the Women's Health Initiative Study suggest a doubling in the risk of haemorrhagic stroke amongst post-menopausal SSRI recipients [28]. This nested case–control study aimed to investigate whether SSRI use was associated with an increased risk of haemorrhagic stroke [29].

4 Real-World Data Sources

Two of the three case studies presented in Sect. 3.2 were conducted in more than one data source. EHRs, population-based registries and health insurance administrative databases are now being used extensively via linkage to other data sources or via a network across many countries for pharmacoepidemiological studies [30]. These systems take advantage of record linkage to provide rapid access to thousands of patients and thus reduce the time and expense required to explore relationships between drug exposure and outcomes. Collaborations for multi-database studies have been embraced by regulators, marketing authorisations and researchers alike in providing real-world data for the generation of decision-grade evidence for benefit–risk assessment of licensed medicines. For example, DARWIN EU is a federated network involving several databases that is supported by the EMA and designed to engage in rapid analytics of safety concerns identified by the EMA that warrant urgent investigation [31].

The European Network of Centres for Pharmacoepidemiology and Pharmacovigilance (ENCePP) is an initiative that brings together expertise and resources in pharmacoepidemiology and pharmacovigilance across Europe. ENCePP is coordinated by the EMA, and its aim is to strengthen the monitoring of the benefit:risk balance of medicinal products. This is achieved by facilitating the conduct of high-quality, multicentre, independent PASS with a focus on observational research. ENCePP is composed of research centres and networks referred to as 'ENCePP partners', and participation in ENCePP is voluntary. ENCePP is globally acknowledged for its expertise and outputs [32]. A meta-data catalogue (the ENCePP Resources Database) was developed as a publicly available electronic index of available European research organisations, networks and data sources, in the fields of pharmacoepidemiology and pharmacovigilance [33]. It included information on expertise and research experience across the region and serves as a hub for both researchers and study sponsors seeking to identify organisations and datasets for conducting specific pharmacoepidemiology and pharmacovigilance studies in Europe. This has been replaced in 2024 by the new EMA-HMA Catalogues of data sources and non-interventional studies.

According to the ENCePP methodological guide [30], the advantages of using multi-database designs over single databases include:

- An increase in the *size* of the study populations. This especially facilitates research on rare events, drugs used in specialised settings or when the interest is in subgroup effects.
- Exploitation of the *heterogeneity* of treatment options across countries, which allows studying the effect of different drugs used for the same indication or specific patterns of utilisation.
- Exploitation of the differences in outcome/event rates across countries/regions.
- Provision of additional knowledge on the *generalisability* of results and on the *consistency of association*, for instance whether a safety issue can be identified in several countries.
- Engagement of experts from various countries addressing case definitions, terminologies, coding in databases and research practices provides opportunities to increase *consistency of results* of observational studies.
- In the case of primary data collection, *shortening the time* needed for obtaining the desired sample size and therefore accelerating investigation of drug safety issues or other outcomes.

Disadvantages relate to data access due to data protection rules as well as the need for standardisation and harmonisation of data architecture to support the pooling of data (or results). Over the last decade, the number of common data models (CDM) that facilitate such harmonisation has grown [34]. An example of a collaborative research network that includes EU databases that uses a generalised CDM is Observational Health Data Sciences and Informatics (OHDSI) (www.ohdsi.org). Through an open science community (European Health Data & Evidence Network (EHDEN) www. www.ehden.eu), many EU databases that participate within OHDSI have been mapped according to the Observational Medical Outcomes Partnership (OMOP) CDM used by OHDSI independent of a study, supported by rigorous quality assurance procedures [27]. When a study is required, a common protocol is developed and a centrally created analysis programme is created that runs locally on each database to extract and analyse the data. The output of the common programmes shared may be an analytical dataset or study estimates, depending on the governance of the network [34].

5 A Prospective Look at Pharmacoepidemiology: Quality, Transparency and Reproducibility

During one's career as a healthcare professional, for making decisions about appropriate use of medicines for a patient, one must evaluate published evidence and guidelines and has to make decisions on what constitutes reliable quality evidence on the safety of medicines. With the increasing availability of EMR, there has been a global expansion of observational research. However, in parallel, there have been numerous examples of failures due to poor quality research that has cast a huge shadow on the acceptability of evidence from observational studies [35, 36].

As we navigate the journey from real-world data to real-world evidence, one needs to establish confidence that the evidence is of sufficient quality, so we must ask ourselves questions such as the following: Given imperfect data, how do we know if the data are of sufficient quality and fit for purpose? Are the generation, recording, verification, analysis and reporting of results accurate enough? Has quality been managed through all stages of the study?

However, quality is not a singular concept that can be directly observed, and researchers must still make judgements about the reliability of study findings. Methods must be developed to measure and manage quality. The ideal is to have in place a quality management system that can apply a risk-based approach—both at the system level (e.g. the computerised system) and at the study level (e.g. are the data to be used and is the study design appropriate to answer the research question). There is no singular definition for quality; however, one can consider the attributes (Box 9.4) that describe quality along the continuum of evidence creation [37].

Box 9.4 Desired Attributes of Reliable Quality Evidence [37]

Repeatable	*For the same question, one gets identical results when applying the same analysis to the same data by the same researcher*
Reproducible	*For the same question, a different researcher should get the same results as another researcher when applying the same analysis to the same data*
Replicable	*For the same question, the same (or a different researcher) should get similar results when applying the same analysis to a different dataset data*
Generalisable	*For the same question conducted across several databases, similar results are observed when applying the same analysis, despite anticipated heterogeneity*
Robust	*For the same question, results are not overly sensitive to subjective choices made within an analysis*
Calibrated	*The performance of any evidence-generating system should be verified*

With many stakeholders having a vested interest in generating quality evidence from pharmacoepidemiological studies, the construction and harmonisation of processes supporting the continuum are firmly underway. What follows are summary descriptions of only a few notable initiatives in the EU; there are many others, and it is beyond the scope of this chapter to present them all.

5.1 The European Network of Centres for Pharmacoepidemiology and Pharmacovigilance (ENCePP) Guide on Methodological Standards

The ENCePP Guide is a document that provides guidance on methodological standards for conducting studies in pharmacoepidemiology and pharmacovigilance. For each topic covered, direct links to internationally agreed recommendations, key points from important guidelines, published articles and textbooks are provided. Where relevant, gaps in existing guidance are addressed with what ENCePP considers good practice. This guide is regarded fundamentally as the best practice standard for the conduct of pharmacoepidemiological observational studies and their application as PASS and is now in its 11th revision. It is maintained by the ENCePP Research Standards and Guidance working group under EMA's coordination and updated annually by structured review to maintain its dynamic nature [30].

5.2 The European Network of Centres for Pharmacoepidemiology and Pharmacovigilance (ENCePP) Checklist for Study Protocols

The Checklist for Study Protocols aims to stimulate researchers to consider important epidemiological principles when designing a pharmacoepidemiological study and writing a study protocol; promote transparency regarding methodologies used in pharmacoepidemiological studies and increase awareness about developments in science and methodology in the field of pharmacoepidemiology [38].

The Checklist is intended to promote the quality of studies and not their uniformity and is aligned with scientific and regulatory developments relevant to pharmacoepidemiology. GVP module VIII on PASS recommends that the Checklist is included as an annex to study protocols [12].

5.3 The Real-World Evidence Transparency Initiative

This is a collaboration between the International Professional Society for Health economics and outcomes research (ISPOR), the International Society for Pharmacoepidemiology (ISPE), the Duke-Margolis Center for Health Policy in the US and the National Pharmaceutical Council in the US with the objective of establishing a culture of transparency for study analysis and reporting of RWE studies [39]. ISPOR (www.ispor.org) was established in 1995 with a mission to promote health economics and outcomes research excellence to improve decision-making for health globally. ISPE (www.pharmacoepi.org) is also an international organisation dedicated to advancing the health of the public by providing a global forum for the open exchange of scientific information and for the development of policy, education and advocacy for the field of pharmacoepidemiology, including such areas as pharmacovigilance, drug utilisation research, comparative effectiveness review and therapeutic risk management. Both societies are multi-stakeholder organisations of a wide variety of healthcare stakeholders, including researchers and academicians, assessors and regulators, payers and policy-makers, the life sciences industry, healthcare providers and patient engagement organisations. As part of the RWE Transparency initiative, they advocate for a culture of transparency to build trust in secondary data study analysis and reporting of hypotheses in regulatory decision-grade studies of comparative effectiveness or safety.

The Initiative has published several position papers, including a list of seven recommendations of good practices covering study registration, replicability and stakeholder involvement [40]. Other remarkable publications that support these recommendations include the HARPER Protocol Template the purpose of which is to create a shared understanding of intended scientific decisions through a common text, tabular and visual structure. The template provides a set of core recommendations for clear and reproducible RWE study protocols and is intended to be used as a backbone throughout the research process from developing a valid study protocol, to registration, through implementation and reporting on those implementation decisions [41]; and structured frameworks that provide processes for the design of studies and feasibility assessments of fit-for-purpose data [42–44].

6 Summary and Conclusions

This chapter has provided a glimpse of how pharmacoepidemiology is an important part of pharmacovigilance, navigating basic principles of concepts and study design through to current best practice for standardisation and harmonisation. Case studies have been presented that explore considerations in the application of three common epidemiological techniques in support of addressing emergent safety issues. Observational pharmacoepidemiological studies are now routinely used to generate real-world evidence on the safety of medicines. The expansion of use of RWD has been profound with regulatory acceptability of such studies being enhanced through multiple initiatives that drive and assure quality suitable for decision-making.

7 Case Studies

The following case studies have been selected to allow the reader to explore how observational study designs have been applied in regulatory decision-making. They are presented in a question-and-answer format, exploring why a particular design was chosen, a particular issue relevant to that design and what a limitation might be.

7.1 Case Study 1: Use of Cross-Sectional Studies in Regulatory Decision-Making

Background	A drug utilisation study using a cross-sectional design aimed to examine whether the impact of European Medicines Agency (EMA) recommendations to restrict use or stop prescribing fluoroquinolones altogether because of safety concerns as implemented throughout 2018–2019 had an impact on fluoroquinolone monthly prescribing trends, overall and to certain age groups [22].
Q1. Why would a cross-sectional study be suitable for understanding trends in drug utilisation patterns?	Cross-sectional studies can collect drug use data on study population at one single time point or multiple points of time. In this example, the hypothesis was that the trend in prescribing would be decreasing suggesting prescribers have been compliant with recommendations. However, the actual results suggested little change after recommendations were introduced.
Q2. The study used electronic healthcare records from six European countries between 2016 and 2021. Why would these types of data sources be appropriate?	Cross-sectional studies often use data from entire populations and also from sub-populations of interest (e.g. vulnerable patients such as elderly). In order for the results to be meaningful, the data needs to be representative of the populations to which one wishes to apply the results to. In this example, each of the data sources are considered to adequately reflect primary care health provision and collect sufficiently granular health-related information for each individual patient, in their respective country.
Q3. The study found that while changes in fluoroquinolone prescriptions were observed over time across countries, these were inconsistent and did not seem to be temporally related to EMA interventions. The authors' conclusion was that the regulatory action associated with the 2018 referral did not seem to have relevant effects on fluoroquinolone prescribing in primary care. What might be some limitations of this study that might have contributed to this conclusion?	Information bias, i.e. missing or inaccurate measurement or recording of a variable, for example, a disease or characteristic, or information from a prescription is a key limitation in cross-sectional studies. In this study, recorded data on prescriptions may not equate to actual use. Knowing if a drug is stopped prematurely and a new one started and the reason for these choices may not be recorded in the medical records. Thus, there may have been under- or over-recording of use by month. Selection bias is also possible, since the study population did not include patients prescribed the antibiotic within the secondary care setting. This means the results may not reflect overall total use within each country.

7.2 Case Study 2: Use of Cohort Study Design for Contextualisation of Safety Signals

Background	By May 2021, four COVID-19 vaccines had been granted conditional marketing authorisation by the European Medicines Agency. After millions of vaccine doses were given in large-scale immunisation campaigns, a safety signal was noted from spontaneous reporting schemes of thrombotic events with concurrent thrombocytopenia (TTS) occurring often after the first dose. A retrospective cohort study using existing electronic healthcare records databases aimed to quantify the incidence of thrombosis, thrombocytopenia or TTS over 28 days following the first dose of an adenovirus-based COVID-19 vaccine or mRNA-based COVID-19 vaccine and compare them to historical, pre-pandemic rates estimated for UK general population. Rates were also estimated following COVID-19 infection [24]
Q1. Why would a cohort study be suitable for studying the risk associated with a medicinal product?	The cohort study design allows one to estimate risk and/or rates of multiple adverse events in one cohort defined by a particular characteristic (e.g. drug or vaccine) and compare those findings to another cohort that does not have that particular characteristic. This approach is an efficient way to get a measure of whether the characteristic increases, decreases or has no effect on multiple risks, and to inform on when those risks occur over time from the first exposure
Q2. For each event of interest, a method of indirect standardisation to the general population was used to estimate the number of events expected to have seen post-vaccination cohort if their outcome experience was the same as that of the general population. Standardised incidence ratios (SIRs) with 95% confidence intervals (CIs) were estimated. Why is such adjustment needed?	The comparison of adverse event rates may be misleading when there are differences in the populations being compared with respect to certain underlying characteristics that can directly (and independently) affect the overall rate, for example, there may be differences in the age structure. Standardisation is a method for overcoming the effect of confounding by age and address the imbalance in age structure that exists
Q3. In this study, one of the results was that more occurrences of TTS were observed than expected following the first dose of the adenovirus-based vaccine (16 compared to 12 events; SIR 1.38 [0.85–2.26]). This meant rates were no higher than expected based on pre-pandemic rates. What might be an important limitation of this study that might have contributed to this observation?	A limitation is that residual confounding may exist. In this study, the standardised rates represent a weighted average of the age-specific rates taken from the pre-pandemic population and are not actual rates. However, age may not be the only confounder. Notably, the time period studied covered the initial phases of vaccination when certain sub-populations were prioritised such as vulnerable people with higher prevalence of other comorbidities than the general population. Although there is no clear relationship between age and risk of TTS according to spontaneous reports, a selection bias towards older population in this study could mitigate the relative difference towards the null

7.3 Case Study 3: A 'Nested' Case–Control Study for Safety Signal Strengthening

Background	Selective serotonin re-uptake inhibitors (SSRI) are associated with an increased risk of bleeding disorders at a number of sites. It is currently unclear whether they increase the risk of haemorrhagic stroke, with conflicting results reported. This nested case–control aimed to investigate whether SSRI use was associated with an increased risk of haemorrhagic stroke. This study was nested in a cohort of antidepressant users using electronic healthcare records from the United Kingdom General Practice Research Database (CPRD) between 1992 and 2006 [29]. Risk associated with tricyclic antidepressant (TCA) exposure was also evaluated
Q1. Why would a case–control study be suitable for studying the risk of an adverse event following exposure to a drug?	The case–control design is based on a comparison of the use of a drug among those with the adverse event (cases) to the use of the drug among people without the adverse event (controls). In this study, the source population is a cohort of antidepressant users, hence the term 'nested'. This design aims to capture all cases and therefore is suitable for rare events. It facilitates exploration of multiple risk factors that could be important in understanding causality
Q2. The authors report that this was a matched case–control study nested in a cohort of GPRD-registered patients who had been prescribed an antidepressant at some time. Why is matching needed?	Sampling of the controls is important as they represent the background use of the drug in the population from which cases arise. The exact same in- and exclusion criteria should be applied to controls as for cases, including no prior history of the outcome. Matching is a method that ensures controls are sampled so that they can be considered a representative subset of the underlying cohort. In this study, five controls (people with no diagnosis of haemorrhagic stroke at any time) were selected per case matched on age (within 2 years), sex, practice and current registration within CPRD on the date of diagnosis of their matched case (index date)
Q3. In this study, the primary analysis showed no evidence of an association between current SSRI or TCA use and haemorrhagic stroke [current use of an SSRI versus no use: adjusted OR 1.11 (95% CI 0.82, 1.50) and current use of TCA versus no use: adjusted OR 0.73 (0.52, 1.02)]. What might be an important limitation of this study that might have contributed to this observation?	Although this study was nested in a cohort of antidepressant users to limit the effects of confounding by indication (since depression is associated with haemorrhagic stroke), these products are used for indications other than depression. Subjects with these indications may be different to those treated for depression, and those characteristics may not have been fully identified for data capture. Thus residual confounding is possible

References

1. Lenz W. KindlicheMissbildungennachMedikament -Einnahmewahrend der Graviditat? Dtsch Med Wochenschr. 1961;86:2555–6.
2. European Medicines Agency. Pharmacovigilance: overview. Available at: Pharmacovigilance: overview | European Medicines Agency (europa.eu). Accessed 20 Aug 2023.
3. Committee on Safety of Drugs. Report for 1969 and 1970. London: HMSO; 1971.
4. House of Commons—Health—Minutes of Evidence (parliament.uk). Available at: https://publications.parliament.uk/pa/cm199899/cmselect/cmhealth/549/99072714.htm. Accessed 21 Aug 2023.
5. Wright P. Untoward effects associated with practolol administration: oculomucocutaneous syndrome. Br Med J. 1975;1(5958):595–8.
6. Anon. Prescription-event monitoring: a new system for assessing drug safety. Reactions. 1983;86(1):2.
7. Layton D. Developments and future directions of prescription-based observational cohort pharmacovigilance. In: Bate A, editor. Chapter 6. Evidence-

based pharmacovigilance: clinical and quantitative aspects. 1st ed. Humana Press; 2018. p. 105–34.
8. European Medicines Agency. Guideline on good pharmacovigilance practices (GVP): Module V—Risk management systems (Rev 1); 2014.
9. European Medicines Agency. Risk Management. Available at: https://www.ema.europa.eu/en/human-regulatory/marketing-authorisation/pharmacovigilance/risk-management. Accessed 15 May 2023.
10. European Commission. Volume 9A—Pharmacovigilance for medicinal products for human use. September 2008. Available at: http://ec.europa.eu/enterprise/pharmaceuticals/eudralex/vol-9/pdf/vol9a_09-2008.pdf. Accessed 15 May 2023.
11. European Medicines Agency. Risk Management. Available at: https://www.ema.europa.eu/en/human-regulatory/post-authorisation/pharmacovigilance/good-pharmacovigilance-practice. Accessed 15 May 2023.
12. European Medicines Agency. Guideline on good pharmacovigilance practices (GVP) Module VIII—post-authorisation safety studies (Rev 3). EMA/813938/2011. 2017 Oct 9. Available at: https://www.ema.europa.eu/en/documents/scientific-guideline/guideline-good-pharmacovigilance-practices-gvp-module-viii-post-authorisation-safety-studies-rev-3_en.pdf. Accessed 15 May 2023.
13. European Medicines Agency. Guideline on good pharmacovigilance practices. Module VI—management and reporting of adverse reactions to medicinal products. (Rev 2). EMA/873138/2011 2017 July 28. Available at: https://www.ema.europa.eu/en/documents/regulatory-procedural-guideline/guideline-good-pharmacovigilance-practices-gvp-module-vi-collection-management-submission-reports_en.pdf. Accessed 15 May 2023.
14. Edlavitch SA, Tilson HH. For consideration by pharmacoepidemiologists. Pharmacoepidemiol Drug Saf. 2021;30(12):1619–20. https://doi.org/10.1002/pds.5365.
15. International Society of Pharmacoepidemiology. About Pharmacoepidemiology. Available at https://www.pharmacoepi.org/about-ispe/about-pharmacoepidemiology/date. Accessed 2 May 2024.
16. Strom BL, Kimmel SE, Hennessy S, editors. Textbook of pharmacoepidemiology. 3rd ed. John Wiley & Sons Ltd.; 2021.
17. Nohr EA, Liew Z. How to investigate and adjust for selection bias in cohort studies. Acta Obstet Gynecol Scand. 2018;97(4):407–16. https://doi.org/10.1111/aogs.13319.
18. FitzGerald GA, Patrono C. The coxibs, selective inhibitors of cyclooxygenase-2. N Engl J Med. 2001;345(6):433–42.
19. Layton D, Souverein PC, Heerdink ER, Shakir SA, Egberts AG. Prescriber adoption of newly approved COX-2 selective inhibitors. Pharmacoepidemiol Drug Saf. 2008;17(12):1168–74.
20. Clarke DWJ, Layton D, Shakir S. Do some inhibitors of COX-2 increase the risk of thromboembolic events? Linking pharmacology with pharmacoepidemiology. Drug Saf. 2004;27(7):421–50.
21. Key C, Layton D, Shakir SAW. Results of a postal survey of the reasons for non-response by doctors in a Prescription Event Monitoring study of drug safety. Pharmacoepidemiol Drug Saf. 2002;11:143–8.
22. Ly NF, Flach C, Lysen TS, Markov E, van Ballegooijen H, Rijnbeek P, Duarte-Salles T, Reyes C, John LH, Karimi L, Reich C, Salek S, Layton D. Impact of European Union label changes for fluoroquinolone-containing medicinal products for systemic and inhalation use: post-referral prescribing trends. Drug Saf. 2023;46(4):405–16.
23. Greifer N, Stuart EA. Matching methods for confounder adjustment: an addition to the epidemiologist's toolbox. Epidemiol Rev. 2022;43(1):118–29. https://doi.org/10.1093/epirev/mxab003.
24. Burn E, Li X, Delmestri A, Jones N, Duarte-Salles T, Reyes C, Martinez-Hernandez E, Marti E, Verhamme KMC, Rijnbeek PR, Strauss VY, Prieto-Alhambra D. Thrombosis and thrombocytopenia after vaccination against and infection with SARS-CoV-2 in the United Kingdom. Nat Commun. 2022;13(1):7167.
25. Ernster VL. Nested case-control studies. Prev Med. 1994;23(5):587–90. https://doi.org/10.1006/pmed.1994.1093.
26. O'Brien KM, Lawrence KG, Keil AP. The case for case-cohort: an applied epidemiologist's guide to reframing case-cohort studies to improve usability and flexibility. Epidemiology. 2022;33(3):354–61. https://doi.org/10.1097/EDE.0000000000001469.
27. Dalton SO, Sørensen HT, Johansen C. SSRIs and upper gastrointestinal bleeding: what is known and how should it influence prescribing? CNS Drugs. 2006;20(2):143–51.
28. Smoller JW, Allison M, Cochrane BB, Curb JD, Perlis RH, Robinson JG, Rosal MC, Wenger NK, Wassertheil-Smoller S. Antidepressant use and risk of incident cardiovascular morbidity and mortality among postmenopausal women in the Women's Health Initiative study. Arch Intern Med. 2009;169(22):2128–39.
29. Douglas I, Smeeth L, Irvine D. The use of antidepressants and the risk of haemorrhagic stroke: a nested case control study. Br J Clin Pharmacol. 2011;71(1):116–20.
30. European Network of Centres of Excellence for Pharmacoepidemiology and Pharmacovigilance (ENCEPP). Guide on Methodological Standards in Pharmacoepidemiology (Revision 11) EMA/95098/2010 July 2023. Available at: https://www.encepp.eu/standards_and_guidances/documents/01.ENCePPMethodsGuideRev.10_Final.pdf. Accessed 21 Aug 2023.
31. European Medicines Agency. Data Analysis and Real World Interrogation Network (DARWIN EU). Available at: https://www.ema.europa.eu/en/about-us/how-we-

work/big-data/data-analysis-real-world-interrogation-network-darwin-eu. Accessed 15 May 2023.
32. ENCePP Home Page. What is ENCePP. Available at: https://www.encepp.eu/structure/index.shtml. Accessed 21 Aug 2023.
33. European Network of Centres of Excellence for Pharmacoepidemiology and Pharmacovigilance (ENCEPP). Resources Database. Available at: https://www.encepp.eu/encepp/resourcesDatabase.jsp. Accessed 15 May 2023.
34. Observational Health Data Sciences and Informatics. Standardized Data: The OMOP Common Data Model. Available at: https://www.ohdsi.org/data-standardization/. Accessed 15 May 2023.
35. Flaherty DK. The vaccine-autism connection: a public health crisis caused by unethical medical practices and fraudulent science. Ann Pharmacother. 2011;45(10):1302–4.
36. Benchimol EI, Moher D, Ehrenstein V, Langan SM. Retraction of COVID-19 pharmacoepidemiology research could have been avoided by effective use of reporting guidelines. Clin Epidemiol. 2020;12:1403–20.
37. Ryan P, Duke J. Evidence quality. Chapter 14. The book of OHDSHI. 2021. Available at: https://ohdsi.github.io/TheBookOfOhdsi/. Accessed 15 May 2023.
38. European Network of Centres of Excellence for Pharmacoepidemiology and Pharmacovigilance (ENCEPP). ENCePP checklist for study protocols. Available at: https://www.encepp.eu/standards_and_guidances/checkListProtocols.shtm. Accessed 15 May 2023.
39. The International Professional Society for Health eConomics and outcomes research (ISPOR). Real-world evidence transparency initiative. Available at: https://www.ispor.org/strategic-initiatives/real-world-evidence/real-world-evidence-transparency-initiative. Accessed 15 May 2023.
40. Berger ML, Sox H, Willke RJ, et al. Good practices for real-world data studies of treatment and/or comparative effectiveness: recommendations from the Joint ISPOR-ISPE Special Task Force on Real-World Evidence in Health Care decision making. Value Health. 2017;20(8):1003–8.
41. Wang SV, Pottegård A, Crown W, Arlett P, Ashcroft DM, Benchimol EI, Berger ML, Crane G, Goettsch W, Hua W, Kabadi S, Kern DM, Kurz X, Langan S, Nonaka T, Orsini L, Perez-Gutthann S, Pinheiro S, Pratt N, Schneeweiss S, Toussi M, Williams RJ. HARmonized Protocol Template to Enhance Reproducibility of hypothesis evaluating real-world evidence studies on treatment effects: a good practices report of a Joint ISPE/ISPOR task force. Value Health. 2022;25(10):1663–72.
42. Gatto NM, Reynolds RF, Campbell UB. A structured preapproval and postapproval comparative study design framework to generate valid and transparent real-world evidence for regulatory decisions. Clin Pharmacol Ther. 2019;106(1):103–15.
43. Gatto NM, Campbell UB, Rubinstein E, Jaksa A, Mattox P, Mo J, Reynolds RF. The structured process to identify fit-for-purpose data: a data feasibility assessment framework. Clin Pharmacol Ther. 2022;111(1):122–34.
44. Gatto NM, Vititoe SE, Rubinstein E, Reynolds RF, Campbell UB. A structured process to identify fit-for-purpose study design and data to generate valid and transparent real-world evidence for regulatory uses. Clin Pharmacol Ther. 2023;113(6):1235–9. https://doi.org/10.1002/cpt.2883.

Spontaneous Reporting Systems

10

Jan Petracek and Marcela Fialova

Abstract

Systems of spontaneous reporting were developed in the 1960s. Nowadays, there are worldwide systems for processing millions of individual case safety reports per year. Despite the significant underreporting bias, the amount and quality of information collected through spontaneous reporting are sufficient for justification of the large number of regulatory actions taken to minimise risks associated with medicinal products.

Spontaneous reports still represent an irreplaceable source of information for pharmacovigilance. They have been significantly strengthened by the new technology of mobile phone apps, social media, and artificial intelligence applications in healthcare. Essential rules of implied causality and acceptance of patient reports, paired with the emphasis on the quality of reports and their validation at source, have further improved the usefulness of the collected information for signal detection, assessment, and regulatory decision-making.

Efforts to integrate data from spontaneous reports with other types of reports and available data in healthcare systems are ongoing on a larger scale. Data science techniques are also being further developed to improve the quality of data and its interpretation. This may lead to even quicker risk minimisation, including predicting adverse drug reactions to new medicinal products. Clinicians benefit from the lower thresholds for reporting and quicker sharing of new knowledge.

Keywords

Spontaneous reporting system · Pharmacovigilance · Signal · Adverse drug reaction · Adverse event · Individual case safety report · Post-marketing · Database system · Causality

Learning Objectives

- Understand the main features of spontaneous reporting systems, including design, strengths, and weaknesses.
- Explain the concepts associated with spontaneous individual case safety reports.
- Understand the origins, present, and future of spontaneous reporting systems.

J. Petracek (✉)
Institute of Pharmacovigilance,
Prague, Czech Republic
e-mail: jan.petracek@pharmacovigilance.institute

M. Fialova
Institute of Pharmacovigilance,
Prague, Czech Republic

iVigee, a.s., Prague, Czech Republic

J. Jose et al. (eds.), *Principles and Practice of Pharmacovigilance and Drug Safety*,
https://doi.org/10.1007/978-3-031-51089-2_10

- Acquire actionable knowledge that may help with spontaneous reporting from own clinical practice.

Key Points
- Spontaneous reporting systems serve as a pillar of pharmacovigilance worldwide.
- The reporting systems represent a key service to clinical practice, allowing both healthcare professionals and consumers to share their experience with medicinal products and learn from the collected information.
- Quality and validity of spontaneous reports greatly influences the utility of them.
- Both industry and regulatory authorities have developed advanced systems for processing individual case safety reports from any source, including spontaneous reports.
- Spontaneous reports from healthcare professionals as well as patients/public are important in the success of the spontaneous reporting system.
- New technology is allowing for quicker and more precise collection of information via both spontaneous and solicited sources of individual case safety reports.

1 Introduction

Spontaneous reports remain an important source of safety signals following the market approval of a drug. This chapter sets out the key attributes of a spontaneous reporting system, using key examples of such systems, their operation, and their utility. It also includes the history and function of spontaneous reporting systems internationally. The assessment and utility of the data documented in spontaneous reporting systems are covered. The implications of regulatory decisions from the National Pharmacovigilance Systems in clinical practice are discussed.

The ability to communicate and learn from mistakes is essential for the success of any system. The suboptimal communication between those who observe adverse drug reactions (ADRs) and those in charge of benefit–harm assessments and decisions may lead to unnecessary harm caused by medicines. Shortly after the thalidomide tragedy, the essential pharmacovigilance feedback loop was created, working with spontaneous reports from healthcare professionals (Fig. 10.1).

The essential pharmacovigilance feedback loop ensures that clinicians can share their patients' observations of suspected adverse reactions with regulatory authorities or public institutions in charge of pharmacovigilance. Data collected at one central database are then available for more advanced analysis, including signal

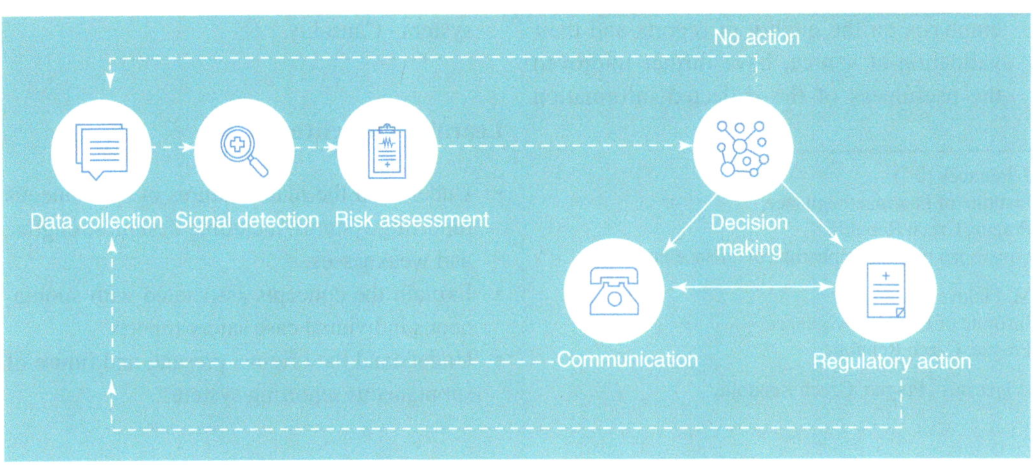

Fig. 10.1 Essential pharmacovigilance feedback loop

detection and risk assessment. The new knowledge could be shared with clinicians quickly through ad-hoc communication and label updates. Regulatory authorities may also withdraw medicinal products with unfavourable benefit–harm profiles from the market.

Since their conception in the 1960s, spontaneous reporting systems have developed worldwide, allowing any user to contribute and learn from the collected data. The system remains to be a significant pillar of pharmacovigilance. Its further improvements, thanks to technology, legal environment, globalisation, and transparency, offer growing opportunities for its continuous use in future.

2 The Concept of Spontaneous Reporting

Pharmacovigilance's spontaneous reporting systems allow clinicians and patients to share their observations of adverse experiences with a medicinal product via the reporting of suspected ADRs. The systems exist globally and locally, use variable technologies, and are increasingly linked at regional and international levels to ensure no information is lost.

Any person can report an adverse experience with a medicinal product via these systems and do so without any limitations to the content. Therefore, spontaneous reports represent the only completely uncurated source of information available in pharmacovigilance.

A reporter may have some choice of where to send her/his report. National regulatory agencies and pharmaceutical companies must accept these reports, while in many countries, the national regulatory authority is the preferred destination by law. The incoming reports are often acknowledged and processed into pharmacovigilance databases, including data coding, translations, assessments, interpretations, and follow-ups. The spontaneous reporting system covers all medicines used within a whole population for an unlimited time, encompassing each medicine's entire product life cycle.

2.1 Spontaneous Versus Solicited Reporting

The motivation of the reporter to share information is critical for the correct interpretation of the report. The circumstances under which the reporter sends the report determine whether it would be considered a spontaneous or solicited report.

Motivation for a solicited report is a request to the reporter to share a particular type of information, such as within an organised data collection scheme. Clinical trials are examples of the most stringent schemes. Nevertheless, even post-authorisation uses of medicinal products, such as named patient use, special access programmes, patient support programmes, observational studies, and similar, represent circumstances under which collected reports are considered solicited.

> *Solicited reports are those derived from organised data collection systems, which include clinical trials, registries, post-approval named patient use programs, other patient support and disease management programs, surveys of patients or healthcare providers, or information gathering on efficacy or patient compliance. Adverse event reports obtained from any of these should not be considered spontaneous. (ICH E2D) [1]*

Motivation for a spontaneous report is not based on any specific request. It is the reporter's own decision to share the information, even though it might be supported by a general legal obligation to report in a particular country. Typical motivation for spontaneous reporting is a striking case about which the reporter wants to learn more or a case where the reporting healthcare professional might feel it is a piece of new information they want to share with others. Patients may feel that they should share their experiences with the expectation that regulatory authorities should know what is happening.

Following the same logic, literature reports are also considered spontaneous. The authors publish cases so their colleagues can also learn from them. Literature case reports are the older and traditional way of sharing information among the medical community. Nowadays, a limited number of medical journals would accept individual case reports for publication. Sharing them through a spontaneous reporting system is considered more efficient in most situations, since the publication of a case report can take many months. Aggregated data can serve the advanced analysis better than individual publications.

> *A spontaneous report is an unsolicited communication by a healthcare professional or consumer to a company, regulatory authority or other organisation (e.g. WHO, Regional Center, Poison Control Center) that describes one or more adverse drug reactions in a patient who was given one or more medicinal products and that does not derive from a study or any organised data collection scheme. (ICH E2D) [1]*

Stimulated reporting can occur in certain situations, such as notification by a 'Direct Healthcare Professional Communication' letter, publication in the press, or questioning healthcare professionals by company representatives. These reports are spontaneous, as no specific request has been made to a particular healthcare professional to collect information.

Stimulated reporting may cause reporting bias or false signals. For proper signal detection and validation, information about the context of such stimulated reporting is invaluable and should always be well understood before reaching any conclusions.

2.2 Individual Case Safety Reports

The term individual case safety report (ICSR) encompasses all kinds of reports describing safety experience(s) with a medicinal product(s) in a person at a particular time. ICSRs may include reports of ADR(s), adverse event (AE)s, or special situations from any source. The ICSR is the fundamental unit of pharmacovigilance reporting systems. The International Council for Harmonisation of Technical Requirements for Pharmaceuticals for Human Use (ICH) has developed a standard ICSR format (Fig. 10.2) to allow for the electronic exchange of the ICSRs between all involved stakeholders worldwide.

2.3 Concepts of Seriousness and Expectedness

Clinicians are typically very busy people. Resources available to pharmacovigilance systems are also limited. Therefore, various prioritisation systems have been developed and implemented for spontaneous reporting systems. Of those prioritisation concepts, seriousness and expectedness are the most used for spontaneous ICSRs.

Serious ICSRs are those that have one of the following outcomes:

1. Death of the patient
2. Life-threatening
3. Hospitalisation of the patient or extension of existing hospitalisation
4. Persistent or significant disability or incapacity
5. Congenital anomaly
6. Medically serious as considered by the reporting physician or a medical reviewer

The serious ICSRs are prioritised for reporting. Globally, a 15-day reporting rule applies to them, meaning that pharmaceutical companies and regulatory authorities must process and report these cases further within 15 calendar days.

The concept of expectedness relates to the nature and severity of the described reactions in the case. Every approved medicinal product has an official label describing its adverse reactions. Those are considered 'expected' adverse drug reactions, as their nature and severity align with the current knowledge described in the label. If at least one of the reactions in the ICSR is unexpected, then the ICSR is considered unexpected too. Unexpected ICSRs may also be prioritised for reporting and signal detection approaches.

CIOMS FORM

SUSPECT ADVERSE REACTION REPORT	

I. REACTION INFORMATION

1. PATIENT INITIALS (first, last)	1a. COUNTRY	2. DATE OF BIRTH Day Month Year	2a. AGE Years	3. SEX	4-6 REACTION ONSET Day Month Year	8-12 CHECK ALL APPROPRIATE TO ADVERSE REACTION
7 + 13 DESCRIBE REACTION(S) (including relevant tests/lab data)						☐ PATIENT DIED ☐ INVOLVED OR PROLONGED INPATIENT HOSPITALISATION ☐ INVOLVED PERSISTENCE OR SIGNIFICANT DISABILITY OR INCAPACITY ☐ LIFE THREATENING

II. SUSPECT DRUG(S) INFORMATION

14. SUSPECT DRUG(S) (include generic name)		20 DID REACTION ABATE AFTER STOPPING DRUG? ☐ YES ☐ NO ☐ NA
15. DAILY DOSE(S)	16. ROUTE(S) OF ADMINISTRATION	21. DID REACTION REAPPEAR AFTER REINTRODUCTION? ☐ YES ☐ NO ☐ NA
17. INDICATION(S) FOR USE		
18. THERAPY DATES (from/to)	19. THERAPY DURATION	

III. CONCOMITANT DRUG(S) AND HISTORY

22. CONCOMITANT DRUG(S) AND DATES OF ADMINISTRATION (exclude those used to treat reaction)
23. OTHER RELEVANT HISTORY (e.g. diagnostics, allergies, pregnancy with last month of period, etc.)

IV. MANUFACTURER INFORMATION

24a. NAME AND ADDRESS OF MANUFACTURER		
	24b. MFR CONTROL NO.	
24c. DATE RECEIVED BY MANUFACTURER	24d. REPORT SOURCE ☐ STUDY ☐ LITERATURE ☐ HEALTH PROFESSIONAL	
DATE OF THIS REPORT	25a. REPORT TYPE ☐ INITIAL ☐ FOLLOWUP	

Fig. 10.2 CIOMS I Form for reporting of ICSR (cioms.ch/cioms-i-form)

3 Origins of Spontaneous Reporting Systems

While the history of pharmacovigilance is as old as the human civilisation, the spontaneous reporting system is a relatively recent component. Various players developed multiple versions of spontaneous reporting in response to the thalidomide tragedy in the 1960s.

Chemie Grünenthal developed thalidomide in Germany shortly after the Second World War. It first entered the German market in 1957 as a sedative and mild hypnotic, available even without a prescription. It was widely marketed for morning sickness in pregnancy with great commercial success. By 1960, thalidomide was sold in 46 countries [2].

In 1961, Dr. WG McBride, based in Australia, sent a letter to Lancet (Fig. 10.3) announcing his observation 'that the incidence of multiple severe abnormalities in babies delivered of women who were given the drug thalidomide ('Distaval') during pregnancy as an anti-emetic or as a sedative, to be almost 20%, asking whether anybody else has observed similar abnormalities' [3].

At the same time, during a Paediatric Convention in Germany, Dr. Lenz suggested a correlation between malformations and thalidomide. His suspicion was published in a German Journal (*Welt am Sonntag*) [4].

Chemie Grünenthal formally withdrew the drug on 26 November 1961 in Germany and other European countries. In the USA, the drug was never approved thanks to the very cautious assessor at US FDA—although this was not because of concerns about birth defects [5]. Nevertheless, it took many years for thalidomide to be eventually removed from the market worldwide, as it was marketed under various names, by many pharma companies, and in developing countries. More than 10,000 babies have been born with phocomelia and other anomalies, affecting millions of people, including families, caregivers, and many communities.

At the time, there was no single place where the suspicions of adverse effects of medicines could be reported. It took many years before the observations of individual physicians were put together and an association could be hypothesised.

The legal amendment in the United States of America (USA) (1962) required drug safety and efficacy data before marketing approval was passed. Since then, the safety data must include teratogenicity tests in different animals [6]. In 1964, the United Kingdom (UK) introduced the

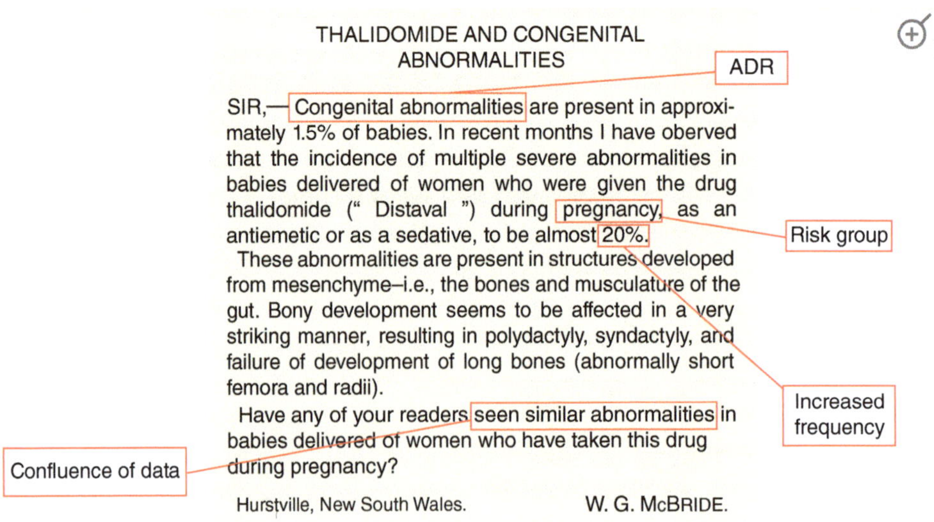
THALIDOMIDE AND CONGENITAL ABNORMALITIES

SIR,—Congenital abnormalities are present in approximately 1.5% of babies. In recent months I have oberved that the incidence of multiple severe abnormalities in babies delivered of women who were given the drug thalidomide (" Distaval ") during pregnancy, as an antiemetic or as a sedative, to be almost 20%.

These abnormalities are present in structures developed from mesenchyme–i.e., the bones and musculature of the gut. Bony development seems to be affected in a very striking manner, resulting in polydactyly, syndactyly, and failure of development of long bones (abnormally short femora and radii).

Have any of your readers seen similar abnormalities in babies delivered of women who have taken this drug during pregnancy?

Hurstville, New South Wales. W. G. McBRIDE.

Fig. 10.3 McBride's letter and important elements forming spontaneous reporting [3]

'Yellow Card' system. The Yellow Card is a specific form for collecting a spontaneous report of suspected ADRs [7].

In Europe (1965), the disaster of thalidomide stimulated the development of European legislation with the EC Directive 65/65. It established the foundations of pharmacovigilance and development of ADR reporting systems.

In 1966, a pilot study of the Boston Collaborative Drug Surveillance Program started [8]. It was the first group to conduct epidemiologic research to quantify the potential adverse effects of drugs. Paper-based in-hospital monitoring and early utilisation of computers played an essential role in developing and applying methods in drug epidemiology, broadly informing the design of pharmacovigilance systems.

In 1968, the World Health Organization (WHO) established a Programme for International Drug Monitoring. Ten member states initially piloted the programme (Australia, Canada, Czechoslovakia, Federal Republic of Germany, Ireland, Netherlands, New Zealand, Sweden, the UK, and the USA). Today, over 170 members contribute to one central database of ICSRs—VigiBase [9].

4 National and Global Spontaneous Reporting Systems

The organisation of spontaneous reporting systems varies around the world. Health professionals, and sometimes patients or consumers, may send reports of adverse experiences to one or more specified locations. These locations can be the drug regulatory authority, an academic or hospital-based pharmacovigilance centre, or the drug manufacturer.

Member states of the WHO Programme for International Drug Monitoring share information with the Uppsala Monitoring Centre (UMC) that operates the programme for WHO. All the reports are available in VigiBase, the world's richest source of pharmacovigilance data. Regulatory authorities may access VigiBase fully. Selected services and datasets are also available to other interested parties.

5 Types of Individual Case Safety Reports

5.1 Adverse Events and Adverse Drug Reactions

The level of suspicion for the causal relationship between the exposure to the medicinal product and the described adverse experience determines whether the ICSR would be considered an AE or an ADR.

While there are many local variations of definitions of AEs and ADRs, the ICH guidelines is a good source of definitions for global applications.

> *An adverse event (AE) is any untoward medical occurrence in a patient administered a medicinal product and which does not necessarily have to have a causal relationship with this treatment. An adverse event can therefore be any unfavourable and unintended sign (for example, an abnormal laboratory finding), symptom, or disease temporally associated with the use of a medicinal product, whether or not considered related to this medicinal product. (ICH E2D)*

> *Adverse Drug Reaction is a noxious and unintended response to a medicinal product related to any dose. The phrase "response to a medicinal product" means a causal relationship between a medicinal product and an adverse event is at least possible. (ICH E2D)*

In contrast to an AE, an ADR is characterised by a suspected causal relationship between the drug and the occurrence. In many countries, the term 'suspected adverse drug reaction' is used to further stress the uncertainty around causality to protect reporting parties from potential legal consequences associated with communication about this information. Thus, communicating about suspected ADRs does not mean the parties acknowledge the causal relationship.

5.2 Special Situations

Special situations are observations that provide valuable safety information about the medicinal product while not meeting the definition of an AE or ADR. They are the third category of ICSRs, other than ADRs and AEs, that may be reported via spontaneous systems. However, in some regions (e.g. EEA) they should be reported only in case they are related to an ADR.

Definition of special situations may vary between regions. Globally, they include the following concepts:

- Overdose
- Off-label use
- Drug abuse
- Drug misuse
- Medication errors
- Lack of efficacy
- Use of product in pregnancy or breast-feeding
- Occupational exposure

Figure 10.4 provides an overview of special situations according to different terms of reference [10].

All spontaneous reporting systems must acknowledge reports of special situations and be able to process them accordingly.

5.3 Implied Causality of Spontaneous Individual Case Safety Reports

A spontaneous reporter's motivation to share an ICSR is not solicited but related to some suspicion that an event is related. As the effort to report is not insignificant, the pharmacovigilance regulatory environment acknowledges this effort by considering all spontaneously reported ICSRs as having some level of implied causality.

Therefore, all spontaneously reported ICSRs are classified as reports of suspected ADRs. While pharmaceutical companies and regulatory authorities may provide their own causality

Special situations	GVP	MedDRA	FDA	Health Canada
Overdose	✓	✓	✓	✓
Off-label use	✓	✓		
Drug abuse	✓	✓	✓	
Drug misuse	✓	✓	✓	
Medication errors	✓	✓	✓	✓
Lack of Efficacy (LOE)/ Lack of Therapeutic Efficacy	✓	✓		
Pregnancy				✓
Occupational exposure	✓	✓		✓
Drug addiction			✓	
Use of medicinal product in a paediatric or elderly population	✓	✓		
Use of medicinal product during pregnancy or breastfeeding	✓			
Product quality issues			✓	
Discontinued products				✓
Unusual failure to Efficacy (only applies to new drugs)				✓

GVP-Good Pharmacovigilance Practice, MedDRA- Medical Dictionary for Regulatory Activities, FDA- Food and Drug Administration, Health Canada- Drug regulatory agency of Canadian government

Fig. 10.4 Overview of special situations according to different terms of reference (example from iViReg system, 2023) [10]

assessment of the reported cases, they cannot dispute the implied causality of spontaneous reports to distribute the report further.

5.4 Individual Case Safety Reports Linked with Product Quality Defects or Falsified Medicines

Should an ICSR be connected with a product quality complaint, the marketing authorisation holder (MAH) shall investigate whether the product met the approved quality criteria. If not, the ICSR is marked as related to product quality and shall not be used in pharmacovigilance assessment.

Pharmacovigilance systems are primarily designed for the situation where medicinal products are of good quality, and still, an adverse experience is observed. If the adverse experience is explainable by substandard quality or exposure to a falsified medicine, then product manufacturing quality departments shall attend to the issue immediately.

6 Sources of Spontaneous Individual Case Safety Reports

6.1 Healthcare Professional Reports and Consumer (Patient) Reports

Spontaneous ICSRs originate at the point of medical care. Healthcare professionals or patients may report them via various channels. These include traditional paper reports via post, fax, email, web, or mobile phone applications. Many countries have designed their forms in official languages, mostly based on the CIOMS form (Fig. 10.2).

While some spontaneous reporting systems were once restricted only to reports from healthcare professionals, there has been growing recognition of the importance of patient reports. Many systems now accept patient-generated reports. For example, Italy, Denmark, Netherlands, and Sweden have accepted patient reports since the early 2000s, while Australia has accepted them since 1964. The USA, which has accepted consumer ICSRs since 1969, developed the MedWatch programme in 1993 to facilitate AE reporting from patients and healthcare professionals [11]. Nonetheless, even in 2012, some countries with highly developed regulatory systems were not actively collecting patient reports. Of the 50 countries with developed drug regulatory systems surveyed in 2013, 44 had direct patient reporting systems, 17 of which were started only in 2012 or 2013 [12].

There is no internationally recognised definition of a 'patient report'. ICH E2D defines a '*consumer*' as '*a person who is not a healthcare professional such as a patient, lawyer, friend, or relative of a patient*' and notes that '*consumers*' can submit AE reports. There is growing evidence that patient reports are a valuable source of information. They often contain more details than reports generated by healthcare professionals and can serve to complement those reports [13].

A study of the UK's Yellow Card system, which allows spontaneous reporting by healthcare practitioners and patients, found that reports generated by patients had a higher median number of suspected ADRs per report. They also had a higher median word count, more detailed information about symptoms, and more description of the emotional and social impact of the AE [14].

A study comparing AE reports submitted by patients and those submitted by healthcare professionals to the Dutch National Pharmacovigilance Centre, Lareb, found that patient reports were comparable to those from health professionals for causality analysis [15]. Similarly, a UMC–Lareb collaboration assessed the contribution of patient reports to global signal detection in VigiBase. It concluded that patient reports provide unique information valuable in signal assessment and recommended their inclusion in signal detection processes [16]. Publications also show that in at least one pharmaceutical company's AE database, signals were detected earlier when patient reports were included than when only reports from healthcare providers were included [17].

Given the potential importance of patient reporting, efforts have been made to encourage and simplify it. In 2012, WHO published a guide for countries to use in setting up a reporting system for the general public, which recommends that a patient reporting system ideally be established in an existing spontaneous reporting system. The patient reporting form may be a dedicated one or the same form used by health professionals, but it should be understandable by a layperson. Education of the public on the importance of patient reporting and training of pharmacovigilance staff in assessing patient reports is recommended.

A discussion on the active involvement of patients in medication safety is elaborated in Chap. 12.

6.1.1 Reporting from Clinical Practice

Process of reporting ADRs in clinical practice may vary significantly and needs to consider local requirements. Many countries have set up local pharmacovigilance centres, often teaching hospitals coordinating the local efforts. All leading physicians should ensure juniors are well trained in differential diagnoses that include ADRs as potential cause of the patient's condition. When a suspicion is raised, the reporting should be as easy as possible, with procedural and technical support given to healthcare professionals. In addition to the physicians, other healthcare professionals who actively involve in the spontaneous reporting are pharmacists, nurses, and dentists. Clinical pharmacists and clinical pharmacologists are the professionals who usually initiate and coordinate ADR reporting programmes within the hospital setup, and the same supports the national pharmacovigilance activities.

Culture influences the willingness to talk about ADRs and sharing experience about them. Open and transparent culture leads to much higher likelihood of clinicians sharing the information and learning from it.

Pharmaceutical industry has a very significant role in continuous education including pharmacotherapy. It should be performed observing high standards of ethics, as cited in many internal and external documents, including guidance from the WHO [18].

6.2 Individual Case Safety Reports from Social Media

Social media includes a wide, and constantly changing, range of computer-based technologies that allow the creation [18] and sharing of information, ideas, photographs, and other messages via electronic communication. User-generated content is a defining feature of social media. This content can be made available to others via computer-based networks that connect one user with the other users or groups to form social networks. Given the widespread use of the internet and social media for health-related topics, there is interest in whether social media can be a source of drug safety signals or otherwise shed light on ADRs [19].

Because social media posts describe individual experiences, they can also describe adverse reactions to medicines. The use of social media for pharmacovigilance presents both opportunities and challenges. With an estimated 2.5 billion social media users worldwide, including in parts of the world where formal pharmacovigilance programmes are not highly developed, social media can be a source of patient- and consumer-generated information about AEs. The ability to tap into this potential source of information is especially relevant, given the growing importance of, and attention to, patient- and consumer-generated reports in pharmacovigilance.

The use of social media for pharmacovigilance is an area of active research to address these challenges. Current research focuses on using natural language processing and other techniques, such as supervised machine learning and large language model (LLM) on identifying drug-related AEs in social media. One of the biggest challenges in this regard is the distinction of drug mentions associated with an AE from those with no association with an AE [20].

Another area of research is determining the utility of social media in pharmacovigilance. In 2014, the Innovative Medicines Initiative (IMI), a public–private partnership between the European Union and the European Federation for Pharmaceutical Industries and Associations, launched WEB-RADR: Recognising Adverse Drug Reactions to develop new technology tools to facilitate the detection and analysis of potential ADRs in social media sites. It also aimed to create a mobile phone app for reporting suspected ADRs to regulatory authorities in the European Union (in the context of traditional AE reporting). One of several planned outgrowths of these efforts is establishing a regulatory framework for social media mining for ADRs.

7 Quality of Individual Case Safety Reports

The quality of reports in pharmacovigilance varies significantly. Despite standardisation, differences in training, national healthcare cultures, languages, tools, technologies, pharmacovigilance practices, and many other factors influence the quality of reports. Poor quality reports may lead to flawed data analysis and delays or fails to detect signals of potential harm. A commonly used phrase to describe this problem is ‘rubbish in, rubbish out’.

Reporting clinicians should provide as much relevant information for the proper assessment of the case that may be available to them. There is very low threshold of reporting enabling a maximum of initial reports to be captured. The initial reports are then followed up to collect as much relevant information as possible (Sect. 7.2), with a focus on those of a more serious nature.

7.1 Validity of Individual Case Safety Reports

The first crucial qualitative requirement is a so-called report’s validity. Only valid reports are exchanged between the parties in the national and global pharmacovigilance system. Invalid reports are stored by the first receiver, who must attempt follow-up to validate the ICSR.

Four minimum criteria are required for ICSR validation:

1. One or more identifiable reporter
2. One single identifiable patient
3. One or more suspected substance/medicinal product
4. One or more suspected adverse reaction

7.2 Follow-Up of Individual Case Safety Reports

Follow-up means contacting the reporter for further information about the case. The first receiving party usually performs a follow-up of a spontaneous ICSR. Typically, follow-up questions are prepared for the telephone, email, or letter conversation with the reporter.

All invalid ICSRs must be followed up until validated or until further attempts are considered futile. Most authorities and pharmaceutical companies perform between zero and three attempts to follow up on spontaneous ICSRs, based on their internal prioritisation system.

8 Processing of Spontaneous Individual Case Safety Reports

Both industry and regulatory authorities have developed advanced systems for processing ICSRs from any source, including spontaneous reports. As technology progresses and the industry prepares for technological changes, the harmonisation of case processing approaches has reached a new level of maturity.

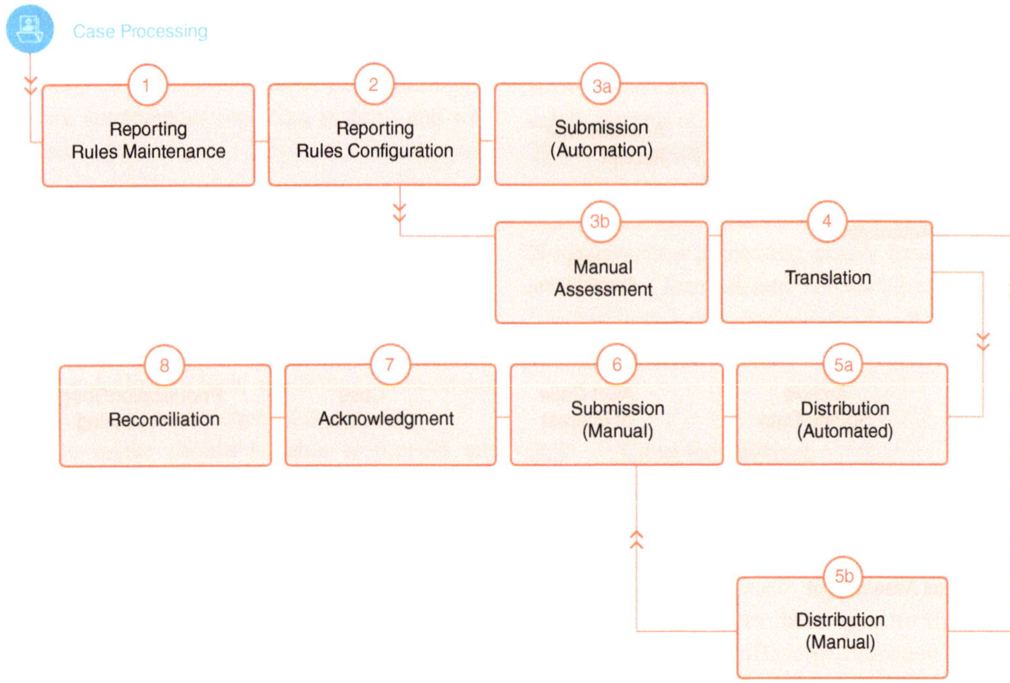

Fig. 10.7 Case reporting flowchart (developed by Transcelerate)

Examples of national reporting systems and databases include the Blue Card system (Australia); Canada Vigilance (Canada); the Canadian Adverse Events Following Immunization Surveillance System (CAEFISS) database (Canada); the French Pharmacovigilance Spontaneous Reporting System database (France); the Adverse Drug Reaction Information Management System of the Pharmaceutical and Medication Devices Agency, Ministry of Health, Labor, and Welfare (Japan); the Lareb database (Netherlands); the BiSi database (Sweden); the MHRA ADR database (UK); the FDA Adverse Event Reporting System (FAERS) database (USA); and the Vaccine Adverse Event Reporting System (VAERS) database (USA).

At the international level, there are two central database systems. The European Medicines Agency (EMA) runs EudraVigilance in the European Union, and VigiBase pools data from more than 170 member countries of the WHO International Drug Monitoring Programme (run by the UMC). VigiBase is also the system used as the national database by around 70 pharmacovigilance centres around the world.

Understanding the unique features of the database when used as a source for analysis is critical for the correct choice of methodology and result interpretation. Coding the suspected medicinal products and adverse event/reaction terms in the same way for all reports is one of the significant considerations. Many databases code drugs according to a local or national standard drug dictionary, while others use a standard international dictionary, such as WHO Drug Dictionary (WHODrug Global). Medical Dictionary for Regulatory Activities (MedDRA) is used in the ICH regions to code AE/ADR terms.

9 Strengths of Spontaneous Reporting Systems

Spontaneous reports are an invaluable resource for signal detection. Most safety issues in the post-authorisation life of medicinal products have been discovered due to spontaneous reports first and then complemented by evidence from other sources.

motivation for creating most existing healthcare records introduces significant biases that spontaneous reports usually do not have. It makes electronic healthcare records complementary to spontaneous reporting systems. In fact, they may enrich each other.

Spontaneous reports with automatically attached data from electronic healthcare records, including laboratory, radiologic, and other diagnostic test results, can significantly improve the quality of data available in spontaneous reporting systems [29].

With new advanced medicinal products, monitoring post-marketing benefits and risks is increasingly necessary. Spontaneous reporting systems will continue to be the cornerstone of this effort because of their unique advantages. As social media, active surveillance, and the use of large healthcare databases begin to play a role in drug safety surveillance, demonstrate their utility, and realise their potential, they could become valuable adjuncts to existing pharmacovigilance reporting systems worldwide.

12 Summary and Conclusions

Early systems of spontaneous reporting were developed in the second half of twentieth century. Now, these systems are worldwide systems for processing millions of ICSRs per year in highly advanced databases. Despite the significant underreporting bias, the amount and quality of information collected are sufficient to inform a large number of regulatory actions to minimise harms associated with medicinal products.

Spontaneous reports still represent an irreplaceable source of information for pharmacovigilance, not least because of the inherent implicit potential suspicion of causation in the mind of the reporter. They have been significantly strengthened by the new technology of mobile phone apps, social media, and AI applications in healthcare. Essential rules of implied causality and acceptance of patient reports, paired with the emphasis on the quality of reports and their validation at source, have further improved the usefulness of the collected information for signal detection, assessment, and regulatory decision-making.

Data integration of spontaneous reports with other types of reports and available data in healthcare systems is ongoing on a large scale. Data science techniques are being further developed to improve the quality of data and its interpretation. This may lead to even quicker risk minimisation, including the prediction of ADRs to new medicinal products.

13 Case Studies

Two cases which illustrate the importance, advantages, disadvantages, limitations, and interpretation of spontaneous report data are described below.

13.1 Case Study 1: Dabigatran

Dabigatran is an oral direct thrombin inhibitor approved in the US in October 2010 to reduce the risk of stroke and systemic embolism in patients with nonvalvular atrial fibrillation. It was the first oral anticoagulant approved for this indication since warfarin had been approved for a similar indication.

In the clinical trial that supported dabigatran's approval, 6076 patients were randomised to dabigatran 150 mg twice daily, and 6022 were randomised to warfarin treatment. The rates of major bleeding were 3.3 per 100 person-years in dabigatran-treated patients and 3.6 per 100 person-years in warfarin-treated patients (hazard ratio 0.93, 95% confidence interval (CI) 0.81–1.07). The corresponding rates for life-threatening bleeds were 1.5 per 100 person-years and 1.9 per 100 person-years in the dabigatran and warfarin groups, respectively (hazard ratio 0.80, 95% confidence interval 0.66–0.98). Gastrointestinal bleeding was more common in dabigatran-treated than in warfarin-treated patients (1.6% vs 1.1%, hazard ratio 1.5, 95% confidence interval 1.2–1.9) [30].

In the first 14 months after dabigatran's approval, the US FDA received 2347 case reports of bleeding with dabigatran (348 with a fatal outcome), compared to 647 case reports of bleeding with warfarin (46 with a fatal outcome) [30].

This disparity in report numbers between the two agents suggested that dabigatran might be responsible for more bleeding in clinical practice. This finding was contrary to the preapproval observations. These numbers also raised the possibility of increased mortality with dabigatran relative to warfarin. A population-based analysis using administrative claims data found that the bleeding rates associated with dabigatran use were no higher than those associated with warfarin use [31].

A subsequent study using data from the US Medicare system found that, in clinical practice settings, dabigatran was associated with a lower risk of ischaemic stroke, intracranial haemorrhage and death, and a higher risk of major gastrointestinal bleeding relative to warfarin. These findings were consistent with the preapproval clinical trial data [32].

This example illustrates some important limitations concerning using aggregate spontaneous report data to estimate population-based risk or relative risk of an AE between two drugs. A comparison of raw numbers of AE reports generally cannot be used to estimate the relative frequency of the AE in a population between two drugs. Population-based rates of an AE generally cannot be estimated from spontaneous reporting data because of underreporting and lack of a reliable measure of population exposure.

Notably, there often is a differential extent of reporting of AEs across a product's marketed life (Weber effect, see above). Thus, even though a newly approved drug may not be widely used, more spontaneous AE reports may be received for the newer drug compared to an older, widely used drug, even if there is no actual difference in risk.

13.2 Case Study 2: Peginesatide

Peginesatide is a synthetic peptide considered a significant breakthrough for treating anaemia in patients with dialysis-dependent chronic kidney disease, approved by US FDA. It was withdrawn from the market in 2012, within months of becoming commercially available, when the manufacturer received a surprising number of case reports of fatal anaphylaxis [33].

Subsequent analyses suggested that the root cause of the reactions may have been a preservative present in the commercially available multiple-use vials [34]. This excipient was not used in the single-use formulation in clinical trials [35].

Anaphylaxis is a rare, unpredictable adverse reaction that can occur within minutes of exposure to an agent. The risk of such reactions must be minimised. If no effective risk minimisation measures are available, the medicinal product will struggle to demonstrate a positive benefit–risk balance and need to be withdrawn from the market.

Fatal anaphylaxis is a rare occurrence with a strong temporal relationship between a triggering exposure and the onset of severe symptoms. It represents an excellent example of the type of ADR for which spontaneous reporting systems are well suited to inform timely signal detection. Although the decision to withdraw peginesatide from market was relatively swift, the results of subsequent nonclinical analyses suggesting an unexpected root cause illustrate the importance of a thorough investigation, including the product quality [36].

References

1. International conference on harmonisation of technical requirements for registration of pharmaceuticals for human use. POST-APPROVAL SAFETY DATA MANAGEMENT: DEFINITIONS AND STANDARDS FOR EXPEDITED REPORTING E2D. Current Step 4 version dated 12 November 2003. https://database.ich.org/sites/default/files/E2D_Guideline.pdf.
2. Vargesson N. Thalidomide-induced teratogenesis: history and mechanisms. Birth Defects Res C Embryo Today. 2015;105(2):140–56. https://doi.org/10.1002/bdrc.21096.
3. McBride WG. Thalidomide and congenital abnormalities. [Letter to the Editor]. Lancet. 1961; 2:1358.

4. Lenz W, Knapp K. Foetal malformations due to thalidomide. In: Problems of birth defects. Springer; 1962. p. 200–6.
5. Kelsey FO. Thalidomide update: regulatory aspects. Teratology. 1988;38(3):221–6. https://doi.org/10.1002/tera.1420380305.
6. Fornasier G, Francescon S, Leone R, Baldo P. An historical overview over Pharmacovigilance. Int J Clin Pharm. 2018;40(4):744–7. https://doi.org/10.1007/s11096-018-0657-1.
7. Yellow Card | Making medicines and medical devices safer. n.d.. https://yellowcard.mhra.gov.uk/.
8. Boston Collaborative Drug Surveillance Program—Medical Technology Assessment Directory—NCBI Bookshelf. n.d.. https://www.ncbi.nlm.nih.gov/books/NBK218319/.
9. Programme for International Drug Monitoring. n.d.. https://www.who.int/teams/regulation-prequalification/regulation-and-safety/pharmacovigilance/health-professionals-info/pidm.
10. IVigee, iViReg. Technology. https://www.ivigee.com/technology.ivireg.
11. Kessler DA. Introducing MEDWatch. A new approach to reporting medication and device adverse effects and product problems. JAMA. 1993;269(21):2765–8. https://doi.org/10.1001/jama.269.21.2765.
12. Margraff F, Bertram D. Adverse drug reaction reporting by patients: an overview of fifty countries. Drug Saf. 2014;37(6):409–19. https://doi.org/10.1007/s40264-014-0162-y.
13. Inácio P, Cavaco A, Airaksinen M. The value of patient reporting to the pharmacovigilance system: a systematic review. Br J Clin Pharmacol. 2017;83(2):227–46. https://doi.org/10.1111/bcp.13098.
14. Avery AJ, Anderson C, Bond CM, Fortnum H, Gifford A, Hannaford PC, Hazell L, Krska J, Lee AJ, McLernon DJ, Murphy E, Shakir S, Watson MC. Evaluation of patient reporting of adverse drug reactions to the UK 'Yellow Card Scheme': literature review, descriptive and qualitative analyses, and questionnaire surveys. Health Technol Assess. 2011;15(20):1–234. https://doi.org/10.3310/hta15200.
15. Rolfes L, van Hunsel F, van der Linden L, Taxis K, van Puijenbroek E. The quality of clinical information in adverse drug reaction reports by patients and healthcare professionals: a retrospective comparative analysis. Drug Saf. 2017;40(7):607–14. https://doi.org/10.1007/s40264-017-0530-5.
16. Watson S, Chandler RE, Taavola H, Härmark L, Grundmark B, Zekarias A, Star K, van Hunsel F. Safety concerns reported by patients identified in a collaborative signal detection workshop using VigiBase: results and reflections from Lareb and Uppsala monitoring centre. Drug Saf. 2018;41(2):203–12. https://doi.org/10.1007/s40264-017-0594-2.
17. Hammond IW, Rich DS, Gibbs TG. Effect of consumer reporting on signal detection: using disproportionality analysis. Expert Opin Drug Saf. 2007;6(6):705–12. https://doi.org/10.1517/14740338.6.6.705.
18. World Health Organization. Ethical criteria for medicinal drug promotion. WHO Publications Center USA Distributor; 1988.
19. Sloane R, Osanlou O, Lewis D, Bollegala D, Maskell S, Pirmohamed M. Social media and pharmacovigilance: a review of the opportunities and challenges. Br J Clin Pharmacol. 2015;80(4):910–20. https://doi.org/10.1111/bcp.12717.
20. Convertino I, Ferraro S, Blandizzi C, Tuccori M. The usefulness of listening social media for pharmacovigilance purposes: a systematic review. Expert Opin Drug Saf. 2018;17(11):1081–93. https://doi.org/10.1080/14740338.2018.1531847.
21. Weber J. Epidemiology of adverse reactions to nonsteroidal anti-inflammatory drugs. In: Rainsford KD, Velo GD, editors. Side-effects of anti-inflammatory drugs, advances in inflammation research. Raven Press; 1984. p. 1–7.
22. McAdams MA, Governale LA, Swartz L, Hammad TA, Dal Pan GJ. Identifying patterns of adverse event reporting for four members of the angiotensin II receptor blockers class of drugs: revisiting the Weber effect. Pharmacoepidemiol Drug Saf. 2008;17(9):882–9. https://doi.org/10.1002/pds.1633.
23. Hoffman KB, Dimbil M, Erdman CB, Tatonetti NP, Overstreet BM. The Weber effect and the United States Food and Drug Administration's Adverse Event Reporting System (FAERS): analysis of sixty-two drugs approved from 2006 to 2010. Drug Saf. 2014;37(4):283–94. https://doi.org/10.1007/s40264-014-0150-2.
24. Hazell L, Shakir SA. Under-reporting of adverse drug reactions: a systematic review. Drug Saf. 2006;29(5):385–96. https://doi.org/10.2165/00002018-200629050-00003.
25. McGettigan P, Golden J, Conroy RM, Arthur N, Feely J. Reporting of adverse drug reactions by hospital doctors and the response to intervention. Br J Clin Pharmacol. 1997;44(1):98–100. https://doi.org/10.1046/j.1365-2125.1997.00616.x.
26. Perlík F, Slanar O, Smíd M, Petrácek J. Attitude of Czech physicians to adverse drug reaction reporting. Eur J Clin Pharmacol. 2002;58(5):367–9. https://doi.org/10.1007/s00228-002-0476-z.
27. Wallerstedt SM, Brunlöf G, Johansson M-L, Tukukino C, Ny L. Reporting of adverse drug reactions may be influenced by feedback to the reporting doctor. Eur J Clin Pharmacol. 2007;63(5):505–8. https://doi.org/10.1007/s00228-007-0270-z.
28. Salas M, Petracek J, Yalamanchili P, Aimer O, Kasthuril D, Dhingra S, Junaid T, Bostic T. The use of artificial intelligence in pharmacovigilance: a systematic review of the literature. Pharmaceut Med. 2022; https://doi.org/10.1007/s40290-022-00441-z.
29. Harpaz R, Vilar S, Dumouchel W, Salmasian H, Haerian K, Shah NH, Chase HS, Friedman C. Combing signals from spontaneous reports and electronic health records for detection of adverse drug reactions. J Am Med Inform Assoc.

2013;20(3):413–9. https://doi.org/10.1136/amiajnl-2012-000930.
30. McConeghy KW, Bress A, Qato DM, Wing C, Nutescu EA. Evaluation of dabigatran bleeding adverse reaction reports in the FDA adverse event reporting system during the first year of approval. Pharmacotherapy. 2014;34(6):561–9. https://doi.org/10.1002/phar.1415.
31. Southworth MR, Reichman ME, Unger EF. Dabigatran and postmarketing reports of bleeding. N Engl J Med. 2013;368(14):1272–4. https://doi.org/10.1056/NEJMp1302834.
32. Graham DJ, Reichman ME, Wernecke M, Zhang R, Southworth MR, Levenson M, Sheu TC, Mott K, Goulding MR, Houstoun M, MaCurdy TE, Worrall C, Kelman JA. Cardiovascular, bleeding, and mortality risks in elderly Medicare patients treated with dabigatran or warfarin for nonvalvular atrial fibrillation. Circulation. 2015;131(2):157–64. https://doi.org/10.1161/circulationaha.114.012061.
33. Bennett CL, Jacob S, Hymes J, Usvyat LA, Maddux FW. Anaphylaxis and hypotension after administration of peginesatide. N Engl J Med. 2014;370(21):2055–6. https://doi.org/10.1056/NEJMc1400883.
34. Weaver JL, Boyne M, Pang E, Chimalakonda K, Howard KE. Nonclinical evaluation of the potential for mast cell activation by an erythropoietin analog. Toxicol Appl Pharmacol. 2015;287(3):246–52. https://doi.org/10.1016/j.taap.2015.06.009.
35. Kotarek J, Stuart C, De Paoli SH, Simak J, Lin TL, Gao Y, Ovanesov M, Liang Y, Scott D, Brown J, Bai Y, Metcalfe DD, Marszal E, Ragheb JA. Subvisible particle content, formulation, and dose of an erythropoietin peptide mimetic product are associated with severe adverse postmarketing events. J Pharm Sci. 2016;105(3):1023–7. https://doi.org/10.1016/s0022-3549(15)00180-x.
36. Hermanson T, Bennett CL, Macdougall IC. Peginesatide for the treatment of anemia due to chronic kidney disease—an unfulfilled promise. Expert Opin Drug Saf. 2016;15(10):1421–6. https://doi.org/10.1080/14740338.2016.1218467.

Further Reading

Strom BL, Kimmel SE, Hennessy S, editors. Pharmacoepidemiology. John Wiley & Sons Ltd.; 2021.

Stephens MD. The dawn of drug safety. Hampshire, UK: George Mann; 2010.

Communicating Drug Safety

11

Marco Tuccori, Irma Convertino, Sara Ferraro, Marco Bonaso, Giulia Valdiserra, and Emiliano Cappello

Abstract

Promoting safety of medications is imperative for optimal use, and the communication of the risk is entrusted to communicators. The communication of the risk of medicine requires peculiar expertise that is different from communications about its benefit. The identification of a risk related to a medicinal product is a dynamic process that involves the acquisition of information that progressively transforms into knowledge. In the initial stages of this process, the risk is often only potential but this uncertainty still requires caution. Uncertain risks are frequently matter of communication, and the magnitude of this uncertainty often drives the risk communication itself as the main subject. A message has to be tailored to the attitude and concerns of the target audience for achieving the best effects. Otherwise, uncertainties and hesitancies could persist even after the confirmation of the absence of a risk or could spread throughout media with consequent possible inappropriate use of drugs or therapeutic failure of medicines. In this regard, case studies such as measles vaccination and autism and the COVID-19 infodemic are paradigmatic examples. In risk communication about medicines, it is important to identify the subjects involved, define their roles (senders or receivers) and characteristics, to build the message and its content, and choosing the appropriate media for conveying the message. Several expertise is also required, including rhetoric, ethics, social sciences, and pharmacoepidemiology.

Keywords

Drug safety · Risk communication · Infodemic · Risk perception · Social media · Rhetoric

Learning Objectives

- Describe the principles and definitions of the risk communication on drugs.
- Understand how to build effective risk communication strategies.
- Discuss the multidisciplinary approaches involved in risk communication on medicines.
- Analyze the ethical and legal framework in risk communication on medicines.

M. Tuccori (✉)
Unit of Pharmacology and Pharmacovigilance, Department of Clinical and Experimental Medicine, University of Pisa, Pisa, Italy

Unit of Adverse Drug Reactions Monitoring, University Hospital of Pisa, Pisa, Italy
e-mail: m.tuccori@ao-pisa.toscana.it

I. Convertino · S. Ferraro · M. Bonaso · G. Valdiserra
E. Cappello
Unit of Pharmacology and Pharmacovigilance, Department of Clinical and Experimental Medicine, University of Pisa, Pisa, Italy

J. Jose et al. (eds.), *Principles and Practice of Pharmacovigilance and Drug Safety*,
https://doi.org/10.1007/978-3-031-51089-2_11

Key Points

- The attention to the communication of risk on medicinal products has grown in the recent years, when the experiences with rofecoxib, thalidomide, and H1N1 influenza vaccine brought regulatory authorities and all professionals to the awareness that preventing and managing risk needs an improvement in transparency and compliance with the recommendations, meaning a quick and effective risk communication.
- Constructing an effective risk communication strategy requires not only specific expertise but also a structured process, tailored to the condition for ensuring its benefit. This includes the identification and characterization (e.g., level of understanding) of subjects involved in the communication process (senders or receivers), the designation of the message and its content, and the determination of the media for conveying the message in a quick way, for stemming fake news and uncertainties from rapid expansion.
- A risk can occur whenever a patient takes a drug. However, to distinguish from fears, uncertainties, and fake beliefs, it is required that after the identification of risk and the classification as potential risk through the observations of evidence from clinical practice or findings from observational studies, the risk has to be confirmed and communicated leading to an impact on clinical practice.

1 Introduction

The Swiss physician, alchemist, and philosopher Paracelsus (1493–1541) considered to be the father of modern toxicology, argued that "*Omnia venenum sunt: nec sine veneno quicquam existit. Dosis sola facit, ut venenum non fit*" (Everything is poison, and nothing exists without poison. Only the dose prevents the poison from taking effect) [1]. The sentence in modern times was intended as "every drug is a poison. It is just a matter of dose." Although he referred in a broad sense to all substances, somehow and perhaps unwittingly, with this admonition, Paracelsus ventured into a sort of proto-communication of the risk of medicinal products. From the perspective of rhetoric, the combination of the two words "poison" and "drug" can condition the attitude of the recipients of the message to move with caution toward substances, thus acting on their perception of risk. The sentence by Paracelsus was probably very effective in communicating the risk of medicine to people of the Renaissance period, but today things are much more complicated.

While in the time of Paracelsus, medical information traveled only on medical treatises and was intended for the medical elite, today the means of communication are much more universal and accessible. The safety of medicines is now a matter of public concern. People are increasingly interested in transparency around medication safety-related matters. Clear communication of the facts relating to drug safety is entrusted to communicators, who can make use of various tools to best exercise their role as mediators. The communication of the risk of medicinal products must therefore take into account many factors and in particular the centrality of the patient in the management of treatments [2]. In the 1980s, the doctor, the patient, and medical information were identified as the three essential elements of *evidence-based medicine* and their optimal interaction is considered the key to ensure the effectiveness of treatments under the maximum safety conditions [3]. The principles of *evidence-based medicine* can now be extended to all communication processes of information on medicines, involving all the stakeholders of modern pharmacovigilance and in particular governments, regulatory agencies, pharmaceutical companies, healthcare professionals, and patients.

In this chapter, we will illustrate the general principles of risk communication on medicinal products starting from the definitions to arrive at the construction of effective communication strategies based on multidisciplinary approaches, passing through some case studies from which we have learned important lessons.

2 The Scope of Communicating Risk About Medicinal Products

The purpose of risk communication of medicinal products is to inform and educate the stakeholders about the potential benefits and harms of using a certain medicinal product and to facilitate the decision-making process based on the best available evidence. Risk communication is an integral part of quality risk management, which is a systematic process for the assessment, control, communication, and review of risks to the quality of medicinal products [4]. Risk communication also supports pharmacovigilance significantly [5].

3 Risk and Risk Perception About Medicinal Products

The risks of a medicinal product, or its ability to cause harm to the patient, are usually linked to the active substance (more rarely to its excipients or contaminants). In some cases, we can identify specific susceptibility of the patient who takes it (e.g., genetics, concomitant diseases, concomitant treatments). However, in many cases, the determinants of a risk may be unknown or undetectable, and in these cases the damage may be unpredictable and not preventable. The risk can also be generated by the circumstances in which the drug is taken (e.g., misuse, errors in therapy management). The lack of efficacy, regardless of the cause, also falls within the concept of risk since it can cause damage that in certain situations can be particularly relevant (life-threatening diseases, vaccines, contraceptives) [6].

Although there is a conceptual difference between harm and risk, in the general language the word risk is used to define both terms. While harm can be defined as an actual injury to someone's goods (e.g., house, car, money) or values (e.g., family, health, freedom), a risk refers to the probability or potentiality or uncertainty that something negative could happen to that goods or values, whatever the magnitude of this probability. In this context, risk communication for medicinal products can be defined as the not necessarily mutual transfer of information about the probability (risk) that a certain clinically adverse event may occur with the intake of a medicinal product in relation or not to an expected benefit (including any measures to be taken to minimize this probability), between two or more subjects, usually a communicator (or sender) and a target audience (receiver) (doctor and patient, regulatory authority and population, pharmaceutical industry and regulatory authority). It is important to underline that the communication of the risk of medicinal products can almost never be separated from that of the expected benefit (benefit–risk balance) and that the evaluation and communication of benefits require specific expertise, different from that of risks [6].

The identification of a risk related to a medicinal product is a process developing through various degrees of certainty, from a risk that can be defined as "potential" up to the confirmation of the risk itself. The hypothesis of the existence of a risk can be generated in a theoretical and speculative way starting from the knowledge surrounding the biological mechanisms with which the drug is supposed to act. Much more often, it is generated by anecdotal reporting of events observed in clinical practice (see, e.g., the case of thalidomide) [7]. More rarely, the signals may be generated by clinical trials or observational studies. The latter are more useful for confirming a risk, but intrinsic limitations of the observational studies themselves (limited study power, statistical assumptions, residual confounding) may produce results that must still be interpreted with caution [8].

Risk communication of medicinal products more often deals with potential risks than with confirmed risks. This means that uncertainties are often the subject of the communication and can affect the characteristics and outcomes of the communication itself. The uncertainties may concern diagnostic and clinical or epidemiological aspects but very often they are related to causality. The description of uncertainties is an element of risk communication that affects the communicator's credibility and must be handled with the utmost transparency [9].

People may have various concerns about taking medicines. These concerns derive from the personal beliefs of individuals and are influenced by education, religious belief, politics, morality, and in general by the environment in which one grows up and by the people who associate with one another. These aforementioned factors determine the individual perception of risk, that is, the cognitive process involved in various daily activities and which guides people's behavior in the face of decisions involving potential risks [9]. The effectiveness of a message may depend on how closely it is tailored to the recipient's possible concerns. Concerns may persist for a long time even when the risk has been definitively excluded, as in the case of autism "fraudly" associated with measles vaccination [10]. Even simple rumors and fake news can fuel or limit worries and, given the popularity of modern means of communication such as social media, the effects can be significant and on a large scale. The main consequences may be the failure to use medicines effectively (resulting in therapeutic failure) or inappropriate use, with the possibility of developing adverse events in the face of a non-existent benefit. In this regard, the COVID-19 pandemic has produced important examples both before and after the advent of vaccines, from which it is essential to learn lessons for the future (see Sect. 8) [11].

4 Essential Elements of Risk Communication for Medicinal Products

Communication refers in common language to the complex interplay of messages, tools, and processes necessary for the transfer of information between different parties in order to achieve certain objectives. Mapping the communication model is recommended for building effective communication (Fig. 11.1). In particular, it is important to identify the subjects involved and define their roles (*senders* or *receivers*), the message and its *content*, the media through which the message is conveyed, and the information transfer flows.

The *content* of the communication refers to the information conveyed. The information describes facts provided or learned from something or someone (source) and is related to knowledge or data. The information is not necessarily in verbal or written form but can also be made in images or sounds. It can contain numerical data to favor cognitive processes of quantification useful for transforming uncertain situations into more certain, in order to favor the decision-making process toward any choices. In the case of medicinal products risk communication, the information is intrinsically uncertain (Sect. 2), the quality of the content and its presentation are highly variable, and the passage of the message can be easily confused or hindered by external elements (rumors and fake news). Therefore, the cognitive process can be particularly challenging for individuals [12].

In the context of the risk communication of medicinal products, the subjects most often involved are patients (also understood as citizens), caregivers, regulatory authorities, the pharmaceutical industry, academia, and organizations of these subjects. However, given today's accessibility to the media, political and religious leaders, governments, journalists, teachers, judges, lawyers, bloggers, film makers, fiction writers, and artists can often be involved in the debate on drug safety [6]. Depending on the situation, all these subjects can be either communicators (*senders*) or target audience (*receivers*).

The drug communication model can be developed through four main levels that can overlap and be more or less defined: (1) the interpersonal level: it is most important for the patient and concerns direct communication of patients with caregivers (doctor, pharmacist, and nurse); (2) the intra-group (or intra-organization) level: patients and caregivers can communicate within groups that include other patients (self-help groups) or

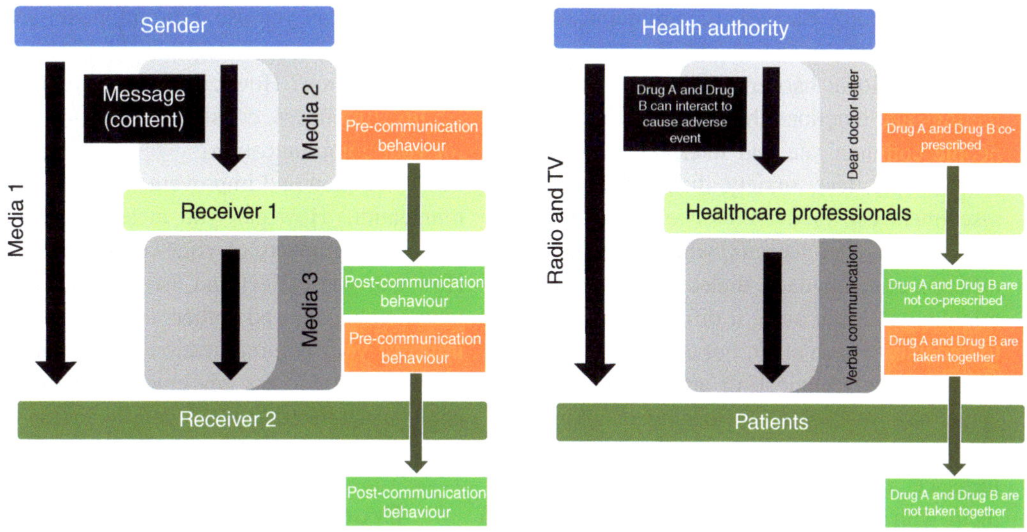

Fig. 11.1 Map of the communication model. This figure presents an example of a risk communication map. In the general flowchart, the roles and paths of communication are identified and defined. In the specific example, the regulatory agency (sender) communicates the risks of a possible interaction between drug A and drug B (message). The receivers are healthcare professionals and patients. Communication takes place through two distinct media: a general one (radio and TV) that reaches all recipients, and a specific one, dear doctor letter, for healthcare professionals. The languages of the two messages can be the same or tailored for the recipient. In this case, recipient 1 (healthcare professionals) acts as an amplifier and in turn becomes a sender toward the patient through verbal communication during the visit. The measurable outcome of the communication process is the change in the behavior of both types of recipients

other health professionals (departmental teams, professional organizations, scientific societies, and scientific board); (3) the inter-group (or inter-organization) level: refers to communications between groups such as pharmaceutical industry, regulatory authorities, patient organizations; (4) mass level: messages are publicly disseminated using universally accessible means of communication (social media threads, newspapers, scientific journals, newsletters, and bulletins) [13].

Referring to socio-ecological models, communication can also be classified into three different spheres of relevance: the private sphere, the community sphere, and the social sphere [14]. The communicative interaction can take place in several spheres simultaneously and at different levels. For example, communication between doctor and patient may occur on an interpersonal level in the private sphere, but some information may be shared with other caregivers of the medical department in the community sphere and furthermore interpersonal communication contributes to (and is influenced by) both general culture and from the infrastructure of the health system into the social sphere. Levels and spheres essentially describe the dimensions of communicative events and are interrelated in particular for public communication events [6].

Since drug safety communication may have different audiences, taking into account the characteristics of these audiences in the development of a communication strategy is the key element for achieving an effective communication [15]. Some of the key considerations for communicating drug safety information to different audiences are:

- The purpose and goals of the communication: What are the main messages and actions that you want to convey and achieve with your communication? How do they align with the needs and expectations of your audience?
- The characteristics and preferences of the audience: Who are they? What are their backgrounds, knowledge levels, attitudes, beliefs, values, and motivations regarding drug safety? How do they prefer to receive and process information? What are their *barriers* and facilitators in understanding and acting on your

communication? Barriers to communication should be carefully considered. Barriers could be (a) emotional barriers, which refer to the feelings and emotions that can affect the way people communicate and interpret messages. For example, fear, anxiety, distrust, anger, or resentment can hinder effective communication; (b) language barriers, which refer to the differences in language, dialect, accent, or terminology that can make it difficult for people to understand each other. For example, the use of unfamiliar, technical, or ambiguous words can create confusion or misunderstandings. Numbers may also represent an element of disturbance in communication and replacing them with easily understandable graphic can be a successful choice; (c) physical barriers, which refer to the material or environmental obstacles that can interfere with the transmission or reception of messages. For example, background noise, geographical distances, closed doors, or faulty equipment can reduce the quality or accessibility of communication; (d) cultural barriers, which refer to the differences in values, beliefs, norms, or habits that can influence the way people communicate and perceive messages. For example, different expectations, preferences, or conventions regarding verbal and non-verbal language can cause misunderstandings or conflicts; (e) attitudinal barriers, which refer to the biases, stereotypes, or discriminations that can affect the way people communicate and relate to others. For example, arrogance, presumption, resistance to change, or lack of respect can hinder open and constructive communication.

- The content and format of the communication: What are the most relevant and credible sources of information for your audience? How can you present the information in a clear, accurate, balanced, and engaging way? How can you use language, visuals, stories, examples, and other elements to enhance your communication? How can you tailor your communication to suit different audiences or contexts?
- The channels and methods of communication: What are the most effective and appropriate ways to reach and interact with your audience? How can you use different media, platforms, tools, and strategies to deliver your communication? How can you ensure accessibility, timeliness, consistency, and feedback for your communication?
- The evaluation and improvement of the communication: How can you measure the outcomes and impacts of your communication? How can you collect and use feedback from your audience and other stakeholders to improve your communication? How can you monitor and address any emerging issues or challenges related to your communication?

5 Drug Safety Communication Research

5.1 Study Design

A risk communication event usually can trigger a risk modification (worsening or improvement) through certain "changes" that are expected to be implemented by the receivers. A communication can therefore be more or less effective in generating this risk modification, and it is appropriate to identify indicators (outcomes) to be able to measure it. When the risk communication strategy is intended with the aim of obtaining a risk mitigation, and the effectiveness of the same is not observed to be that expected, the entire communication process can be studied to identify its weaknesses and introduce improvements.

The evaluation of the effectiveness of a risk communication has traditionally been carried out through surveys and expert assessments [16], but the trend in recent years is to rely on more robust and reliable analytical studies. These studies can measure risk outcomes before and after the introduction of the communication itself by integrating different data sources and are able to consider and subsequently control different variables simultaneously [6]. To improve the reliability of the results, it is recommended that research protocols to study the impact of drug risk communication be designed using a multidisciplinary approach, involving the contribution of pharmacoepidemiologists and experts in social sciences, rhetoric, media, and cognitive and behavioral sciences [17].

Systematic reviews, which outline the state of the art evidence from interventional (e.g., randomized clinical trials) and observational studies (e.g., cohort, case–control, and case series designs) [18], show that the available studies to assess the impact of risk communication of medicinal products have been conducted taking into account a single perspective, often that of the health system or the regulatory one. This is far enough from an integrated view of the disciplines, which should include, for example, the behavior of the population among the outcomes, to give a comprehensive view of the impact of a risk communication intervention [6, 19].

5.2 Outcome Assessment

To assess risk communication and design-specific studies, the definition of outcomes of interest is essential. These outcomes can be classified as intended or unintended. The first category concerns outcomes that try to interpret the effect of predetermined communication events that have the purpose of avoiding or realizing the object of the communication. The second includes general positive and negative outcomes regardless of any communication objectives [6]. An example of unintended negative outcomes could be the situation in which following a certain communication, the patient decides to voluntarily discontinue the drugs they are taking without medical support. In this case, the outcome of interest could be the percentage of subjects who stop treatment in the population in a defined period following the date of the communication of interest. An unintended positive outcome is characterized by positive behavior achieved by patients as a result of communication. This positive attitude, deriving from the communication related to a specific drug, affects the awareness of the management of all the drugs taken by the patient [20]. In light of the above, the first outcome of the communication that should be measured corresponds to the purpose of the communication itself, and that is the behavior and not the impact on health. The latter is in fact the result of the change in behavior stimulated by communication. Actually, the flow of information and the associated effects give light to a labyrinthine environment, whereby communication can lead to several concomitant and interconnected outcomes, which inevitably change over time and within different groups of the population. Table 11.1 proposes a classification of the outcomes that could allow the overcoming of heterogeneities and obtain comparable results from a multidisciplinary standpoint [6].

Table 11.1 Examples of outcomes to assess risk communication effectiveness [6]

Type of outcome	Study question	Outcome (Endpoints)
Exposure to message	How many subjects did the communication touch?	Amount of person receiving the message (number of message receipt received) Amount of person receiving a video communication (number of visualizations or number of people connected to a direct broadcast on social media)
Debate	Was the communication interesting for the target audience?	Volume of debate on social media (number of people sharing message in social media, number of comments, and number of emoticons) Volume of debate on journals (number of articles, volumes of articles, and page in which the information is given) Volume of debate on TV (number of TV shows or TV news which dedicates time for the message)
Risk knowledge	What is the level of knowledge in the target audience about the risk object?	Knowledge about risk using questionnaires and survey (number and percentage of people aware about the risk, number and percentage of people aware of the correct behavior to avoid the risk)
Attitude	Did the communication affect the behavior of the target audience?	Behavior following communication (number and percentage of target audience following recommendations and trends in dataflow)

5.3 Investigating Social Media

Over the past two decades, communication via the internet and social media has increased significantly. According to the latest "Digital 2022" report from the "We Are Social" agency, global internet users rose to 4.95 billion at the beginning of 2022, to include more than 4.6 billion social media users, 58.4% of the world population [21]. Billions of people interacting with the internet can therefore generate traces of important information that can be aggregated and analyzed for research purposes. While most of this research was conducted for marketing purposes, social media can be an interesting source of information for health research as well. The communication of the risk of medicinal products also uses the social media channel extensively. In particular, a great deal of daily social media discussions is about health and disease information, as well as biomedical and medical products that address these conditions (medicines, devices, vitamins, supplements, etc.) [22]. Many of these health-related discussions are patient-generated and include a large body of free-text narratives that can be leveraged for health-specific research [22]. A specific line of pharmacovigilance research was born and developed to conduct signal detection research using these data, developing a specific methodology. These studies can be very interesting for measuring the perception of the risk of medicinal products in the population, the response of the population to certain communication stimuli, and also for building communication strategies that are based on the needs of the population itself. In particular, for example, the exchange of information between users of a patient community can be studied to understand their feelings in relation to the therapies they use (enthusiasm for efficacy, complaints about adverse events) and develop a communication that helps them to better manage the therapies according to their need [6, 23].

Social media is a privileged observatory for exploring the use of drugs in the real world. They can help identify safety problems and risk factors and can offer additional information not typically captured by existing reporting systems, such as benefits, misuse, or lack of effectiveness. Furthermore, online discussions among patients about medicines often extend to broader aspects of use, such as off-label use (i.e., use not in accordance with the terms of the marketing authorization), as well as problems with product quality, formulation, handling, disposal, sensitive or stigmatized topics (e.g., events involving the sexual sphere), and reluctance to adhere to treatment due to bothersome adverse reactions experienced by the patient [6, 24–26]. A very interesting approach to measure the risk communication response of medicinal products could be sentiment analysis, a semantic technique that evaluates in posts shared by the community the combination of words that express positive, negative, or neutral feelings in combination with the medicinal products subject of the communication itself [6, 24–26]. Of course, there is still a long way to go, but undoubtedly the potential offered by these approaches in the field of risk communication for medicinal products is enormous.

6 Building a Medicinal Product Risk Communication Strategy: A Multidisciplinary Approach

Building an effective risk communication strategy for medicinal products can require the contribution of different expertise. Similarly, a communicative event can be analyzed from different perspectives. In the next paragraphs, we will briefly analyze the main disciplines that can play a key role in the construction and analysis of a risk communication strategy for medicinal products.

6.1 Rhetoric

Rhetoric is the art and science of persuading and influencing others through language. Rhetoric can impact the communication of safety of medicinal products in different ways, both positive and negative. For this reason, it is important to analyze the language used in different sources and situations of communication of safety of medicinal products, to evaluate its quality, credibility, and effectiveness.

Rhetorical analysis is the study of the ways in which language is used to persuade and influence others. In the context of communication of safety of medicinal products, rhetorical analysis can serve to evaluate the quality and credibility of the sources of information on medicinal products, verifying their competence, reliability, and impartiality. This helps to identify the arguments and evidence used to support the claims on the benefits and risks of medicinal products, verifying their validity, consistency, and relevance; to recognize the emotional appeals and persuasive techniques used to influence the attitudes and behaviors of the users of medicinal products, verifying their appropriateness, ethics, and transparency; and to compare and contrast the different perspectives and positions of the stakeholders involved in the communication of safety of medicinal products, verifying their representativeness, balance, and dialogue.

Some practical examples of rhetorical analysis in the communication of safety of medicinal products are analyzing the language used in the leaflets of medicinal products, to verify if it is clear, understandable, and suitable for the public to whom it is addressed; analyzing the language used in the information campaigns on medicinal products, to verify if it is informative, educational, and motivational; analyzing the language used in the reports of adverse events by patients and health professionals, to verify if it is accurate, complete, and timely [27, 28].

6.2 Pharmacoepidemiology

Risk communication finds its backbone in pharmacoepidemiology, the science that evaluates the utilization of drugs in the populations and the related health determinants and outcomes [29–31]. Pharmacoepidemiology overcomes several limitations of clinical trials and provides a picture of the real world of drug usage [32]. By applying elaborated methods to control biases and confounding, the aim of pharmacoepidemiology is to provide robust evidence of the causal association between drug exposure and outcomes, featured by the balance of statistics, clinical, and pharmacology fields [33, 34]. The communication of the risks and the safe use of drugs based on pharmacoepidemiologic findings is a tricky process since this has to answer to the need to communicate to the public the health hazards found in the studies, switching from scientific to divulgation language, and share decisions made by stakeholders accordingly. Several variables have to be taken into account in communicating the findings of a pharmacoepidemiology study, such as the quality, the accuracy, and the robustness of the study performed, as well as the clinical and health implications. These variables are classified as dependent variables of the risk communication. Examples of independent variables are instead the intervention on drug usage and prescription, the patients' adherence or the spontaneous adverse drug reaction reporting, and the spread of information through the different media [35–39]. Guidelines on transparency, funding, and conflicts of interest for disseminating pharmacoepidemiologic evidence have been outlined by the European Network of Centres for Pharmacoepidemiology and Pharmacovigilance (ENCePP) [32], and adherence to these guidelines can be helpful to achieve a good quality management of risk communication processes.

In a broad cyclic vision, pharmacoepidemiology research and risk communication on medicinal products are intimately connected [6]. Indeed, the goal of good risk communication on medicinal products, a whole meal of the risk minimization measures, is the reduction of the exposure of patients to specific risks related to medicine intakes and consequently of the related adverse reactions [40, 41]. Thereby the risk communication itself is a determinant of the exposure to drugs [42].

6.3 Cognitive and Behavioral Sciences

In the construction and study of drug-related risk communication, an important contribution comes from the cognitive and behavioral sciences.

The cognitive sciences have shown the importance of the distinction between real risk and how it is perceived, and how in reality it is the latter that has a decisive impact on people's behavior.

While cognitive sciences explore which factors influence risk perception, behavioral sciences have developed numerous theories on how risk perception can affect behavior. The purpose of these models is to predict people's behavior and the factors that determine it. The common thread of these models is the importance of the subjective perception of danger and efficacy or the perception of one's ability to implement a protective action.

In building an effective communication of the risk of a medicinal product with the patient, the objective must be to put them in a position to make decisions and adopt behaviors with respect to that drug that do not involve avoidable risks for their health. In this sense, it can be important to know the heuristics, or mental paths, often called "shortcuts," which allow you to make decisions in uncertain situations or that cannot be fully understood. The decision you make is not necessarily the right one, but it is certainly satisfactory enough. Usually these paths are guided by the experience of everyday life and by the observation of what happens to the people close to us. Let us discuss some examples.

In the **heuristic of representativeness**, one tends to consider a valid sample of experiences as the representativeness of one's own knowledge, leaving out fundamental details for fully understanding a problem. For example, a patient may be reluctant to take a drug because the neighbor who took it had a stroke. In this case, the patient neglects various elements necessary to reach an informed decision such as, for example, the number of subjects who take that drug without problems or the fact that the neighbor had important risk factors for stroke. In this case, the doctor must provide the patient with the missing information in a very simple way in order to obtain greater compliance.

In the **availability heuristic**, the patient tends to attribute frequency to an event on the basis of how often he receives information about that event and the emotional impact of the information provided. For example, a patient may not want to be vaccinated because the media have very often reported in the last week that the vaccine caused a fatal case of thrombosis in a 40-year-old patient, father of two children. This unique case is "amplified" many times based on how many times it has been heard of (media hype) and as the effect increases, the greater the empathy developed so that in the end its frequency is perceived as very probable. Also in this case, the doctor must clearly provide information on the frequency of the event (number of subjects with thrombosis and number of subjects treated, the use of infographics can be useful) and use the frequencies of "emotionally similar" events in subjects not vaccinated.

In the **anchoring heuristic**, the probability of an event is influenced by terms of comparison that are also far from the context of interest but as close as possible to everyday experience. In the previous example, in order to support the patient in the understating of the magnitude of the risk of thrombosis with the vaccine, it could be useful to provide a comparison with the risk of thrombosis associated with exposures that are commonly experienced (e.g., use of oral contraceptives), not recommended but socially accepted (e.g., cigarette smoking) or even linked to desirable situations (travel with long flights).

The complexity of the processes underlying people's behavior toward their own health problems has made it necessary to implement specific research methods and approaches to evaluate the ways of communicating on the safety of drugs. Research in this field is divided into **formative research** and **evaluative research**. **Formative research** examines people's perceptions and understanding of risks and preferences regarding drug safety information. This type of research can be conducted through qualitative and quantitative studies in the area of social and behavioral sciences. In a classic example of educational research, participants in these studies are interviewed before and after having undergone a certain information campaign in order to understand users' preferences in terms of risk communication. **Evaluation**

research, on the other hand, operates through analytical studies and compares the effectiveness of various tools and strategies in obtaining a change in preferences or behavior.

Effective risk communication on drug use requires going beyond the simple "knowledge deficit communication model" [43, 44], that is, with a simple statement of facts. Communication strategies should be instead dynamically designed taking into account the point of view and needs of the person receiving the information.

6.4 The Social Sciences

Social research is a method used by social scientists and researchers to learn about people and societies with the aim of designing products/services that meet their specific needs. Social research is conducted following a systematic strategy that includes different observation methods that can also be applied to risk communication on medicinal products. In particular, qualitative, investigative, and quasi-experimental methods commonly used in the social sciences can greatly contribute to the creation of generalizable knowledge to inform the development of new risk communication approaches and to evaluate established ones [6].

The choice of research method must be appropriate to the type of question. In general, we can distinguish qualitative approaches, surveys, experimental and quasi-experimental methods, and mixed approaches. Qualitative methods are suitable for understanding perspectives through open and conversational discussions between people (listening) with the aim of generating theoretical concepts. In particular, the results of this method are accurate and can be the basis for generalization. They are effective in incorporating emotional, ethical, and cognitive aspects of risk communication. Surveys are useful for studying the prevalence (e.g., of attitudes toward the types of risk communication or the resulting behaviors) and correlations (e.g., perception of risk in relation to the severity of the health problem) through the use of questionnaires [6]. Experimental and quasi-experimental methods are suitable for measuring the effect of a risk communication intervention or of some of its elements or modalities. Finally, mixed-approach studies that combine investigative and qualitative methods are particularly suitable for evaluating established risk communication interventions, combining breadth and depth. Indeed, mixed-method research can provide the in-depth and contextualized data of qualitative research along with the predictive power of quantitative research. It is important to emphasize that these studies could take a long time to be conducted and generate non-overlapping evidence [6].

In recent years, there has been a growing involvement of patients and the public in research processes. Indeed, the importance of their participation is becoming increasingly recognized, and social science methods should be further developed for their efforts as co-researchers in data collection, analysis, and dissemination. Paying more attention to patient and public involvement in research will undoubtedly in itself lead to studies that more effectively address the social and emotional context of the disease and treatment. While numerous challenges remain to be addressed, there is great potential in increased collaboration between researchers in pharmacovigilance and social sciences to improve the study of drug risk communication and thus improve the services that professionals and organizations provide to patients, clients, families, and the global public [6].

6.5 Media Science

Drugs and vaccines information are increasingly being reported in the media, such as the press, television, radio, websites, and social media; therefore, the media are an important source of information for the public, patients, and healthcare professionals. However, the sheer size of the media offering can make it quite difficult for patients and healthcare professionals to discern valid and relevant information from unreliable information. For the same reason, it can be difficult for regulatory agencies and other pharmacovigilance stakeholders to speak out clearly to provide information on the safe use of medicinal products [6]. Communication on COVID-19 vaccines is certainly a recent example of how important it is to be able to manage all these aspects [45, 46].

It becomes essential to understand how the news media deals with drug-related topics and how they provide information to their target audience. In a rapidly evolving media landscape, media science-based research can make an essential contribution to drug risk communication, particularly in informing media communication strategies, optimizing interactions with journalists, and evaluating communication outcomes in the light of specific contents. In recent years, much has been learned from academic studies and professional practice about how media channels inform, educate, and persuade people, including healthcare professionals, about the benefits, risks, and use of drugs [6].

For drug risk communication research, media science applies a number of methods, many from the social sciences. These methods include both qualitative and quantitative approaches, ranging from individual interviews to large-scale monitoring of traditional and social media content and product mentions [6]. Most of these methods have been described in the section devoted to social sciences (Sect. 5.3). Future work on communicating information on drug risks is likely to focus heavily on information that can be gleaned from social media discussions and traditional media analysis.

7 Ethical Frameworks

Bioethics is a discipline that deals with moral issues related to biological research and medicine [47]. The four principles of bioethics such as autonomy, beneficence, non-maleficence, and justice must also be applied in the communication of the risk of medicinal products. Autonomy recognizes the individual's right to self-determination and identifies respect for the individual's ability to make informed decisions about personal matters. According to the principle of beneficence, healthcare professionals should make decisions aimed at gaining patient interest in the clinical setting. The principle of non-maleficence, on the other hand, underlines the importance of not causing harm to the individual. When considering this principle for possible harm caused by a drug, the risk/benefit ratio remains an important factor to be considered. Justice guarantees the same patients to be treated with the same treatment and different patients to be treated with different treatments if those differences are relevant to obtain the best individual interest. The application of the principle of justice becomes critical when resources are limited and not sufficient to cover the needs of all patients requiring clinical treatment [47].

Appropriate communication on the risks and safe use of medicines is associated with several ethical challenges. Providing patients with relevant information can help them realize their authentic preferences, thus fostering independent choices. However, correct communication is essential to avoid sending the wrong messages to citizens that could lead to harmful actions. In this case, the outcome of the communication (decisions and behaviors) can be conditioned by factors such as literacy and psychological reactance. Psychological reactance is a situation where some people have a cognitive bias in the way they perceive the social order and their place within it. This is why they are resistant to following rules, guidelines, or patterns. They find it more motivating to follow a different path [48].

When considering the risks of drug treatments, expert opinion from stakeholders and regulatory agencies is based on observation of the evidence. The quantity and quality of evidence, together with the risk–benefit profile described for a drug establish the level of uncertainty surrounding the safe use of drugs. Uncertainty can generate ethical tensions in drug safety communication. For example, experienced scientists face both the duty to tell the truth and the concerns of possible public reactions. Strategies for overcoming this tension include the concealment of uncertainty or the clear transmission of uncertainty [49, 50]. This is a clear example of a moral problem communicators face in communicating the risk and safe use of drugs during public debates.

8 Examples on Communicating Drug Safety from Regulatory/Marketing Authorization Holder's Perspective

8.1 Rofecoxib

The withdrawal of rofecoxib represented an epochal event for pharmacovigilance, especially because it involved a market of about 80 million users worldwide [51]. The official US Food and Drug Administration (FDA) statement attributing many deaths to this drug due to cardiovascular causes [52] produced a general loss of confidence for the population toward the regulatory agency perceived as too close to the interests of the pharmaceutical industry, so much so as to request greater transparency in the conduct of clinical trials and clearer post-surveillance safety plans [53, 54]. Some English media declared the failure of the regulatory process for approval of marketing authorization for drugs, insinuating that the FDA had "hidden" unfavorable data [55, 56]. While prescribers relied on guidelines issued by regulatory agencies and discussed them in scientific journals, citizens needed to be reassured [57].

Newspapers reported the story of rofecoxib from its commercialization until its withdrawal using sensational and frightening headlines. The fearful attitude of patients and prescribers automatically extended to drugs in the same class [58]. Several studies conducted after the suspension of rofecoxib showed that users of COX-2 inhibitors discontinued treatment four times more than users of similar analgesic drugs. The problem is that patients switched to non-selective NSAIDs without considering the risk of gastrointestinal bleeding or opioids in case of chronic illness [59]. The "reaction" times to communication were quite rapid, but the speed depends a lot on media hype. In 2013, the milder communication about the increased risk of cardiovascular effects with diclofenac compared to other non-selective NSAIDs such as naproxen did not produce visible effects on the diclofenac market [60]. However, in 2015, naproxen prescription increased from 20% to 55%, demonstrating that the message had been received by prescribers with a certain delay [61].

This case emphasizes the importance of transparency in maintaining public confidence in the regulatory agency. It is important to involve both healthcare professionals and patients in the safety communication process to avoid dangerous behaviors such as the decision to suspend or change treatment without medical supervision.

8.2 Thalidomide Re-introduction

The tragedy of thalidomide [7], always used as a paradigmatic example of the need to monitor drug safety, had a strong emotional impact on public opinion, generating a distrust of this drug (and probably drugs in general) that was very difficult to overcome. Yet a few years after its withdrawal, it was realized that the use of thalidomide could have important applications, especially in oncology [62].

In the early 2000s, the FDA approved thalidomide for the treatment of multiple myeloma. To minimize the risk of teratogenicity, thalidomide access is restricted through the System for Thalidomide Education and Prescribing Safety (STEPS) program [63]. The new drug authorization has elicited opposing reactions among adults who developed phocomelia with thalidomide and cancer patients who hoped for treatment with thalidomide. This has put regulatory authorities in what is called "ambiguity" in terms of risk governance [64]. The European Medicine Agency brought together the two organizations to comment on the thalidomide risk management plan with the result of a re-approval of the drug in 2008. During the meeting, a harsh pregnancy prevention program (PP) was also drawn up [6].

In this case, risk communication had to aim on one hand to overcome the demonization of the drug and on the other hand to discourage its use in risky conditions (e.g., "off-label" uses). The strategy involves transmitting fundamental information such as, for example, that a single administration is sufficient for devastating damage to occur to the fetus. Patients must be instructed on the importance of following drug label warnings and prescriber-recommended precautions. It is important to consider that about 50% are unplanned pregnancies and that the communication target must be all users of childbearing age. Mistrust must instead be overcome by communicating that injuries to the fetus caused by thalidomide are absolutely preventable if the recommendations are respected [63].

8.3 H1N1 Influenza Vaccine

In the spring of 2009, the H1N1 A influenza virus spread around the world, causing a pandemic which, according to WHO data, caused 18,156 deaths [65]. Thanks to the early identification of the new virus and the contingency plans developed for years to contain a possible pandemic, a vaccine was rapidly developed [66]. In December 2009, the immunization campaign began in Europe and the USA [67, 68].

The management of communication on the H1N1 A influenza pandemic in France had some problems. The information campaign for vaccination stimulated the entire population on the need to be vaccinated with many messages in the media, but the limited availability of the vaccine required prioritization of at-risk subjects only [69]. Family doctors and pediatricians were not included in the priority populations, fueling skepticism about the vaccine and reducing collaboration by healthcare professionals [70]. This emergency management has created confusion in the population who have begun to underestimate the risk of the virus [69]. The media also had ample space for information on alleged safety problems of a vaccine developed too quickly, promoting doubtfully pertinent information such as the safety of adjuvants and the comparison with "historical" epidemics of adverse vaccine events such as that of Guillain–Barré syndrome in the H1N1 vaccination campaign of 1976 in the United States [71]. With increasing distrust in vaccines and decreasing infection pressure on the population, public attitudes toward vaccination have been reduced to a minimum. As a result, only about 11.1% of the overall population was immunized [70].

The events in France during the vaccination campaign are an example of how difficult it is to communicate uncertainties when the population perceive a disagreement between health authorities and experts. The experience with the H1N1 pandemic has been useful for developing integrated communication strategies for vaccination campaigns, which take into account the social, behavioral, and media aspects and the influences that these elements could have on the perception of risk in the population [72, 73]. During a pandemic, where fear takes the place of logic, it is imperative that public health agencies communicate very quickly and effectively not only with the population (especially those at high risk of developing serious disease) but also with journalists and healthcare professionals who can amplify the message effectively, but also distort it [6].

8.4 The COVID-19 Infodemic

Declared a pandemic by the WHO in March 2020, the COVID-19 disease caused by the SARS-CoV-2 virus has had a profound impact on the lives of millions of people and has changed the economic and social status of many countries around the world. This important event still represents an exceptional challenge for the communication of health risk and could lead to the understanding of new concepts related to the perception of risk and the pursuit of health by people.

The spread of the new coronavirus has been accompanied by the uncontrolled spread of an enormous amount of information that the WHO has defined as an "infodemic" [74]. This chaotic stream of information has touched all the problems related to the disease, from the characteristics of transmissibility to possible treatments. In a context of great uncertainty where scientific research needed time to acquire evidence-based knowledge, the infodemic incorporated contradictory messages, misinformation, and fake news, making it difficult for both decision-makers and the public to develop an adequate risk perception for the disease. In a situation of zero or extremely limited scientific knowledge on the disease, with the population frightened and threatened in its daily freedoms, numerous positions of thought and behavior, even extreme ones, have emerged. For example, some misinformation campaigns pointed toward denial of the actual existence of the virus. Behaviors that are very sensitive to risk communication, such as the adoption of correct social distancing measures and the acceptance or not of vaccination, have had a decisive impact on the spread of the virus and on the possibility of developing severe forms of the disease.

It is possible to frame two different moments of the pandemic to study risk communication: the COVID-19 pre-vaccine period and the COVID-19 post-vaccine period.

In the pre-vaccine COVID-19 period, especially in the early stages of the pandemic, the lack of effective therapies to fight the disease immediately triggered a test run of already available drugs that could have an effect in fighting the disease or alleviating its symptoms. As researchers struggled to identify and test therapies, news spread uncontrollably about the alleged effectiveness of many drugs. This news triggered expectations in both the population and healthcare workers, leading to a hoarding rush and a depletion of stocks, which on the one hand exposed users to the risk of adverse events without there being an established benefit and on the other hand deprived of the cure for those patients who used the drug for its approved indications. The most important example is that of hydroxychloroquine [11].

With the advent of COVID-19 vaccines, the infodemic has produced new emotional conflicts in the population exhausted by several months of restrictions on daily freedom. On one hand, the key to get out of the pandemic nightmare was presented; on the other, there was fear of the low efficacy and possible side effects of rapidly developed vaccines and, in the case of mRNA vaccines, with immunization mechanisms that have not been previously tested in humans. This has resulted in vaccination hesitancy even among health professionals. The situation became complicated with the identification of thrombosis with vaccine thrombocytopenia as a possible adverse effect of the ChAdOx1-S/nCoV-19 vaccine in April 2021.

The Australian network called "Collaboration on Social Science and Immunization" (COSSI) has published useful recommendations on how to effectively communicate the risk of COVID-19 vaccines. The recommendations took into account the vaccine-induced thrombosis with thrombocytopenia emergency and the availability of vaccines at that time in Australia (ChAdOx1-S/nCoV-19 vaccine was immediately available while for mRNA vaccines it was necessary to wait) [75]. The approach takes into account the physician's need to establish a constructive dialogue with the patient to obtain informed consent. To encourage patients to get vaccinated, doctors should encourage patients to express their doubts and concerns and show empathy and understanding toward them. They should involve the patients in the decision-making process through an open dialogue on the pros and cons of vaccination. Doctors should also transparently share information between themselves and the patients on vaccine-related risks. To motivate patients to accept vaccination, doctors should consider the patient's values. They should define options, pros, and cons for both vaccination and non-vaccination. Finally, doctors should leave the door open to review the patient's positions if the epidemiological picture worsens.

COSSI also proposes some guidelines on public disclosure of vaccine risks by authorities such as making a transparent and frequent communication, leveraging on people's values, and using clear messages taking into account the differences in understanding people may have compared to healthcare professionals. Further, it was required to ensure that the communications are not over-reassuring especially in situations of uncertainty, to diversify communication channels, identify fake news and disinformation, and to try to deny them point by point, to use spokespersons with established scientific credibility that people appreciate, and to monitor the effectiveness of communication campaigns through surveys and analyses, and acting on the results. Well-structured communication strategies, such as those proposed by COSSI, might have played an important role in reducing vaccination hesitation and in maintaining high vaccination rates, which during the period of the pandemic contributed to improving the epidemiological picture.

9 Legal Framework

The communication of the risk of medicinal products is subjected to specific rules and requirements that are established mainly by the principle of transparency of information that serves to ensure informed choices for users [6]. These rules may vary from country to country. In the European Union, the package leaflet, summary of product characteristics and package labeling are required by law [68]. These documents contain the mandatory information of a medicine, including safety features. Regulatory authorities may require marketing authorization holders to provide additional risk management materials or to undertake communications. Both patients and doctors should be aware of the risks associated with administering a drug. The description of the indication, posology, adverse effects, contraindications, drug interactions, and the finding of new evidence on the risks of the drug are of fundamental importance for correct information on the product and, consequently, for responsibility in case of any damage related to the use of the drug.

In health policy, the precautionary principle is applied to take preventive measures in order to avoid any damage, even if there is no certainty about the nature and probability that the damage will actually occur [76]. When a new possible unexpected adverse reaction to the drug is identified, pharmaceutical companies and regulators are asked to address the matter immediately and carry out all necessary scientific research to generate evidence that can confirm or reject the new association. In particular, pharmacovigilance systems play a key role in investigating possible safety problems. According to the precautionary principle, measures must be taken promptly to avoid potential risks and there is a legal obligation to communicate the measures taken. For criminal law, waiting for evidence is considered negligent behavior and may result in the attribution of responsibility for damages related to failure to communicate [6]. When planning and preparing a risk communication intervention, it is important to have clear obligations and legal provisions of all participants in the communication process, so that responsibilities can be defined in case there are consequences.

10 Summary and Conclusions

In conclusion, the communication of a risk is essential together with the communication of benefit of medicinal products. Both aspects require specific expertise, but different approaches. Building an effective risk communication strategy requires the tailoring of communication based on the identified potential risks and on the audience characteristics. A multidisciplinary approach and the timeliness are also essential for quickly overcoming the spreading of fears and fake beliefs and for confirming the risk. The structured process of the risk communication encompasses the identification of the target audience, the construction of an appropriate message, and the choice of media used for delivering the communication. We learned from some experiences (e.g., COVID-19 infodemic, rofecoxib) that all of these aspects are essential to ensure an effective communication and avoid or control the risk. The implementation of the discipline of risk communication in medicine and the subsequent education of all stakeholders involved in the management of medicinal products is very essential. This will improve the dialogue between caregivers and patients and between healthcare institutions and the population toward a safer and more informed use of medications.

11 Case Studies

To illustrate the importance of appropriate communication on risks of medicines to patients as well as to address their concerns on risk with medications, two cases are provided below in the form of dialogue between clinician and patient/care giver.

11.1 Case Study 1: Fear of Adverse Drug Reaction

Dialogue	Comment
Doctor: I looked at your tests and decided to give you risperidone, an antipsychotic drug that can help control your symptoms.	Inform the patient that your decision is individualized on his/her specific clinical picture.
Patient: Risperidone? But isn't that what causes pituitary tumor? I remember reading about it while I was searching various treatment options for my condition.	Patients may have information on some scaring adverse effects.
Doctor: I understand your concern. I assure you that the risk of developing pituitary tumor is very low and only occurs in a small percentage of patients who take risperidone for long periods of time.	Do not minimize patient's fears Try to illustrate the patients the magnitude of risk (infographics can help).
Patient: And how long should I take it?	Patients are often scared of chronic treatments.
Doctor: It depends on your response to treatment and the severity of your symptoms. In general, it is recommended that risperidone be continued for at least six months after symptoms have resolved, to prevent relapse.	Clearly explain why adherence to therapy is important to control the diseases. Provide him information about the possibility of interrupting the treatment (if any).
Patient: What if I feel better sooner?	Patients can be tempted to self-manage resulting in treatment interruption.
Doctor: You must not stop risperidone without consulting me, as it may have unwanted side effects, such as insomnia, anxiety, nausea or tremor. If you want to reduce or stop the dosage, we must do it gradually and under my supervision.	Inform the patient about the problems (symptoms or conditions) connected with abrupt interruption (if any). Reassure the patient about your continued support and supervision.
Patient: But I don't want to take this drug forever. I'm afraid it will hurt me.	Patients can be scared about important effects of prolonged exposure.
Doctor: I understand you, but I ask you to trust me. Risperidone is a relatively safe and effective drug, which can improve your quality of life and help you manage your disease. I assure you that I will carefully monitor your clinical situation and the effects of the drug, and that I will have you undergo periodic tests to check your hormone levels and pituitary function. If I should notice any abnormalities or any signs of intolerance to risperidone, I would be ready to change your treatment.	Inform the patient that the process of monitoring will greatly help preventing the occurrence of serious complications. Inform the patient that you will be ready to stop and modify the treatment at the first occurrence of an alarming signal.
Patient: What if it doesn't work?	Patients are usually reassured by having alternative treatment options.
Doctor: There are other treatment options available for your case, but before trying them we have to give risperidone a chance. I only ask you to be patient and cooperative, and to follow my directions. I am sure that together we will be able to find the best solution for you.	Reassure the patient about the possibility of alternative treatments in case of failure of the one you proposed as best option. Consider the patient as a teammate for the success of the treatment.

11.2 Case Study 2: Vaccine Safety Discussed with a Mother

Dialogue	Comment
Pediatrician: Today I wanted to talk to you about something important. Are you aware that the vaccine against COVID -19 has been available for children aged 5–11 from a few weeks?	Explore patient's knowledge about the vaccine and give him/her the possibility to report any concern.
Mom: Yes, I've heard of it.	The patient can be informed.
Pediatrician: Good. I advise you to vaccinate your child as soon as possible. The vaccine is safe and effective and may protect your baby from a potentially serious disease and its complications.	State your priority about the immunization of child, illustrating the risks of not receiving the vaccine.

Dialogue	Comment
Mom: But doctor, I'm a little worried. I read on the internet that the vaccine can cause serious side effects in children, causing heart disease. And then I don't know if the vaccine has been tested enough on children. I don't want there to be any long-term risks.	Patient's perception of the magnitude-specific risk can be amplified by media claim. Patient can be concerned about uncertain evidence.
Pediatrician: I understand your fears, but I assure you that they are unfounded. Let me explain what I know. The vaccine has undergone rigorous clinical trials involving thousands of children and which have demonstrated its safety and efficacy. Side effects are rare and mild and resolve within a few days. Heart disease have been reported only in very few cases and have not had serious consequences. Furthermore, the vaccine has no negative impact on children's development or fertility.	Do not minimize patient's fears. Share your knowledge with the patient in the attempt of removing barriers related to fear of uncertain or unproven risks and benefits. Try to reduce the influence of media claims on patient's thoughts.
Mom: But doctor, wouldn't it be better to wait a little longer and see how it goes with the other children who get vaccinated? Maybe there are effects that only show up after months or years.	The patient could think that "doing nothing" is a safer solution than "doing anything" (omission bias).
Pediatrician: No, I don't think think it would be better. Waiting means exposing your child to an unnecessary and unjustified risk. The alternatives to the vaccine are very limited and not as effective. There are only few drugs used to treat COVID-19 in children and have little evidence of benefit. Children who get sick with COVID-19 could develop permanent damage to lungs, heart or brain. Not to mention that unvaccinated children can transmit the virus to other more fragile or vulnerable people, such as the elderly or the chronically ill.	Illustrate the possible consequences of "doing nothing". Illustrate the limitation of alternatives to vaccine, including the limitations and risks of possible solutions in case of infection.
Mom: But doctor, I'm afraid of hurting my baby.	The mother can consider only harmful effects of the vaccine because the benefit is not visible since the child is healthy at present.
Pediatrician: I do not consider that you harm your child if you vaccinate him. On the contrary, you do good for your child and for the whole community. The vaccine is the most powerful weapon we have to fight this pandemic and get back to normal. I ask you to trust me and science and not to be influenced by false or misleading information circulating on the internet or on social media. I'm here to help you take the best decision for your child's health	Explain that vaccination means protection and not harming. Help the patient to identify external elements (positive and negative) that may have an influence on his/her decision. Let the patient feel he/she is the only one who will finally take a decision.

References

1. Michaleas SN, Laios K, Tsoucalas G, Androutsos G. Theophrastus Bombastus Von Hohenheim (Paracelsus) (1493–1541): the eminent physician and pioneer of toxicology. Toxicol Rep. 2021;8:411–4. https://doi.org/10.1016/j.toxrep.2021.02.012.
2. King A, Hoppe RB. "Best Practice" for patient-centered communication: a narrative review. J Grad Med Educ. 2013;5:385–93. https://doi.org/10.4300/jgme-d-13-00072.1.
3. Evidence-Based Medicine Working Group. Evidence-based medicine. A new approach to teaching the practice of medicine. JAMA. 1992;268:2420–5. https://doi.org/10.1001/jama.1992.03490170092032.
4. European Medicine Agency. ICH Guideline Q9 on quality risk management. September 2015. https://www.ema.europa.eu/en/documents/scientific-guideline/international-conference-harmonisation-technical-requirementsregistration-pharmaceuticals-human-use-ich-guideline-q9-quality-risk-management-step-5-first-version_en.pdf. Last accessed January 30th, 2024.
5. World Health Organization. What is Pharmacovigilance. WHO website. https://www.who.int/teams/regulation-prequalification/regulation-andsafety/pharmacovigilance#:~:text=Pharmacovigilance%20is%20the%20science%20and,they%20are%20authorized%20for%20use. Last Accessed January 30th, 2024.
6. Bahri P. Communicating about risks and safe use of medicines: real life and applied research. Springer; 2020. p. 1–504. https://doi.org/10.1007/978-981-15-3013-5.
7. Stephens TD, Brynner R. Dark remedy: the impact of thalidomide and its revival as a vital medicine. Perseus Pub; 2001.
8. Fischoff B, Brewer N, Downs J. Communicating risk and benefits: an evidence-based users' guide. Food and Drug Administration; 2011.

9. Aronson JK. Risk perception in drug therapy. Br J Clin Pharmacol. 2006;62:135–7. https://doi.org/10.1111/j.1365-2125.2006.02739_1.x.
10. Flaherty DK. The vaccine-autism connection: a public health crisis caused by unethical medical practices and fraudulent science. Ann Pharmacother. 2011;45:1302–4. https://doi.org/10.1345/aph.1Q318.
11. Tuccori M, Convertino I, Ferraro S, et al. The impact of the COVID-19 "Infodemic" on drug-utilization behaviors: implications for pharmacovigilance. Drug Saf. 2020;43:699–709. https://doi.org/10.1007/S40264-020-00965-W/FIGURES/2.
12. Gugerty L, Link DM. How heuristic credibility cues affect credibility judgments and decisions. J Exp Psychol Appl. 2020;26:620–45. https://doi.org/10.1037/xap0000279.
13. Littlejohn S, Foss K, Oetzel J. Theories of human communication. 11th ed. Long Grove, IL: Waveland Press Inc; 2016.
14. Batel S, Castro P. A social representations approach to the communication between different spheres: an analysis of the impacts of two discursive formats. J Theory Soc Behav. 2009;39:415–33. https://doi.org/10.1111/j.1468-5914.2009.00412.x.
15. Vogt EM. Effective communication of drug safety a new look. Drug Saf. 2002;25:313–21.
16. Academies C of C. Health product risk communication: is the message getting through? 2015. https://cca-cac.flywheelsites.com/reports/health-product-risk-communication-is-the-message-getting-through/. Accessed 6 Jun 2022.
17. Kesselheim AS, Campbell EG, Schneeweiss S, et al. Methodological approaches to evaluate the impact of FDA drug safety communications. Drug Saf. 2015;38:565–75. https://doi.org/10.1007/S40264-015-0291-Y.
18. Murad MH, Asi N, Alsawas M, Alahdab F. New evidence pyramid. BMJ Evid-Based Med. 2016;21:125–7. https://doi.org/10.1136/EBMED-2016-110401.
19. Goedecke T, Morales DR, Pacurariu A, Kurz X. Measuring the impact of medicines regulatory interventions—systematic review and methodological considerations. Br J Clin Pharmacol. 2018;84:419–33. https://doi.org/10.1111/bcp.13469.
20. Pang A. Dealing with external stakeholders during the crisis: managing the information vacuum. Handb Res Cris Leadersh Organ. 2013:209–30. https://doi.org/10.4337/9781781006405.00020.
21. Kemp S. Digital 2022: Global overview report—global digital insights. In: DataReportal; 2022. https://datareportal.com/reports/digital-2022-global-overview-report. Accessed 18 May 2022.
22. Powell GE, Seifert HA, Reblin T, et al. Social media listening for routine post-marketing safety surveillance. Drug Saf. 2016;39:443–54. https://doi.org/10.1007/S40264-015-0385-6.
23. Smart Patients Inc. Smart patients. In: Smart patients; 1995. https://www.smartpatients.com/about. Accessed 17 May 2022.
24. Caster O, Dietrich J, Kürzinger ML, et al. Assessment of the utility of social media for broad-ranging statistical signal detection in pharmacovigilance: results from the WEB-RADR Project. Drug Saf. 2018;41:1355. https://doi.org/10.1007/S40264-018-0699-2.
25. Convertino I, Ferraro S, Blandizzi C, Tuccori M. The usefulness of listening social media for pharmacovigilance purposes: a systematic review. Expert Opin Drug Saf. 2018;17:1081–93. https://doi.org/10.1080/14740338.2018.1531847.
26. Rees S, Mian S, Grabowski N. Using social media in safety signal management: is it reliable? Ther Adv drug Saf. 2018;9:591–9. https://doi.org/10.1177/2042098618789596.
27. Dan B. Medical rhetoric and rhetoric medicine. Dev Med Child Neurol. 2014;56:916.
28. Lingard L, Haber RJ. Teaching and learning communication in medicine: a rhetorical approach. Acad Med. 1999;74:507–10. https://doi.org/10.1097/00001888-199905000-00015.
29. Evans SJW. Pharmacoepidemiology. Br J Clin Pharmacol. 2012;73:973–8. https://doi.org/10.1111/J.1365-2125.2012.04248.X.
30. Lapeyre-Mestre M, Sapède C, Moore N, et al. Pharmacoepidemiology studies: what levels of evidence and how can they be reached? Therapie. 2013;68:247–52. https://doi.org/10.2515/THERAPIE/2013038.
31. Wettermark B. The intriguing future of pharmacoepidemiology. Eur J Clin Pharmacol. 2013;69(Suppl. 1):43–51. https://doi.org/10.1007/S00228-013-1496-6.
32. Kurz X, Perez-Gutthann S. Strengthening standards, transparency, and collaboration to support medicine evaluation: ten years of the European Network of Centres for Pharmacoepidemiology and Pharmacovigilance (ENCePP). Pharmacoepidemiol Drug Saf. 2018;27:245–52. https://doi.org/10.1002/PDS.4381.
33. Bakhriansyah M, Souverein PC, de Boer A, Klungel OH. Gastrointestinal toxicity among patients taking selective COX-2 inhibitors or conventional NSAIDs, alone or combined with proton pump inhibitors: a case-control study. Pharmacoepidemiol Drug Saf. 2017;26:1141–8. https://doi.org/10.1002/PDS.4183.
34. Carson JL, Strom BL, Soper KA, et al. The association of nonsteroidal anti-inflammatory drugs with upper gastrointestinal tract bleeding. Arch Intern Med. 1987;147:85–8. https://doi.org/10.1001/ARCHINTE.1987.00370010087021.
35. Blind E, Dunder K, De Graeff PA, Abadie E. Rosiglitazone: a European regulatory perspective. Diabetologia. 2011;54(2):213–8. https://doi.org/10.1007/S00125-010-1992-5.
36. Hernandez JF, Mantel-Teeuwisse AK, van Thiel GJMW, et al. A 10-year analysis of the effects of media coverage of regulatory warnings on antidepressant use in The Netherlands and UK. PLoS One. 2012;7 https://doi.org/10.1371/JOURNAL.PONE.0045515.

37. Radawski C, Morrato E, Hornbuckle K, et al. Benefit-Risk Assessment, Communication, and Evaluation (BRACE) throughout the life cycle of therapeutic products: overall perspective and role of the pharmacoepidemiologist. Pharmacoepidemiol Drug Saf. 2015;24:1233–40. https://doi.org/10.1002/PDS.3859.
38. Vandenbroucke JP, Rosing J, Bloemenkamp KWM, et al. Oral contraceptives and the risk of venous thrombosis. N Engl J Med. 2001;344:1527–35. https://doi.org/10.1056/NEJM200105173442007.
39. Weatherburn CJ, Guthrie B, Dreischulte T, Morales DR. Impact of medicines regulatory risk communications in the UK on prescribing and clinical outcomes: systematic review, time series analysis and meta-analysis. Br J Clin Pharmacol. 2020;86:698–710. https://doi.org/10.1111/BCP.14104.
40. Pitts PJ, Le LH, Moride Y, Conti RM. 21st century pharmacovigilance: efforts, roles, and responsibilities. Lancet Oncol. 2016;17:e486–92. https://doi.org/10.1016/S1470-2045(16)30312-6.
41. Potts J, Genov G, Segec A, et al. Improving the safety of medicines in the European Union: from signals to action. Clin Pharmacol Ther. 2020;107:521. https://doi.org/10.1002/CPT.1678.
42. Sheiner LB. Learning versus confirming in clinical drug development. Clin Pharmacol Ther. 1997;61:275–91. https://doi.org/10.1016/S0009-9236(97)90160-0.
43. Tong V, Raynor DK, Blalock SJ, Aslani P. Consumer interpretation of ramipril and clopidogrel medication risk information—implications for risk communication strategies. Patient Prefer Adher. 2015;9:983. https://doi.org/10.2147/PPA.S86414.
44. Trevena LJ, Zikmund-Fisher BJ, Edwards A, et al. Presenting quantitative information about decision outcomes: a risk communication primer for patient decision aid developers. BMC Med Inform Decis Mak. 2013;13:1–15. https://doi.org/10.1186/1472-6947-13-S2-S7/FIGURES/1.
45. Ministero della Salute (Italia). Fake news. In: Salut; 2022. https://www.salute.gov.it/portale/nuovocoronavirus/archivioFakeNewsNuovoCoronavirus.jsp?lingua=italiano&tagId=881. Accessed 28 Jun 2022.
46. Steinert JI, Sternberg H, Prince H, et al. COVID-19 vaccine hesitancy in eight European countries: prevalence, determinants, and heterogeneity. Sci Adv. 2022;8:9825. https://doi.org/10.1126/SCIADV.ABM9825/SUPPL_FILE/SCIADV.ABM9825_SM.PDF.
47. Beauchamp TL, Childress JF. Principles of biomedical ethics. New York: Oxford University Press; 1979.
48. Resnik DB. Ethical dilemmas in communicating medical information to the public. Health Policy (New York). 2001;55:129–49. https://doi.org/10.1016/S0168-8510(00)00121-4.
49. Folker AP, Sandøe P. Leaping "Out of the Doubt"—nutrition advice: values at stake in communicating scientific uncertainty to the public. Heal Care Anal. 2008;16(2):176–91. https://doi.org/10.1007/S10728-007-0054-8.
50. Goodwin J, Honeycutt L. When science goes public: from technical arguments to appeals to authority. Stud Commun Sci. 2009;9:19–30.
51. Sukkar E. Still feeling the Vioxx pain. Pharm J. 2014; https://pharmaceutical-journal.com/article/feature/still-feeling-the-vioxx-pain. Accessed 28 Jun 2022
52. Greener M. First do no harm. Improving drug safety through legislation and independent research. EMBO Rep. 2008;9:221–4. https://doi.org/10.1038/EMBOR.2008.17.
53. Eichler HG, Bloechl-Daum B, Brasseur D, et al. The risks of risk aversion in drug regulation. Nat Rev Drug Discov. 2013;12:907–16. https://doi.org/10.1038/NRD4129.
54. Goldacre B, Gray J. OpenTrials: towards a collaborative open database of all available information on all clinical trials. Trials. 2016;17:517–29. https://doi.org/10.1186/S13063-016-1290-8.
55. Doran J. US officials 'knew of Vioxx threat' | The Times. In: The Times; 2004. https://www.thetimes.co.uk/article/us-officials-knew-of-vioxx-threat-cbm56jt657p. Accessed 28 Jun 2022.
56. Laurance J. Drug giants "ignored dangers of painkiller in pursuit of profits" | The Independent. In: India; 2004. https://www.independent.co.uk/life-style/health-and-families/health-news/drug-giants-ignored-dangers-of-painkiller-in-pursuit-of-profits-543009.html. Accessed 28 Jun 2022.
57. BBC. Arthritis drug removed for safety. In: BBC News website; 2004. http://newsimg.bbc.co.uk/1/hi/health/3704640.stm. Accessed 28 Jun 2022.
58. Hawkes N. Bestselling drug axed over fears that it increases heart attack risk | The Times. In: The Times website; 2004. https://www.thetimes.co.uk/article/bestselling-drug-axed-over-fears-that-it-increases-heart-attack-risk-hkzftpmm92n?region=global. Accessed 28 Jun 2022.
59. Sukel MPP, van der Linden MW, Chen C, et al. Large-scale stopping and switching treatment with COX-2 inhibitors after the rofecoxib withdrawal. Pharmacoepidemiol Drug Saf. 2008;17:9–19. https://doi.org/10.1002/PDS.1508.
60. McGettigan P, Henry D. Use of non-steroidal anti-inflammatory drugs that elevate cardiovascular risk: an examination of sales and essential medicines lists in low-, middle-, and high-income countries. PLoS Med. 2013;10:e1001388. https://doi.org/10.1371/JOURNAL.PMED.1001388.
61. University of Oxford. EBM DataLab 2017. In: Openprescribing.net; 2017.
62. World Health Organization. Leprosy. In: who.int website; 2017. https://www.who.int/news-room/fact-sheets/detail/leprosy. Accessed 28 Jun 2022.
63. Rehman W, Arfons LM, Lazarus HM. The rise, fall and subsequent triumph of thalidomide: lessons learned in drug development. Ther Adv Hematol. 2011; https://doi.org/10.1177/2040620711413165.
64. Renn O. Stakeholder and public involvement in risk governance. Int J Disaster Risk Sci. 2015; https://doi.org/10.1007/s13753-015-0037-6.

65. World Health Organization. Pandemic (H1N1) 2009—update 104. In: who.int website; 2009. https://www.who.int/emergencies/disease-outbreak-news/item/2010_06_11-en. Accessed 28 Jun 2022.
66. Chan M. WHO | World now at the start of 2009 influenza pandemic. WHO; 2010.
67. CDC. Summary of 2009 Monovalent H1N1 Influenza vaccine data--vaccine adverse event reporting system. In: wonder.cdc.gov website; 2010. http://vaers.hhs.gov. Accessed 28 Jun 2022.
68. European Medicines Agency. 15th pandemic pharmacovigilance update. In: ema.europa.eu website; 2010. www.ema.europa.eu. Accessed 28 Jun 2022.
69. Raude J, Caille-Brillet AL, Setbon M. The 2009 pandemic H1N1 influenza vaccination in France: who accepted to receive the vaccine and why? PLoS Curr. 2010;2 https://doi.org/10.1371/CURRENTS.RRN1188.
70. Vaux S, Van Cauteren D, Guthmann JP, et al. Influenza vaccination coverage against seasonal and pandemic influenza and their determinants in France: a cross-sectional survey. BMC Public Health. 2011;11:30. https://doi.org/10.1186/1471-2458-11-30.
71. Pollack A. Swine Flu fears of 1976 offer lessons, and concerns, today—the New York Times. In: New York Times; 2009. https://www.nytimes.com/2009/05/09/health/09vaccine.html. Accessed 28 Jun 2022.
72. Brewer NT, Chapman GB, Rothman AJ, et al. Increasing vaccination: putting psychological science into action. Psychol Sci Public Interest. 2017;18:149–207. https://doi.org/10.1177/1529100618760521.
73. MacDougall DM, Halperin BA, MacKinnon-Cameron D, et al. The challenge of vaccinating adults: attitudes and beliefs of the Canadian public and healthcare providers. BMJ Open. 2015;5:e009062. https://doi.org/10.1136/BMJOPEN-2015-009062.
74. Zarocostas J. How to fight an infodemic. Lancet (London, England). 2020;395:676. https://doi.org/10.1016/S0140-6736(20)30461-X.
75. Leask J, Carlson SJ, Attwell K, et al. Communicating with patients and the public about COVID-19 vaccine safety: recommendations from the Collaboration on Social Science and Immunisation. Med J Aust. 2021;215:9–12.e1. https://doi.org/10.5694/MJA2.51136.
76. World Health Organization. United Nations Conference on Environment and Development; 1992.

Patient and Public Involvement in Pharmacovigilance

12

Florence van Hunsel, Manal M. Younus, and Anthony R. Cox

Abstract

Patient involvement has become increasingly important in pharmacovigilance in recent years. There should be an active and collaborative interaction between patients and other stakeholders. Decision making should be guided by patients' contributions as partners, recognising their unique perspective, experiences, values, and expertise.

In pharmacovigilance, direct patient reporting was an important first step in including the patient perspective in drug safety monitoring. Direct patient reporting has been shown to add value to pharmacovigilance, by contributing to signal detection and helping to uncover blind spots of pharmacovigilance, such as safety of the herbal medicines. Direct patient reporting also plays an important role in vaccine pharmacovigilance, as was highlighted during the COVID-19 pandemic.

Patient-reported information can give us insight into the burden of adverse drug reactions (ADRs) and the course of ADRs. This is information that is relevant to patients and is not always readily available. In addition to their role as reporters, patients should have a role in regulatory decision making. This is something that regulatory agencies have focused more on in recent years. Engagement from patients requires sustained engagement strategies, since pharmacovigilance is a relatively unknown area for them. Patient involvement should be a two-way street with pharmacovigilance benefiting from patient-reported information, but also ensuring relevant information is relayed to patients and that they are involved in decision making.

Keywords

Patient involvement · Public involvement · Patient engagement · Pharmacovigilance · Spontaneous reporting · Patient reporting

F. van Hunsel (✉)
Netherlands Pharmacovigilance Centre Lareb, 's-Hertogenbosch, The Netherlands

Faculty of Science and Engineering, FarmacoTherapie, Epidemiologie en Economie Groningen Research Institute of Pharmacy, Groningen, The Netherlands
e-mail: f.vanhunsel@lareb.nl

M. M. Younus
Iraqi Pharmacovigilance Center, Ministry of Health and Environment, Baghdad, Iraq

International Society of Pharmacovigilance, Patient Engagement SIG, London, UK

A. R. Cox
Clinical Pharmacy and Drug Safety, School of Pharmacy, College of Medical and Dental Sciences University of Birmingham, Birmingham, UK

J. Jose et al. (eds.), *Principles and Practice of Pharmacovigilance and Drug Safety*,
https://doi.org/10.1007/978-3-031-51089-2_12

Learning objectives

- Recognising the important contribution patients can make to pharmacovigilance and how to engage with them.
- Learning about guidance and legislation that anchor the patient's role in pharmacovigilance.
- Recognising the importance of good communication towards patients and the public and the provision of patient-friendly educational materials.

Key Points

- Patient reporting brings a unique perspective to pharmacovigilance and can strengthen pharmacovigilance.
- Decision making should be guided by patients' contributions as partners, recognising their unique perspective, experiences, values, and expertise.
- Pharmacovigilance organisations should make efforts to engage with patients and their organisations and to have a clear communication strategy towards patient and the general public.

1 Introduction

Patient and public involvement has become increasingly important in pharmacovigilance in recent years [1–3]. The patient is the one who experiences the adverse drug reaction (ADR) if it occurs and therefore is often best placed to give an insightful first-hand description of the ADR. As society has moved from a more paternalistic medical model to one based on shared decision making, denying a role to patients in pharmacovigilance is untenable.

1.1 The Changing Landscape of Patient Involvement

The changing landscape of patient involvement in pharmacovigilance is being shaped by a number of factors, including:

- The rise of digital health: Digital health technologies, such as electronic health records (EHRs), patient portals, and social media, are providing new opportunities for patients to participate in pharmacovigilance. For example, EHRs can be used to mine data for potential ADRs, and social media can be used to monitor patient descriptions of ADRs [4].
- The increasing focus on patient-centred care: There is a growing recognition that patients should be active partners in their own healthcare, including in the monitoring of the safety of the medicines they take. This has led to a greater emphasis on patient involvement in pharmacovigilance [5].
- The evolving regulatory landscape: Regulatory bodies around the world are developing new guidelines and requirements for patient involvement in pharmacovigilance. For example, the European Medicines Agency (EMA) now requires pharmaceutical companies to submit patient experience plans (PEPs) for all new medicines. PEPs describe how the company will involve patients in the monitoring and assessment of the safety of the medicine [6].

As digital health technologies continue to develop and patient-centred care becomes more widespread, we can expect to see even more innovative and effective ways for patients to participate in the monitoring and assessment of the safety of medicines.

1.2 Scope of Patients Involvement: From Development to Monitoring

The Council for International Organizations of Medical Sciences (CIOMS) Working Group XI on 'Patient involvement in the development, regulation and safe use of medicines' was launched in April 2018. It included participants from patient organisations, industry, regulators, academia, and the World Medical Association. A report on their work was published in 2022 and describes the issues around the involvement of patients throughout the life journey of medicines, including post-marketing safety monitoring [7].

The CIOMS Working Group report 'Patient involvement in the development, regulation and safe use of medicines' defined the patient community as 'patients are a wider group of people than just those taking medicines. The term can include patient organizations, patients' families, patients' carers and patient representatives in various forums. All of these are said to make up the "patient community"' [7]. More broadly consumers or the general public can sometimes be used instead of 'patient'. For instance, in preventive vaccination campaigns in healthy individuals the term 'patient' might be seen as too narrow. However, for simplicity the remainder of the chapter will largely refer to patients and patient involvement.

The CIOMS Working Group report also defined 'Involvement' as the active and collaborative interaction between patients and other stakeholders where decision making is guided by patients' contributions as partners, recognising their unique perspective, experiences, values, and expertise. 'Involvement' and 'engagement' are sometimes used interchangeably [7].

The CIOMS report is a landmark document that provides a comprehensive overview of the benefits of patient involvement and existing initiatives, gives many examples and recommendations, and addresses the remaining challenges and practice gaps. The report highlights the importance of systematically involving patients throughout a medicine's life cycle, from its early development through the regulatory process to ongoing monitoring and safe use in everyday healthcare [7].

1.3 International Experience with Patient Reporting

The notion that patients should be involved throughout the medicine's life—from their development, through regulation to ongoing safe use in everyday healthcare—is widely promoted [7]. In pharmacovigilance, direct patient reporting was an important step towards more patient involvement and a means to get more data on ADRs, which are chronically underreported [8]. Ideally, pharmacovigilance organisations would receive relevant reports of ADRs which give a good insight of the safety of medicines in daily practice and which allow for the detection of (aspects of) previously unknown adverse events.

In an international survey of the state of patient reporting from 2016, 107 of 141 countries, or 76% of those surveyed, do allow patients to report ADRs directly. This is a positive development, as it allows patients to play a more active role in their own safety and in the safety of other patients. However, 24% of participating countries indicated that patients were not yet able to report ADRs directly [9]. According to the study, patient reports are used to detect new ADRs and to monitor the safety of medicines. However, some countries collect patient reports, but do not actively use them. This is a missed opportunity, as patient reports can provide valuable insights into the safety of medicines and help to identify new safety risks. Moreover, barriers to create a reporting culture among patients and using their information are primarily financial constraints, but also the lack of education among the patient population in their country [9].

Inacio et al. [10] investigated the influence of 42 global sociodemographic and economic factors for 44 countries on the patient reporting rate of ADRs. They found that health investment indicators, such as per capita public health expenditure, were the relevant factors responsible to discriminate between countries that have higher patient reporting rates [10].

Both studies stress the importance of having adequate finances in place in order to build and maintain a patient reporting scheme. Furthermore, these international comparisons of barriers help us grasp reasons for underreporting by patients and the public at country level and that the under reporting is unequally distributed across conditions, medicines, and population groups. A systematic review of factors associated with underreporting of ADRs found that patient's age and level of education were the most commonly reported factors. Older age groups and individuals with higher level of education were more likely to report ADRs. Underreporting was related to knowledge, attitudes, and excuses for not reporting [11]. Another systematic review on this topic found that in addition to poor awareness, factors such as confusion about who should report the ADR, difficulties with reporting procedures, lack of feedback on submitted reports, mailing costs, ADRs being resolved, and prior negative reporting experiences affected patient reporting [12]. While behavioural determinants that influence patient and public reporting of ADRs have been studied [13], less is known about the effects of having to deal with multimorbidity and use of multiple medicines, and the nature and severity of a patient's indication on reporting behaviour.

2 Patient Involvement in Pharmacovigilance

2.1 Start of Patient Reporting Schemes in Pharmacovigilance

Although there have been pharmacovigilance centres worldwide where patients have been able to report since the start, such as in the United States, Canada, and Australia since the 1960s, it was still unusual in many countries in the early 2000s to accept reports directly from the public. In 1983, following the withdrawal of benoxaprofen, a Committee on Safety of Medicines working group considered patient reporting, but concluded it was essential to have the expert medical opinion of the treating doctor [14]. As recently as 2002, an editorial in the *Lancet* argued that 'without careful thought this latest move to involve patients in health care could end up overwhelming an already struggling system, and risk being seen as politically rather than scientifically driven' [15].

Arguments against patient reporting were that the reports would be of relatively lower quality than those from healthcare providers, that patients would report only non-serious ADRs, and that a large bulk of non-serious and well-known ADRs would interfere with actual signal detection [15]. This view on signal detection implies taking pertinent information from noise, with an implicit connotation that some reporting is more valid than others. However, allowing patients to report was described by others as a new step in pharmacovigilance that could have beneficial effects [16–18].

2.2 Current Patient Reporting Schemes in Pharmacovigilance

Direct patient reporting in pharmacovigilance is an essential method for collecting information on ADRs directly from patients or their caregivers. By involving patients actively in the monitoring process, it enhances the comprehensiveness and accuracy of drug safety data. Some examples of the implementation and impact of direct patient reporting in pharmacovigilance globally are listed below:

1. European Union: In the European Union (EU), direct patient reporting has gained momentum as an integral part of pharmacovigilance systems. The EMA supports patient reporting through the 'Strengthening Collaboration for Operating Pharmacovigilance in Europe' (SCOPE) project [19]. Various studies have investigated the utility and potential benefits of patient reporting [20–22]. This led to the implementation of European (EU)-wide legislation, making it mandatory in the EU to have direct patient reporting schemes in place. Patient reports are collected in EudraVigilance, the system for managing and analysing information on suspected ADRs to medicines which have been authorised or being studied in clinical trials in the European Economic Area and operated by EMA [23].
2. United Kingdom: The Medicines and Healthcare products Regulatory Agency (MHRA) launched patient reporting in 2005 as

a pilot programme, and patients can now report online, by phone, or by completing paper forms available at GP surgeries and pharmacies. Direct patient reporting through the Yellow Card Scheme is valued by users as a way to provide their unique perspective on ADRs, which can benefit pharmacovigilance [24].

3. United States: In the United States, the Food and Drug Administration (FDA) has been actively encouraging patient reporting through their MedWatch programme. The FDA recognises that patients can provide unique insights into ADRs due to their direct experience with medications [25]. A study by Golder et al. evaluated the patient reporting programme at the FDA, finding that patients reported a substantial number of ADRs not captured through healthcare professionals (HCPs) reporting alone [26]. This emphasised the importance of patient involvement in pharmacovigilance efforts.
4. Canada: Health Canada, the regulatory authority responsible for drug safety in Canada, also recognises the importance of patient reporting. The Canada Vigilance Program encourages patients to report ADRs directly using the online reporting form [27].
5. Global Initiatives: The World Health Organization (WHO), through the International Drug Monitoring Program, actively promotes patient reporting as part of global pharmacovigilance efforts. VigiBase, the WHO global database for the individual case safety reports, maintained by the Uppsala Monitoring Center in Sweden, also accepts non-HCPs like consumers, patients, and caregivers reports alongside those from HCPs. Currently, reports from patients in 141 countries constitute around 32% of the total number of reports in the VigiBase, which contains more than 36 million reports. Across the years, there was an increase in the number of reports received from patients submitted to the VigiBase as shown in Fig. 12.1. The accelerated increase in reporting in 2021 and 2022 is related to a large influx of reports on COVID-19 vaccines.

2.3 Clinical Quality of Patient Reports

If we focus on ADR reporting in a spontaneous reporting system, good documentation of clinical information is important for a proper assessment of an ADR report. A Dutch study investigated the clinical information of duplicate cases of ADRs reported by both patients and HCPs. A total of 197 cases were included, and in 54.3% of these cases, patients and HCPs reported a similar quality of clinical information. Statistical analysis demonstrated no overall differences between patients and HCPs in the presence of clinical information [21]. However, a study in France, investigating 16 key elements of information in reports, found that patient reports often need to be completed on key elements of information that were required for case assessment. For instance, data on medical history and concomitant medication were missing in 75% of the initial reports. Contacting the reporter helped to increase the informativeness of most elements of information for more than 90% of the reports [28].

2.4 Differences with Healthcare Professional Reports

Studies have found both differences and similarities in the reporting patterns of patients and HCPs. An analysis of the European ADR database Eudravigilance® found that patients were more likely than HCPs to report for genito-urinary, hormonal, and reproductive indications. Patients reported more general disorders and administration site conditions, whereas HCPs reported more ADRs related to investigations. It should, however, be noted that 13 of the 20 reactions most frequently reported by patients were also among the top 20 reactions reported by HCPs [18]. A review study by Inch et al. [22] from 2012 found that in the Netherlands and the UK, ADR reports by patients and HCPs were about similar drugs, with medicines such as statins and proton pump inhibitors in the top five

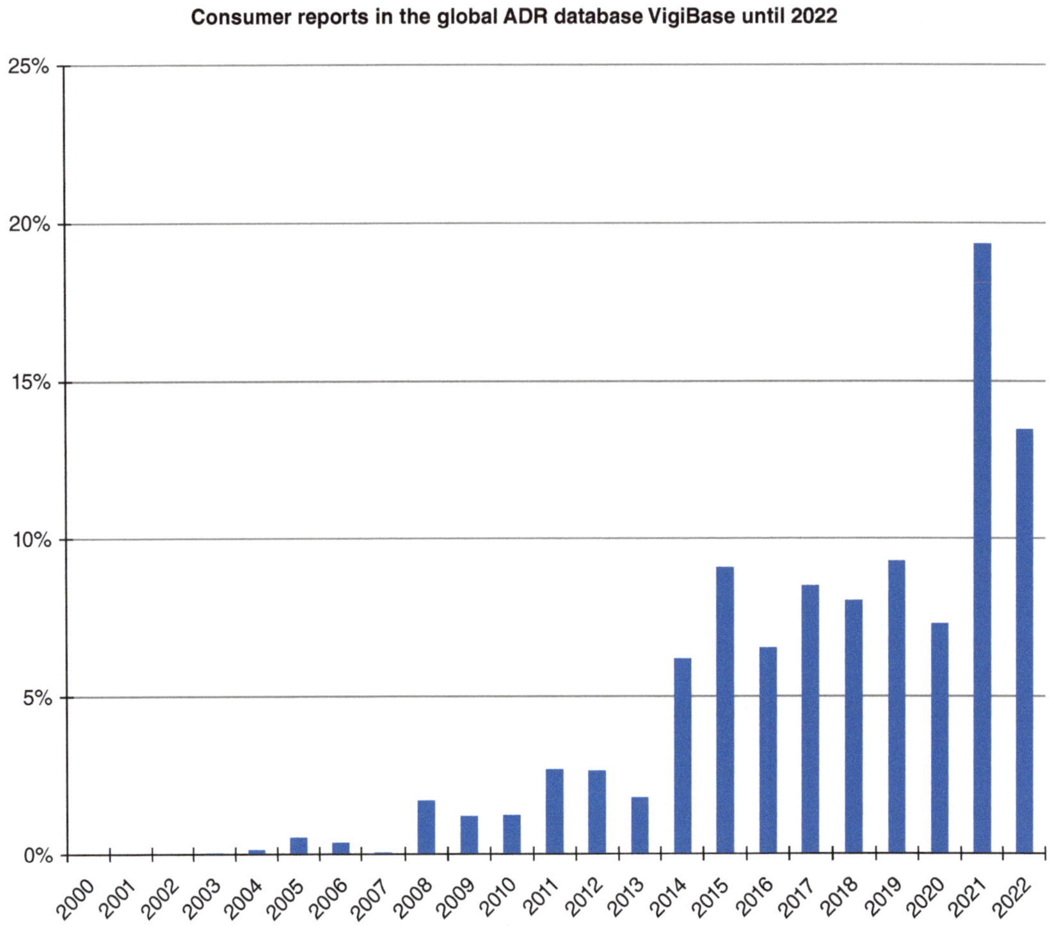

Fig. 12.1 Patients reports across the years in the VigiBase (source: VigiBase)

drugs. Patients and HCPs reported ADR about different organ classes. Table 12.1 shows the differences between patient ADR reports and those of HCPs.

2.5 Understanding the Burden of Adverse Drug Reactions

The influence of ADRs on daily life, the so-called burden of an ADR, is information that is considered important by patients and patients also report about this more often than HCPs [29, 30]. Research has shown that the decrease in quality of life due to ADRs can be mapped in a structured way and used by pharmacovigilance centres [31, 32].

Recently a thematic analysis [28] identified themes associated with ADR burden in patient-reported information consisting of 'effect on medication prescription,' 'impact on appearance,' 'impact on autonomy,' 'impact on daily life,' 'psychological consequences,' 'distressing aspects of ADR,' and 'physical consequences.' This study concluded that patients describe perceived ADR burden in both physical and psychological themes, which was comparable with HCP-reported information. However, HCP perspective put more focus on psychological impact, which is only part of the burden that patients describe themselves [33]. In addition to information on the burden of ADRs, aspects characterising the course of ADRs from the patient

Table 12.1 The differences between patient ADR reports and those of HCPs

Characteristics	Patient ADR reports	HCPs ADR reports
Source of information	Patient's own experience, family, friends, and other patients	HCPs observations of ADRs in their patients
Level of detail	May include information about lifestyle and habits, course of the ADR, and adherence	May provide a higher level of clinical details, includes a medical history and lab results
Medical terminology	Patient reports may use less medical terminology	HCP reports may use more medical terminology
Completeness	Patient reports may be incomplete, as patients may not be able to provide all of the relevant information	HCP reports may be more complete, as HCPs have access to medical records and other clinical information
Impact	May include more detailed information on the impact or burden of an ADR on the patient's life	Generally includes less information on impact and burden
Causality	May perceive the ADR's cause differently than HCP	HCP perspective on causality with clinical expertise
Perspective	Personal experience and symptoms. Report on ADRs that are important to them	Clinical and medical expertise, often focused on serious, new, or rare ADRs

perspective could be information that is useful for patients and HCPs and not always readily available. Recently, a framework was developed based on common themes in the course of ADRs identified from patient descriptions in patient-reported ADRs. The identified themes could be used for improving the systematic data collection of more extensive details about ADRs from patients [34].

One problem is that ADR reports in pharmacovigilance databases often contain coded information and, in addition, large amounts of unstructured or semi-structured information in plain text format. Harnessing and using this information could help to give more insight in the patient perspective on ADRs. Analysis techniques designed for free text analysis could be helpful in identifying topics in these reports [35].

2.6 Impact of Patient-Reported Adverse Drug Reactions on Pharmacovigilance

Patient-reported ADRs play a vital role in pharmacovigilance. They can help identify new safety signals, which can lead to improved patient safety. 'A "Safety Signal" is defined as information on a new or known adverse event that is potentially caused by a medicine and that warrants further investigation. Signals are generated from several sources such as spontaneous reports, clinical studies, and the scientific literature [36].' For example, a study found that patient reports accounted for 26.3% of all ADR reports in Dutch drug safety signals between 2010 and 2015 [24]. There are signals that are based entirely on reports from healthcare providers. However, there are also a number of signals that would not have been found without the input of patients [24]. For instance, patient reports were essential in identifying a safety signal for high-dose vitamin B6 products and the development of neuropathy, which led to a regulatory action in the Netherlands to restrict the maximum dosage of vitamin B6 in vitamin supplements [27].

Patient-reported ADRs can also help to identify safety concerns for medications that are not typically monitored by pharmacovigilance systems, such as herbal products and over-the-counter medications [25, 26]. It should be noted that a signal is more than just a 'new' ADR; it could also relate to a previously unknown aspect of an ADR, such as risk factors or severity of the reaction. This is information that is often missing from official patient information leaflets. For healthcare providers and patients, this information is important for making choices and expectations about the use of medicines. The reporting of ADRs should not be limited to the unknown, serious ADRs.

Patient-reported ADRs are a valuable source of information for pharmacovigilance systems. They can help identify new safety signals, improve our understanding of the safety of medications, and lead to regulatory actions to protect patients.

2.7 Patient Experiences on Social Media

Multiple attempts have been made to find utility in the patient experience of medicines shared on the internet [37–39]. The widespread uptake of social media following the growing use of smartphones intensified interest in this area, for instance for signal detection or signal strengthening purposes. However, knowledge of the mere existence of this unstructured information has also presented problems, since it has at times been in danger of creating an impossible obligation for market authorisation holders to scan for potential harms from their products [40]. A 3-year-long EU project called WEB-RADR explored the value of social media in finding new ADRs through signal detection. Despite developing some novel analytical tools to utilise such data, they were unable to find evidence that Twitter (nowadays rebranded as X) and Facebook added value compared to existing spontaneous reporting systems, although there may be niche usage cases (such as pregnancy-related outcomes or drug abuse) [38].

Similarly, an FDA study looking at the combined use of FDA Adverse Event Reporting System data and Twitter data found that while spontaneous data improved the signal from Twitter, Twitter did not add value to the use of spontaneous data [41]. It should be noted that both projects were performed some years ago and data mining techniques are quickly advancing. During the COVID-19 pandemic, the WHO invested in technology for digital real-time online listening, the Peek Platform which is an early warning system for COVID-19 vaccine-related events. This platform uses artificial intelligence (AI) to identify information on COVID-19 vaccine-related events on the internet and public social media platforms and news outlets in English, Spanish, and Russian [42]. This event-based surveillance system, which serves as a complement to information from other routine surveillance systems, was used to detect a potential ADR of nephrotic syndrome following the administration of the second dose of the COVID-19 vaccine in early 2022. Researchers from the Uppsala Monitoring Centre had detected a similar signal in the global adverse event database VigiBase nearly a year before, where IgA nephropathy was linked to the COVID-19 vaccine. The alert provided by this PEEK early warning system gave more context on this signal, helping them see the bigger clinical picture for this ADR and the vaccine [43]. While there may be future refinements and opportunities in the use of social media data, continuing instability of platforms, including researcher access to data, and format changes may mean that future work in this area is hampered.

3 Role of Patient Reporting in Vaccine Pharmacovigilance

3.1 The Significance of Patient Reports of Vaccine Safety Issues

Patient reports of adverse events following immunisation (AEFIs) are essential for monitoring the safety of vaccines and identifying potential safety signals. Nowadays, in the Netherlands, for instance, the majority of AEFI on the childhood immunisation programme and the yearly influenza vaccination programme are reported by parents or care-takers and vaccinated persons themselves [38]. Also for new vaccines, patients can help to elucidate the safety profile of a vaccine; the spreading of the MPox (previously known as monkeypox) virus in 2022 led to a vaccination campaign in the Netherlands for individuals at high risk of infection. Vaccinated persons were actively encouraged to report any AEFI to the spontaneous reporting system and almost all reports on this new vaccine were made by vaccinated persons themselves, including reports on serious AEFIs [44]. Patient reports can provide valuable insights into the types of AEFIs that are occurring and the populations that are most affected. This information can be used to [45]:

- **Identify new AEFIs:** Patient reports can help to identify safety signals for AEFIs, for example, those with a longer time-to-onset and especially those for which medical attention is generally less often sought but are important from a patient perspective.
- **Monitor the safety of vaccines in real-world settings:** Patient reports can provide insights into the safety of vaccines in real-world settings, where people are receiving vaccines in combination with other vaccines and may have underlying health conditions. This information can be used to monitor the safety of vaccines over time and identify new safety risks.
- **Improve the understanding of the impact of AEFIs on patients' lives:** Patient reports can provide valuable insights into the impact of AEFIs on patients' lives, including the impact on their quality of life, work productivity, and relationships. This information can be used to inform decision-making about risk management and to develop interventions to help patients cope with AEFIs.

In addition to the traditional spontaneous reporting system, cohort event monitoring studies, using Patient-Reported Outcomes (PROs), have made an important contribution to vaccine pharmacovigilance over the years. This type of study has been used, for instance, in the monitoring of the H1N1 vaccine in 2010 [46], influenza vaccines [47], and COVID-19 vaccines [48, 49].

3.2 The COVID-19 Pandemic and Patient Reporting

The pandemic has affected patient reporting of adverse effects. Early in the pandemic, there was a decrease in patient reporting, likely due to concerns about COVID-19 exposure and disruptions to healthcare services. A similar decrease was seen, for instance, in France, for HCP reports [50]. However, the COVID-19 vaccination campaign has resulted in a surge in the number of ADR reports from the general public in many countries. In the Netherlands, over 250,000 reports were received in the first 1.5 years after the first vaccines were registered, with the majority being reported by vaccinated persons themselves [51]. Consumers report on ADRs that concern them, such as was seen by a huge number of reports on menstrual disorders after COVID-19 vaccination which led to a subsequent signal and addition of heavy menstrual bleeding as an ADR to the Summary of Product Characteristics for the commonly used mRNA vaccines in Europe [52].

3.3 Building Public Confidence in COVID-19 Vaccines

Effective communications are essential with regard to medicines safety. A good example of this is the management of the public communications about COVID-19 vaccines. While there have been concerns about a lack of knowledge on the process of vaccine and medicines development for patients and the general public, both the UK's MHRA and the EU's EMA had prepared extensive pharmacovigilance plans for the vaccines in the months prior to their launch [53]. These focused on ensuring the safety of the vaccines, but also on seeking to ensure there was public confidence in the regulatory systems that monitored safety. Both agencies tried to be open and transparent about the reported harms of vaccines, while setting up new safety studies to actively look for harms.

Both the UK and EU also regularly published contextualised reports on spontaneous reports related to COVID-19 vaccines and held public panels on safety issues as they arose. In the UK, discussions on vaccine benefit and harms were held live on television with experts from the MHRA, the health service, and the committee in charge of vaccines, leading to open discussion about benefits and harms of the vaccines. This was also the case in the Netherlands, where the media attention and public interest for vaccines were unprecedented. This also meant that many patients actively sought information on vaccine safety. In 2021, there were more than 4.6 million visits to the Lareb website, where a dedicated section was made covering safety information for COVID-19 vaccines [54]. Compared to 2020, before COVID-19 vaccines were registered, this was a 500% increase in access. Lareb's active media contributions also rose from 52 in 2020 to 288 in 2021 [54].

In addition to the efforts of the UK's MHRA and the EU's EMA, the International Society of Pharmacovigilance Special Interest Group on Medicinal Product Risk Communication (ISoP CommSIG), as an expert group on medicinal product risk communication, contributed to the development of infographics for patients; one on the safe use of medicines during the pandemic and a later one on the safety of COVID-19 vaccines [55].

3.4 Overcoming Misinformation and Increasing Public Trust in Pharmacovigilance

Misinformation, for instance on social media, has been an issue pharmacovigilance had to deal with, although during the initial vaccination campaign, uptake was high. A lot of misinformation was seemingly generated by a very small number of sources [56]. In this light, quickly identifying and addressing public concern about vaccination should be a priority. Patient involvement should be a two-way street, where organisations involved in pharmacovigilance should strive towards providing comprehensive information for patients to make an informed decision on vaccination in a timely fashion, instead of only involving patients by receiving their reports [7, 57].

4 Patients Involvement in Regulatory Decision-Making

4.1 The Journey Towards Consistent Patient Engagement

From the beginning of the twenty-first century, more and more countries started accepting patient reports, with Denmark, the Netherlands, and the UK became the first countries within the EU in 2003 [27].The first scientific articles from the Netherlands [21, 58], Denmark [59], and the UK [20] showed that patients were able to make high-quality reports. A well-designed (online) report form, through which patients are guided and know which data elements they have to fill in, is a precondition for this [27]. In 2012, a handbook for consumer reporting of ADRs was developed as part of the 'Monitoring Medicines project' [60], funded by the FP-7 EU framework. This guidance aimed to provide practical guidelines on how to set up national systems for consumers to report adverse reactions to medicines and was published by the WHO [61].

A breakthrough in the acceptance of patient participation came in 2012 when new European pharmacovigilance legislation made it possible for patients in all EU Member States to report adverse reactions directly to the national adverse drug reaction centre [62]. This gave patients a permanent role in monitoring the safety of medicines. The number of patient reports in the European Eudravigilance® database rose from a total of 53,130 patient reports in the 3 years preceding the legislation operation period to 113,371 reports in the 3 years after. However, there are still large differences in the number of patient reports between the various EU Member States. Member states contributing the most patient reports to the European ADR database (Eudravigilance®) were the Netherlands, the UK, Germany, France, and Italy [23].

4.2 Frameworks for Patient and Consumer Engagement

In recent years, more attention has been paid to involving the patient's perspective in decisions about the registration and monitoring of medicines. In Europe, representatives for patients have been involved in the European Pharmacovigilance Risk Assessment Committee (PRAC) since 2012. Patient representatives sit as full members of the Committee. As a result, patients are now fully involved with the difficult assessments of benefit–risk that sit at the heart of the regulatory process [63]. In 2017, the first public hearing where European citizens representing patients, carers, HCPs, and academia shared their experience with valproate occurred [64]. As input from patients and HCPs to regulatory assessments is increasingly essential for benefit–risk management of medicines, *Bahri and Pariente* studied the ways to obtain patient input in different risk scenarios [65]. Their proposed decision guide aims at ensuring systematic and consistent engagement across regulatory assessments, to effectively obtain real-world input for regulatory decision making [65].

In 2019, *Bahri and Brown* published a first conceptual and methodological framework for 'Engagement of patients and healthcare professionals in regulatory pharmacovigilance' [66], and EMA has published an engagement framework in 2022. This framework describes the objectives and methodologies for EMA's engagement with patients, consumers, and their organisations in relation to medicines for human and veterinary use [67]. In addition to the European efforts that are being made to involve patients, there have also been national initiatives. In the Netherlands, the Dutch Medicines Evaluation Board appointed a new board member for Patient and Consumer Perspective in 2015 [68].

Despite increasing efforts to involve patients in pharmacovigilance, a qualitative study has noted the level of actively involving patients as rather low and scattered across the different phases of the lifecycle of medicines [69]. The authors describe barriers which hamper the transitioning of patient involvement from theory to practice [69]. In order to overcome some of these barriers, best practices in patient involvement in pharmacovigilance were studied based on a qualitative multi-stakeholder interview study across Europe, including representatives of patient organisations, regulators, and pharmaceutical companies at both the national and European level. Best practices involved patient education and empowerment, engagement from the start, structured involvement and guidelines, patients as same-level partners, face-to-face communication, and setting common goals (Fig. 12.2) [70].

4.3 The Patient's Role in Decision Making

Patients carry not only the risk of harms from medicines but also the benefits of medicines. While there has been a move away from a paternalistic framework when using medicines to a shared decision-making model at an individual level, regulatory agencies still operate by making decisions at a population level—using a public health model. However, decisions to withdraw drugs are not always universally welcomed. There will be a set of patients who are deriving benefits from the withdrawn medicine, without adverse effects, or at least willing to accept the risks that the regulator has deemed too high at a population level.

When benoxaprofen was withdrawn in the United States in the 1980s, the FDA received hundreds of letters from doctors and patients asking if benoxaprofen would still be available to them [71]. In the UK, the famous playwright Dennis Potter, who lived with psoriatic arthritis for most of his life, complained that he had been left 'high and dry' following the withdrawal [72]. Following the withdrawal of alosetron in 2000, which had been associated with severe ADRs such as ischaemic colitis and death, the FDA and GlaxoSmithKline were lobbied by thousands of patients to keep the drug on the market. The drug was made available again under a risk management programme run by GlaxoSmithKline in 2002 [73].

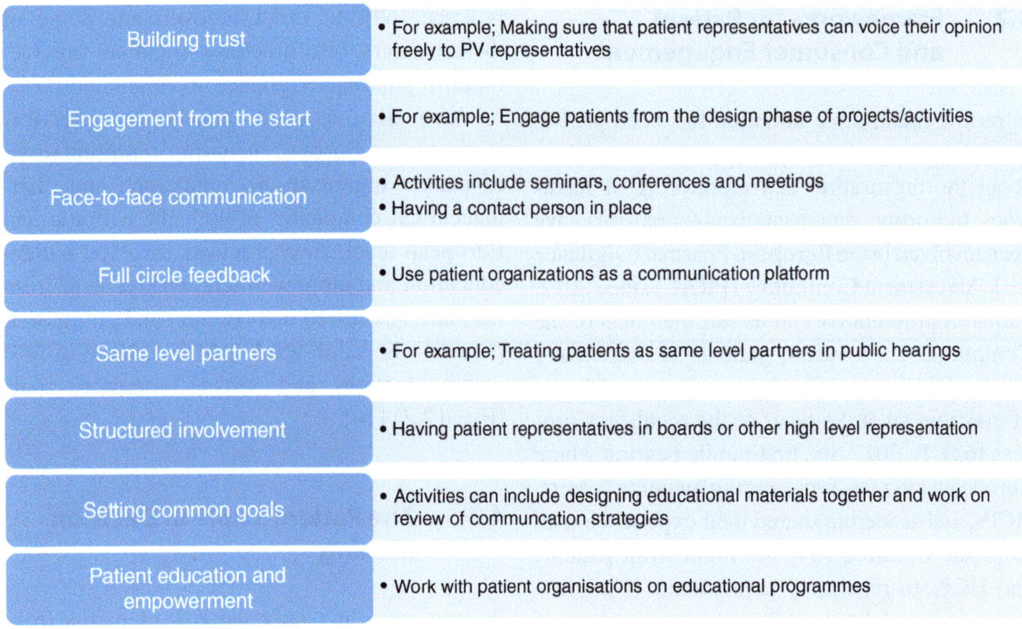

Fig. 12.2 Best practices in pharmacovigilance for patient involvement and the activities that relate to them

The case study of the conditional approval of bevacizumab for use in breast cancer in the United States is a particularly interesting intersection of public views on benefits and harms, compared to a regulator's assessment. Following the withdrawal, over 450 public submissions arrived at the FDA, mostly asking for the drug to remain on the market. Such differences of opinion can be driven by differing interpretations of evidence, differing expectations and values, risk/benefit weightings which are shaped by socio-cultural processes, trust, hope and their rootedness in vulnerability and a need to cope, and lastly, newspaper reporting of drug benefits.

Clarity in public communications by regulators towards the public and media have been suggested to increase alignment of the public and regulators [74]. However, patients' experiences, knowledge, opinions, and preferences about medicines were not always considered as important as those of other stakeholders in answering questions about the risks and benefits of medicines [63].

4.4 Getting Engagement

Awareness that ADRs can be reported and that it is important to do so is not always optimal among patients or the general public. During the annual 'MedSafetyWeek', the Uppsala Monitoring Centre teams up with medicine regulatory authorities and national pharmacovigilance centres across the world to run a social media campaign that raises awareness of ADRs [44]. Although, for some countries the mass vaccination campaigns in 2021/2022 resulted in more awareness and reports in patient reporting schemes, overall, there is still much to gain in informing patients and the general public about the possibility to report. It would also be helpful if reporting functions would be integrated into functionalities that patients already use, such as apps [75, 76], preferably those which are already used to manage their disease.

4.5 The Role of Patient Organisations

One of the ways to create a more optimal reporting culture among patients is to get engagement from patient organisations. Patient organisations, either umbrella organisations or targeted towards specific diseases, can have an important role in encouraging patients to talk with their doctors/pharmacists about ADRs experienced or to help patients report the ADRs to the pharmacovigilance systems [45]. Patient organisations can help enable effective communication of ADRs to a relevant audience, for instance, through social media posts. As an example, a signal on levothyroxine and panic reactions was communicated via the Dutch thyroid organisation's digital newsletter, social media channels, website, and print magazine. The social media post generated the most engagement [46].

However, barriers to being involved in pharmacovigilance for patient and patient organisations also still exist and include a lack of awareness, a lack of resources and/or budget, and support from regulators [45]. Strategies to stimulate patient-organisation participation are, among others, the creation of more awareness campaigns, more research that creates awareness, education for patient organisations, and a more proactive approach from national competent authorities [47].

5 Future Steps

5.1 Challenges and Opportunities in Patient Involvement

Patient and public engagement in pharmacovigilance is essential for ensuring the safety of medications. However, there are a number of challenges that can make it difficult for patients to participate in this process [13]. One of the biggest challenges is that patients may not be aware of the importance of pharmacovigilance or how to report ADRs. Patients may also be hesitant to report ADRs because they are worried about being labelled as a 'difficult patient' or because they believe that their report will not make a difference. Another challenge is that patients may not have the time or resources to report ADRs. Patients may be busy with work, family, and other commitments, and they may not have access to the internet or other resources needed to report ADRs. Finally, some patients may not be able to recognise ADRs or may not understand the relationship between their adverse events and the medications they are taking. This can be particularly challenging for patients who are taking multiple medications or who have complex medical conditions. In addition, patients may just accept ADRs as part of their illness trajectory. Such stoicism may be linked to their disease condition but also to age or gender.

Despite these challenges, there are a number of strategies for promoting patient engagement in pharmacovigilance [12]. First, it is important to educate patients about the importance of pharmacovigilance and how to report ADRs. This can be done through public awareness campaigns, development of patient education materials, and healthcare provider training. Additionally, it is important to make it easy for patients to report ADRs. This can be done by providing patients with easy-to-use reporting tools and by making sure that healthcare providers are aware of and willing to accept patient reports. Finally, it is important to support patients who report ADRs by providing them with feedback on their reports and by following up on their concerns. This helps to ensure that patients feel valued and respected and that they are more likely to report ADRs in the future.

5.2 Leveraging Patient-Reported Information and Patient-Reported Outcomes in Pharmacovigilance

Patient-reported information (PRI) and patient-reported outcomes (PROs) are valuable sources of data for pharmacovigilance because they give a unique view of the patient. PRI and PROs can be collected through a variety of sources, such as patient surveys, social media, and electronic patient records. PRIs and PROs can help find new safety signals, check the safety of medicines in real-life situations, track how well safety measures are working, monitor the effectiveness of safety interventions, and create better safety measures [77–79]. Further information could be found in Case Study 1.

5.3 Patient Engagement Special Interest Group

The International Society of Pharmacovigilance (ISoP), an international non-profit scientific organisation, which aims to foster pharmacovigilance both scientifically and educationally and enhance all aspects of the safe and proper use of medicines, has recently established the Patient Engagement Special Interest Group (PatEG-SIG) to describe, develop, and promote patient engagement in pharmacovigilance. The vision of this SIG is to enhance the core role of patients in medication safety, which will '*ultimately result in best practices that can be integrated into operational everyday pharmacovigilance both in healthcare and at the health policy level, and hence contribute to enabling informed therapeutic choices and keeping patients safe*' [57].

5.4 Medication Safety in Clinical Practice

While the involvement of patients in pharmacovigilance has been the focus of this chapter, it should not be forgotten that patients are a key stakeholder in the wider healthcare system. When it comes to their own health, patients have to make benefit-harm judgements to consent to treatment, have a high awareness of the potential harms of the medication, and can be the last line defence in the case of an error. The role of the patient in clinical safety has been categorised into three main areas [80].

1. Interventions to directly support patient safety (e.g. challenging healthcare staff when they see a medication error).
2. Contributing to self-management (e.g. self-adjustment of warfarin or insulin dosing).
3. To provide feedback on the quality of care (e.g. reporting of medication errors or ADRs).

A review of current evidence of patient engagement in healthcare safety found that while there was good evidence for a number of interventions (self-management of anticoagulants, adverse event monitoring, and medical record accuracy) that these were not widely implemented [81]. The review also found that adherence to medication could be improved by patient engagement with patient education programmes, self-management, and online access to medical notes. As well as confirming the role of patients in pharmacovigilance reporting, there was also some positive impact of patient reporting of medication errors.

A systematic review of patient and family strategies to improve medication safety found over 19 studies targeted at mainly older adults [82]. These were based on either patient education or medicines reconciliation—the latter including medication lists, drug safety information, bringing medications to appointments, and checking procedures when patients arrive at healthcare centres. While patients, the public, and families appear to be generally well disposed to medication safety, some have argued that the evidence remains poor. Patients may be concerned about damaging relationships with healthcare professionals [82].

A patient-centred framework for primary care found a number of contributory factors for medications errors in primary care [83]. Key contributing factors for medication errors were related to communication issues, patient- and carer-related factors, HCP factors, computer systems and programmes, and supply of medication and appliances. A Patient Medication Safety Framework (P-MEDs) was created with communication issues at the centre, since failures of communication were common—particularly across primary and secondary care interfaces [83].

In the hospital sector, there is some evidence that both patients and HCPs would welcome better patient involvement in medication safety [84], and there have been attempts to create patient-centred medication measure concepts for that sector in order to orientate future research into patient-centred activity [85]. These were aligned to health system-orientated safety measures, such as improved patient reporting of adherence, reporting of drug–drug interactions, side effects, and medication errors, and enabling patients to report on the treatment burden they are carrying. Others were more patient centred, including patient preferences on communication methods, ensuring that patient medication goals are understood in the context of preferences and any patient concerns about safety.

6 Summary and Conclusions

It is clear that the patient and public involvement in pharmacovigilance adds value. However, actually normalising this practice goes beyond allowing patient reporting, with much work to be done to increase actual patient involvement in the wider arena of pharmacovigilance. Patients make a clear contribution in giving information about the impact of the ADR on their daily life and this information could be more routinely used in pharmacovigilance.

With increasing numbers of direct patient reports, it is crucial to look towards new methodologies in pharmacovigilance to make the best use of patient-reported information. This also means that our methods and systems used for collecting, coding, and analysing patient reported information need to be further developed. Patient involvement should be a two-way street where pharmacovigilance benefits from patient-reported information, but also provides relevant information back to patients and involves them in decision making.

7 Case Studies

7.1 Case Study 1: Developing Patient-Reported Outcome Measures to Capture and Track Patients' Experiences with Medications

1. *What are patient-reported outcome measures (PROMs)?*

   They are tools used to capture patients' perspectives on their health and well-being.
2. *What is the purpose of developing PROMs?*

   PROMs can be used to track patients' experiences with medications, including side effects, efficacy, and quality of life. This information can be used to improve patient care, inform pharmacovigilance efforts, and support research and the development of new medications [78, 86–90].
3. *Describe the steps involved in developing PROMs to capture patients' experiences with medications?*

   There are a number of steps involved in developing PROMs to capture patients' experiences with medications [78, 86–90]. These steps include:

   (a) Identifying the patient population of interest and the specific medication experiences that are important to measure: This can be done through literature reviews, focus groups with patients, and interviews with patients and HCPs.

   (b) Generating items for the PROM: Items should be clear, concise, and relevant to the patient population of interest. They should also be easy to read, understand, and complete.

   (c) Evaluating the PROM for content validity: This can be done by having a panel of experts review the PROM items to ensure that they are relevant, comprehensive, and appropriate for the intended use.

   (d) Pilot testing the PROM in a small sample of patients to assess its feasibility, acceptability, and psychometric properties: This may involve making changes to the PROM items or format to improve

their usability. Qualitative research may play an important role here as what the experts reflect upon may not represent what the burden and experience is of the patient.
(e) Validating the PROM in a larger sample of patients to assess its reliability and responsiveness: This can be done by comparing the PROM scores to other measures of the same construct, such as clinical outcomes or clinician ratings.

4. *How could we involve patients in the development of PROMs?*

   It is important to involve patients in all stages of the PROM development process. This helps to ensure that the PROM is relevant to patients' needs and concerns and that it is easy to understand and complete. Patients can be involved in generating items for the PROM, evaluating the PROM for content validity, and pilot testing the PROM.

5. *Provide an example of a PROM to capture patients' experiences with medications:*

   The Patient-Reported Outcomes Measurement Information System (PROMIS) is a set of validated PROMs that can be used to measure a wide range of patient-reported outcomes, including medication experiences [78, 86–90].

   The PROMIS Medication Experience Module (PEM) is a 10-item PROM that can be used to assess patients' experiences with medications, including side effects, efficacy, and quality of life.

   The PEM items are:

   (a) In the past week, how often have you had any side effects from your medications?
   (b) In the past week, how much have your side effects bothered you?
   (c) In the past week, how much did your side effects limit your activities?
   (d) In the past week, how often did you take your medications as prescribed?
   (e) In the past week, how confident were you that your medications were working?
   (f) In the past week, how satisfied were you with the overall effect of your medications?
   (g) In the past week, how much did your medications improve your quality of life?
   (h) In the past week, how much did your medications make it difficult to do your job or go to school?
   (i) In the past week, how much did your medications make it difficult to manage your daily activities?
   (j) In the past week, how much did your medications make it difficult to enjoy your life?

The PEM items are rated on a 5-point Likert scale, with higher scores indicating more severe side effects, lower efficacy, and lower quality of life. The PEM has been validated in a number of studies and has been shown to be reliable and responsive to changes in patients' medication experiences [78, 86–90].

7.2 Case Study 2: Creating Patient-Friendly Educational Materials on Pharmacovigilance

Pharmacovigilance is the process of monitoring the safety of medicines after they have been marketed. However, many patients are not aware of the importance of pharmacovigilance or how to recognise and report ADRs. It is important to involve patients in pharmacovigilance so that they can recognise and report ADRs.

1. *What is the purpose of patient-friendly educational materials on pharmacovigilance?*

   Patient-friendly educational materials can be used to inform patients about the importance of pharmacovigilance and how to recognise and report ADRs.

2. *What are the basic characteristics of patient-friendly educational materials on pharmacovigilance?*

   These materials should be written in clear and concise language, and they should be easy to understand for patients with all levels of health literacy [91–94].

3. *Describe the steps for developing patient-friendly educational materials on pharmacovigilance:*
   (a) Identify the target audience and their needs: What do patients need to know about pharmacovigilance and ADRs? What level of health literacy do patients have?
   (b) Develop learning objectives: What do patients need to be able to do after reading the educational materials? For example, patients should be able to define pharmacovigilance, identify ADRs, and report ADRs to the appropriate authorities.
   (c) Choose the right format: What format of educational materials will be most effective for the target audience? For example, educational materials could be in the form of brochures, leaflets, infographics, posters, videos, or online resources.
   (d) Write and design the educational materials: The educational materials should be written in clear and concise language, and they should be visually appealing. It is also important to use plain language and avoid jargon.
   (e) Pilot test the educational materials: The educational materials should be pilot tested with a small yet diverse group of patients to ensure that they are easy to understand and effective.
   (f) Disseminate the educational materials: Once the educational materials have been finalised, they should be disseminated to the target audience. This could be done through clinics, hospitals, pharmacies, and other healthcare settings.
4. *Provide examples of patient-friendly educational materials on pharmacovigilance:*
   (a) Brochures that explain what pharmacovigilance is, why it is important, and how to report ADRs.
   (b) Videos that explain pharmacovigilance in a clear and engaging way.
   (c) Infographics that provide easy-to-understand information on pharmacovigilance.
   (d) Websites of regulatory authorities with a dedicated section on pharmacovigilance for patients.

References

1. Rolfes L. Patient participation in pharmacovigilance. Thesis. Rijksuniversiteit Groningen; 2018.
2. Smith MY, Benattia I. The patient's voice in pharmacovigilance: pragmatic approaches to building a patient-centric drug safety organization. Drug Saf. 2016;39(9):779–85. https://doi.org/10.1007/s40264-016-0426-9.
3. Smith MY, Hammad TA, Metcalf M, Levitan B, Noel R, Wolka AM, et al. Patient engagement at a tipping point—the need for cultural change across patient, sponsor, and regulator stakeholders: insights from the DIA conference, "patient engagement in benefit risk assessment throughout the life cycle of medical products". Ther Innov Regul Sci. 2016;50(5):546–53.
4. Naik N, Hameed BMZ, Sooriyaperakasam N, Vinayahalingam S, Patil V, Smriti K, et al. Transforming healthcare through a digital revolution: a review of digital healthcare technologies and solutions. Front Digit Health. 2022;4:919985. https://doi.org/10.3389/fdgth.2022.919985.
5. What is patient-centered care? Catal Carryover. 2017;3(1) https://catalyst.nejm.org/doi/full/10.1056/CAT.17.0559.
6. European Medicines Agency (EMA). Patient Experience Data (PED)—update on progress. 2023. https://www.ema.europa.eu/en/documents/presentation/presentation-patient-experience-data-ped-update-progress-r-gonzalez-quevedo-ema_en.pdf. Accessed 30 Oct 2023.
7. CIOMS Working Group report. Patient involvement in the development, regulation and safe use of medicines. Geneva, Switzerland: Council for International Organizations of Medical Sciences (CIOMS); 2022.
8. Hazell L, Shakir SA. Under-reporting of adverse drug reactions : a systematic review. Drug Saf. 2006;29(5):385–96.
9. Matos C, Harmark L, van Hunsel F. Patient reporting of adverse drug reactions: an international survey of national competent authorities' views and needs. Drug Saf. 2016;39(11):1105–16.
10. Inácio P, Gomes JJ, Airaksinen M, Cavaco A. Exploring sociodemographic and economic factors that promote adverse drug reactions reporting by patients. Health Policy. 2018;122(3):263–8. https://doi.org/10.1016/j.healthpol.2017.10.004.

11. Costa C, Abeijon P, Rodrigues DA, Figueiras A, Herdeiro MT, Torre C. Factors associated with underreporting of adverse drug reactions by patients: a systematic review. Int J Clin Pharm. 2023; https://doi.org/10.1007/s11096-023-01592-y.
12. Al Dweik R, Stacey D, Kohen D, Yaya S. Factors affecting patient reporting of adverse drug reactions: a systematic review. Br J Clin Pharmacol. 2017;83(4):875–83. https://doi.org/10.1111/bcp.13159.
13. Shafei L, Mekki L, Maklad E, Alhathal T, Ghanem R, Almalouf R, et al. Factors that influence patient and public adverse drug reaction reporting: a systematic review using the theoretical domains framework. Int J Clin Pharm. 2023;45(4):801–13. https://doi.org/10.1007/s11096-023-01591-z.
14. Medicines CoSo. Report of the working party on adverse reactions: Part I. London: DHSS; 1983.
15. Anonymous. Improving ADR reporting. Lancet. 2002;360(9344):1435.
16. van Grootheest K, de Graaf L, de Jong-van den Berg L. Consumer adverse drug reaction reporting: a new step in pharmacovigilance? Drug Saf. 2003;26(4):211–7.
17. Medawar C, Herxheimer A, Bell A, Jofre S. Paroxetine, Panorama and user reporting of ADRs: consumer intelligence matters in clinical practice and post-marketing drug surveillance. Int J Risk Saf Med. 2002;15(3–4):161–9.
18. Medawar C, Herxheimer A. A comparison of adverse drug reaction reports from professionals and users, relating to risk of dependence and suicidal behaviour with paroxetine. Int J Risk Saf Med. 2004;16:5–19.
19. Radecka A, Loughlin L, Foy M, de Ferraz Guimaraes MV, Sarinic VM, Di Giusti MD, et al. Enhancing pharmacovigilance capabilities in the EU regulatory network: the SCOPE joint action. Drug Saf. 2018;41(12):1285–302. https://doi.org/10.1007/s40264-018-0708-5.
20. Avery AJ, Anderson C, Bond CM, Fortnum H, Gifford A, Hannaford PC, et al. Evaluation of patient reporting of adverse drug reactions to the UK 'Yellow Card Scheme': literature review, descriptive and qualitative analyses, and questionnaire surveys. Health Technol Assess. 2011;15(20):1–iv.
21. de Langen J, van Hunsel F, Passier A, de Jong-van den Berg L, van Grootheest K. Adverse drug reaction reporting by patients in the Netherlands : three years of experience. Drug Saf. 2008;31(6):515–24.
22. Sienkiewicz K, Burzyńska M, Rydlewska-Liszkowska I, Sienkiewicz J, Gaszyńska E. The importance of direct patient reporting of adverse drug reactions in the safety monitoring process. Int J Environ Res Public Health. 2021;19(1) https://doi.org/10.3390/ijerph19010413.
23. Banovac M, Candore G, Slattery J, Houÿez F, Haerry D, Genov G, et al. Patient reporting in the EU: analysis of EudraVigilance data. Drug Saf. 2017;40(7):629–45. https://doi.org/10.1007/s40264-017-0534-1.
24. Anderson C, Krska J, Murphy E, Avery A. The importance of direct patient reporting of suspected adverse drug reactions: a patient perspective. Br J Clin Pharmacol. 2011;72(5):806–22. https://doi.org/10.1111/j.1365-2125.2011.03990.x.
25. Blenkinsopp A, Wilkie P, Wang M, Routledge PA. Patient reporting of suspected adverse drug reactions: a review of published literature and international experience. Br J Clin Pharmacol. 2007;63(2):148–56.
26. Golder S, Smith K, O'Connor K, Gross R, Hennessy S, Gonzalez-Hernandez G. A comparative view of reported adverse effects of statins in social media, regulatory data, drug information databases and systematic reviews. Drug Saf. 2021;44(2):167–79. https://doi.org/10.1007/s40264-020-00998-1.
27. van Hunsel F, Harmark L, Pal S, Olsson S, van Grootheest K. Experiences with adverse drug reaction reporting by patients: an 11-country survey. Drug Saf. 2012;35(1):45–60.
28. Kheloufi F, Default A, Rouby F, Laugier-Castellan D, Boyer M, Rodrigues B, et al. Informativeness of patient initial reports of adverse drug reactions. Can it be improved by a pharmacovigilance centre? Eur J Clin Pharmacol. 2017;73(8):1009–18. https://doi.org/10.1007/s00228-017-2254-y.
29. Rolfes L, van Hunsel F, Wilkes S, Grootheest KV, van Puijenbroek EV. Adverse drug reaction reports of patients and healthcare professionals-differences in reported information. Pharmacoepidemiol Drug Saf. 2015;24(2):152–8. https://doi.org/10.1002/pds.3687.
30. van Hunsel F, Passier A, van Grootheest K. Comparing patients' and healthcare professionals' ADR reports after media attention: the broadcast of a Dutch television programme about the benefits and risks of statins as an example. Br J Clin Pharmacol. 2009;67(5):558–64. https://doi.org/10.1111/j.1365-2125.2009.03400.x.
31. Rolfes L, van Hunsel F, Taxis K, van Puijenbroek E. The impact of experiencing adverse drug reactions on the patient's quality of life: a retrospective cross-sectional study in the Netherlands. Drug Saf. 2016;39(8):769–76.
32. Rolfes L, Haaksman M, van Hunsel F, van Puijenbroek E. How do adverse drug reactions influence the patient's daily life? Qualitative analysis on spontaneous reports by patients. Drug Saf. 2017;40(10):964.
33. Westerink HJ, Kosse LJ, Jessurun NT, Tubergen AV, Vonkeman HE, Nurmohamed MT, et al. Patients' and health-care professionals' perspectives on adverse drug reaction burden attributed to the use of biological DMARDs: a qualitative study. Expert Opin Drug Saf. 2023;22(5):417–24. https://doi.org/10.1080/14740338.2023.2134344.
34. van Lint JA, Sonnenberg M, Vonkeman HE, van den Bemt BJF, van Puijenbroek EP, Jessurun NT. Development of a framework structuring themes in the course of adverse drug reactions from a patient's perspective. Drug Saf. 2023; https://doi.org/10.1007/s40264-023-01343-y.

35. Lösch L, Brown P, van Hunsel F. Using structural topic modelling to reveal patterns in reports on opioid drugs in a pharmacovigilance database. Pharmacoepidemiol Drug Saf. 2022;31(9):1003–6. https://doi.org/10.1002/pds.5502.
36. European Medicines Agency (EM). Safety signal; 2021. https://www.ema.europa.eu/en/glossary/safety-signal. Accessed 23 Feb 2021.
37. Butt TF, Cox AR, Oyebode JR, Ferner RE. Internet accounts of serious adverse drug reactions: a study of experiences of Stevens-Johnson syndrome and toxic epidermal necrolysis. Drug Saf. 2012;35(12):1159–70. https://doi.org/10.1007/bf03262001.
38. van Stekelenborg J, Ellenius J, Maskell S, Bergvall T, Caster O, Dasgupta N, et al. Recommendations for the use of social media in pharmacovigilance: lessons from IMI WEB-RADR. Drug Saf. 2019;42(12):1393–407. https://doi.org/10.1007/s40264-019-00858-7.
39. Brosch S, de Ferran AM, Newbould V, Farkas D, Lengsavath M, Tregunno P. Establishing a framework for the use of social media in pharmacovigilance in Europe. Drug Saf. 2019;42(8):921–30. https://doi.org/10.1007/s40264-019-00811-8.
40. Edwards IR, Lindquist M. Social media and networks in pharmacovigilance: boon or bane? Drug Saf. 2011;34(4):267–71. https://doi.org/10.2165/11590720-000000000-00000.
41. Li Y, Jimeno Yepes A, Xiao C. Combining social media and FDA adverse event reporting system to detect adverse drug reactions. Drug Saf. 2020;43(9):893–903. https://doi.org/10.1007/s40264-020-00943-2.
42. World Health Organization (WHO). Technical meeting report. 'Unmasking safety signals during a pandemic'; 2021. https://cdn.who.int/media/docs/default-source/medicines/pharmacovigilance/unmasking-safety-signals-in-an-infodemic_technical-report.pdf?sfvrsn=5890874b_1&download=true.
43. Uppsala Monitoring Centre (UMC). Uppsala reports: could social media vigilance aid pharmacovigilance? 2023. https://www.uppsalareports.org/articles/could-social-media-vigilance-aid-pharmacovigilance/. Accessed 27 Nov 2023.
44. van der Boom M, van Hunsel F. Adverse reactions following MPox (monkeypox) vaccination: an overview from the Dutch and global adverse event reporting systems. Br J Clin Pharmacol. 2023;89(11):3302–10. https://doi.org/10.1111/bcp.15830.
45. CIOMS. CIOMS guide to vaccine safety communication—report by topic Group 3 of the CIOMS Working Group on Vaccine Safety. Geneva, Switserland: CIOMS; 2018.
46. Harmark L, van Hunsel F, Hak E, van Grootheest K. Monitoring the safety of influenza A (H1N1) vaccine using web-based intensive monitoring. Vaccine. 2011;29(10):1941–7. https://doi.org/10.1016/j.vaccine.2010.12.123.
47. Slingerland P, van Hunsel F, Lieber T, van Balveren L, Duijster JW. The effect of sex on the incidence, latency, duration and perceived burden of adverse events following seasonal influenza vaccination in the Netherlands. Drug Saf. 2023; https://doi.org/10.1007/s40264-023-01356-7.
48. Raethke M, van Hunsel F, Thurin NH, Dureau-Pournin C, Mentzer D, Kovačić B, et al. Cohort event monitoring of adverse reactions to COVID-19 vaccines in seven European countries: pooled results on first dose. Drug Saf. 2023;46(4):391–404. https://doi.org/10.1007/s40264-023-01281-9.
49. Osibogun AO, Shuaib FM, Adeyeye CM, Onajole AT, Ejembi CL, Banwat ME, et al. Cohort event monitoring for safety signal detection in adult individuals 18 years and above after immunisation with coronavirus disease 2019 vaccines in Nigeria. Niger Postgrad Med J. 2023;30(1):18–24. https://doi.org/10.4103/npmj.npmj_299_22.
50. de Germay S, Singier A, Salvo F, Pariente A. Impact of Covid-19 vaccination on spontaneous pharmacovigilance reporting in France. Drug Saf. 2023; https://doi.org/10.1007/s40264-023-01359-4.
51. Oosterhuis I, Scholl J, van Puijenbroek E, Kant A, van Hunsel F. Optimizing safety surveillance for COVID-19 vaccines at the National Pharmacovigilance Centre Lareb: one year of COVID-19 vaccine experience. Drug Saf. 2023;46(1):65–75. https://doi.org/10.1007/s40264-022-01253-5.
52. Duijster JW, Schoep ME, Nieboer TE, Jajou R, Kant A, van Hunsel F. Menstrual abnormalities after COVID-19 vaccination in the Netherlands: a description of spontaneous and longitudinal patient-reported data. Br J Clin Pharmacol. 2023; https://doi.org/10.1111/bcp.15799.
53. Durand J, Dogné JM, Cohet C, Browne K, Gordillo-Marañón M, Piccolo L, et al. Safety monitoring of COVID-19 vaccines: perspective from the European Medicines Agency. Clin Pharmacol Ther. 2023;113(6):1223–34. https://doi.org/10.1002/cpt.2828.
54. Lareb. Jaarverslag 2021. 2021. https://www.lareb.nl/media/afyfia5u/lareb-jaarverslag-2021.pdf. Accessed 24 Oct 2023.
55. Bahri P, Bowring G, Edwards BD, Anton C, Aronson JK, Caro-Rojas A, et al. Communicating for the safe use of medicines: progress and directions for the 2020s promoted by the special interest group of the International Society of Pharmacovigilance. Drug Saf. 2023;46(6):517–32. https://doi.org/10.1007/s40264-023-01285-5.
56. National Public Radio (NPR). All things considered: just 12 people are behind most vaccine hoaxes on social media, research shows; 2021. https://www.npr.org/2021/05/13/996570855/disinformation-dozen-test-facebooks-twitters-ability-to-curb-vaccine-hoaxes. Accessed 27 Nov 2021.
57. Younus MM, Alkhakany M, Bahri P, Caro A, Rostom H, Ndagije HB, et al. The ISoP PatEG-SIG for promoting patient engagement in pharmaco-

vigilance: a change of paradigm is needed. Drug Saf. 2023;46(7):619–23. https://doi.org/10.1007/s40264-023-01313-4.

58. van Grootheest AC, Passier JL, van Puijenbroek EP. Direct reporting of side effects by the patient: favourable experience in the first year. Ned Tijdschr Geneeskd. 2005;149(10):529–33.
59. Aagaard L, Nielsen LH, Hansen EH. Consumer reporting of adverse drug reactions: a retrospective analysis of the Danish adverse drug reaction database from 2004 to 2006. Drug Saf. 2009;32(11):1067–74.
60. Pal SN, Olsson S, Brown EG. The monitoring medicines project: a multinational pharmacovigilance and public health project. Drug Saf. 2015;38(4):319–28. https://doi.org/10.1007/s40264-015-0283-y.
61. World Health Organization (WHO). Safety monitoring of medicinal products—reporting system for the general public; 2012. https://www.who.int/publications/i/item/9789241503198.
62. Borg JJ, Aislaitner G, Pirozynski M, Mifsud S. Strengthening and rationalizing pharmacovigilance in the EU: where is Europe heading to? A review of the new EU legislation on pharmacovigilance. Drug Saf. 2011;34(3):187–97.
63. European Medicines Agency (EMA). The patient's voice in the evaluation of medicines; 2013. http://www.ema.europa.eu/docs/en_GB/document_library/Report/2013/10/WC500153276pdf.
64. European Medicines Agency (EMA). EMA's first public hearing: giving EU citizens a voice to help reduce the risk of valproate; 2017. https://www.ema.europa.eu/en/news/emas-first-public-hearing-giving-eu-citizens-voice-help-reduce-risk-valproate.
65. Bahri P, Pariente A. Systematising pharmacovigilance engagement of patients, healthcare professionals and regulators: a practical decision guide derived from the international risk governance framework for engagement events and discourse. Drug Saf. 2021;44(11):1193–208. https://doi.org/10.1007/s40264-021-01111-w.
66. Brown P, Bahri P. 'Engagement' of patients and healthcare professionals in regulatory pharmacovigilance: establishing a conceptual and methodological framework. Eur J Clin Pharmacol. 2019;75(9):1181–92. https://doi.org/10.1007/s00228-019-02705-1.
67. European Medicines Agency (EMA). Engagement framework: EMA and patients, consumers and their organisations; 2022. https://www.ema.europa.eu/en/documents/other/engagement-framework-european-medicines-agency-patients-consumers-their-organisations_en.pdf. Accessed 0-6-2022 2022.
68. College ter Beoordeling van Geneesmiddelen. Annemiek van Rensen nieuw Collegelid Patienten-en consumentenperspectief; 2015. https://www.cbg-meb.nl/actueel/nieuws/2015/10/01/annemiek-van-rensen-nieuw-collegelid-patienten-en-consumentenperspectief.
69. Janssens R, van Overbeeke E, Verswijvel L, Meeusen L, Coenegrachts C, Pauwels K, et al. Patient involvement in the lifecycle of medicines according to Belgian stakeholders: the gap between theory and practice. Front Med. 2018;5:285. https://doi.org/10.3389/fmed.2018.00285.
70. van Hoof M, Chinchilla K, Härmark L, Matos C, Inácio P, van Hunsel F. Factors contributing to best practices for patient involvement in pharmacovigilance in Europe: a stakeholder analysis. Drug Saf. 2022;45(10):1083–98. https://doi.org/10.1007/s40264-022-01222-y.
71. Laurence DR. Medicine and the media. Br Med J. 1978;2(6133):350–1. https://doi.org/10.1136/bmj.2.6133.350.
72. Inman WHW. Don't tell the patient : behind the drug safety net. 1st ed. Los Angeles: Highland Park Productions; 1999.
73. Andresen V, Hollerbach S. Reassessing the benefits and risks of alosetron: what is its place in the treatment of irritable bowel syndrome? Drug Saf. 2004;27(5):283–92. https://doi.org/10.2165/00002018-200427050-00001.
74. Vitry A, Nguyen T, Entwistle V, Roughead E. Regulatory withdrawal of medicines marketed with uncertain benefits: the bevacizumab case study. J Pharm Policy Pract. 2015;8:25. https://doi.org/10.1186/s40545-015-0046-2.
75. Pierce CE, de Vries ST, Bodin-Parssinen S, Härmark L, Tregunno P, Lewis DJ, et al. Recommendations on the use of mobile applications for the collection and communication of pharmaceutical product safety information: lessons from IMI WEB-RADR. Drug Saf. 2019;42(4):477–89. https://doi.org/10.1007/s40264-019-00813-6.
76. Bahk CY, Goshgarian M, Donahue K, Freifeld CC, Menone CM, Pierce CE, et al. Increasing patient engagement in pharmacovigilance through online community outreach and mobile reporting applications: an analysis of adverse event reporting for the Essure device in the US. Pharmaceut Med. 2015;29(6):331–40. https://doi.org/10.1007/s40290-015-0106-6.
77. Basch E. New frontiers in patient-reported outcomes: adverse event reporting, comparative effectiveness, and quality assessment. Annu Rev Med. 2014;65:307–17. https://doi.org/10.1146/annurev-med-010713-141500.
78. Banerjee AK, Okun S, Edwards IR, Wicks P, Smith MY, Mayall SJ, et al. Patient-reported outcome measures in safety event reporting: PROSPER Consortium guidance. Drug Saf. 2013;36(12):1129–49. https://doi.org/10.1007/s40264-013-0113-z.
79. Desai S. Patient-reported outcomes: engaging patients as partners for better pharmacovigilance practices; 2016. https://www.clinicalleader.com/doc/patient-reported-outcomes-engaging-patients-as-partners-for-better-pharmacovigilance-practices-0001. Accessed 23 Oct 2023.
80. Lawton R, Armitage G. The role of the patient in clinical safety. In: The Health Foundation; 2012. https://www.health.org.uk/publications/the-role-of-the-patient-in-clinical-safety. Accessed 24 Nov 2023.

81. Sharma AE, Rivadeneira NA, Barr-Walker J, Stern RJ, Johnson AK, Sarkar U. Patient engagement in health care safety: an overview of mixed-quality evidence. Health Aff (Millwood). 2018;37(11):1813–20. https://doi.org/10.1377/hlthaff.2018.0716.
82. Kim JM, Suarez-Cuervo C, Berger Z, Lee J, Gayleard J, Rosenberg C, et al. Evaluation of patient and family engagement strategies to improve medication safety. Patient. 2018;11(2):193–206. https://doi.org/10.1007/s40271-017-0270-8.
83. Giles SJ, Lewis PJ, Phipps DL, Mann F, Avery AJ, Ashcroft DM. Capturing patients' perspectives on medication safety: the development of a patient-centered medication safety framework. J Patient Saf. 2020;16(4):e324–e39. https://doi.org/10.1097/pts.0000000000000583.
84. Mohsin-Shaikh S, Garfield S, Franklin BD. Patient involvement in medication safety in hospital: an exploratory study. Int J Clin Pharm. 2014;36(3):657–66. https://doi.org/10.1007/s11096-014-9951-8.
85. Lee JL, Dy SM, Gurses AP, Kim JM, Suarez-Cuervo C, Berger ZD, et al. Towards a more patient-centered approach to medication safety. J Patient Exp. 2018;5(2):83–7. https://doi.org/10.1177/2374373517727532.
86. Broderick JE, DeWitt EM, Rothrock N, Crane PK, Forrest CB. Advances in patient-reported outcomes: the NIH PROMIS(®) measures. EGEMS (Wash DC). 2013;1(1):1015. https://doi.org/10.13063/2327-9214.1015.
87. US Food and Drug Administration (FDA). Patient-reported outcome measures: use in medical product development to support labeling claims;. 2008. https://www.fda.gov/regulatory-information/search-fda-guidance-documents/patient-reported-outcome-measures-use-medical-product-development-support-labeling-claims. Accessed 24 Oct 2023.
88. Reeve BB, Hays RD, Bjorner JB, Cook KF, Crane PK, Teresi JA, et al. Psychometric evaluation and calibration of health-related quality of life item banks: plans for the Patient-Reported Outcomes Measurement Information System (PROMIS). Med Care. 2007;45(5 Suppl 1):S22–31. https://doi.org/10.1097/01.mlr.0000250483.85507.04.
89. Cella D, Riley W, Stone A, Rothrock N, Reeve B, Yount S, et al. The Patient-Reported Outcomes Measurement Information System (PROMIS) developed and tested its first wave of adult self-reported health outcome item banks: 2005–2008. J Clin Epidemiol. 2010;63(11):1179–94. https://doi.org/10.1016/j.jclinepi.2010.04.011.
90. Hays RD, Bjorner JB, Revicki DA, Spritzer KL, Cella D. Development of physical and mental health summary scores from the patient-reported outcomes measurement information system (PROMIS) global items. Qual Life Res. 2009;18(7):873–80. https://doi.org/10.1007/s11136-009-9496-9.
91. US Food and Drug Administration (FDA). CDER learn training and education. https://www.fda.gov/training-and-continuing-education/cderlearn-training-and-education. Accessed 23 Oct 2023.
92. European Medicines Agency (EMA). Partners and networks, patients and consumers; 2023. https://www.ema.europa.eu/en/partners-networks/patients-consumers#activities-of-patients-and-consumers-section. Accessed 21 Oct 2023.
93. US Food and Drug Administration (FDA). Reporting serious problems to FDA; 2023. https://www.fda.gov/safety/medwatch-fda-safety-information-and-adverse-event-reporting-program/reporting-serious-problems-fda. Accessed 21 Oct 2023.
94. European Medicines Agency (EMA). Partners and networks, training and resources for patients and consumers; 2023. Partners and networks, training and resources for patients and consumers. Accessed 21 Oct 2023.

Further Reading

Avery AJ, Anderson C, Bond CM, Fortnum H, Gifford A, Hannaford PC, et al. Evaluation of patient reporting of adverse drug reactions to the UK 'Yellow Card Scheme': literature review, descriptive and qualitative analyses, and questionnaire surveys. Health Technol Assess. 2011;15(20):1–iv.

CIOMS Working Group XI on Patient involvement. Patient involvement in the development, regulation and safe use of medicines. Geneva, Switzerland: Council for International Organizations of Medical Sciences (CIOMS); 2022.

van Hunsel F, Harmark L, Rolfes L. Fifteen years of patient reporting—what have we learned and where are we heading to? Expert Opin Drug Saf. 2019;18(6):477–84.

13 Collaborative Approaches to Establishing and Implementing Pharmacovigilance Systems

Brian Edwards and Angela Caro-Rojas

Abstract

Pharmacovigilance is neither one single discipline nor is it confined to a single professional group. The concept of pharmacovigilance originated with clinical pharmacologists based on the principles of clinical examination of a patient for evidence of causality and then blending these ideas with epidemiological concepts. This was triggered by the thalidomide catastrophe in the 1960s and the need to identify safety signals for medicines much more promptly. Initially, the main priority was the detection of serious and unexpected adverse reactions primarily through analysis of spontaneous reports. Now it is a multidisciplinary topic which requires collaboration from various stakeholders within a complex system to demonstrate that the benefit–harm arm profiles of healthcare products remain acceptable for millions of patients throughout the life cycle of a medicine. These stakeholders include all types of healthcare providers, industry professionals, regulatory agencies, patients and their families, and the wider public. To optimise the use of medicines, we need to understand the role of each stakeholder and strive towards closer cooperation. This requires a flexible and adaptable approach to implementing pharmacovigilance systems in various settings according to different regulatory requirements and the needs of public health both nationally and internationally. It is important for professionals during their development, throughout their career starting as an undergraduate, to understand and appreciate the steps involved in setting up and collaborating within the pharmacovigilance systems at different levels. As ISO 9001 states, a system is how a certain set of processes operate to work towards a particular goal which for pharmacovigilance is to optimise benefit and mitigate harm of medicinal products to enhance patient safety. Unfortunately, the importance of effective implementation of pharmacovigilance as a system based on organisational science including human factors remains under-recognised by many responsible for education and development. Putting human performance at the heart of the pharmacovigilance system design is critical for success. This chapter charts how our current pharmacovigilance system arose based on principles of surveillance and regulation and discusses

B. Edwards (✉)
Husoteria Ltd., Ashtead, Surrey, UK

International Society of Pharmacovigilance, Geneva, Switzerland
e-mail: husoteriabe@gmail.com

A. Caro-Rojas
Pontificia Universidad Javeriana, Bogotá, Colombia

International Society of Pharmacovigilance, Geneva, Switzerland

J. Jose et al. (eds.), *Principles and Practice of Pharmacovigilance and Drug Safety*,
https://doi.org/10.1007/978-3-031-51089-2_13

what should happen now and in the future using systems thinking based on organisational science using a collaborative approach.

Keywords

Benefit–harm · Complex systems · Human factors · Medication safety · Pharmacovigilance · Collaborative approaches

Learning Objectives

- To understand from where and how pharmacovigilance arose to help explain today's processes and the advances that have occurred over time.
- To gain insight into the fundamental principles, challenges, and barriers for setting up a system with a focus on human performance to ensure safe and proper use of medicines.
- Recognise the importance of international pharmacovigilance guidelines and the need for collaboration and cooperation between multiple stakeholders across the system.
- To define principles of a pharmacovigilance quality system and how each task is part of a process with multiple components, links, and influences.

Key Points

- Pharmacovigilance requires a multidisciplinary approach among patients, healthcare professionals (HCPs), and with others such as the industry and government.
- Pharmacovigilance has moved from passive surveillance to active risk management requiring the cooperation of HCPs, patients, and their families.
- Pharmacovigilance is more than just safety but also about designing a system to improve the use of all medicinal products for the benefit of patients.
- HCPs have a critical role in ensuring adequate quality in pharmacovigilance systems to help meet public health needs for society.
- Together as a team, we can apply the science of human factors and organisational learning in the design of better processes that focus on optimising human performance in the global pharmacovigilance system.

1 Introduction

Pharmacovigilance is neither one single discipline nor is it confined to experts of a single professional group. It is a multidisciplinary topic, which refers to the policies, the regulatory structures, processes, technology, information, resources, and medicinal products requiring collaboration from various stakeholders within a complex global sociotechnical system. All this happens round the clock under the scrutiny of politicians, the public, and, more recently, social media. This chapter will discuss the role of the different participants such as healthcare providers (for example, physicians, pharmacists, nurses, and dentists), industrial professionals, regulatory agencies, academics and patients, their families, and the wider public, and the importance and opportunities for partnership between them.

Setting up pharmacovigilance systems in various areas such as hospitals, industry, and regulatory agencies needs different requirements and approaches. It is important for professionals during their development to understand and appreciate the steps involved in setting up, and collaborating within, pharmacovigilance systems at different levels.

2 Why a Pharmacovigilance System Is Essential to Reassure Society About the Effectiveness and Safety of Medicines

A successful pharmacovigilance system is key to help reassure that medicines are effective and safe regardless of whether they are traditional or natural medicines, generic versions of well-established medicines, or newly developed medicines. What society should be trying to achieve in pharmacovigilance has recently and more eloquently been defined as follows: '*pharmacovigilance monitors how different humans are exposed to a myriad of medicines in different ways, for different reasons, in differing situations, using a variety of methods and doses. The science is about detecting not just harm caused by products and substances themselves but also the effects of errors, irrational use, and other almost limitless variables in how they are consumed. Its mission is to constantly examine and learn from this experience to find out why one outcome is better than another and how to prevent or mitigate problems*' [1].

A fundamental requirement for effective pharmacovigilance is integration into the regulatory system for medicines throughout their life cycle. No medicine should be sold without some form of prior licencing or registration by a government. However, the quality of regulatory practice varies across the world and with different medicines. If product quality cannot be assured, no amount of pharmacovigilance can compensate. Product quality complaints may concern product purity, stability (shelf-life), and potential for transmission of infectious agents. Lack of therapeutic effect for the authorised indication may also indicate quality problems [2]. The relationship between pharmacovigilance and product quality is important and is best illustrated by three examples (Fig. 13.1).

Ideally, for a new medicine, pharmacovigilance should start with the preclinical testing phase through to the pivotal clinical trials required to obtain a marketing authorisation. Each phase of development does not have fixed start and end dates so that preclinical testing and clinical pharmacology studies may be extended into the post-marketing phase. A vital part of pharmacovigilance is communicating information effectively to users and HCPs and taking regulatory action when necessary to protect public health. This is referred to as the Summary of Product Characteristics (in the UK or EU) or Package Insert (in the US) and may be accompanied by a patient information leaflet. This latter requirement is not necessarily fulfilled in low-income countries. Once authorised, a pharmaceutical company (within which will be the marketing authorisation holder [MAH]) can market the medicine, either directly or through partners, and post-authorisation surveillance begins [3].

3 A Brief History of How Our Current Global Pharmacovigilance System Arose

Following the thalidomide crisis in the early 1960s, there was much regulatory activity about how to monitor the safety of medicines with the focus on spontaneous reports of suspected adverse reactions for marketed medicines. However, there was no coordination resulting in different regulations, definitions, and reporting forms with no attention to systems thinking or design as that science was still in its infancy [4, 5]. One problem, among many other challenges, for a country's pharmacovigilance regulator, was what to do with foreign cases and multiple positions were adopted nationally. As a result, during the 1960s and 1970s, each country worked out their own schemes for collecting and managing spontaneous reports for marketed products [6, 7]. Such disjointed procedures consumed much effort and time as legislation had to be drafted for each country with some countries making significant organisational changes. In addition to no harmonisation about what to collect and how to manage data both for marketed and investigational products, there was no agreement about how and when regulatory authorities should be kept informed. That is why in the late 1980s, regulators from the three main regions (US, EU, and Japan) had joined with industry to form the International Council (previously Conference) for Harmonisation of Technical Requirements for Pharmaceuticals for Human Use (ICH). ICH's mission is to achieve greater harmonisation worldwide to ensure that safe, effective, and high-quality medicines are developed and registered in the most resource-efficient manner.

QUALITY EXAMPLE 1: In 1979, a urinary antiseptic called oxalinic acid, was shown to cause rapid resistance in previously sensitive bacteria causing lack of effect. As a result, the licence was suspended.

QUALITY EXAMPLE 2: FDA pools data about product quality obtained from GMP inspections, adverse events, and substandard pharmaceutical bioequivalence issues. As a result, FDA withdrew generic bupropion, and metoprolol in 2014 and methylphenidate in 2015 after reports of subtherapeutic outcomes which is when a product does not perform as expected because of issues with the active pharmaceutical ingredients or excepients or low-quality manufacturing practices.

QUALITY EXAMPLE 3: Between 1998 and 2004, a change in manufacturing led to an increase in pure red cell aplasia (PRCA) associated with erythropoietin alpha which has never been fully explained. The marketing authorisation holders were required to monitor cases classified as lack of effect carefully to capture all PRCA cases in case this important adverse reaction has been missed.

Fig. 13.1 Examples illustrating relation between pharmacovigilance and product quality

Harmonisation is achieved through the development of ICH guidelines through a process of scientific consensus with regulatory and industry experts working side-by-side. Key to the success of this process is the commitment of the ICH regulators to implement the final guidelines. These ICH guidelines form the foundation for international regulatory pharmacovigilance [8]. Based on the recommendations of the Council for International Organizations of Medical Sciences (CIOMS) and ICH, common definitions and standards for reporting for individual cases and aggregate datasets were developed that were then implemented in the ICH regions. However, variations in the detail remained between the regions so that although the principles have been harmonised through ICH, the regulatory details about implementation can still vary, often for reasons which remain obscure.

An important step in harmonising EU-wide multiple national systems was the creation of the EU pharmacovigilance system starting on January 1, 1995, with the European Medicines Agency (previously called EMEA, now EMA) and a central database, EudraVigilance which came later [9]. A further major change in EU pharmacovigilance occurred with a new legislation in 2012 (Directive 2010/84/EU). This legislation established Good Pharmacovigilance Practices (GVP) which are legally binding and are divided into modules covering major pharmacovigilance processes with modules covering product- or population-specific considerations such as vaccines and biologicals. There are special chapters dedicated to pregnancy and breast feeding and the geriatric population. As GVP applies to EU market authorisation holders wherever they market their medicines, this legislation has had global impact either through the affiliates of multinational companies or through the implementation of pharmacovigilance agreements with partners [10, 11].

It is important to remember that even now there are still countries, such as those with a low-income, whose pharmacovigilance systems are at an early phase of development. There are also some countries which have not started talking about medicine safety. That means within the International Society of Pharmacovigilance we often find a lack of understanding amongst HCPs about pharmacovigilance.

4 The Move from Passive Surveillance to Active Risk Management

In the 1990s, there were several high-profile studies showing the extensive harm caused by all forms of medical errors including harm from medicines [12–14]. This led to a recognition that pharmacovigilance needed to be reformed by starting the process earlier before a marketing authorisation is granted, and that a change in philosophy was needed towards demonstrating safety as opposed to looking for harm. This led to the creation of 'risk management' strategies to be applied to the development and marketing of medicines throughout their life cycles. These risk management strategies have common themes including dialogue between stakeholders and the creation and maintenance of risk management or minimisation plans which can be implemented once a marketing authorisation is granted. These ideas were first discussed in an important seminal document produced by US FDA in 1999 entitled 'Managing the Risks from Medical Product Use: Creating a Risk Management Framework'. Recommendations included heightened surveillance of products on the market, further epidemiological studies, and enhanced communication. The report emphasised the need for greater systems integration because risk management is a shared responsibility with industry, HCPs, patients, other government departments, healthcare delivery system, and professional organisations. A safe product is one that has reasonable risks, given the magnitude of the benefit expected and the alternatives available [15].

Throughout the decade from 2000, risk management developed into active planning and risk minimisation and ICH then produced ICHE2E guidelines which have been implemented in each of the main ICH regions [16]. The US emphasised risk minimisation whereas the EU and Japan developed the concept of full risk management. Despite these ICH guidelines and definitions, there is no internationally agreed definition for integrating risk management for both pharmaceuticals and devices together so that separate legislation for their regulatory systems remains. Regionally and nationally, regulators have developed their own practical strategies for blending the collection and analysis of safety information for medicines and devices with measures to reduce risks to patients in their jurisdiction [17]. The US FDA's definition of risk management is useful for all involved with medicines and devices by describing the continuing process of minimising risk throughout the product's life cycle to optimise benefit–harm balance [18]. First, benefits and harms are evaluated, then risks minimised through appropriate interventions, which are evaluated and revised as information is gathered about impact. A risk minimisation tool is a process, or a new system, intended to minimise known risks. This may be enhancing the communication of further guidance about prescribing, dispensing, and/or using product in most appropriate circumstances or patient populations. The categories of tools which can be discussed between stakeholders include:

1. Targeted education and outreach, specifically, to increase knowledge for key people or groups is often used especially if it can be linked to continuing medical education. For the industry, these can be introduced in disease management or patient access programmes.
2. Reminder systems in addition to targeted education that prompt, remind, double check, or otherwise guide HCPs and/or patients in prescribing, dispensing, or receiving products in ways that minimise risk.
3. Performance-linked access systems are those which link access to product to laboratory testing results or other documentation.

Points to consider when choosing a tool to minimise risk require discussion and cooperation between stakeholders to try and ensure that the optimal tools are selected and implemented for each healthcare system. These tools should maintain widest access to a medicine while creating the least burden on both the healthcare system and relationships between HCPs and patients. This means that sponsors of such tools, which are usually MAHs, should obtain input from key groups about the feasibility of implementing and accepting tools in usual healthcare practices, disease conditions, and lifestyles. This includes compatibility of tools with current technology and that they are applicable in both outpatient and inpatient settings with accessibility to patients in diverse localities, including non-urban. Tools should be consistent with existing tools or programmes that have been shown to be effective with similar products, indications, or risks. The MAH for a medicine usually has a responsibility to periodically evaluate the effectiveness of risk minimisation and report to the supervising regulatory authority at agreed intervals [19, 20].

5 Impact of Social Media and the Internet on Pharmacovigilance

One evolving aspect of the global pharmacovigilance system which involves many of us has been the impact of social media and the internet because patients, carers, and their families can generate information concerning safety and effectiveness of medicines. However, such social media data are unstructured and lack quality standards. Key issues around patient self-generated reports on social media are credibility and origin of reports with concerns about inadequate and inconsistent data requiring additional follow-up which in turn is very difficult [21, 22]. It is uncertain how best to integrate social media 'AE' reports with those obtained from more standard sources, especially to identify duplicates and map multi-lingual data which may use colloquial and slang terminology. Another concern is the potential bias due to the reporter population [23]. Of the many social media users, only a small percentage (1%) specifically report adverse events, while most others occasionally contribute or observe. Many elderly individuals, constituting a large demographic of prescription medication users, may not use social media or use it in a different way, creating a strong user bias for pharmacovigilance using social media.

From the published evidence, it appears that many tweets and Facebook postings would have to be examined to identify any important new information relevant to benefits and harms. When social media has been examined and AEs identified, they are usually labelled and non-serious. An occasional new ADR can be found. As described in EU Good Pharmacovigilance Practice module VI, there is EU regulatory consensus about MAH sponsored social media activities so that cases of suspected adverse reactions from the internet or digital media should be handled as spontaneous reports. However, assessment of these cases reveals that it is difficult to identify duplicates and validate individual case components such as 'reporter details', severity, and seriousness which have different meanings with these postings and follow-up is in practice very difficult. As a result, there remains regulatory uncertainty about how to handle information from non-sponsored sources (e.g. social media listening, noncompany website) if information cannot be structured into an individual case safety report or an identifiable product complaint [24].

6 The Importance of Quality Systems and Human Factors for Pharmacovigilance

In pharmacovigilance, there is a need to pay close attention to the design of appropriate processes and quality of those actions required for the collection, collation, and evaluation of good quality information, which can be transformed into good-quality data. A common medical terminology, The Medical Dictionary for Drug Regulatory Affairs (MedDRA), is used by regulatory agencies and the industry for supporting transfer of information [25]. These data form the basis for how the pharmaceutical sector assesses the benefits and harms of a medicine. This up-to-date information needs to be communicated to relevant HCPs and patients in a way so that it can be interpreted unambiguously, which is a huge challenge with variable results across the world [26, 27]. No single system of surveillance such as spontaneous reporting will pick up every problem which is why we require additional epidemiological data to help us, for example, understand the profile of diseases in the intended target population as well as the frequency of serious medical events and mortality rates, which can confound causality assessment of suspected adverse reactions. This epidemiology is especially important for orphan medicines for rare diseases where a low number of patients makes ADRs difficult to distinguish from background adverse events.

Every national pharmacovigilance system will have its own needs based on some fundamental principles that form the basis of the current EU Good Pharmacovigilance Practices and system that are in place today in Europe [28, 29]. However, as with many healthcare areas, there is increasing pressure to do more with less. Every country has limited resources with respect to the size of the pharmacovigilance tasks that face them. This means that we can never achieve everything that we want in pharmacovigilance, so that priorities must be set, and expectations of stakeholders carefully managed. On top of this, there have been numerous advances in developing new medical technologies with a proliferation of new and complex products. This means the system struggles to keep up to date and find the necessary expertise to assess and monitor evidence from new medicines derived from innovative technologies. In addition, there is worldwide shortage of professionals working full time in pharmacovigilance and so available expertise must be used prudently, especially in low-income countries. This makes it imperative for all of us in pharmacovigilance to adopt efficiencies, leverage the work of others, and collaborate across regulatory authorities and institutions to achieve better regulation and oversight over national markets for medicines. Thus, the less money available for a country, the more important good-quality design is for a country's pharmacovigilance system as such a country can ill afford waste and duplication of effort. These challenges led to the understanding that pharmacovigilance should be implemented as a quality system which is flexible, adaptable, and fit for purpose for each organisation and each country [30]. This in turn requires cooperation and collaboration by all participants in a system.

When discussing a system, it is important to examine the relevance of human factors otherwise known as ergonomics. These are both defined as the scientific discipline concerned with the understanding of interactions among humans and other elements of a system, and the profession that applies theory, principles, data, and methods to system design to optimise human well-being and overall system performance [31]. In pharmacovigilance, we consider patient safety includes safety of medicines, which means focusing attention on the patient's quality of life and how it is affected by medicines in real life, beyond the pharmacology of how medicines affect patients. Additionally, we must include those who are managing medications such as HCPs and patients, by examining their limitations, cognitive biases, and ignorance about medication risk. In healthcare, some concepts such as human-centred care and humanism are related and impact safe use of medicines.

Each pharmacovigilance system requires strategies and plans to ensure continuity and enable prompt recovery from any type of disruption such as pandemics, natural disasters, or conflict. Codes of ethics and conduct supported by monitoring and enforcement, including sanctions for misconduct are also important in a pharmacovigilance system. There should not be inconsistencies between different policies across the wider national and international systems as this can result in barriers to implementation and wasted effort. Unfortunately, lack of harmonisation remains a significant issue. Therefore, goals of any pharmacovigilance system should be aligned with the health goals both nationally and internationally which can be summarised as six main components as described in Table 13.1.

Table 13.1 Components of any pharmacovigilance system

I. An adequate and appropriate pharmacovigilance policy with strategic aims to meet the public health needs of a country. This may include the following:
Identification of the existence of current, future, and emerging hazards
Determination of which hazards pose the greatest risks to human health or the environment
Development of effective strategies to manage risks including how to measure the benefits of regulatory action and assess unintended consequences
Allocation of resources rationally and effectively
Stakeholders recognise how their role is involved in the system, what their responsibilities are and act appropriately
II. Pharmacovigilance processes need to be defined in sufficient detail to describe how the main system outputs are created to a pre-defined quality to enable the following:
Effective information management systems that involve efficient case management and filing and archiving of documentation and evidence with timely retrieval
Continuous and timely information on the clinical expression of ADRs
Adequate information on at-risk groups and underlying mechanisms and risk factors such as pharmacogenomics
Analysis of causality based on algorithms, and approaches blending human factors and complex system sciences
Rapid and precise detection of important signals
A sufficiently precise estimate of risk to allow valid benefit-risk evaluations and comparisons of risk
Ability to respond and communicate robustly to important safety concerns with a medicine within a reasonable timeframe, including detailed risk communication and interaction with journalists and media
Actions to minimise the risk, such as educational campaigns and up-to-date information for HCPs and patients or regulatory actions such as a change in authorisation and labelling or access arrangements
III. Definition of scope of product responsibility and areas to be covered including territorial jurisdiction
A system flexible enough to adapt to all therapeutic areas including clinical trial safety, compassionate use, and post-authorisation surveillance; consumer products including nutraceuticals, herbals, natural products, and cosmetics; counterfeit strategy
Appropriate oversight of promotional and marketing activities of the pharmaceutical industry and other sectors to ensure fair and balanced messaging about a medicine

Table 13.1 (continued)

IV. Sufficient staff who are trained and competent working in a motivational and learning culture
Organograms and diagrams of organisational structure to demonstrate accountability and governance relationships
Roles and responsibilities defined in job descriptions
Available expertise in workload, resource, and financial management
Continuous training considering best evidence in pharmacovigilance
V. Ability to monitor and report on pharmacovigilance performance through system reviews, audits, inspections, and investigations when normal processes fail
VI. A fair and risk-proportionate system for regulating the pharmaceutical industry to ensure marketing authorisations are kept up to date with variations and renewals, individual case and periodic reports are assessed, and product risk is adequately managed through communication and other risk minimisation measures

7 The Need for Better Capacity Building in Pharmacovigilance

A large gap remains in pharmacovigilance capacity and expertise from one country to another emphasising the need for cooperation and team working between all stakeholders [32]. Experience from organisations such as the World Health Organization (WHO) shows that capacity develops in phases and over time. Factors such as the level of development and legal basis of the pharmaceutical sector, appropriate regulations, and the availability of trained staff, infrastructure, and financial resources influence the size and sophistication of the pharmacovigilance system and its ability to carry out various pharmacovigilance functions [33, 34]. International experience suggests that pharmacovigilance is often only as strong as the available resources for activities such as training and education the availability of which in turn influences implementing a quality system. Training can be in the form of manuals, videos, workshops, courses, simulation learning, case-based learning, or on-the-job learning. Such training in pharmacovigilance should be incorporated in a country's medical curricula for training of HCPs [35]. Human resource barriers to implementation of a pharmacovigilance system include overburdened staff, a high staff turnover, the mobility of staff between jobs, the mobility of patients between different healthcare facilities, and inadequate allocation of healthcare resource within and between countries. Poorly developed technological infrastructure such as a slow internet can undermine the system.

8 Why Communication, Collaboration, and Cooperation Are Essential for Pharmacovigilance

As already explained above, those of us who work in pharmacovigilance, as in many other aspects of public health, are expected to do more with less. This makes it imperative to adopt efficiencies, leverage the work of others, and collaborate across regulatory authorities, other government departments, healthcare systems and institutions to achieve better pharmacovigilance systems with adequate scientific and regulatory oversight of national markets. That is why the WHO has stressed that we all have a responsibility to strengthen the system by fostering interdependent engagement among countries and national and exogenous stakeholders. We need intelligence and information mechanisms to improve communication between national regulatory authorities, state pharmacovigilance centres, patients, HCPs, policymakers, and the public with respect to supporting the safe use of medicines. At an inter-governmental level, the pharmacovigilance system should interface with the environmental agency pricing and reimbursement and enforcement services including the police and customs. More broadly, pharmacovigilance centres need to interact with the many different parts of the pharmaceutical industry such as parallel importers, distributors, and wholesalers as well as professional bodies for healthcare professionals. All these groups should aim to provide safe and effective medicines to patients and so should be looking for synergies between their own policy or business objectives and be conscious of mixed or conflicting messages about the benefits and harms of medicines.

9 The Role of the Pharmaceutical Industry and Regulators

The pharmaceutical industry consists of more than just the large multinational research and development companies which provide the most familiar image. The industry is a complex arrangement involving distributors and wholesalers, importers under special licence such as parallel imports, as well as vendors such as contract research organisations and consultants. There are multiple industry bodies, and there is no one body that speaks as the 'voice of the industry' or who acts as a leader. Through pharmacovigilance regulation and guidances, industry requires up-to-date clarity from regulatory authorities about their expectations concerning what submissions should occur within what timeframes with timely and constructive regulatory feedback. The pharmacovigilance regulator must optimise the relationship with the industry through mutual respect for their respective roles without the regulator compromising their impartiality and independence. Through constructive dialogue, between all interested parties, practical risk minimisation measures can be designed where they are appropriate.

Clarification of regulatory expectations about how industry should implement pharmacovigilance regulations can be achieved through issuing guidances, newsletters, public presentations, and setting up an information service for industry. The sort of pharmacovigilance topics which can cause uncertainty are expectations for a national qualified person for pharmacovigilance, what reporting should occur between submission of a marketing authorisation and its approval, arrangements for electronic reporting and periodicity of periodic report submission. In addition, the pharmacovigilance regulator can help the industry set its own pharmacovigilance priorities stressing the importance of signal detection and the obligation to report all relevant safety information to a regulator and what relevant means.

Regulatory safety actions may include, in extreme cases, restricting indications, suspension, withdrawal, or revocation of the marketing authorisation. More often these actions involve amendments to the package leaflet, labelling, and summary of product characteristics (SPC) (safety variations) and education about proper use for the HCP and patients [36]. There are multiple organisations in many national systems who influence the safe and effective use of medicines both pre- and post-authorisation. For example, in the United Kingdom, as well as the MHRA, the National Institute for Health and Clinical Excellence makes safety recommendations as do the various National Health Services (NHS), professional bodies such as the Royal Colleges, and professional regulators such as the General Medical Council and General Pharmaceutical Council. However, there is usually just one regulatory authority who issues marketing authorisations and directly regulates MAHs in one market.

To help get the best out of industry, engagement requires having a high-level understanding of how a company commercialises a product to enable better integration of risk minimisation solutions. Such commercial activities include market research, patient support programmes, and product promotion. There is an increasing number of company initiatives concerning patient and public engagement, which should be welcome although processes need to be transparent about objectives, funding, and outcomes. HCPs should better appreciate the heterogeneity and complexity of the industry and their ethical obligations. This will help them understand about who they are dealing with in a company and identify where they have common priorities without compromising ethical behaviour and impartiality in the choice of a medicine [37].

10 Interactions Between the Regulators and the Healthcare System

Those within government with a responsibility for pharmacovigilance regulation would be expected to coordinate across different stakeholders to monitor, evaluate, and reach common decisions about medicines [38, 39]. This includes taking a lead in initiatives relating to electronic information networks, data standards, and terminology to facilitate communication. There may be legitimate differences to explain why the licensing and pharmacovigilance systems do differ [36]. Information about the benefits and harms of a medicine obtained in a certain country (e.g. the country of origin of the drug) may not be relevant to other parts of the world, where circumstances may be different [26]. Safety of a medicine will be impacted by genetics, diet, and traditions of the people. The end finished product may arise from a country outside direct supervision of a regulator. Indeed, components of a medicinal product (such as the carton and other packaging) may come from different sources.

Domestic manufacturers may be operating to a different pharmacopeia resulting in pharmaceutical quality and composition (excipients) of locally produced pharmaceutical products. The package insert for HCPs may differ regarding indications and dose. The use of medicines which are not regulated (e.g. herbal remedies) may create special toxicological problems, when used alone or in combination with other medicines, posing challenges to harmonisation. Thus, socio-political attitudes to how medicines are regulated and how patients and families can access medicines influence the conduct of pharmacovigilance. This makes collaboration between all the stakeholders even more essential for pharmacovigilance systems to function effectively. Additionally, the restricted resources of regulatory agencies, manufacturers, and hospitals, particularly in low-income countries, means it is difficult to enact both vigilance and preventive actions.

Developing national pharmacovigilance systems requires close interaction between the regulatory and the healthcare systems to collect continuous and timely information on the clinical expression of ADRs [39, 40]. This may include setting up centres for the collection and evaluation of suspected adverse reactions and reports of misuse and abuse. Where they exist, toxicology and poisoning centres play an important role as well as being the experts in the management of overdoses. The pharmacovigilance regulator may want more information about underlying mechanisms and at-risk groups for suspected adverse reactions which requires discussions about feasible modes of data collection and study. This may involve collection of biological material such as is required for pharmacogenomics. Agreement is required about how best to record medication errors and what should be public health priorities which in turn will be translated into priorities for the pharmacovigilance system. Should the pharmacovigilance regulator or pharmacovigilance centre identify a safety concern with a medicine, discussion with relevant healthcare stakeholders is needed to identify and implement practical risk minimisation measures. This may include a collaborative approach with HCPs and patients about how best to communicate risk and newly emerging safety issues.

11 The Role of Academia and the Place of Scientific Societies and Professional Bodies of Healthcare Professionals

HCPs and academia provide an important source of expert advice, analysis, and opinion within the pharmacovigilance system especially as many are involved in treating patients or undertaking drug safety and pharmacovigilance research activities. By directly or indirectly working closely with those who use medicinal products, they may be more in tune with real-life clinical use of medicines and may propose original solutions to improve use. They may take a position on safety issues themselves as well which may not be aligned with the regulatory view [41, 42]. However, they have an ethical obligation to ensure that messages for users are evidence-based, coherent, and consistent. In undergraduate healthcare professional training, it is still uncommon in many countries to have a specific module for pharmacovigilance [43, 44]. Where it does appear in training for healthcare professions then it usually involves pharmacology or clinical risk management of patients with inadequate emphasis about the sociotechnical system that supports medication safety [45–47]. A collaborative approach with patients and their families means an active approach can be taken to minimise the risk of adverse effects and if it is possible to prevent irreversible harm which should be the common aim for all.

As regards formal undergraduate and postgraduate training, this is more limited and is usually confined to short courses. Apart from the EU programme in Pharmacovigilance and Pharmacoepidemiology, very few universities offer a Masters or a PhD about pharmacovigilance topics. This means there are few options to develop deeper research into pharmacovigilance to critically evaluate current scientific approaches, and the quality of the system. Indeed, there are only a few academic departments with dedicated research groups who are critically evaluating pharmacovigilance regulations to assess whether their implementation has achieved their public health objectives or whether implementation could be improved.

Collaboration among stakeholders, who manage and use medicines regularly, should produce better-defined information for decision-makers and feed the system with a different and a more elaborate worldview. Academic societies can help with comparative benefit–harm assessments and develop treatment algorithms in a way regulators cannot as they focus on individual MAHs. As HCPs dispense, prescribe, and use medicines, it is important for them to understand how intrinsic human factors, such as cognitive bias, fatigue, and stress, impact decision-making so individuals can mitigate against any unwanted impact on prescribing or using a medicine safely [48, 49]. The inclusion of teaching about human factors and complex systems in academia could help us all to better understand the risks from medicines, not just as a product problem, but as a complex sociotechnical system, and a design challenge as suggested by WHO [35, 46]. Such education and learning would help not just physicians but also all HCPs understand how best to balance productivity at work (such as: working with limited resources of money, time pressures, and adverse human interactions) and the safety of the patients while encouraging optimal use of medicines. Depending on the healthcare institution, the processes should be sensitive to the performance needs of HCPs, balancing costs while minimising unacceptable and avoidable risks for patients. Unfortunately, close attention to culture, systems, and human factors is still insufficiently commonplace in the education of HCPs in many countries which in turn impacts on the effective use of medicines. Countries should examine the experience of the UK and US with the role of medication safety officers to assess whether their healthcare systems would benefit from such a role [50, 51].

Professional bodies for HCPs often produce guidelines which include recommendations about safe product use. They have a responsibility to incorporate pharmacovigilance both within ethical and professional codes and into curricula as well as professional certification and accreditation. Programmes such as Prescribing Safety Assessment are a good example of collaboration between the British Pharmacology Society and the General Medical Council to improve education and training about safe prescribing for doctors in the UK. In addition, there are prescribers who are not physicians such as pharmacists and midwives in the UK. They have the responsibility to develop a basic level of pharmacovigilance competency. In addition, these societies have the possibility to influence public policies and inform the impartial position of experts in various topics to help the government to take decisions. It is important for such societies to have transparent policies about conflict of interest. Some of these societies produce material that may later be adopted by regulators to facilitate dialogue between the regulatory authority and the wider community (such as recommendations for cardiac resuscitation or management of anaphylaxis).

12 The Place of Patient Organisations and Groups

Patient groups and patients are an important stakeholder of increasing importance who should, where possible, be involved in decision-making such as advisory groups. They will expect as much transparency as possible behind the basis of safety decisions. To hear from individual patients either in hospital or the community, directly or indirectly through their HCPs, helps those in pharmacovigilance understand the reality of use for a medicinal product as well as identifying those aspects which are important for them [52–54]. This may refer not only to suspected adverse reactions about a medicine but also the consideration of how the medicine has impacted their quality of life [55]. For example, some patients (particularly in low- and middle-income countries) with HIV continue living with stigmas that do not allow them to have the freedom and confidence to talk about their treatments which in turn risks low knowledge, which could lead to adverse effects too. In addition to the elderly, the frail, and those with sensory impairment of communication, there are groups of patients who may be easily overlooked such as the incarcerated and refugees, who may have special needs and challenges to ensuring access to safe medicines let alone ensure these medicines are used properly.

To open channels of easy and free communication between patients and government helps understand problems arising from the context and reality of use of medicines for patients. By adding such information to the results in clinical trials to help improve decision-making relies on transforming real-world patient experiences into quality data [56]. Sometimes patients find original solutions to optimise use of medicines which is why some hospitals implement peer support to manage patients. For example, when patients collaborate as peers they can educate each other about adverse reactions, how to act in case they suspect an adverse reaction, when they should seek medical advice or when it is better to remain calm and wait. To improve patient engagement must be a priority for understanding what patients need, what they can teach us, and how other stakeholders could contribute to their safety [57, 58]. Recently, CIOMS released a report entitled 'Patient involvement in the development, regulation, and safe use of medicines' which they refer to as a pragmatic handbook summarising our current understanding of best practice [59]. Their assessment is succinctly summarised as follows:

To date, research on the impact of patient and public involvement is sparse and it is not known which strategies are most appropriate. Qualitative and quantitative research is needed to better understand what constitutes meaningful patient and public involvement and how to optimise processes and strategies to obtain the best and most impactful input from patients and members of the public. Patient and public involvement rests mainly on ethical and democratic principles. So even if we do not yet know what works best in different settings and for each different goal, there is no doubt that strengthening patient involvement in all healthcare contexts and taking every effort to make it meaningful is the way to go....'

13 The Place of Those Who Work in Logistics and Sellers of Medicines

Everyone who contributes to the logistics and supply chain has a significant responsibility in ensuring safe use of medicines and appropriate risk management especially concerning product diversion [60]. For example, should a patient develop a very strange and unexpected adverse reaction, the plausibility of which no one can explain, the possibility of a counterfeit, contaminated, or adulterated product should be considered early on. Good distribution practice with tracking and tracing of medicines can help shield patients from the risk of low-quality substituted and counterfeit medicines. For some medicines, such as opiate derivatives, diversion for criminal and abuse purposes is an added risk and additional regulations and safeguards may be needed. All HCPs need to be exceptionally vigilant in checking where and how these medicines are being used and assist in their tracking.

When pharmacists dispense prescribed medicines or sell medicines directly to patients, this is not merely the last step in logistics and distribution. Pharmacists have a key role in providing education to patients to ensure proper use of a medicine, and what they should do in case they develop certain symptoms after taking their therapy which may be a reportable adverse reaction. This would include encouraging them to report concerns through national reporting schemes as has been set up on the portal of the UK Regulatory Authority (https://yellowcard.mhra.gov.uk/).

What do we expect from those who are involved in pharmacovigilance?

To address the shortage in capacity throughout the pharmacovigilance system it requires explaining what we should expect from all those who are engaged in pharmacovigilance as a career. Regardless of the position of the role in the pharmacovigilance system, the authors suggest seeking the following attributes during appointment which are developed once in post (see Fig. 13.2).

Questioning attitude: They should show an interest in problem solving and wanting to find solutions by showing adaptability and flexibility.

Act rigorously and prudently: They should pay close attention to detail with a desire to establish the facts without cutting corners. A sensible and honest approach to decision-making and actions is required in recognising one's own limi-

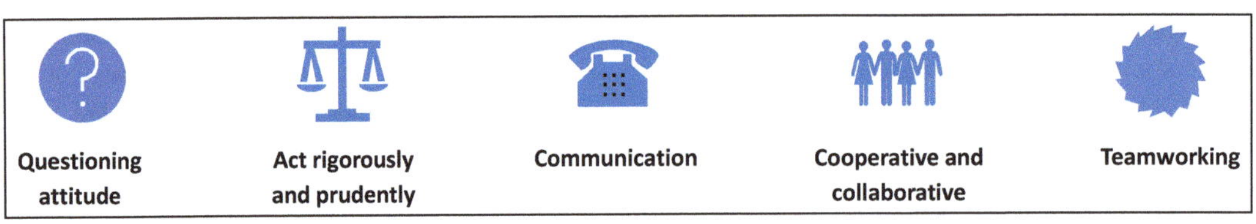

Fig. 13.2 Skills needed for people who work in pharmacovigilance

tations and understanding one's own role and how it fits into the system. Prompt management of errors should be encouraged as well as looking upon them as an opportunity to learn both for the individual and for the team.

Communication: They should be careful and precise with use of terminology such as not confusing an adverse event with an adverse reaction. This means prompt correction and clarification if there is misunderstanding about communications about safety of medicines. Assertiveness is an asset as knowing how to escalate and to whom when operational, compliance, or safety concerns arise. We need individuals who can keep their manager and team appropriately informed.

Cooperative and collaborative: They should engage team members and other organisational members in a positive spirit as recognising interdependent and reliance. Being helpful and polite wherever possible are key attributes in the stressful environment for many in pharmacovigilance.

Teamworking: In pharmacovigilance, we should think of each process in terms of who is in the team and how we can work together to support each other. We should remember the team may well extend beyond our own organisation. Identifying individual and collective strengths and weaknesses is critical so that measures that can mitigate risk can be implemented. Prioritisation on what is important is essential. We need to recognise the importance of a shared mental state, collective orientation, and situational awareness especially when these human factor elements are poorly designed within the processes for those working within an organisation.

14 Elements for Achieving a Good Interaction Among Stakeholders

Collaboration between all these stakeholders that we have mentioned is required for product risk management and effective risk minimisation. This means helping each participant in the system define their role within the system which requires stakeholder engagement. Policy recommendations for government, professional societies, and business to achieve these aims are as follows:

- Influencing professional education and core competency training to include pharmacovigilance and risk management
- Integrating technology with uniform application of healthcare IT and app development with input into design of analytical tools such as for data queries, data entry, and editing
- Developing new methodologies for available datasets such as patient outcomes in electronic health records
- Identifying additional risk minimisation measures for products of public health importance which have risks not manageable through routine activities
- Prioritising surveillance for newly marketed products based on agreed criteria
- Intervening for special risk products such as mandatory education through a register and reminder schemes; restricted distribution and performance-linked access such as pregnancy prevention schemes
- Ensuring there are adequate legislative mechanisms for risk interventions such as authority to suspend marketing authorisations and protection of HCPs should they wish to report adverse reactions
- Arranging regular meetings with stakeholders based on good communication practices

The final point above concerning good communication is critical so it is worth reflecting on what good principles for collaboration across the pharmacovigilance system between different roles might look like:

Open and transparent communication: The ethical, legal, and regulatory environment requires that the interests of each stakeholder should be declared (most of which may be totally legitimate and uncontroversial) with specific conflict of interests being revealed when a particular safety situation is under review.

Confidence to speak up: When interests are declared in a just and fair culture, then this builds confidence between stakeholders to enable frank and open discussion. Such confidence requires time to build, and human interactions and performance should be monitored to ensure that all stakeholders are behaving with transparency, objectivity, and adherence to safety objectives.

Creating a focus on common goals aligned with healthcare priorities: It is important for the stakeholders to define specific goals for their own country and region bearing in mind the following points:

- Although patient safety is the most important goal, different stakeholders may have legitimately different interpretations as to what that means. Ideally, this should be supported with evidence using systematic reviews and real-world studies about effectiveness.
- To understand that every stakeholder has conflict of interests and the best scenario all should seek is a win-win situation requiring sensitive negotiation with attention to detail. Stakeholders should recognise that compromise may be required, or else access to medical products can be impaired and excessive burden on healthcare system introduced with unintended consequences.
- To understand that medication risk is a systemic problem and not solely an individual responsibility.
- Identify and agree on what are avoidable important risks and how much effort should be spent to minimise them.
- To share wherever possible relevant information in the interests of patients recognising that some stakeholders will have genuine proprietary concerns.

15 Summary and Conclusions

The concept, scope, and practice of pharmacovigilance has developed considerably since its inception in the 1960s. We now understand that pharmacovigilance encompasses all aspects of evaluation of drug safety across the life cycle including monitoring clinical investigation as soon as a medicine enters humans and extends into how medicines are used in clinical practice. A proactive, systematic, and investigative approach is necessary in pharmacovigilance using a variety of methods of surveillance and evaluation. At all phases, key objectives of pharmacovigilance remain identification of new hazards or changing safety profiles, taking actions to improve safe use of medicines and communications of all matters concerning drug safety to all end users including patients. These actions underpin benefit/harm assessment as part of clinical safety pre-authorisation, assessment at the time of granting a marketing authorisation and then continues as post-authorisation development including progress to change of legal status from prescription only to pharmacy and over-the-counter status [61].

Although regulation is important and necessary, it alone cannot create good quality pharmacovigilance. We must take a systems approach incorporating all stakeholders with patients at the centre. Such a pharmacovigilance system can be understood as a combination of three subsystems based on information collection/data management, analysis/signal detection, and interventions to manage risk [62]. Thus, our understanding of the scope of pharmacovigilance systems extends beyond the scientific risk of medicines and devices and includes risk when humans in the real world use these products in clinical environments and ambulatory care such as in homes and community residences. This means pharmacovigilance involves more than just the regulator or company who is legally accountable for a medicine's safety but also the wider community in general, including addressing the vision and wishes of patients and their families. Each HCP has a key role in advising and implementing ideas about risk minimisation, how best to communicate among stakeholders the possibility of risk and why measures to protect patients are needed. Finally, it is the patients and their clinicians who should decide ultimately whether a medicine is effective or not, and its safety profile is acceptable. They have a responsibility to know what to do should they suspect an adverse reaction, or a medication error has occurred to a medicine and how they should notify the appropriate authorities.

Despite the considerable progress in pharmacovigilance and risk management, there remain significant questions which require more in-depth and detailed collaboration between stakeholders to help us resolve them. We all know that 'safety is everybody's responsibility' but what does that mean? What is meant by risk-based compliance? What is the basis for an effective safety system? How can we facilitate reporting of meaningful information about medicines? These questions reflect changing values and attitudes in society towards risks and human rights so these must be kept under review. Ultimately, the solutions to many avoidable risks with medicines result from humans working in complex systems, where they will make what appear to be medication errors (or so it may seem although often what we call 'errors' reflect what most people would have done under a certain set of circumstances). This is because ultimately the safe use of medicines and devices depends on human performance. This is not just the performance of the end user, such as the prescribing healthcare professional and their patients, but all who contribute to the pharmacovigilance system from the governing bodies at the top to the end users at the bottom of the hierarchy.

There is now overwhelming evidence that most of what is referred to as non-compliance and unsafe use of a medicine or device can be explained by understanding human factors and system design which can be referred to as organisational science. There is good news as the science around human factors has expanded in the last 20 years so that there is a vast amount of evidence that can be examined [63]. We now better understand the importance and relevance of topics such as situational awareness, leadership, communication, error management, understanding the impact of personality on human performance and safety behaviour, and finally, safe decision-making [63]. In addition, there are already those individual professionals scattered throughout the global pharmacovigilance system with excellent human factors skills who have been struggling individually to make the system more effective when they can exert influence. The problem is that this piecemeal approach means that standards for making human factors the centre of process design have not been systematised or recognised for their importance. Indeed, there are no globally accepted principles to achieve a global system to optimise use of medicines [64]. In the absence of internationally agreed guiding principles, it will remain challenging for the wide array of stakeholders to cooperate and collaborate both within and between national systems for ensuring safe use of medical products.

To our knowledge, there has been little emphasis on system design and organisational sciences in pharmacovigilance curricula and training. Training in the industry and elsewhere concerning safety of medical products is all too often focused only on documented standard operating procedures although these documents are only part of the process and all features of a process require attention in pharmacovigilance. No organisation can afford to ignore human factors given that they are often primarily responsible for many examples of process breakdown. There is an urgent need to optimise human performance within the pharmaceutical sector for patient safety and efficiency with systematic implementation of situational awareness, safety leadership, communication, error management, team working, understanding the impact of personality on human performance and behaviour and finally, safe decision-making.

Human factors encompass all those factors that can influence people and their behaviour in a work context. Human factors include environmental, organisational, and job factors, as well as individual and team characteristics which influence behaviour at work as the basis for safety and efficiency. We strongly believe that through an understanding of the effects of teamwork, tasks, equipment, workspace, culture, organisation on human behaviour, perception, motivation, and overall ability, and the effective application of that knowledge in all pharmaceutical settings and processes, this will enhance performance and maintain safety with a just system that will restore and promote dignity and fairness to all participants.

Human factors training needs to be fully integrated into medical, pharmaceutical, nursing, and other healthcare professional curricula in the teaching and training of tasks and activities. It is *not* an add-on as a 'soft skill' which is 'nice to have'. Such an understanding of human factors is archaic and must be discarded; in reality, effective use of non-technical skills can take great moral courage. An effective human factors approach must similarly apply to all respective regulatory bodies. Systems and organisational science should be developed as a healthcare speciality with sponsorship of research into systems science for safety of healthcare products. Adoption of human factors needs top-down and bottom-up buy-in and needs to be fully embedded in all aspects of healthcare. This includes initial training for the current workforce in the short-term and tighter integration into the training of all future healthcare workers from the outset.

In conclusion, our approach in pharmacovigilance should focus on system design, the product, and all individuals and how human factors affect the functioning of all based on guiding principles. There is more to this than merely regulatory compliance. The fewer the resources, the more important understanding and applying human factors and quality becomes. The cost of not doing so is high.

16 Case Studies

16.1 Case Study 1 [65]

Clozapine is prescribed for severely ill schizophrenic patients who fail to respond adequately to standard drug treatments for schizophrenia. However, through spontaneous reports, it was noted that a life-threatening adverse reaction, agranulocytosis (an absolute neutrophil count <500/cumm), which can lead to fatal sepsis, could occur commonly with a cumulative incidence of 1.3%. But treatment-resistant schizophrenia is a very serious life-threatening condition for both the patient and those around them so measures had to be implemented so that clozapine could be kept on the market safely. Early detection of agranulocytosis and treatment interruption would be the aim of a risk mitigation strategy.

1. *Is there a widely available blood test to detect a fall in white cell count early?*

   Yes, measurement of full blood count is widely available. However, all stakeholders need to be made aware of the strategy. Haematology laboratories need to be able to identify samples from patients on clozapine and put processes in place to feedback white cell count results promptly to pharmacists so they can dispense clozapine.
2. *Can the strategy rely on routine pharmacovigilance or are additional measures required?*

   No, relying on routine practices and surveillance is inadequate. A national patient register is required of patients receiving clozapine typically monitoring for agranulocytosis weekly during the first 3 months after a first prescription or after restarting after a pause following leucopenia. After 3 months, monitoring can be adjusted as the risk falls with further adjustments after 6 months as the risk declines further. The MAHs set up the registry which is approved by the regulatory authority. However, cooperation is essential of prescribing psychiatrists, HCPs who arrange for blood test monitoring, haematology laboratories and pharmacists to ensure the register is a success.
3. *Does the register replace the normal surveillance responsibilities of HCPs?*

   No, HCPs must still be vigilant for worrying and unexpected adverse reactions which they should report to the MAH who is responsible for the register. This means that those who prescribe and dispense clozapine should have the MAH contact details readily available. The MAH must compile periodic reports for its supervising regulatory authority reporting all abnormal white cell counts and other serious or unexpected adverse reactions.

4. *How are HCPs supposed to find out about a clozapine register?*

   MAHs prepare Dear Healthcare Professional communications which must be approved by the supervising regulatory authority. The MAHs often may consult with and inform professional societies and patient groups about their plans for a register to obtain feedback about feasibility and burden. The Summary of Product Characteristics will be kept up to date with monitoring instructions to reduce risk so that HCPs should know where they can access the latest version.

16.2 Case Study 2 [17]

Terfenadine was a non-sedating H1 Receptor antagonist for the relief of allergic rhinitis symptoms, which was very popular as an over-the-counter medicine as its non-sedating properties were widely welcomed so that there were blockbuster sales. Around 1992, studies were published showing that metabolism of terfenadine could be blocked by drugs inhibiting hepatic enzymes metabolising cytochrome P450 (CYP)3A4 and that resultant accumulation of the unmetabolised parent drug led to serious cardiac abnormalities including QT prolongation and torsade de pointes.

1. *What immediate action needs to be taken when new risk evidence occurs for an over-the-counter medicine such as terfenadine?*

   When major risk factors have been identified then advice for prescribers and users should be modified. As a result, in 1992, the existing warning statements in the SPC about concomitant use of terfenadine with ketoconazole or macrolide antibiotics or in hepatically impaired patients were elevated to contraindications. This regulatory action was supported by press releases and HCP communications. For labelling changes alone to reduce risk requires the cooperation of prescribing HCPs, dispensing pharmacists, and patients to check whether the requirements for safe use have changed and what they are expected to do.

2. *Can society rely on spontaneous reporting to monitor the impact of changing the warnings and contraindications in the approved product information?*

   Spontaneous reports are an excellent source for signal generation but cannot be relied upon for monitoring the potential for drug interaction. Epidemiological database studies (such as pharmacy claims and health insurance databases in the US) showed substantial declines in use of contraindicated medicines with terfenadine after the labelling change although concurrent use of terfenadine with contraindicated drugs continued. However, heightened vigilance by HCPs meant spontaneous reports of malignant ventricular arrhythmias and sudden death continued to be reported.

3. *Electrocardiograms (ECGs) can be used to measure QT intervals, and these are widely available so that ECG monitoring should help, shouldn't it?*

   Terfenadine is used in the community so that regular monitoring using ECGs would not be practical. Prevention of high-risk drug interactions was the essential part of managing risk. That is why as spontaneous reports of serious ventricular arrhythmias continued, terfenadine was returned to prescriber only status so that prescriptions could be better controlled.

4. *Medicines with serious risks can often be supported on the market by collaboration between stakeholders. How did the benefit–harm of terfenadine become so negative that revocation of the marketing authorisation was required?*

   The indication for terfenadine, allergic rhinitis, is not a life-threatening or medically serious condition although it can be very distressing for patients Thus, in its own right having life-threatening risks put the medicine under regulatory pressure. However, what really pushed terfenadine off the market was the arrival of safer alternatives. In particular, in 1997, the active metabolite fexofenadine was approved and then plans to withdraw terfenadine announced. The arrival of an alternative product can be a game changer for the benefit–harm evaluation of a medicine already under scrutiny. When there is a comparable access and efficacy but without the known harms, then justification for retaining a product rapidly disappears. Indeed, in reality, regulators rely on prescribers to show good judgement and turn to the safer product(s) which is what happened with terfenadine.

16.3 Case Study 3 [66]

Cisapride was approved in 1993 for nocturnal heartburn in adults with gastrooesophageal reflux disease. However, this specific indication led to extensive off label use for all sorts of heartburn without needing to demonstrate reflux, as well as other gastrointestinal disorders thought to be caused by dysfunctional motility. Through spontaneous reports, serious cardiac arrhythmias (such as torsades de pointes) were identified. Following regulatory requests, the MAH performed preclinical studies which in 1998 showed a direct effect of cisapride on cardiac conduction.

1. *In what way can new approaches from clinical pharmacology help us explain newly identified adverse reactions?*

   The serious cardiac arrhythmias associated with cisapride coincided with our evolving pharmacological understanding of the relation of the hepatic cytochrome system to metabolism and how the effect of medicines on QT interval could be better investigated preclinically. For marketed medicines, new nonclinical and pharmacology data can continue to be produced which can impact causality assessment of spontaneous reports thus strengthening signals.
2. *What were the aims of the initial risk management actions for cisapride?*

   As with terfenadine, the original targets for managing risk with cisapride focussed on strengthening warnings about drug interactions leading to contraindication with drugs known to prolong QT interval or in patients who may have disorders that predispose to QT interval prolongation. This meant HCPs had a critical role in understanding the relevance of this new information and how these changes impacted prescribing and dispensing.
3. *What role did academia play in assessing the effectiveness of risk minimisation actions for cisapride?*

   When the serious cardiac safety concerns were raised for cisapride this motivated development of epidemiological assessment by academia using different healthcare databases and methodologies. Between 1998 and 2000, there were several epidemiology studies assessing whether co-prescribing of cisapride was reduced which reached different conclusions. The pharmacovigilance regulator has an important role in collating epidemiological data and helping drive concepts such as metanalysis and the optimum way to perform this.
4. *How did the changing science about gastrointestinal motility impact the benefit–harm of cisapride?*

   The important role of *Helicobacter pylori* in gastroesophageal disease and the rise of proton pump inhibitors fundamentally changed treatment of upper gastrointestinal disorders. This was especially deleterious for cisapride as the macrolides were treatment of choice for *Helicobacter pylori* and yet they were contraindicated with cisapride. In addition, gastrointestinal motility theories to explain other disorders became less fashionable. As HCPs better understood the science, scientific societies changed their guidelines against the use of cisapride dramatically driving down use. These changing opinions about pathophysiology had a more powerful impact on limiting harm from cisapride than regulatory action on indications, which is often a next step once the options of warnings and contraindications have been exhausted. In the EU, a restricted access register has been created to maintain supply of cisapride to those patients who need it under strictly controlled conditions.

References

1. Hembrow I. Rare events: the inside story of a worldwide quest for safer medicines. Springer; 2022. https://doi.org/10.1007/978-3-031-14981-8.
2. Sardella M, Belcher G, Lungu C, Ignoni T, Camisa M, et al. Monitoring the manufacturing and quality of medicines: a fundamental task of pharmacovigilance. Ther Adv Drug Saf. 2021;12:20420986211038436. https://doi.org/10.1177/20420986211038436.
3. Commission Implementing Regulation (EU) No 520/2012 of 19 June 2012. On the performance of pharmacovigilance activities provided for in Regulation (EC) No 726/2004 of the European Parliament and of the Council and Directive 2001/83/EC of the European Parliament and of the Council. https://eur-lex.europa.eu/LexUriServ/LexUriServ.do?uri=OJ:L:2012:159:0005:0025:EN:PDF (accessed 23 Feb 2023)
4. Fornasier G, Francescon S, Leone R, Baldo P. An historical overview over pharmacovigilance. Int J Clin Pharm. 2018;40(4):744–7. https://doi.org/10.1007/s11096-018-0657-1. (accessed 7 Aug 2022)
5. Penn RG. The state control of medicines: the first 3000 years. Br J Clin Pharmacol. 1979;8:293–305.
6. Rawlins MD. Spontaneous reporting of adverse drug reactions: I: the data. Br J Clin Pharmacol. 1988a;26:1–5.
7. Rawlins MD. Spontaneous reporting of adverse drug reactions: II: uses. Br J Clin Pharmacol. 1988b;26:7–11.
8. Goldsmith DI. The impact of the International Conference on Harmonization (ICH) on pharmacoepidemiology and pharmacovigilance. Pharmacoepidemiol Drug Saf. 1998;7:289–91.
9. Santoro A, Genov G, Spooner A, Raine J, Arlett P. Promoting and protecting public health: how the European Union pharmacovigilance system works. Drug Saf. 2017;40:855–69.
10. Edwards B, Johnson C, Gandhi S. Legal basis—EU. In: Andrews EB, Moore N, editors. Mann's pharmacovigilance. 3rd ed; 2014. https://doi.org/10.1002/9781118820186.ch3. (Chapter 2).
11. Edwards B, Gandhi S. Pharmacovigilance for human medicinal products. In: Regulatory toxicology in the European Union. RSC Books Production Team; 2018. p. 129–62. (Chapter 4).
12. Bates DW, Spell N, Cullen DJ, Burdick E, Laird N, Petersen LA, Small SD, Sweitzer BJ, Leape LL. The costs of adverse drug events in hospitalized patients. Adverse Drug Events Prevention Study Group. JAMA. 1997;277:307–11.
13. Lazarou J, Pomeranz BH, Corey PN. Incidence of adverse drug reactions in hospitalized patients. JAMA. 1998;279:1200–5.
14. Pirmohamed M, James S, Meakin S, Green C, Scott AK, Walley TJ, Farrar K, Park B, Breckenridge A. Adverse drug reactions as a cause of admission to hospital: prospective analysis of 18 820 patients. BMJ. 2004;329:15–9.
15. Goldman SA. Postmarketing pharmacovigilance compliance in the midst of regulatory uncertainty. Food Drug Law J. 2007;62(3):513–28.
16. ICH Harmonised tripartite guideline pharmacovigilance planning E2E; 2004. https://database.ich.org/sites/default/files/E2E Guideline.pdf (accessed 8987 Aug 2022)
17. Huang SM, Booth B, Fadiran EO, Lesko L. What lessons have we learned from the recent market withdrawal of terfenadine and mibefradil? Clin Pharmacol Ther. 2000;67(2):148.
18. FDA's Role in Managing Medication Risks; 2018. https://www.fda.gov/drugs/risk-evaluation-and-mitigation-strategies-rems/fdas-role-managing-medication-risks (accessed 7 Aug 2022)
19. Edwards B, Teeling M, Toivonen M. Chapter 39: Pharmacovigilance and risk management. In: Cartwright AC, Matthews BR, editors. International pharmaceutical product registration. 2nd ed. CRC Press; 2008.
20. Vora P, Artime E, Soriano-Gabarró M. A review of studies evaluating the effectiveness of risk minimisation measures in Europe using the European Union electronic Register of Post-Authorization Studies. Pharmacoepidemiol Drug Saf. 2018;27:695–706.
21. Di Santo Stefano RL, Painter JL, Thomas M, Powell G. Safety assessment and selection bias: who uses social media to communicate about medications? Pharmacoepidemiol Drug Saf. 2015;24(Suppl. 1):547–8.
22. Golder S, Norman G, Loke YK. Systematic review on the prevalence, frequency, and comparative value of adverse events data in social media. Br J Clin Pharmacol. 2015;80(4):878–88.
23. ABPI Guidance notes on the management of safety information and product complaints from digital activities; 2021. https://www.abpi.org.uk/publications/guidance-notes-on-the-management-of-safety-information-and-product-complaints-from-digital-activities/ (accessed 20 Mar 2023)
24. Brosch S, de Ferran A, Newbould V, Farkas D, Lengsavath M, Tregunno P. Establishing a framework for the use of social media in pharmacovigilance in Europe. Drug Saf. 2019;42:921–30.
25. Mozzicato P. MedDRA: an overview of the medical dictionary for regulatory activities. Pharm Med. 2009;23(2):65–75.
26. Cornelius VR, Liu K, Peacock J, Sauze O. Variation in adverse drug reactions listed in product information for antidepressants and anticonvulsants, between the USA and Europe: a comparison review of paired regulatory documents. BMJ Open. 2016;6:e010599. https://doi.org/10.1136/bmjopen-2015-010599.
27. Edwards B, Chakraborty S. Risk communication and the pharmaceutical industry: what is the reality? Drug Saf. 2012;35(11):1027–40.

28. Waller PC, Evans SJW, Beard K. Drug safety and regulation. BMJ. 2005;331:5–6.
29. Waller PC, Evans SJW. A model for the future conduct of pharmacovigilance. Pharmacoepidemiol Drug Saf. 2003;12:17–29.
30. SCOPE Work Package 7 Quality management systems; 2016. Pharmacovigilance quality manual template. https://www.ema.europa.eu/en/documents/other/scope-training-survey-report-resource-management_en.pdf (accessed 7 Aug 2022)
31. International Ergonomics Association. 2000. https://iea.cc/about/what-is-ergonomics/ (accessed 28 Mar 2023)
32. Price J. Pharmacovigilance in crisis: drug safety at a crossroads. Clin Ther. 2018;40(5):790–7.
33. Barry A, Olsson S, Minzi O, Bienvenu E, Makonnen E, Kamuhabwa A, Oluka M, Guantai A, Bergman U, van Puijenbroek E, Gurumurthy P, Aklillu E. Comparative assessment of the national pharmacovigilance systems in East Africa: Ethiopia, Kenya, Rwanda, and Tanzania. Drug Saf. 2020;43:539–50.
34. Edwards B, Tilson HH, West S. Defining the competencies of those conducting pharmacovigilance. Pharmacoepidemiol Drug Saf. 2006;15(3):193–8.
35. World Health Organisation (WHO). Patient safety curriculum guide: multi-professional edition; 2011. https://www.who.int/publications/i/item/9789241501958 (accessed 7 Aug 2022).
36. Onakpoya IJ, Heneghan CJ, Aronson JK. Post-marketing withdrawal of 462 medicinal products because of adverse drug reactions: a systematic review of the world literature. BMC Med. 2019;17:56. https://doi.org/10.1186/s12916-019-1294-9.
37. Peters T, Soanes N, Abbas M, Ahmad J, Delumeau JC, Herrero-Martinez E, Paramananda M, Piper J, Smail-Aoudia F, van der Spuij W, Veizovic T, Winstanley G, On behalf of the EFPIA International Pharmacovigilance Group. Effective pharmacovigilance system development: EFPIA-IPVG consensus recommendations. Drug Saf. 2020;44(1):17–28.
38. WHO. Minimum requirements for a functional pharmacovigilance system; 2010. https://who-umc.org/media/1483/pv_minimum_requirements_2010_2.pdf (accessed 7 Aug 2022).
39. WHO. WHO Drug Information Regulatory collaboration—collaboration, not competition: developing new reliance models. WHO Drug Inform. 2016;30(4):558–66. https://apps.who.int/iris/handle/10665/331005 (accessed 7 Aug 2022)
40. Ampadu HH, Hoekman J, Arhinful D, Amoama-Dapaah M, Leufkens HGM, Dodoo ANO. Organizational capacities of national pharmacovigilance centres in Africa: assessment of resource elements associated with successful and unsuccessful pharmacovigilance experiences. Global Health. 2018;14:109–26.
41. Radley DC, Finkelstein SN, Stafford RS. Off-label prescribing among office-based physicians. Arch Intern Med. 2006;166:1021–6.
42. Wittich CM, Burkle CM, Lanier WL. Ten common questions (and their answers) about off-label. Drug Use Mayo Clin Proc. 2012;87(10):982–90.
43. García MP, Figueras A. Pharmacoepidemiology and drug safety the lack of knowledge about the voluntary reporting system of adverse drug reactions as a major cause of underreporting: direct survey among health professionals. Pharmacoepidemiol Drug Saf. 2011;20(12):1295–302.
44. Hartman J, Härmark L, van Puijenbroek E. A global view of undergraduate education in pharmacovigilance. Eur J Clin Pharmacol. 2017;73:891–9. https://doi.org/10.1007/s00228-017-2237-z.
45. Caro-Rojas A. Health Care communication empowerment: a successful program in Colombia. Drug Saf. 2018b;41:1111.
46. Leveson N, Couturier M, Thomas J, Dierks M, Wierz D, Psaty B, Finkelstein S. Applying system engineering to pharmaceutical safety. J Healthcare Eng. 2012;3(3):391–414.
47. Paudyal V, Al-Hamid A, Bowen M, Hadi MA, Hasan SS, Jalal Z, Stewart D. Interventions to improve spontaneous adverse drug reaction reporting by healthcare professionals and patients: systematic review and meta-analysis. Expert Opin Drug Saf. 2020;19(9):1173–91.
48. Formica D, Sultana J, Cutroneo PM, et al. The economic burden of preventable adverse drug reactions: a systematic review of observational studies. Expert Opin Drug Saf. 2018;17(7):681–95. https://doi.org/10.1080/14740338.2018.1491547.
49. Naseralallah L, Stewart D, Azfar RA, Paudyal V. An umbrella review of systematic reviews on contributory factors to medication errors in health-care settings. Expert Opin Drug Saf. 2022;21(11):1379–99.
50. Institute Safe Medication Practices (ISMP). The case for Medication Safety Officers (MSO); 2018. https://www.ismp.org/sites/default/files/attachments/2018-08/MSOS%20White%20Paper_Final_080318_1.pdf (accessed 7 Aug 2022)
51. Kirk E. Medication safety officer handbook; 2016. https://www.sps.nhs.uk/articles/medication-safety-officer-handbook/ (accessed 7 Aug 2022)
52. Härmark L, Weits G, Meijer R, Santoro F, Noren G, van Hunsel F. Communicating adverse drug reaction insights through patient organizations: experiences from a Pilot Study in the Netherlands. Drug Saf. 2020;43:745–9.
53. Janssens R, Russo S, van Overbeeke E, et al. Patient preferences in the medical product life cycle: what do stakeholders think? Semi-structured qualitative interviews in Europe and the USA. Patient-Patient-Centered Outcomes Res. 2019;12:513–26.
54. Ndagije HB, Manirakiza L, Kajungu D, et al. The effect of community dialogues and sensitization on patient reporting of adverse events in rural Uganda: uncontrolled before after study. PLoS ONE. 2019; https://doi.org/10.1371/journal.pone.0203721.

55. Rolfes L, van Hunsel F, van der Linden L, Taxis K, van Puijenbroek E. The quality of clinical information in adverse drug reaction reports by patients and healthcare professionals: a retrospective comparative analysis. Drug Saf. 2017;40(7):607–14.
56. Faulkner SD, Sayuri S, Pakarinen C. Understanding multi-stakeholder needs, preferences, and expectations to define effective practices and processes of patient engagement in medicine development: a mixed-methods study. Health Expect. 2021;24:601–16.
57. Bahri P, Pariente A. Systematising pharmacovigilance engagement of patients, healthcare professionals and regulators: a practical decision guide derived from the international risk governance framework for engagement events and discourse. Drug Saf. 2021;44(11):1193–208.
58. Cavaller-Bellaubi M, Faulkner SD, Teixeira B, et al. Sustaining meaningful patient engagement across the lifecycle of medicines: a roadmap for action. Ther Innov Regul Sci. 2021;55:936–53.
59. CIOMS Working Group XI Report. Patient involvement in the development, regulation, and safe use of medicines; 2022. https://doi.org/10.56759/iiew8982.
60. Edwards B, Gloor CA, Toussaint F, Guan C, Furniss D. Human factors: the pharmaceutical supply chain as a complex sociotechnical system. Int J Qual Health Care. 2021;32(Suppl. 1):56–8.
61. Evans SJW. Pharmacovigilance: a science or fielding emergencies? Curr Perspect Future Direct Med Stat. 2000;19(23):3199–209.
62. Caro-Rojas A. Patient safety context and its advances in Latin America chapter. In: Papale RM, editor. Manual of good pharmacovigilance practices, Latin American edition.; ISBN 978-987-46704-2-7; 2018a. p. 771–8.
63. Edwards B. Best safety practices now and in the future. In: Pharmacovigilance: critique and ways forward. Switzerland: ADIS; 2017. p. 35–48. (Chapter 5).
64. Edwards B, Olsen AK, Whalen MD, Gold MJ. Guiding principles of safety as a basis for developing a pharmaceutical safety culture. Curr Drug Saf. 2007;2:135–9.
65. Kar N, Barreto S, Chandavarkar R. Clozapine monitoring in clinical practice: beyond the mandatory requirement. Clin Psychopharmacol Neurosci. 2016;14(4):323–9.
66. Quigley EMM. Cisapride: what can we learn from the rise and fall of a prokinetic? J Digest Dis. 2011;12:147–56.

Further Reading

Andrews EB, Moore N, editors. Mann's pharmacovigilance. 3rd ed. Wiley Blackwell; 2014.
Eu2P: European training programme in Pharmacovigilance and Pharmacoepidemiology https://www.eu2p.org/ (accessed 25 Mar 2023).
Good Pharmacovigilance Practices. https://www.ema.europa.eu/en/human-regulatory/post-authorisation/pharmacovigilance/good-pharmacovigilance-practices (accessed 23 Feb 2023).
ICH Efficacy Guidelines. https://www.ich.org/page/efficacy-guidelines (accessed 25 Mar 2023).
Medicines and Healthcare Product Agency Yellow Card reporting site https://yellowcard.mhra.gov.uk/) (accessed 25 Mar 2023).
Prescribing Safety Assessment. https://prescribingsafetyassessment.ac.uk/ (accessed 25 Mar 2023).
Talbot J, Aronson JK, editors. Stephens' detection and evaluation of adverse drug reactions: principles and practice. 6th ed. John Wiley & Sons Ltd.; 2012.

Ethics in Pharmacovigilance

14

Alison Thompson and Ana Komparic

Abstract

Healthcare practitioners play a vital role in facilitating effective and ethical pharmacovigilance, as well as in translating evidence generated through pharmacovigilance activities into clinical practice to improve the care of patients and to improve population health. Physicians, nurses, dentists, pharmacists, and other health practitioners have ethical obligations stemming from their professional obligations to act in their patients' best interests, to protect and promote the public good, and to maintain their professional competence. In turn, these obligations give rise to a host of ethical principles and considerations related to pharmacovigilance and the safe use of pharmaceuticals. This chapter outlines several of these key principles and considerations, including the fiduciary duty, the duty to protect the public from harm, the duty to maintain professional competence, privacy, consent, disclosure, equity, trust, inclusiveness, the duty to report, scientific integrity, the duty to use the highest quality evidence, and conflicts of interest.

Keywords

Professional ethics · Bioethics · Public health ethics · Clinical ethics · Pharmacovigilance ethics · Drug safety · Patient engagement · Equity · Conflict of interest · Integrity · Nocebo effect

Learning Objectives

- To identify ethical concepts of relevance to pharmacovigilance activities.
- To analyze how professional ethics duties intersect with pharmacovigilance activities.
- To understand how public health ethics is relevant to pharmacovigilance and drug use.
- To understand that scientific integrity is an ethical issue related to evidence used in drug safety in clinical practice and drug regulation.

Key Points

- Pharmacovigilance relies on the ethical actions of researchers, healthcare practitioners, industry, patients, and the public; it is not enough to rely on evidence alone when making clinical decisions.
- Healthcare practitioners have ethical duties to patients and to the public that

A. Thompson (✉)
Leslie Dan Faculty of Pharmacy & Dalla Lana School of Public Health, University of Toronto, Toronto, ON, Canada
e-mail: a.thompson@utoronto.ca

A. Komparic
Dalla Lana School of Public Health, University of Toronto, Toronto, ON, Canada

J. Jose et al. (eds.), *Principles and Practice of Pharmacovigilance and Drug Safety*,
https://doi.org/10.1007/978-3-031-51089-2_14

guide pharmacovigilance activities, but healthcare practitioners can encounter ethical dilemmas when faced with conflicting ethical duties, or when legal duties conflict with ethical duties.
- Ethical practice requires ethical deliberations with other professionals, patients, and society more broadly and requires sensitivity to cultural differences.

1 Introduction

Healthcare practitioners play a crucial role in pharmacovigilance and are responsible for identifying and minimizing the risks to patients posed by pharmaceuticals. Increasingly, patients are being asked to help identify potential adverse events that result from their use of pharmaceuticals. There are several ethical considerations pertaining to pharmacovigilance in the context of clinical practice, and this chapter will provide an overview and discussion of the most salient issues facing healthcare practitioners.

While primarily conceived of as a scientific endeavor, pharmacovigilance relies on the ethical actions of researchers, healthcare practitioners, industry, patients, and the public to generate reliable and comprehensive data to keep people safe. And while causation assessment is grounded in science, without taking patients seriously about their experiences with drugs and biologics, we cannot hope to understand the risk/benefit profile of a pharmaceutical product. Recent efforts to engage patients more actively and broadly in potential adverse event reporting and clinical trial design signifies an ethical shift toward valuing the perspectives of patients as partners in pharmacovigilance, and toward a more collaborative model of clinical practice when it comes to pharmaceutical care.

In this chapter, we will explore the ethical landscape in clinical practice with the hope that healthcare practitioners can further explore these issues in a constructive and fair dialogue with colleagues, patients, and the broader community within which they practice. Cultural differences in values can also give rise to different framings of ethical issues, so we do not claim that this chapter is the final word on ethical issues in pharmacovigilance, but rather the start of a dialogue on these issues that must be broadened.

As ethical dilemmas frequently involve tensions between professional obligations or ethical principles, the principles and ethical considerations provided here are meant to inform readers about ethical issues that can arise in practice. However, only through a process of ethical deliberation can healthcare practitioners decide on the best course of action. This will often mean choosing to act on one value or consideration over another. The process of ethical discernment may involve discussions with colleagues and patients, and subsequent actions need to be justified based on ethical arguments that most people would agree are reasonable, even if they do not agree with the substantive decision itself.

The ethical considerations related to pharmacovigilance are listed in Fig. 14.1 and are discussed in detail in the remaining part of the chapter.

Ethical Considerations for Pharmacovigilance

PROFESSIONAL ETHICS	Healthcare providers are guided by codes of ethics that put patient welfare and public health at the centre of their practice
PRIVACY	Respect for patient confidentiality is rooted in their right to privacy
CONSENT	Patient consent for release of personal health information or for participation in pharmacovigilance studies is warranted
DISCLOSURE	Healthcare practitioners often have formal disclosure responsibilities when medication errors or violations occur
EQUITY	Inequitable representation in clinical trial design and big data sets can impact real world drug safety and effectiveness
TRUST	Pharmacovigilance can help bolster public trust, but it also relies on the willing participation of a trusting public
INCLUSIVENESS	It is important to include diverse patient perspectives on drug safety and effectiveness in pharmacovigilance activities
DUTY TO REPORT	This duty is grounded in the need to protect the public from harm by increasing collection of safety and effectiveness data
SCIENTIFIC INTEGRITY	Integrity is important for the validity of the evidence used to inform prescribing and for building patient and public trust

Fig. 14.1 Ethical principles and considerations for pharmacovigilance

2 Professional Ethics

Healthcare practitioners involved in the development, supply, prescribing, administration, and management of pharmaceuticals are members of healthcare professions. Professions are often characterized as being in an implicit contract with society [1]. In other words, healthcare professionals are expected to commit to uphold the *fiduciary duty*—that is, to act in their patients' (or clients') best interests—and to protect and promote the public good, as well as to maintain professional competence. In return, professions are granted certain privileges such as professional autonomy, meaning that the profession is responsible for determining its members' standards of practice and that professionals can exercise their independent, professional judgment in decision-making, and self-regulation. This allows professions to oversee the education, licensing, and disciplining of their members' conduct [1–4]. The ethical obligations that healthcare professionals must abide by with respect to their patients and the public at large are articulated in a profession's code of ethics and underpin the more detailed rules and standards outlined in the laws, regulations, standards, by-laws, and guidelines that govern clinical practice. A professional's ethical obligations often extend beyond the minimum legal standards that they must abide by in the jurisdiction where they practice.

Upholding the fiduciary duty and promoting the public good are vital for building and maintaining the trust of patients and the public at large [4]. Trust is central to an effective therapeutic alliance and to an open patient–clinician relationship. In the absence of trust, patients may be reluctant to seek or follow the advice of healthcare practitioners, or to openly raise concerns with healthcare practitioners, including related to their use of pharmaceuticals and any resulting adverse events [5]. As a result, mistrust or a lack of trust can hamper pharmacovigilance efforts and harm patients.

In addition to being grounded in professional ethics, effective pharmacovigilance in clinical practice requires inter-professionalism, since pharmaceutical prescribing and management often involves inter-professional teams. Accordingly, professionals must make a concerted effort to work with colleagues across the multiple professions that comprise a patient's circle of care to facilitate safe and effective treatment and to address the ethical and professional issues concerning pharmaceutical use that they may encounter in practice.

Many of the ethical considerations and principles related to pharmacovigilance that are outlined in this chapter can be understood as being grounded in, or supportive of, healthcare practitioners' fundamental ethical obligations to act in the patients' best interests and to protect and promote public good. A wider ethics discussion about the relationship between those directly involved in healthcare delivery and those who are in the commercial pharmaceutical industry is out of scope but is touched on in several places in this chapter. However, the influence of industry on prescribing habits and the scholarly literature is not insignificant, and this is important to understand for a fuller picture of society's pharmacovigilance system [6–8].

3 Privacy

The ethical obligation to keep a patient's health information confidential is based on the principle of respect for patient privacy. Most adverse event reporting systems do not require the reporting clinician to violate patient privacy, such as the anonymous reporting in the UK through the government's Yellow Card scheme. However, when identifying information is required for reporting, patients should be asked for their permission.

Having enough information to identify a patient in a report is essential for follow-up for outcome and to help prevent duplication, and this should be explained to the patient. The expectation that patients have around confidentially must be balanced with the need to protect the public, or other patients, from harm. Most codes of professional ethics include an articulation of responsibility in some form to the broader public, whether that be in the form of a responsibility to maintain public trust in their respective profession, or in a duty to warn, or a duty to care. Many jurisdictions will have laws articulating when a patient's privacy may or ought to be breached to protect others, or to report abuse of pharmaceuticals. Not many, however, have a clear articulation of when to prioritize the public's health over patient confidentiality outside of the reporting of infectious diseases. It could be argued, however, that the duty to report adverse drug events trumps a patient's right to privacy if and only if there is no way to report the event that can maintain patient confidentiality—for example, in the case where the population of drug users is so small that it is likely that the patient could be identified, as can happen with orphan medicines, or where identifying information about the patient is crucial to reporting the adverse event.

The digital transformation of pharmacovigilance is aimed at improving adverse event reporting and safety signal identification, but the protection of private health information will remain central to the ethical use of digital technologies. Data sources include voluntary adverse event reporting applications for mobile devices, mobile health technologies and applications, internet-based surveys of patient experiences with drugs, and machine learning algorithms that aid in the identification of safety signals by mining sources of patient information such as electronic health records, health information technologies, and pharmacovigilance database systems. Commercial entities, insurance companies, and even law enforcement and immigration authorities are all potential parties who could have an interest in these data. Protecting privacy will not only encourage reporting, but it will also ensure that these data are not used in ways that might violate dignity or disadvantage individuals and/or groups of people who may already be disadvantaged or stigmatized. Private, for-profit, third parties are often hired to manage and collect these data [9], which raises issues around data privacy, especially in light of healthcare data breaches. A recent study revealed that "hacking/IT incidents are the most prevalent forms of attack behind healthcare data breaches, followed by unauthorized internal disclosures" and that healthcare data are deemed highly valuable, with the result that "the frequency of healthcare data breaches, magnitude of exposed records, and financial losses due to breached records are increasing rapidly" [10]. Balancing the promise of digital technologies to improve pharmacovigilance activities with vigilance over patient privacy and the appropriate uses of these data sources to improve drug safety and effectiveness will require that patients be not just informed of the risks, but that they are actively engaged in conversations around privacy and digital health technologies.

4 Consent

Informed consent is a fundamental ethical principle and is grounded in the principle of respect for persons—that is respect for patients and/or research participants—and their right to autonomy or self-determination. Consent from patients for treatment or research participation should be considered on a spectrum from no consent to fully informed consent (Fig. 14.2), which raises some challenging ethical issues related to reporting adverse events spontaneously without jeopardy and to pharmacovigilance research.

In clinical practice, patients must consent to treatment, and this typically requires the full disclosure of the risks and benefits associated with a course of treatment. Where risks are unknown or there is uncertainty about benefit, this ought to be disclosed to patients. Concerns that sharing information with patients about the possible side effects of medication would bias patient reports of side effects (and thereby taint pharmacovigilance studies that include patient reported side effects) do not seem to have been born out in the literature [11]. There is some concern that full disclosure to patients might "manifest as nocebo-effect," where an adverse event results from the belief that an intervention will cause harm, but that "concerns about the undesirable effects should not deter the active involvement of patients in pharmacovigilance activities" [11]. The tension for healthcare practitioners is that in respecting patient autonomy and seeking informed consent—which normally entails full disclosure of possible side effects—the clinician is actually causing harm [12]. For public health, there are also significant costs related to subsequent clinical management of nocebo effects in addition to the potential impact of this effect on adverse event reporting [13]. However, one proposal for mitigating the possible harms from full disclosure of side effects is to seek to attain "contextualized informed consent" [12], where nocebogenic information is not disclosed to the patient. Vague, nonspecific side effects like fatigue, dizziness, or nausea are more likely than drug-specific side effects to contribute to a nocebo effect. Drug-specific side effects should be disclosed to patients, it is argued, because "they may result in more debilitating symptoms/conditions and thus may be more important for the patient's full informed consent" [12] as well as for their decision-making about whether or not to switch to a drug with a better side effect profile. In this approach, the consideration whether or not to disclose the information

Approaches to Informed Consent in Data-Generating Activities

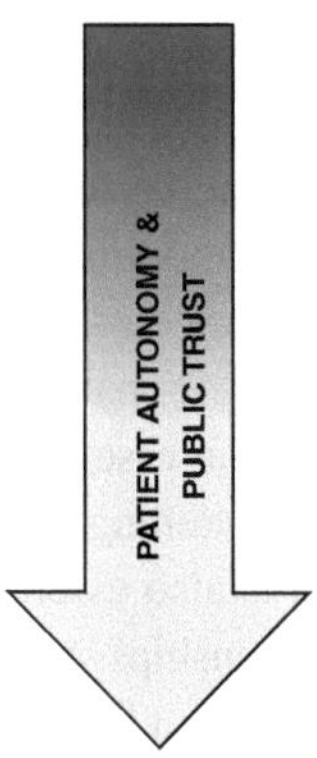

1. **Fully informed consent:** patients are given all information required for them to freely make decisions where they understand and appreciate the consequences of taking a particular medication, of participating in a research study, or allowing their health information to be shared
2. **Integrated consent:** usually used in the context of pragmatic trials where the clinical consent process is integrated with the research consent process
3. **Contextualized consent:** clinicians make decisions based on their knowledge of the patient and the patient's condition about how much information to provide to maximize patient autonomy whilst simultaneously minimizing the risk of harms from disclosing potential nocebogenic information
4. **Consent waiver:** in some circumstances and jurisdictions, the need to obtain consent is waived when consent can negatively impact data validity and quality, create major practical problems, and/or distress participants

Fig. 14.2 The continuum of approaches to informed consent in data-generating activities

on side effects in both nonspecific and drug-specific side effects will be influenced by the nature, severity and seriousness of possible side effects, its likely impact on medication adherence and the patient's daily life. This model of contextualized informed consent requires healthcare practitioners to take into consideration who the patient is, what they are treating, and how their relationship with the patient plays a role in how patients take up information about side effects to maximize patient autonomy without causing harm in the process.

Recent methodological developments in drug comparative effectiveness research, such as cluster randomized trials of prescribing policy, pragmatic trials, or when data are anonymized, are generally considered to be low risk to patients, but questions about whether individual informed consent from patients is necessary have been raised [14, 15]. Because seeking individual consent from each patient/participant contributes to the costs of such studies, as well as potentially negatively impacting study enrollment, some have proposed an opt-out, rather than opt-in approach to enrollment for studies that are low risk and where there is genuine clinical equipoise or where community consent is more appropriate [14, 16]. However, whether or not this is permissible will depend on the jurisdiction where the research is being conducted and whether or not the jurisdiction has something comparable to the Common Rule in the United States that articulates the situations in which consent can be exempt from ethical review [17]. A proposal for "integrated consent" for pragmatic trials that integrates the clinical consent process with the research consent process avoids the ethically problematic proposal to not seek consent at all for pragmatic trials [18], which would involve deceiving patients. International research ethics guidelines vary on this, and the Good Clinical Practice guidelines that govern clinical trials do not allow for waivers of informed consent [19]. Ultimately, the clinician has a fiduciary duty to the patient to act in a trustworthy manner, and failure to disclose research participation to patients may well damage the therapeutic alliance between provider and patient. This is unlike reporting of adverse events in most jurisdictions, which is not considered a violation of patient confidentiality, such as in the UK's Yellow Card system, and therefore does not require patient consent to report. In the context of research, there is, of course, mandatory reporting of adverse events which also does not require explicit consent from research participants.

Pharmaceutical companies continue to evolve into information gathering companies through their ownership of online medical practices that systematically collect patient data and through data mining activities [20, 21]. Patients use applications on their smartphones and other devices to monitor and collect their own health data that is then mined often without their informed consent because of the impenetrability of the legalese in app agreements or because there is no express privacy or tracking agreement [22–24]. Where pharmacovigilance activities use these data, or where healthcare professionals use mobile applications to store or collect patient data, care must be taken to ensure data were collected ethically, and in keeping with relevant privacy and consent laws.

5 Disclosure

In addition to duties to disclose information to patients to facilitate their ability to make informed decisions, healthcare practitioners often have formal disclosure responsibilities when medication errors or violations occur. Harms from medications are sometimes the result of human error, system error, or even negligence and recklessness such as deliberate off-label use or administration. Violations can also occur when behavior leads to neglect of safety monitoring, which can be motivated by cost-cutting or disregard for monitoring or reporting requirements. The importance of disclosing medication errors and violations for patient safety has been widely recognized as an essential part of preventing future errors, maintaining the trust of patients and the public, and is also essential for repairing therapeutic relationships and patient/family healing [25]. It is typically a formal process of communication between a clinician and/or organization and the patient or their family members. Ethically, a clinician has a duty to warn in particular situations, and disclosure of medical error is at least partly about warning others about potential systemic or root causes of medication errors so that they can be prevented in the future. If an institution does not have a culture of error reporting that is nonpunitive, it will discourage the transparent disclosure of medication errors, which in turn has a negative impact on patient safety [26, 27]. In the case of deliberate violations or reckless disregard for protocols, sanctions may well be appropriate in addition to disclosure.

In addition to having a duty to warn others of potential drug safety issues related to error and deliberate violations, healthcare practitioners have a fiduciary responsibility to patients that is rooted in their obligation to act in the best interests of the patient. When medication errors or violations occur, healthcare practitioners are accountable to patients for their actions and the need for healthcare practitioners to be honest with patients and not withhold the truth about an error, or even a near-miss incident, requires disclosure. While most errors are related to decision-making mistakes, institutional factors can also contribute to errors [27] and also possibly deliberate violations if cost-cutting and lack of time are issues. Disclosure to colleagues and others in institutions where there are institutional or systemic causes of error would also be important for creating a culture of safe medication use.

Globally, there are disparities between high-income countries and low-income countries with respect to the prevalence and quality of pharmacovigilance: patients living in low-income countries experience twice as many disability-adjusted life years lost due to medication-related harm than those in high-income countries [28], and this is partly attributable to lack of global cooperation around pharmacovigilance [29]. Given that most medication errors are avoidable, this presents an opportunity for high-income countries to share data and resources for error reporting and medication safety incidents with low-income countries, who may lack the resources and systems to monitor and redress adverse events and errors. Despite the comparative lack of infrastructure and/or resources, innovative uses of disease monitoring systems for reporting adverse events and South-South collaboration are promising to improve pharmacovigilance systems and capacity in the Global South [30].

6 Equity

Healthcare practitioners can also help protect their patients and the public by being vigilant about how inequities in clinical trial design might impact real-world safety and effectiveness of drugs and vaccines (Fig. 14.3). This might require that study populations in clinical trials be examined to identify the potential need for targeted monitoring in the post-market context because a lack of diversity in clinical trials can make existing health inequalities worse or create new inequalities [31]. There are gaps in our knowledge that result from the failure to recruit diverse populations for inclusion in clinical trials, and this can result in clinical blind spots about how drugs, devices, and behavioral interventions affect different groups of people—and often they are the people most affected by a particular disease or condition [32]. A recent review of studies reporting on randomized clinical trials revealed that little progress has been made in increasing the reporting and representation of participants' racial and socioeconomic status, despite the fact that reporting of their sex has increased [33]. Healthcare practitioners involved in clinical trials are being urged to collect and report data "in ways that allow them to be aggregated in systematic reviews of the literature" [34].

Equity issues are not limited to representation and reporting issues in clinical trials, however. Given the challenges of running trials that are diverse and large enough to generate statistically valid observations about sub-populations, partnering with people from poorly and underserved groups in society so that their unique perspectives can be brought to bear on study design is equally important [34]. Partnership in study design is relatively new to clinical trial research but is increasingly recognized to be important from an ethical perspective, especially in the context of global health research where it is important to account for diverse experiences and perspectives concerning research practices as well as accessing and using pharmaceuticals [35, 36].

As pharmacovigilance goes digital and relies increasingly on big data and algorithms to iden-

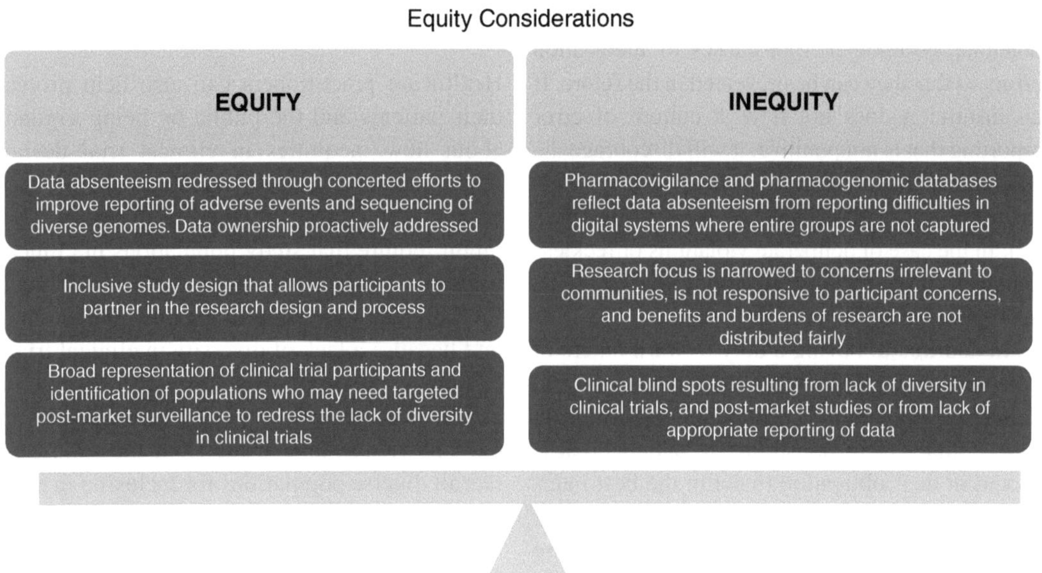

Fig. 14.3 Contributing factors to equitable or inequitable clinical trial design

tify safety and effectiveness issues, the gaps in knowledge of how drugs impact underrepresented and/or marginalized populations are replicated as issues of "data absenteeism" in pharmacovigilance databases (where certain populations may be entirely absent), as well as in pharmacogenomic databases [37, 38]. In the context of disparities in access to digital reporting technologies, patient reporting of adverse drug reactions (ADRs) can be difficult, and this can create gaps in reporting. As these databases are mined for information about safety, effectiveness, and idiosyncratic drug reactions related to genetic makeup, it is important to ensure that data absenteeism is recognized and actively addressed to prevent or at least not exacerbate health inequities. Such inequities can be reflected as missing information in the risk management plan a pharmaceutical company must produce for new medicines.

Pharmacogenetics also raises concerns about how populations are screened for genetic predispositions to adverse drug effects. The creation of categories of risk in the population based on stratification of such things as race or multigenerational ancestry has become accepted in clinical practice, but such an approach risks reaffirming socially constructed categories of race which do not match the biological reality that intrapopulation genetic variation can be greater than inter-population variation. Decision-making in pharmacogenomic practice may over-rely on racial categories that are fluid and socially constructed and mistakenly use categories such as White or Asian as surrogates for actual data about genetic variation that can be generated through universal testing [39]. The need for diversity in pharmacogenomic data is compelling and needs to be done thoughtfully in order to avoid worsening existing health disparities by excluding marginalized populations, while not overgeneralizing based on misguided notions of race [40]. Issues of consent for data collection, data ownership, and usage (particularly in Indigenous communities) need to be ethically addressed prior to expanding databases.

7 Trust

Recruitment of diverse populations for research and inclusion in databases that can be used in pharmacovigilance activities can be a challenge because of historical issues of mistrust in science, scientists, healthcare practitioners, or other authorities by people who have been subject to systemic racism, sexism, or other forms of discrimination by society or within the healthcare system in particular [32]. This mistrust can spill over into the clinical encounter, as systemic forms of discrimination are also present in the clinic. In the context of prescribing, being transparent about what is known about a drug and its side effects, as well as what is not known can go some way to helping healthcare practitioners build trust with their patients. As discussed above in the section about the importance of disclosure, the need to be truthful with patients can sometimes conflict with the desire to be able to conduct health systems level research. However, since patient trust is so central to the clinical and therapeutic relationship and is enshrined in the clinician's fiduciary duty, the impact of clinical decisions on patient trust should be top of mind. Not only can trust in the clinician be undermined when important information about side effects or patient involvement in data collection is not disclosed or is not accessible to the patient, public trust in a health profession as a whole can be undermined. As discussed further below, healthcare practitioners ought to also be aware of how actual or perceived conflicts of interest can impact patient and public trust in the safety of pharmaceuticals and the integrity of prescribers and researchers. In systems with publicly funded pharmaceutical insurance, access to medicines can be limited to those that meet pharmacoeconomic criteria (e.g., cost-effectiveness) for reimbursement. In some cases, this can result in patients receiving less effective medications, or not being able to access medicines available to those who can pay out of pocket. These situations can be perceived by some as limiting choice, which may also potentially impact public trust. Public trust in health professionals and in science itself is crucial for effective health systems and for research participant recruitment for drug trials and even adverse event reporting [41]. Pharmacovigilance can help bolster public trust, but it also relies on the willing participation of a trusting public.

8 Inclusiveness

As a counterpoint to the equity issues created by a lack of inclusiveness or representation of diverse patient populations in clinical trials, patient engagement in pharmacovigilance activities is growing. As "citizen science" has become increasingly valued in many areas of science, there has been increasing engagement of patients and the broader public in pharmacovigilance and pharmacoepidemiology and there are now guidelines on engaging patients in research across the drug life cycle [42]. Drug safety monitoring systems are being designed to receive patient-reported outcomes, and internet-based surveys about adverse events can be administered to patients directly with relative ease, and countries engaging patients this way see these data to be of scientific value [43]. Not only does this illustrate an improvement in how adverse event data can be collected, but it also indicates a change in how pharmacovigilance researchers, clinical trialists, and healthcare practitioners value the patient perspective [44].

As sociologist Nicky Britton has observed, there are several reasons why this is significant. The first is that respect for persons involves taking patients seriously, otherwise "interactions with professionals can be profoundly damaging" [45]. Patients are not empty vessels to be filled with information from their healthcare practitioners: how patients respond to the advice of their healthcare practitioners is crucial to the effectiveness of treatment, but they will have their own "ideas, experiences, concerns and so on…" [45]. And lastly, engaging with publics during the research process "can help to ensure that academics attend to issues of importance to patients, which may also affect the delivery of health care" [45]. Respect for persons, which is the underlying ethical principle in patient autonomy, requires healthcare practitioners to attend to their patients' stories, especially when something their physician has prescribed (recently or in the past) might have harmed them in some way. Expanding notions of harm to include patient perspectives on, and the social context around, how drugs impact their quality of life, and expanding our notions of effectiveness to include patient perspectives on what they think is effective is crucial to improving our understanding of how drug effectiveness is understood and assessed, and what role drugs ought to play in the treatment of health conditions [46, 47]. Recognition of the importance of engaging with and elevating patient perspectives for patient safety in the use of medicines is exemplified by the establishment of the first ever Patient Safety Commissioner for England—a role which aims to provide an independent point of contact for patients to voice their concerns and to elevate patients' concerns and interests to health systems decision-makers [48].

9 Duty to Report

It has been estimated that over 90% of adverse drug events go underreported [49], including due to forgetfulness or time constraints, as discussed further below. While systems would be overwhelmed if every suspected or even expected event were reported, effective pharmacovigilance requires the cooperation of industry, regulators, researchers, healthcare practitioners, and patients. Healthcare practitioners are especially well positioned to identify and report ADRs that are worrying and unexpected given their close relationships with patients [50]. In addition to the duty of disclosure of medication errors and safety events to patients, healthcare practitioners have a public health duty to report suspected ADRs to the appropriate regulatory and/or scientific bodies, even if they lack an explicitly stated, corresponding legal duty in the jurisdiction in which they practice [51]. This ethical duty is grounded in healthcare practitioners' professional obligations to protect and promote the public's health, which involves taking measures to protect the public from harm. Analogous ethical duties to report exist in the reporting of certain infectious diseases by healthcare practitioners to public health authorities. Although ADR reporting can be burdensome for healthcare practitioners due to the time, effort, administrative challenges associated with reporting, and the potential lack of compensation, emphasis on the importance of the duty to report for patient safety and contributing to the evidence base for medicines may help mitigate these barriers. Efforts to digitize and streamline reporting processes as well as opportunities to educate patients on patient-led and "citizen science" reporting initiatives can help healthcare practitioners uphold this important public health duty [51].

The duty to report is also grounded in healthcare practitioners' professional ethical obligations to contribute to professional and scientific excellence, which they can uphold through contributing to building the base of scientific evidence available to inform clinical, public health, and regulatory decision-making. Adverse event reporting is key to building a high-quality body of real-world evidence concerning the safety and effectiveness of pharmaceuticals, which contributes to informing future clinical decisions and acting in patients' best interests and thus benefits both patients who take medications as well as the healthcare practitioners who prescribe and manage the use of medications.

Spontaneous ADR reporting also contributes to identifying safety signals that may not have been identified in pre-market clinical trials for various reasons, including due to limited sample sizes, nonrepresentative study populations, limited trial periods, and the use of surrogate end points [46]. Identifying safety signals is important both for protecting the public from harm and for equity. In particular, groups that are systematically underrepresented in pre-market trials may be at greater risk of ADRs just by virtue of the fact that they have been excluded from trials, and as a result, there is very limited or no evidence concerning the safety or efficacy of the pharmaceutical product for them [46, 52]. Moreover, groups that are often excluded from pre-market trials may be at greater risk of pharmaceutical-related harms due to one or multiple genetic, biological, behavioral, or social factors that affect their morbidity and mortality, how they metabolize or react to pharmaceuticals, as well as their capability to access pharmaceuticals or adhere to pharmaceutical regimens. Failing to increase the availability and quality of pharmaceutical safety and effectiveness information available for these groups may contribute to or exacerbate health inequities faced by certain groups.

Healthcare practitioners' duties to report are stronger in cases where there is greater evidentiary uncertainty. For example, pharmaceuticals used to treat rare diseases, pharmaceuticals used in populations that are underrepresented in clinical trials, pharmaceuticals used in public health emergencies, and other instances in which there is limited evidence of safety and effectiveness, are all cases where healthcare practitioners' contributions to building the real-world evidence base, especially within the first 5 years of market use, are especially vital to help inform and facilitate safe pharmaceutical use. Furthermore, the duty to report supports healthcare practitioners' integrity-related obligations, discussed below, concerning the use of the highest quality evidence to inform clinical decision-making.

10 Scientific Integrity

As users of, and contributors to the generation of evidence concerning the safety and effectiveness of pharmaceuticals, healthcare practitioners ought to demonstrate integrity. Integrity is a virtue, or an ethically desirable character trait, which requires that healthcare practitioners be dependable in their actions and decision-making, and that their actions and decision-making be consistent with the ethical principles and obligations to which they are bound as healthcare professionals [53–55]. With respect to pharmacovigilance, healthcare practitioners can demonstrate integrity in at least two main ways: first, by using the highest quality evidence possible to inform their pharmaceutical prescribing and management decisions; and second, by identifying, avoiding, and managing conflicts of interest that arise in practice and pharmacovigilance activities (Fig. 14.4). Integrity is important for contributing to the validity of the evidence used to inform pharmaceutical use (such as by reducing the potential for bias in the collection, analysis, and reporting of data), thus helping

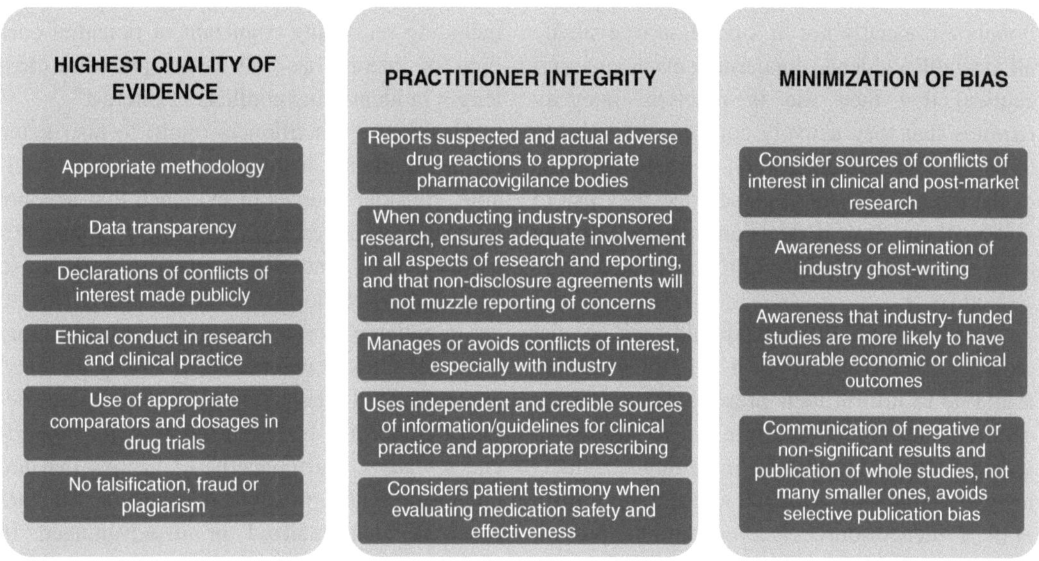

Fig. 14.4 Aspects of scientific integrity

mitigate key factors contributing to medication errors. It is also important for building and maintaining patient and public trust in healthcare practitioners and the safety and effectiveness of the pharmaceuticals they take. Some initiatives of note are the American and Canadian Choosing Wisely recommendations, and the UK's Prescribing Safely Assessment [56, 57]

10.1 Duty to Use the Highest Quality Evidence

Healthcare practitioners use pharmaceutical safety, efficacy, and effectiveness data from pre- and post-market studies to inform pharmaceutical prescribing and management decisions. Prescribers have an ethical obligation to use the highest quality data possible in their practices [58]. As discussed in the preceding section, this duty is complimented by healthcare practitioners' duties to contribute to professional and scientific excellence by reporting suspected ADRs to build the real-world evidence base concerning pharmaceutical safety, especially for new pharmaceuticals. While individual healthcare practitioners are usually not in a position to evaluate all available evidence concerning every pharmaceutical that they use in practice, integrity requires that they actively consider the validity of the data and the credibility, or trustworthiness of the data source for evidence that they use to inform their clinical decision-making [59]. In other words, the integrity of the science itself is also an issue.

Healthcare practitioners should seek out the most complete and highest quality evidence available to inform their prescribing and medication management decisions. The ability to appraise clinical evidence, including considering the validity of evidence and the credibility of the evidence source, is a foundational professional competency for healthcare professionals; this competency is grounded in professionals' ethical obligation to maintain professional competence, or to ensure that their professional skills and knowledge remain up-to-date with the latest evidence and accepted standards of practice [60].

Clinical appraisal skills include assessing the methodological soundness of clinical trials and post-market studies as well as of resulting analyses and practice recommendations; to aid them in this endeavor, healthcare practitioners should seek out independent sources or organizations where (ideally independent) groups of experts and methodologists review and assess the quality of evidence—including the methodological soundness of research studies—to inform practice recommendations. Examples of sources include Cochrane, vetted clinical practice guidelines or evidence syntheses or reviews developed by professional or specialty organizations, organizations such as Choosing Wisely, or health technology assessment organizations specializing in evidentiary assessment such as the United Kingdom's National Institute for Health and Care Excellence (NICE) or Canada's Canadian Agency for Drugs and Technologies in Health (CADTH), and patient safety organizations. However, even in these contexts, and as discussed further below, healthcare practitioners ought to do their due diligence by considering the credibility of the source of the review or guidelines that they consult, including remaining cognizant of potential conflicts of interest, as well as the potential challenges in identifying conflicts of interest.

Healthcare practitioners ought to also listen to their patients' testimonies, and where available, consider sources of evidence that account for patient experiences concerning pharmaceutical use, safety, and effectiveness [61]; doing so contributes both to better understanding how to act in patients' best interests as well as to more equitable clinical practice [62]. Taking patients' experiences of medication use seriously is especially important for ensuring that the experiences, values, and concerns of groups that are underrepresented in clinical trials, or who are otherwise marginalized or disadvantaged in healthcare, are not overlooked or discounted in ways that can create or exacerbate health inequities. Not reporting suspected adverse events also can compromise the knowledge base in pharmacovigilance.

10.2 Conflicts of Interests

Healthcare practitioners ought to be aware of how conflicts of interest can arise and impact clinical decision-making, both with respect to the generation of the pharmaceutical safety and effectiveness evidence that they use, as well as in their own pharmaceutical prescribing and management decisions and interactions with industry representatives and stakeholders [63, 64]. Conflicts of interest arise when a person in a position of trust has a secondary interest (e.g., a financial, professional, or personal interest) that could reasonably be assumed to unduly influences their decision-making with respect to the primary professional interest. Healthcare practitioners' primary interests include the duty to act in patients' best interests and the duty to protect and promote the public good, while for healthcare practitioners and researchers, primary interests include protecting research participants and upholding scientific integrity [3, 4]. Identifying and taking measures to avoid or manage actual or perceived conflicts of interest are ethically important as conflicts of interest can impact clinical decisions in ways that are harmful to patients and public health. Furthermore, conflicts of interest can undermine patient and public trust both in the integrity of healthcare practitioners, professions, regulators, and industry, as well as in the safety of the pharmaceutical products that they use.

As discussed in the preceding section, the duty to use the highest quality evidence possible requires that physicians consider how stakeholders' vested interests can influence pre- and post-market study outcomes and resulting clinical practice recommendations [7]. As discussed above, healthcare practitioners should seek evidence, or evidence assessments and syntheses, from credible, independent sources, rather than primarily relying on information from pharmaceutical manufacturers and industry representatives and sources. Moreover, healthcare practitioners ought to assess the credibility of data sources by considering whether the sources have relationships with industry or other vested interests in particular study outcomes. Healthcare practitioners should also be aware that identifying and assessing conflicts of interest may be difficult due to practices such as medical ghost-writing, where pharmaceutical manufacturers or industry stakeholders hire medical writers, academics, and healthcare professionals to write and publish scientific articles in scientific journals in order to influence the evidence base and clinical practice [65].

Industry influence can occur in the context of assessing the safety, effectiveness, and especially the comparative-effectiveness of pharmaceuticals, such as when so-called "me-too" pharmaceuticals offering only marginal improvements in effectiveness over first-in-class or existing products, but often at a far greater cost, are presented as novel or safer and more effective than existing products [66]. Although prescribing pharmaceuticals that are not first-in-class can offer clinical benefits to patients, it is important that physicians consider the quality and certainty of the evidence concerning the risk–benefit profile of a product carefully, including patient accounts of side effect profiles. In addition to potentially being harmful to patients where newly marketed products pose safety risks to patients, prescribing less effective or cost-effective pharmaceuticals can be harmful to both patients, who may face financial burdens due to higher out-of-pocket costs or co-pays or deductibles, as well as to insured individuals and society as it increases the financial burden to payers, whether public or private.

Integrity requires that physicians identify and take steps to avoid or manage conflicts of interest that arise in their prescribing and pharmaceutical management. This requires critically evaluating under which circumstances it is appropriate, and beneficial to patients, to interact with industry representatives or attend industry-sponsored events or learning activities, including in the course of continuing professional education and development activities aimed at maintaining professional competence around drug safety and effectiveness [8]. Healthcare practitioners should be aware of their obligations with respect to conflicts of interests and interactions with industry as outlined in codes of ethics and professional guidelines in their jurisdiction (e.g., related to accepting compensation, professional development, advising industry, or investing in industry). Healthcare practitioners should also be cognizant of the fact that industry associations may also have guidelines or codes governing industry representatives' and organizations' interactions with healthcare practitioners [67–69].

11 Summary and Conclusions

Healthcare practitioners play a vital role in facilitating effective and ethical pharmacovigilance, as well as in translating evidence generated through pharmacovigilance activities into clinical practice to improve the treatment and care of patients and improve population health. Healthcare practitioners have ethical obligations grounded in their obligations to act in their patients' best interests, to protect and promote the public good, and to maintain their professional competence; in turn, these obligations give rise to a host of ethical principles and considerations related to pharmacovigilance and the safe use of pharmaceuticals. This chapter has outlined several of these key principles and considerations, including: the fiduciary duty, the duty to protect the public from harm, the duty to maintain professional competence, privacy, consent, disclosure, equity, trust, inclusiveness, the duty to report, scientific integrity, the duty to use the highest quality evidence, and conflicts of interest.

Notably, pharmacovigilance requires healthcare practitioners to attend to their obligations to, and the immediate needs of, the individual patients that they treat and care for in their day-to-day practice; however, pharmacovigilance also requires healthcare practitioners to take seriously their broader obligations to upholding public safety, as well as to contribute to the broader endeavor of supporting professional and scientific excellence by contributing to generating high-quality, real-world pharmaceutical evidence. As a result, pharmacovigilance is an area of clinical practice that spans both clinical practice and public health and thus raises ethical issues and considerations pertaining to both domains in ways that other areas of clinical practice may not. Given the complexity of clinical practice, and the interplay between obligations to individual patients and to public health, healthcare practitioners may encounter ethical dilemmas in which they are tasked with discerning between competing ethical obligations or duties and courses of action. Safe and ethical pharmaceutical prescribing and management requires that healthcare practitioners engage in ethical reasoning and reflection to determine the appropriate course of action when treating and caring for their patients and executing their public health-related duties. Reflecting upon the ethical principles and considerations outlined in this chapter, and deliberating about difficult cases with colleagues, including in inter-professional teams, can aid in reasoning through challenging scenarios and contribute to a more robust process of ethical deliberation.

12 Case Studies

12.1 Case Study 1

The opioid crisis in Canada and other countries has claimed many lives due to opioid overdoses and has disproportionately impacted marginalized people. According to the Public Health Ontario, more than 2800 Ontarians died from opioid-related causes in 2021 alone [70]. Naloxone, a Schedule II medication according to Canada's *National Food and Drugs Act*, is used to reverse opioid overdose and can be distributed to the public free of cost without prescription, provided that a pharmacist provides education on its use, on how to identify overdoses, and on how to perform resuscitation.

In 2019 in a small town in Ontario, Canada, a pharmacist was distributing naloxone kits door-to-door with the help of nonpharmacist employees. These employees received training on how to use the kits and provide education to those receiving the kits, but they were not legally permitted to distribute the kits. The pharmacist was motivated to put these kits into the hand of community members after visiting a shelter for homeless people that refused to allow him in to provide education to its clients. He was also aware that illicit drug use comes with stigma and claimed he was concerned that this stigma represents a significant barrier to accessing naloxone as well as the services of a pharmacist for an already marginalized group of people. The pharmacist distributed kits at community events and door-to-door at several businesses in the vicinity of the shelter with the help of his employees, who were not always directly supervised by him as is required by law.

The pharmacist was subject to a disciplinary hearing by the Ontario College of Pharmacists, the provincial regulator, for dispensing naloxone kits without regard to individual need and/or clinical appropriateness and for improperly directing or permitting nonpharmacist employees or agents to dispense naloxone kits to patients in the community. The pharmacist pleaded guilty. The College Panel found that he failed to "maintain a standard of practice of the profession; failed to provide an appropriate level of supervision to a person or persons whom he was professionally obligated to supervise; failed to carry out or abide by an undertaking given to the College; and engaged in conduct or performed an act relevant to the practice of pharmacy that, having regard to all the circumstances, would reasonably be regarded by members of the profession as unprofessional" [2]. Additionally, the disciplinary panel argued that "integrity and trust are paramount to the profession of pharmacy, as pharmacists are held in high regard for their role in the provision of healthcare in Ontario. The Panel observed that Member's conduct tarnished the reputation of the profession" [71].

There was a controversy at the time in Ontario about access to the life-saving naloxone kits. Many harm reduction advocates claimed that it was too hard to access the drug, especially given that drug-overdose deaths were highest in rural settings where pharmaceutical care is more difficult to access than in urban centers, and where issues of stigma might be greater given the higher likelihood of being known to healthcare professionals.

The pharmacist said to the press, "I am guilty of misconduct...Despite that, I have certainly saved lives with what I did" [72].

1. *What are the key ethical and legal issues in this case?*

   This case illustrates the difference between ethics and the law. It is clear that this pharmacist was aware that the drug he was distributing should not have been distributed outside of the pharmacy context and to people who are not technically considered patients of the pharmacy as was specified in the legal regulations governing these types of medications. His decision to ignore the law and to provide naloxone to the public in the community near his pharmacy was informed by his belief in the ethical primacy of saving lives, and possibly also a commitment to equity and justice for marginalized populations. While aiming to save the lives of a marginalized population is ethically admirable and even justifiable, the pharmacists' actions raise questions about who the patient is in community pharmacy practice, as well as whether he adequately considered his professional duty to do no harm.

2. *What are the possible negative consequences of this pharmacist's actions?*

   Naloxone has been shown to drastically reduce deaths from overdoses in the community when distributed to people living with addiction and when they are taught how to administer it correctly. However, it is possible that harm may have been done because the community outreach was conducted by people not empowered to teach the correct administration of naloxone. By distributing the drug outside of the pharmacy, the pharmacist also forwent an opportunity to connect patients with the formal healthcare system and the help it can provide to persons living with addiction. Do these possible harms outweigh the harms possibly avoided by the pharmacist's actions?

Additionally, one must consider the implications of these actions for the public's trust in both the pharmacist and the profession as a whole. What might this pharmacist's other patients think about his actions, and how might this have impacted their therapeutic relationship with the pharmacist? If the pharmacist is someone who disregards the law and professional standards of practice, are they still behaving in a trustworthy manner? And might these actions tarnish the reputation of the profession as a whole? These are additional potential harms that must be weighed in this case.

3. *What is the role of the professional regulatory body in addressing public health crises such as the opioid crisis?*

   While the main goal of professional regulatory bodies is to govern the behavior of their members, they are also charged with maintaining public trust in their members and the profession as a whole. Many healthcare professionals prioritize the dyadic relationship between themselves and their patients as a result of their fiduciary duty. However, many codes of ethics for health professionals also indicate that they are committed to promoting the health of the broader population or society. Additionally, many professional bodies articulate competencies for their healthcare providers that include competency in advocacy. One could argue that there is a conflict of commitment here between maintaining the reputation of the profession and engaging in advocacy work that could redress public health crises and expand access to potentially life-saving medications to a marginalized population.

4. *What alternative actions could have been taken to achieve the same goal of saving lives?*

   The pharmacist in this case could have engaged in advocacy that may not have had such an immediate impact on the crisis, but that would have allowed them to stay within the boundaries of their professional ethics and the law. For example, advocating for changes to how naloxone is accessed in communities with very high illicit drug usage rates, providing safe needle exchanges, or even providing education in the community could all be longer term but effective strategies. However, given the significant rise in overdose rates at the time, one could argue that this would not be enough to make a difference to overdose rates in the short term and that too is ethically problematic.

   The Ontario College of Pharmacists could also engage in advocacy around improving access to care for people living with addiction, providing more training for its members in addiction management and prevention, and lobbying for legislative changes that could improve the health of this marginalized population. Naloxone continues to become more available in some jurisdictions as governments weigh the harms from overdose against the harms of incorrect administration and restricted access to this life-saving drug.

12.2 Case Study 2

In recent years, prescribing of antidepressants for subsyndromal levels of depression has been identified as an area where widespread overprescribing occurs, especially for elderly patients. In recent systematic surveys, only 15% of adults ≥65 years of age who were taking antidepressants had met criteria for major depressive disorder (MDD) during the prior year [74].

You are designing a multicenter, cluster-randomized clinical trial to compare the effectiveness of providing nudges to healthcare practitioners via email and electronic health records to encourage physicians to consider alternatives to prescribing SRI medication and prevent potentially inappropriate or prolonged prescribing in antidepressant-naïve patients who have fewer than 5 of the 9 symptoms for MDD.

Healthcare practitioners will not be masked to the arm of the trial they are participating in. Because the study is deemed to be of minimal risk to patients, they will not be asked to provide consent and will not even be made aware that they are participating in a trial. To ensure patients are receiving appropriate care, healthcare practitioners will ask that patients attend the clinic for administration of the diagnostic questionnaire for MDD at least one additional time in the next 4 months.

Healthcare practitioners will be randomized to different arms of the trial: (1) control group; (2) group where they are given the prescribing guidelines and asked to justify their decision to prescribe in the electronic health record and; (3) group where they are given the prescribing guidelines and a weekly email in which their prescribing rates are compared to other healthcare practitioners'; (4) group where they receive both the guidelines and emails as well as being asked to justify their decisions on the electronic health record.

1. *How might this trial impact patients' autonomy and/or dignity?*

   We should ask ourselves when designing trials like this one whether patient choice in treatment options is being limited in some way. As models of care move toward shared decision-making, a trial like this presumes that prescribers are always making decisions without input from patients. It is worth asking whether that is appropriate for this class of medications, or for this (potential) condition. Are there some medications and/or conditions where shared decision-making is more or less important? What if a patient really wants the medication and is unwilling or unable to engage in clinically proven alternative methods to improve low mood, such as exercise? Are we respecting the dignity of patients when we ask healthcare practitioners to withhold information from their patients about research that involves them and their personal health information (e.g., about their health outcomes)?
2. *Is the burden on patients insignificant?*

   This trial is likely not terribly onerous for most patients given that they are being asked to return to the clinic only once within 4 months. So, the nonclinical risks and burdens have been deemed low enough to proceed without obtaining explicit consent of the patients. But what about the patient who lives far away, or the patient who cannot afford to pay for parking, or the patient who works two jobs and cannot take time off work easily? It is important that we do not make assumptions about the extent of patients' nonclinical risks and burdens, as these are often subjective and can vary across sociodemographic groups, including in ways that disproportionately burden already disadvantaged groups.
3. *Will all patients benefit equally from this trial or its findings?*

   Related to the question above, we need to ask if the risks and burdens from this trial might fall disproportionately on patients who are already socially disadvantaged. Where exercise is prescribed instead of medication, it is important to note that not all patients have access to safe places to walk in their neighborhoods, just as some might not have the time to exercise due to having to work long hours or care for children or elderly relatives. While the trial findings may help low-income patients who can avoid having to pay for an unnecessary prescription medication, is it possible that those who are more socially advantaged will benefit more? As such, does the trial risk exacerbating existing inequities in access to care or health outcomes between certain sociodemographic groups?
4. *Is it fine not to disclose to patients that they are participating in this trial?*

   While some research is sufficiently low risk that it is accepted that patients do not need to be informed, particularly in situations where study recruitment could be a challenge, some healthcare practitioners might find not disclosing the trial to patients ethically problematic. This stems from healthcare practitioners' professional ethics duty to respect patient autonomy and their right to provide informed consent. However, healthcare practitioners could also be concerned that patients' trust in their providers might be compromised if patients were to find out that they were unwitting participants in research, even if it is low risk. So, although it might not be a legal requirement to disclose trial participation to patients, some healthcare practitioners might deem it ethically necessary. However, this could cause problems in the context of a multicentre trial where adherence to protocols is necessary to provide consistency across trial sites.

Acknowledgments Alison Thompson would like to thank the Canadian Institutes for Health Research for funding prior research into the ethical dimensions of drug safety and effectiveness.

Ana Komparic would like to thank the Fondation Brocher in Hermance, Switzerland, where she had the opportunity to work on this chapter during a visiting research stay.

References

1. Public Health Ontario. Interactive Opioid Tool. Opioid-related morbidity and mortality in Ontario. [cited 2022 Dec 15]. Available from: https://www.publichealthontario.ca/en/Data-and-Analysis/Substance-Use/Interactive-Opioid-Tool.
2. Ontario (College of Pharmacists) v. Newman. 2020 [cited 2022 Dec 15]. Available from: https://canlii.ca/t/jg953.
3. Weeks C. Ontario pharmacist facing disciplinary action for distributing naloxone kits door-to-door says he will keep distributing; Case highlights tensions over the province's distribution program and whether current practices are working to ensure enough of the drug is getting into the right hands. The Globe and Mail (Breaking News); 2019 Sep 17 [cited 2022 Dec 15]. Available from: http://global.factiva.com/redir/default.aspx?P=sa&an=GMBN000020190917ef9g0002t&cat=a&ep=ASE.
4. Safer DJ. Overprescribed medications for US adults: four major examples. J Clin Med Res. 2019;11(9):617–22.
5. Cruess RL, Cruess SR. Expectations and obligations: professionalism and medicine's social contract with society. Perspect Biol Med. 2008;51(4):579–98.
6. Swick HM. Toward a normative definition of medical professionalism. Acad Med J Assoc Am Med Coll. 2000;75(6):612–6.
7. Cruess SR, Johnston S, Cruess RL. "Profession": a working definition for medical educators. Teach Learn Med. 2004;16(1):74–6.
8. McCullough LB. Taking the history of medical ethics seriously in teaching medical professionalism. Am J Bioeth. 2004;4(2):13–4.
9. Taber JM, Leyva B, Persoskie A. Why do people avoid medical care? A qualitative study using national data. J Gen Intern Med. 2015;30(3):290–7.
10. Sismondo S, Doucet M. Publication ethics and the ghost management of medical publication. Bioethics. 2010;24(6):273–83.
11. Lexchin J. Those who have the gold make the evidence: how the pharmaceutical industry biases the outcomes of clinical trials of medications. Sci Eng Ethics. 2012;18(2):247–61.
12. Mintzes B, Lexchin J, Sutherland JM, Beaulieu MD, Wilkes MS, Durrieu G, et al. Pharmaceutical sales representatives and patient safety: a comparative prospective study of information quality in Canada, France and the United States. J Gen Intern Med. 2013;28(10):1368–75.
13. Fung AE, Rosenfeld PJ, Reichel E. The International Intravitreal Bevacizumab Safety Survey: using the internet to assess drug safety worldwide. Br J Ophthalmol. 2006;90(11):1344–9.
14. Seh AH, Zarour M, Alenezi M, Sarkar AK, Agrawal A, Kumar R, et al. Healthcare data breaches: insights and implications. Healthc Basel Switz. 2020;8(2):E133.
15. Jose J, AlHajri L. Potential negative impact of informing patients about medication side effects: a systematic review. Int J Clin Pharm. 2018;40(4):806–22.
16. Wells RE. To tell the truth, the whole truth, may do patients harm: the problem of the Nocebo effect for informed consent. Am J Bioeth. 2012;12(3):22–9.
17. Barsky AJ, Saintfort R, Rogers MP, Borus JF. Nonspecific medication side effects and the nocebo phenomenon. JAMA. 2002;287(5):622–7.
18. Rogers A, Craig G, Flynn A, Mackenzie I, MacDonald T, Doney A. Cluster randomised trials of prescribing policy: an ethical approach to generating drug safety evidence? A discussion of the ethical application of a new research method. Trials. 2020;21(1):477.
19. Kalkman S, van Thiel GJMW, Grobbee DE, Meinecke AK, Zuidgeest MGP, van Delden JJM. Stakeholders' views on the ethical challenges of pragmatic trials investigating pharmaceutical drugs. Trials. 2016;17(1):419.
20. Cassell J, Young A. Why we should not seek individual informed consent for participation in health services research. J Med Ethics. 2002;28(5):313–7.
21. 45 CFR 46.104—Exempt research. [cited 2023 Apr 21]. Available from: https://www.ecfr.gov/current/title-45/subtitle-A/subchapter-A/part-46/subpart-A/section-46.104.
22. Kim SY, Miller FG. Informed consent for pragmatic trials—the integrated consent model. N Engl J Med. 2014;370(8):769–72.
23. Vijayananthan A, Nawawi O. The importance of good clinical practice guidelines and its role in clinical trials. Biomed Imaging Interv J. 2008;4(1):e5.
24. Drucker PF. Innovation and entrepreneurship: practice and principles. Harper & Row; 1985. 296 p

25. Team DDW. Data mining in the pharmaceutical industry. Drug Discovery World (DDW); 2001 [cited 2023 May 10]. Available from: https://www.ddw-online.com/data-mining-in-the-pharmaceutical-industry-814-200110/.
26. Alfawzan N, Christen M, Spitale G, Biller-Andorno N. Privacy, data sharing, and data security policies of women's mHealth apps: scoping review and content analysis. JMIR Mhealth Uhealth. 2022;10(5):e33735.
27. Grundy Q, Chiu K, Held F, Continella A, Bero L, Holz R. Data sharing practices of medicines related apps and the mobile ecosystem: traffic, content, and network analysis. BMJ. 2019;364:l920.
28. Tangari G, Ikram M, Ijaz K, Kaafar MA, Berkovsky S. Mobile health and privacy: cross sectional study. BMJ. 2021;373:n1248.
29. Hebert PC. Disclosure of adverse events and errors in healthcare: an ethical perspective. Drug Saf. 2001;24(15):1095–104.
30. Denny DBAD, Shinners C. Medical error reporting, culture, and infrastructure. J Clin Oncol. 2018;36(Suppl. 30):245.
31. Naseralallah L, Stewart D, Azfar Ali R, Paudyal V. An umbrella review of systematic reviews on contributory factors to medication errors in health-care settings. Expert Opin Drug Saf. 2022;21(11):1379–99.
32. WHO. Medication without harm—global patient safety challenge on medication safety. Geneva: World Health Organization; 2017. [cited 2022 Jul 4]. Report No.: Licence: CC BY-NC-SA 3.0 IG. Available from: https://www.who.int/publications-detail-redirect/WHO-HIS-SDS-2017.6.
33. Ünal A, Seren IŞ. Scientific view of the global literature on medical error reporting and reporting systems from 1977 to 2021: a bibliometric analysis. J Patient Saf. 2022;
34. Innovative approaches for improving drug & vaccine safety. [cited 2023 Apr 21]. Available from: https://tdr.who.int/our-work/research-for-implementation/innovative-approaches-for-improving-drug-vaccine-safety.
35. Chen MS Jr, Lara PN, Dang JHT, Paterniti DA, Kelly K. Twenty years post-NIH Revitalization Act: enhancing minority participation in clinical trials (EMPaCT): laying the groundwork for improving minority clinical trial accrual. Cancer. 2014;120(S7):1091–6.
36. National Institutes of Health. Diversity and Inclusion in Clinical Trials. National Institute on Minority Health and Health Disparaties. [cited 2022 Jul 7]. Available from: https://nimhd.nih.gov/resources/understanding-health-disparities/diversity-and-inclusion-in-clinical-trials.html.
37. Alegria M, Sud S, Steinberg BE, Gai N, Siddiqui A. Reporting of participant race, sex, and socioeconomic status in randomized clinical trials in general medical journals, 2015 vs 2019. JAMA Netw Open. 2021;4(5):e2111516.
38. Equity must be baked into randomized controlled trials. Nature. 2022;606(7915):624.
39. Solarin O, Mohammed SI, Ndlovu N, Vanderpuye V, Olaiya V. Partnerships and Collaborations: the right alliances for clinical trials in Africa. JCO Glob Oncol. 2020;6:954–8.
40. De Las ND, Hacker K, DiGirolamo A, Hicks LS. A systematic review of community-based participatory research to enhance clinical trials in racial and ethnic minority groups. Health Serv Res. 2012;47(3 Pt 2):1363–86.
41. Wesson P, Hswen Y, Valdes G, Stojanovski K, Handley MA. Risks and opportunities to ensure equity in the application of big data research in public health. Annu Rev Public Health. 2022;43(1):59–78.
42. Planelles B, Margarit C, Inda MD, Ballester P, Muriel J, Barrachina J, Ajo R, Esteban MD, Peiró AM. Gender based differences, pharmacogenetics and adverse events in chronic pain management. Pharmacogenomics J. 2020;20(2):320–8.
43. Goodman CW, Brett AS. Race and pharmacogenomics—personalized medicine or misguided practice? JAMA. 2021;325(7):625–6.
44. Magavern EF, Gurdasani D, Ng FL, Lee SSJ. Health equality, race and pharmacogenomics. Br J Clin Pharmacol. 2022;88(1):27–33.
45. Resnik DB. Scientific research and the public trust. Sci Eng Ethics. 2010;17(3):399–409.
46. CIOMS Working Group XI. Patient involvement in the development, regulation and safe use of medicines. Geneva: Council for International Organizations of Medical Sciences; 2022.
47. van Hunsel F, Härmark L, Pal S, Olsson S, van Grootheest K. Experiences with adverse drug reaction reporting by patients: an 11-country survey. Drug Saf. 2012;35(1):45–60.
48. Rolfes L, van Hunsel F, van der Linden L, Taxis K, van Puijenbroek E. The quality of clinical information in adverse drug reaction reports by patients and healthcare professionals: a retrospective comparative analysis. Drug Saf. 2017;40(7):607–14.
49. Britten N, Maguire K. Lay knowledge, social movements and the use of medicines: personal reflections. Health (N Y). 2016;20(2):77–93.
50. Komparic A, Smith MJ, Thompson A. An ethical justification for expanding the notion of effectiveness in vaccine post-market monitoring: insights from the HPV Vaccine in Canada. Public Health Ethics. 2016;9(1):78–91.
51. Mohammed MA, Moles RJ, Chen TF. Medication-related burden and patients' lived experience with medicine: a systematic review and metasynthesis of qualitative studies. BMJ Open. 2016;6(2):e010035.
52. First ever Patient Safety Commissioner appointed. GOV.UK. [cited 2023 May 10]. Available from: https://www.gov.uk/government/news/first-ever-patient-safety-commissioner-appointed.
53. Hazell L, Shakir SAW. Under-reporting of adverse drug reactions: a systematic review. Drug Saf. 2006;29(5):385–96.
54. Lopez-Gonzalez E, Herdeiro MT, Figueiras A. Determinants of under-reporting of adverse

drug reactions: a systematic review. Drug Saf. 2009;32(1):19–31.
55. Klein E, Bourdette D. Postmarketing adverse drug reactions: a duty to report? Neurol Clin Pract. 2013;3(4):288–94.
56. Smith M, Komparic A, Thompson A. Deploying the precautionary principle to protect vulnerable populations in Canadian post-market drug surveillance. Can J Bioeth. 2020;3(1):110–8.
57. Levinson W, Ginsburg S, Hafferty FW, Lucey CR. Integrity and accountability. In: Understanding medical professionalism. New York, NY: McGraw-Hill Education; 2014. [cited 2023 May 10]. Available from: accessmedicine.mhmedical.com/content.aspx?aid=1105135170.
58. Edgar A, Pattison S. Integrity and the moral complexity of professional practice. Nurs Philos Int J Healthc Prof. 2011;12(2):94–106.
59. Tyreman S. Integrity: is it still relevant to modern healthcare? Nurs Philos Int J Healthc Prof. 2011;12(2):107–18.
60. Recommendations. Choosing Wisely Canada. [cited 2023 May 10]. Available from: https://choosingwiselycanada.org/recommendations/.
61. PSA. [cited 2023 May 10]. Available from: https://prescribingsafetyassessment.ac.uk/#intro.
62. Thompson A, Komparic A, Smith MJ. Ethical considerations in post-market-approval monitoring and regulation of vaccines. Vaccine. 2014;32(52):7171–4.
63. Upshur R. Making the grade: assuring trustworthiness in evidence. Perspect Biol Med. 2009;52(2):264–75.
64. Ilic D. Assessing competency in evidence based practice: strengths and limitations of current tools in practice. BMC Med Educ. 2009;9:53.
65. Anderson C, Krska J, Murphy E, Avery A, Yellow Card Study Collaboration. The importance of direct patient reporting of suspected adverse drug reactions: a patient perspective. Br J Clin Pharmacol. 2011;72(5):806–22.
66. Fickweiler F, Fickweiler W, Urbach E. Interactions between physicians and the pharmaceutical industry generally and sales representatives specifically and their association with physicians' attitudes and prescribing habits: a systematic review. BMJ Open. 2017;7(9):e016408.
67. Fleischman W, Agrawal S, King M, Venkatesh AK, Krumholz HM, McKee D, et al. Association between payments from manufacturers of pharmaceuticals to physicians and regional prescribing: cross sectional ecological study. BMJ. 2016;354:i4189.
68. Flaherty DK. Ghost- and guest-authored pharmaceutical industry-sponsored studies: abuse of academic integrity, the peer review system, and public trust. Ann Pharmacother. 2013;47(7–8):1081–3.
69. Aronson JK, Green AR. Me-too pharmaceutical products: history, definitions, examples, and relevance to drug shortages and essential medicines lists. Br J Clin Pharmacol. 2020;86(11):2114–22.
70. 2022 Code of Ethical Practices. Innovative Medicines Canada. [cited 2023 May 10]. Available from: https://innovativemedicines.ca/resources/all-resources/2022-code-of-ethical-practices/.
71. Code on Interactions with Health Care Professionals. [cited 2023 May 10]. Available from: https://phrma.org/resource-center/Topics/STEM/Code-on-Interactions-with-Health-Care-Professionals.
72. ABPI 2021 Code of Practice. 2023 [cited 2023 May 10]. Available from: https://www.abpi.org.uk/reputation/abpi-2021-code-of-practice/.

Part II

Safer Prescribing and Drug use in Practice

15 Medication Errors in Healthcare

Myungsun Ro, Daniel Degnan, and John Hertig

Abstract

Medication errors occur throughout the medication use process and carry the potential to cause severe patient harm. This chapter discusses various types of medication errors, methods of detection, components of error, and strategies for risk mitigation. Terminology frequently used in medication safety such as "adverse drug event," "adverse drug reaction," and "near miss" or "close call" is defined, and James Reason's Swiss Cheese Model is explained as relating to active and latent failures. Various error detection methods such as voluntary error reporting, trigger tools, direct observation, and technology-generated data as well as diverse factors that contribute to medication errors are presented. Medication safety officers play a critical role in preventing medication errors by implementing proactive and retrospective strategies such as failure modes and effects analysis and root cause analysis. Additionally, the importance of patient education, human factors and systems engineering, and the safety culture of an institution cannot be underestimated. Patients have a right to safe care, and providers must first do no harm. Special attention is given to understanding, practicing, and systematically employing the tools and concepts presented in this chapter.

Keywords

Medication error · Medication errors · Adverse event · Adverse drug reaction · Adverse drug event · Near miss · Medication use process Medication safety · Drug safety · Patient safety · Pharmacovigilance

Learning Objectives

- Define medication error and other terms frequently used in medication safety.
- Explain the medication use process and the Swiss Cheese Model as they relate to active and latent failures in the systems process.
- Identify various methods to detect errors and factors that contribute to medication errors.
- Describe the position of a medication safety officer and their role in preventing and mitigating medication errors.
- Recognize the impact of patient education, human factors and systems engineering, and culture on medication safety.

M. Ro (✉)
Patient Safety Authority, Harrisburg, PA, USA
e-mail: mro@pa.gov

D. Degnan
Purdue University College of Pharmacy, West Lafayette, IN, USA

J. Hertig
Butler University College of Pharmacy and Health Sciences, Indianapolis, IN, USA

J. Jose et al. (eds.), *Principles and Practice of Pharmacovigilance and Drug Safety*,
https://doi.org/10.1007/978-3-031-51089-2_15

Key Points

- Medication errors can occur during various stages of the medication use process. It is important to recognize the potential safety gaps that healthcare providers may encounter during the process.
- It is essential to distinguish between commonly used terms in medication safety, such as *medication error, adverse drug event, adverse drug reaction*, and *near miss,* when describing a medication error event.
- The Swiss Cheese model is a conceptual framework that illustrates how multiple layers of defense within healthcare systems can fail, leading to errors reaching patients. Errors could be due to active and latent failures, and addressing latent failures is crucial for preventing errors from reaching patients.
- Healthcare professionals have an important role in remaining vigilant for potential errors. Different types of methods that are used in healthcare to detect errors include incident reporting systems, trigger tools, direct observation, and technology-generated data.
- There are several components to a medication error, such as technology failures, human error, at-risk behavior, and reckless behavior. An understanding of the ten key elements of medication use will help healthcare providers identify the root causes of a medication error event.
- Healthcare providers are encouraged to find an improvement methodology that is appropriate for their practice setting and workflow. It is vital to consider implementing error mitigation strategies with a focus on patient and consumer education, risk reduction strategies in healthcare settings, human factors and system engineering, medication error classification, risk analysis assessments, and error reporting culture.

1 Introduction

The field of medication safety as it relates to the formalized study of medication errors dates back to the work of Michael Cohen and Kenneth Barker, both of whom were influenced by Avedis Donabedian. Dr. Donabedian became renowned following the publication of a lengthy paper titled *Evaluating the Quality of Medical Care* in 1966. This seminal work introduced the concepts of structure, process, and outcome to the evaluation of healthcare quality [1]. Subsequently, in 1981, Cohen published a leading textbook in the area of medication errors, while Barker established the first research methods for studying medication errors, still used widely today [2]. Also, in the late 1980s, a Harvard-trained physician, Lucian Leape, discovered an alarming number of medical errors in his research on the utilization of cardiac procedures [3]. This work led him to focus on medical errors, culminating in the Institute of Medicine (IOM, now the National Academy of Medicine) report, *To Err is Human: Building a Safer Health System* [4]. This report introduced the concept that medication errors are the result of faulty systems and not solely due to human mistakes. The IOM report describes the widespread problem of medication errors, the barriers preventing improvement, and the strategies needed to make healthcare safer for all patients. These concepts were influenced by the advances in safety demonstrated by areas outside of healthcare, such as the aviation and automobile industries [5]. A comparison of risk in healthcare with respect to other safety industries is shown in Fig. 15.1.

The World Health Organization (WHO) estimates that at least one death every day and 1.3 million injuries occur per year in the United States as a result of medication errors [6]. Although the rates of medication error may be similar in low- and middle-income countries compared with high-income countries, the number of years of healthy life lost may be approximately twice as high based on the available data [6]. In addition to the lives lost, the economic cost of medication errors has been estimated at US$42 billion [6].

The Joint Commission (TJC) and other accrediting agencies acknowledged the harmful implica-

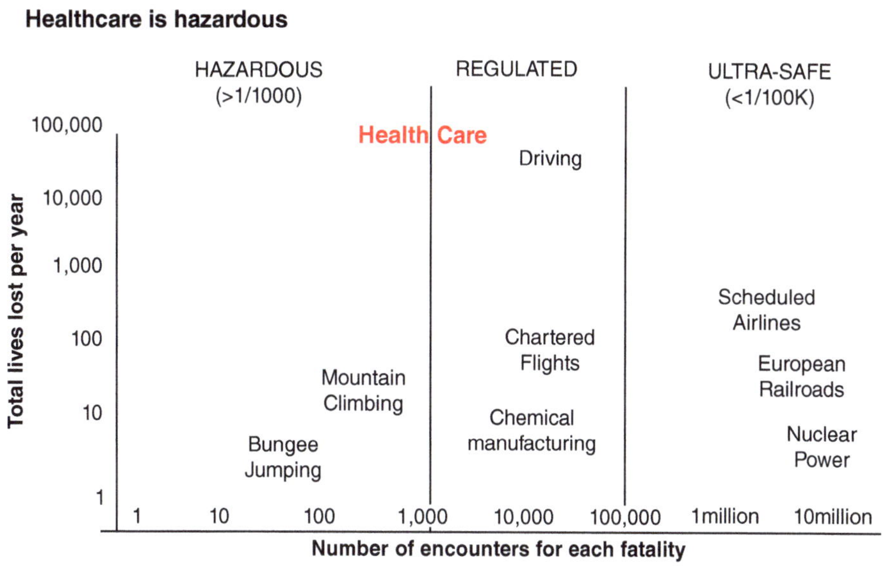

Fig. 15.1 Comparison of healthcare to other safety industries. Healthcare is generally highly regulated, yet relatively dangerous when compared to other industries. Reproduced with permission (See acknowledgment section). The figure extrapolates from earlier work by: R Amalberti. The paradoxes of almost totally safe transportation systems Saf Sci, 37 (2001), pp. 109–126

tions of medication error and required hospitals to establish programs to identify and prevent medication errors and adverse drug events (ADEs). To meet these regulatory requirements, programs have been developed, often led by Departments of Pharmacy and pharmacists to review medication errors and work with various disciplines (physicians, nurses, and administrators) to design interventions to increase medication error reporting and reduce harmful events. Most hospitals did not have specific medication safety programs, and the programs that were in place were centered on medication processes instead of the broad medication use system (e.g., procurement and inventory management, nursing unit processes, and physician prescribing) [7]. Given the challenge to ensure medication safety is a priority in all aspects of care delivery, combined efforts of interdisciplinary teams are frequently used to prevent patient harm. To assist in an interdisciplinary focus and to promote fundamental understanding of data, a variety of definitions, tools, and resources can help pharmacy and other health professionals as they take leadership roles in medication safety [8].

Describing differences among the various definitions used in medication safety became such a prevalent issue that scholars have frequently highlighted the problem as hindering progress in improving care. Yu et al. attempted to categorize a hypothetical event using various definitions on publicly available websites [9]. The process identified more than 119 definitions for 25 medication safety-related terms. In the study, there were 10 definitions for *adverse drug event*, 11 different definitions for *adverse drug reaction*, and 7 different definitions collected for the term *medication error*. Although the authors were quick to point out that some of these were functionally the same, the issue of developing a common definition of key terms used in medication safety is a fundamental tenement to improving the systems around medication use.

In order to create a safe medication use process for all patients around the world, it is essential to understand related definitions, identification of errors, and practices to analyze and mitigate harm. Medication errors are common throughout all healthcare systems and occur during all stages of the use of a medicine, such as prescribing, dispensing, and administration. This chapter will cover the etiology of medication errors and the burden they produce on patients and healthcare systems. It will outline the operation of key medication error systems. It will also focus on the methods of learning from error, at an international, national, and local level.

2 The Medication Use Process

Originally developed through TJC to evaluate the use of medications in hospitals, the medication use process (Fig. 15.2) has since been established as a systematic way to measure the effectiveness of the use of medications and to review potential safety mitigation strategies. Generally, the five steps of the medication use process can be defined as prescribing, transcribing, dispensing, administration, and monitoring. With the advent of computerized provider order entry (CPOE), the step of transcribing may be combined with the prescribing step of the process [10]. As supply chain issues have become more prevalent with regard to medication safety, the step of medication procurement has been added by some organizations when evaluating the medication use process.

A classic pair of studies completed in 1995 attempted to identify the frequency of ADEs in each segment of the medication use process [11, 12]. The two frequently cited studies identified the incidences of breakdown of events occurring in each segment of the medication use process at a major US medical center as: ordering (39–49%), administering (26–38%), transcribing (11–12%), and dispensing (11–14%). It is important to note that the prevalence may vary depending on the therapeutic areas, as observed in one study that attributed 78% of all medication errors involving direct-acting oral anticoagulants to the prescribing stage [13]. The studies were conducted before any significant adoption of CPOE technology. Using the conceptual framework of the medication use process can help to identify complimenting medication event mitigation strategies. The two studies identified underlying system errors associated with the medication use process. In the Leape study, the most common system failures identified included the inadequate availability of patient information and the poor dissemination of drug knowledge throughout the medication use process [10]. The Bates study found that ADEs most frequently occurred in the ordering and administering stage of the medication use process and were often preventable according to the definitions used in the study [11].

2.1 Medication Safety Terminology

A fundamental element of improving a system or a process is the need to quantify or measure the progress. In the field of healthcare improvement, particularly in medication safety, a challenge exists in providing accurate comparators and definitions. The international multitude of definitions related to medication safety-related terms and the resulting confusion have led to challenges in developing evidence associated with specific improvement strategies. The problem of a lack of common taxonomy for medication-related events and the harm

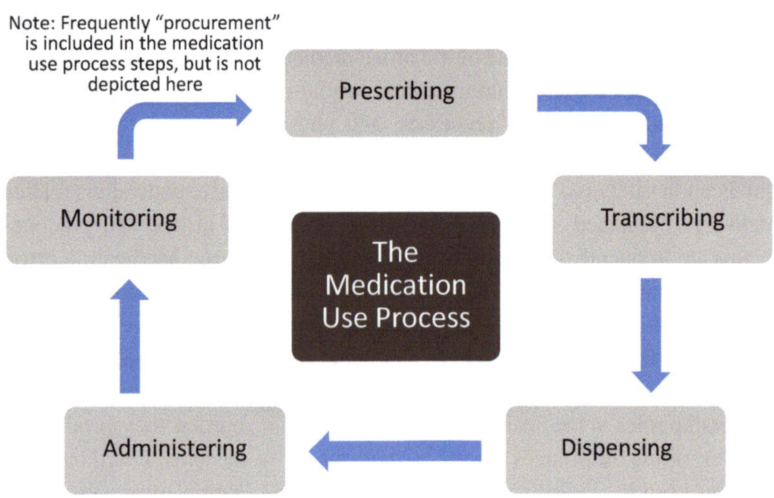

Fig. 15.2 The medication use process. The medication use process consists of (procurement), prescribing, transcribing, dispensing, administering, and monitoring

caused to patients is an important component of evidence analysis. When definitions are operationalized by individual healthcare organizations and even healthcare practitioners, as well as the pharmaceutical industry and regulatory agencies, additional taxonomy drift can occur.

The confusion that exists when analyzing medication safety-related terms is not new. As early as 1989, Dr. Henri Manasse described the challenges that existed with regard to "terminology associated with the negative effects of drugs" [14]. The problem with regard to definitions related to medication safety has been perpetuated to date and identified by authors such as Yu and Lisby [9–16]. In the case of Yu, more than 119 definitions for medication safety terms were encountered when reviewing 33 safety-related websites. Both authors identified frequently used definitions across a variety of sources and then applied case-based scenarios to identify commonalities and differences among the definitions used.

A frequently used definition for the term *medication error* is provided by the American organization, the National Coordinating Council for Medication Error Reporting and Prevention (NCC MERP), an independent body composed of 27 national and international organizations [17]. A key aspect of the NCC MERP definition is that a medication error can be identified by asking three questions:

1. Was this a preventable event?
2. Could the event cause harm or lead to inappropriate medication use or patient harm?
3. Was the medication in the control of a healthcare professional, the patient, or the consumer?

Outside of the United States, the European Medicines Agency (EMA) is well known for establishing its own definition of the term *medication error* and issuing guidance on pharmacovigilance and reporting of errors in Europe [18].

Adverse drug reaction is another frequently used term in medication safety. The definition commonly used by healthcare practitioners was one that was proposed by the WHO in 1972 and widely accepted by other healthcare groups [19]. The term *adverse drug reaction* and its associated definitions have undergone scrutiny and attempts at modification since its inception [20, 21]. The International Council for Harmonisation of Technical Requirements for Pharmaceuticals for Human Use (ICH) has established its own definition and guidance on *adverse drug reaction* that are widely accepted in Europe, especially for pre-marketing and post-marketing clinical safety in the regulatory and pharmaceutical sectors [22].

Perhaps the broadest proposed definition of a medication safety-related term is that of *adverse drug event* which has its historical roots in the 1999 report, *To Err is Human,* where it is described as "any injury resulting from medical intervention related to the drug." This definition was further refined and discussed by Nebecker in 2004 using the definition "any injury resulting from the use of a drug." This is by nature a broad definition and encompasses primary questions:

1. Was the medication administered to the patient?
2. Did patient injury or harm, in any form, result from the use of the medication?

It is important to note that *ADEs* are not always preventable using the definition expanded upon by Nebecker. In addition, the ICH, with input from the WHO Collaborative Centre, defines adverse event or adverse experience (AE) as *any untoward medical occurrence that may present during treatment with a medicine, but which does not necessarily have a causal relationship with this treatment* [22].

A near miss medication event, sometimes also called a close call event, is a medication situation that did not produce patient injury but was prevented by active intervention or chance detection. A common source for this definition comes from the Agency for Healthcare Research and Quality (AHRQ) in the United States [23]. It should be noted that a near miss event could also be defined as a medication error using the NCC MERP definition of a medication event that could have led to harm but never reached the patient.

While the four basic definitions used in the taxonomy of medication safety are medication error, adverse drug reaction, adverse drug event,

Table 15.1 Common definitions used in medication safety [24]

Medication safety term	Common definition
Medication error	Any preventable event that may cause or lead to inappropriate medication use or patient harm while the medication is being handled by the healthcare professional, patient, or consumer
Adverse drug event	Patient harm (injury) that resulted from the use of a medication
Adverse drug reaction	A response to a medicine which is noxious and unintended at doses normally used in man for prophylaxis, diagnosis, or therapy of disease or the modification of physiologic function
Near miss event or close call event	Any medication event that could have had adverse consequences for the patient but did not

Table 15.2 Other terms frequently used in medication safety

Adverse event	Medical error
Adverse medication event	Medication incident
Adverse reaction	Medication-related problem
Associated factor	Potential adverse drug event
Contributory factor	Potential adverse event
Drug problem	Potential error
Drug-related problem	Risk factor
Error	Root cause
Incident	Side effect

and near miss event or close call event, other medication safety-related terms are pervasive in practice and the literature [9, 25–27]. These terms and definitions can be seen in Tables 15.1 and 15.2.

2.2 The Swiss Cheese Model and Active and Latent Failures

Human errors can occur throughout the various steps of the medication use process and are most likely to occur when (1) an individual healthcare practitioner makes a mistake, (2) the process subsequently fails to deliver the desired outcome, and (3) a high-risk procedure is involved. This is frequently explained using James Reason's "Swiss Cheese Model" of human error, as shown in Fig. 15.3 [28]. The Swiss Cheese Model is based on the premise that each process step in a system is prone to varying likelihood of error. As each process step is completed, there may be a hole (similar to a hole identified in Swiss cheese) where a potentially harmful event can be perpetuated and move on to the next step of the process.

Often these environmental factors result in process step failures and errors that may ultimately affect a patient. These failures can occur in each step—pieces of Swiss cheese—of any process and are represented by the holes in each piece of cheese. When the holes in each piece of cheese all align perfectly, harmful patient events can occur.

Using Reason's model, there are two general strategies for reducing errors. *The first* strategy is to *prevent the initial source of the error.* This is not always possible given the desired outcome. *The second*, and more commonly used, strategy is to *find and fix the system problems*. In this case, additional pieces of Swiss cheese are added, and the holes in each piece are made smaller. In other words, strategies are employed to decrease the probability of failure at each step. Examples of failure reduction strategies for each step in the medication use process will be evaluated later on in this chapter.

Thinking of healthcare processes as multiple pieces of Swiss cheese—with holes representing the potential for errors that may result in harm to the patient—is the basis for a healthcare improvement model known as "Systems Thinking." Systems Thinking requires the evaluation of the whole process rather than focusing on just one step or individual. This approach suggests all process parts are interrelated, and adverse outcomes are comprised of both *active failures* and *latent failures*. Active failures are errors committed at the "sharp end," usually inadvertently by healthcare practitioners and staff. These take the forms of slips, lapses, mistakes, and procedural violations [29]. Unlike active failures that are more apparent and obviously attributable to the error, latent failures are underlying weaknesses in the structure of the system, environment, or equipment that are hidden and much more difficult to detect, known as the "blunt end" of errors. Latent failures will always be present in a process, and therefore the entire system must be

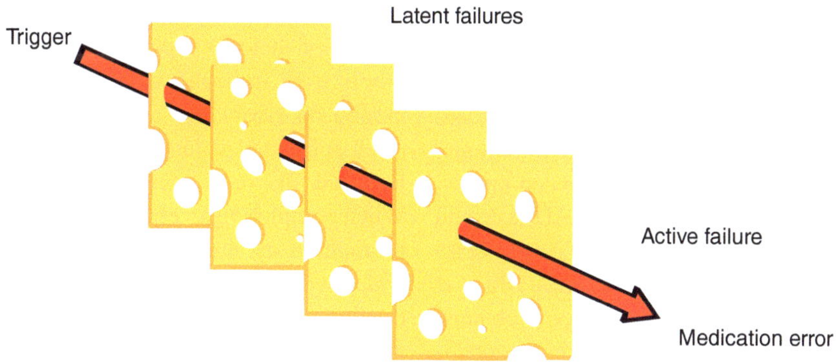

Fig. 15.3 Swiss cheese model. James Reason proposed that individual holes of the Swiss cheese represent failures and that multiple failures must align for a medication error to reach the patient

evaluated to ensure all identified points of both active and latent failures can be reduced or eliminated altogether [29]. An example of a latent failure would be storing the hydroxyzine and hydralazine medications next to one another without any obvious identifiable differences on the bottles; this circumstance is an accident waiting to happen. The active failure, then, is the human action of selecting and filling the wrong medication. "Systems Thinking" involves evaluating this situation in its entirety, assessing both active and latent failures inherent in a system, and then employing strategies to reduce the likelihood of either occurring.

3 Detection of Errors in Healthcare

3.1 The Case of Betsy Lehman

In Boston, Massachusetts, United States, sits a patient safety center called Betsy Lehman Center, which is named after a former healthcare reporter for the newspaper *The Boston Globe*. Betsy Lehman, the mother of two young daughters, sought treatment for metastatic breast cancer at the Dana-Farber Institute, which is also located in Boston. In December 1994, Betsy Lehman died as a result of the treatments she received. The reasons for Ms. Lehman's death were not initially known and were thought to have been a result of her cyclophosphamide treatments. A subsequent but routine review of the medication administered noted that Ms. Lehman received a fourfold overdose of cyclophosphamide which induced cardiac damage and resulted in her tragic death.

Significant lessons in safe medication systems and improvement strategies have occurred since Betsy's death in 1994 [30–32]. Both significant awareness regarding the need to seek out the reporting of medication errors and near misses, and the technology and analytical capabilities to detect medication errors have grown significantly. In fact, during the improvement journey at Dana-Farber Institute, a former executive at the facility, James Conway, identified the need to continually and actively seek out medication errors with an eye for improvement. Conway elaborated that the work of creating safe care is a continual journey and that comprehensive, multidimensional error detection methods are an important component [33]. No one error detection method will identify all medication errors, and they should be used in combination to be truly effective.

3.2 Medication Error Detection Methods

A variety of sources should be used to determine the relative safety of the medication use process. It is important to identify and collect many data in order to obtain a comprehensive picture of medication safety. Data may include (1) voluntary error reports submitted through formal reporting programs; (2) automated trigger tools—such as the administration of reversal agents following the administration of opioids; (3) direct observation of process errors; (4) peer review of electronic or paper-based medical records; and (5) information from technology applications and hardware such as bar code medication administration (BCMA) systems, smart infusion pumps, automated dispensing cabinets (ADCs), and CPOE systems. There are strengths and weaknesses with each of these data sources, which is why multiple strategies are necessary to obtain a more accurate assessment of safety in an organization [34]. Four common collection methods are voluntary error reports, trigger tools, direct observation, and technology-generated data as described below. Their advantages and disadvantages are listed in Table 15.3.

Table 15.3 Advantages and disadvantages of drug event detection methods

Drug event detection method	Advantages	Disadvantages
Voluntary error report	• Frequently detects harmful patient errors	• Labor-intensive process • May not be effective without a healthy reporting culture
Automated trigger tool	• Efficiently collects information without human intervention	• Provides nonspecific information which may require follow-up
Direct observation	• Frequently provides comprehensive process data	• Labor-intensive process that requires trained observers
Technology-generated data	• Expensive to implement • May not have end user buy-in regarding accuracy and efficiency	• Cover multiple areas of the medication use process • Produce large amounts of data to compensate for weaknesses

3.2.1 Voluntary Error Reports

Voluntary incident reporting systems are commonly used in health systems to collect information on errors that occur. These reports are often submitted voluntarily by those who were involved in, or witnessed, the actual event. When completing an error report, it is important to include as much information as possible, which will aid in the review and possible investigation of the incident. Many reporting systems allow the reporter to remain anonymous; however, providing contact information can help enable follow-up and evidence gathering. Voluntary reporting systems traditionally have resulted in significant underreporting of medication errors [35]. Thus, voluntary error reporting data should be supplemented with information from other sources [36].

3.2.2 Trigger Tools

The use of automated trigger tools to detect ADEs was originally reported by Classen in 1991 [37]. An ADE trigger can be defined as a “clue” that an ADE may have occurred. The original tool was adapted and further refined by the Institute for Healthcare Improvement (IHI). In 2003, Rozich and colleagues suggested additional ADE detection methods and categories using electronic triggers. Rozich also suggested that trigger tools could be an efficient method to collect ADE information within an organization [38]. Trigger tools can be identified using a wide variety of electronic information to retrospectively examine particular errors without examining the actual event specifically. Another advantage to the use of trigger tools is that it removes the reporting burden from an individual practitioner. Examples of triggers that might be used by a hospital can be found in Table 15.4.

While the automated collection of trigger data is frequently utilized at healthcare institutions, manual methods are also available to detect similar types of events. The specific trigger data often gathered from retrospective review of patient charts can be manually characterized and organized. The data is presented in three formats: adverse events per 1000 patient days, adverse

Table 15.4 Examples of electronic adverse drug event triggers and their possible associated events

Example of an electronic adverse drug event trigger	Possible associated event
Prothrombin time (PTT) >100 seconds	Excessive dose of heparin administered to patient
Serum glucose <50 mg/dL	Administration of an oral hypoglycemic agent and insulin without proper monitoring of the patient's serum glucose
Naloxone administration	Combination opioid therapy administered to a patient or suspicion of opioid overdose
International normalized ratio (INR) >6	Excessive dose administration of warfarin or improper dose calculation
Diphenhydramine administration for the treatment of rash	A possible allergic reaction to medication administration

events per 100 admissions, and percent of admissions with an adverse event. The most commonly used metric is "adverse events per 1000 patient days." The manual collection of trigger tool data can be labor-intensive but can be useful data to monitor over time to identify trends and patterns.

3.2.3 Direct Observation

Direct observation is a method used to monitor the medication use process in real time, recording data as actions are taken. Traditionally, the direct observation method employs independent, trained observers to watch a medication administration take place and document the process with standardized forms. Typically, an observer will watch 50–100 doses be dispensed or administered while documenting any observed findings. These notes then are reconciled against the original orders to determine if there are any discrepancies between the intended therapy and the medications actually given to the patient. These discrepancies are validated, categorized, and recorded as errors. Albeit resource-intensive and possibly subject to the Hawthorne effect, the direct observation method helps identify trends, creating an objective and quantitative set of safety data [39].

3.2.4 Technology-Generated Data

Information from medication safety technology can be used both proactively and retrospectively to identify potential errors that could or may have resulted in patient harm. CPOE systems with decision support can be used to identify the frequency with which allergies and drug–drug interaction alerts are activated and lead to modifications in therapeutic regimens. This type of data can be used to proactively design formulary alternatives and electronic schemes for presenting preferred medications to prescribers.

BCMA systems can generate a variety of near miss and operational dose omission data. A study conducted at a teaching hospital in London concluded that the implementation of CPOE and BCMA resulted in more legible and coherent prescriptions by prescribers and more detected errors identified by pharmacists [40].

Smart infusion pumps, especially those that are connected to the medical record, can provide organizations access to valuable patient safety-related data. The data can identify near miss situations in which a smart infusion pump was programmed incorrectly. The dose error reduction software (DERS) is an integral component of smart infusion pumps that prevents users from delivering too much or too little of a medication or fluid. Multiple sources of data can be used to monitor the patient safety aspects of smart pump use [41].

4 Components of a Medication Error

There are many factors that create and heighten the potential for a medication error. Throughout the complex stages of the medication use process, medications are handled through numerous hands of interdisciplinary healthcare team members and vetted by technology, human factors, systems design, and safety culture, to name a few, until they finally reach the patient. Some errors may remain unnoticed or undetected, while some may cause serious harm to patients and must be investigated for causes in order to prevent their future recurrence. Therefore, identification of the components of a medication error serves to not only rectify patient harm but also ascertain significant knowledge and strategies for risk reduction.

4.1 Institute of Safe Medication Practices' 10 Key Elements of Medication Use

The Institute for Safe Medication Practices (ISMP) classifies components of medication error into the following ten key elements [42, 43]. The key elements and their associated potential medication errors are listed in Table 15.5. An understanding of these key elements is useful when investigating all potential causes and contributors of medication error and developing their associated risk mitigation strategies.

The first element in Table 15.5, documentation of wrong patient information, can inevitably lead to the downstream occurrence of medication errors. Examples of patient-specific information include age, weight, allergies, medical history, lab results, and contraindications related to individual medication use, e.g., pregnancy status for medications with teratogenic potential. Updated documentation of renal status for patients taking direct oral contraceptives has been shown to prevent medication errors in a UK-based study [44]. An analysis of event reports submitted to the Pennsylvania Patient Safety Reporting System (PA-PSRS) revealed that incorrect or missing documentation of patient's weight led to several types of medication errors such as overdose, underdose, and wrong rate of administration [45]. Five of the 10 most commonly reported medications in the study were considered high alert, meaning that they carry a heightened risk of causing significant harm when used in error [45, 46]. Some of the recorded types of weight-based errors included confusion between pounds versus kilograms, wrong documentation of weight, missing weight, incorrect estimated weight, and calculation error [45].

A special patient population that particularly depends on weight-based dosing of medications are pediatric patients. They face a heightened risk for medication errors due to a multitude of unique factors. These include pharmacokinetic parameters that differ at various stages of development, use of extemporaneous compounding due to the lack of available certain dosage forms and concentrations for pediatric patients, inability for very young children to communicate adverse effects, and requirement of specialized knowledge required by the healthcare providers [47–49]. Unofficial temporary naming of newborns [50] and shared last names between the mother and the child [51] pose additional safety risks that are unique to the pediatric population.

The second key element in Table 15.5, maintaining easily accessible up-to-date and accurate drug information, is critical for identifying, preventing, and mitigating potential for error. These may include institution-specific guidelines, electronic health record (EHR) order sets, literature-based references, and drug information resources such as Lexicomp or Micromedex. Medication-specific information such as adverse effects, drug interactions, maximum dose, typical dose, precautions, special populations, and contraindications are necessary for all stages of the medication use process, including prescription, verification, preparation, administration, and monitoring of safe and effective medication use [43].

A combination of the first and third key elements in Table 15.5, which pertains to documentation, communication, and transmission of accurate information about the medications, applies to the example of medication reconciliation. Medication reconciliation, informally known as *med rec*, is defined by the American Pharmacists Association (APhA) as "the comprehensive evaluation of a patient's medication regimen any time there is a change in therapy" [52]. Medication reconciliation requires collaboration by patients and interdisciplinary providers as well as clear and consistent communication across all levels of care and points of care transitions [53]. According to one study, 68% of medication discrepancies during admission to an emergency department were found to be significant, serious, or life threatening [54]. In order to improve patient safety and outcomes, TJC has identified medication reconciliation as a major

Table 15.5 Key elements of medication use and associated potential medication errors [42, 43]

ISMP's key element of medication use	Examples of associated areas for potential errors
1. Patient information	Patient name, age, weight, allergies, past medical history, lab values, and insurance status
2. Drug information	Contraindication, warning, adverse effects, drug interactions, cross-allergies, storage, preparation, administration, and requirement of delivery device
3. Communication related to medications	Communication of drug orders, communication dynamics, confused abbreviations, illegible prescriptions, and misheard verbal orders
4. Drug labeling, packaging, and nomenclature	Unlabeled medications, look-alike/sound-alike medications, confusing labels on medications, and poorly positioned labeling components that obscure important drug information
5. Drug standardization, storage, and distribution	Storage proximity to look-alike/sound-like medications, failure to properly dilute or reconstitute medications prior to administration, multiple available concentrations leading to wrong selection, and nonstandard medication administration times
6. Medication delivery device acquisition, use, and monitoring	Unfamiliarity with medication delivery devices, pump programming errors, use of inappropriate measuring device for oral liquids, and line mix-ups leading to wrong route administration
7. Environmental factors	Inadequate staffing, noise, lighting, physical space, work schedules, interruptions, and sensory distractions
8. Staff competency and education	Orientation training, education, competency assessment, certifications, practice drills and simulations, and off-site education
9. Patient education	Low health literacy, lack of patient counseling, discharge instructions, complex dosing schedules, cultural and language barrier, lack of resources or access to information, and improper selection of medications (e.g., duplication of active ingredients exceeding recommended dose) due to lack of knowledge
10. Quality processes and risk management	Leadership, culture, error reporting, safety strategies, focus on blaming individuals rather than improving system, and operating without a medication safety officer

area for healthcare improvement in the National Patient Safety Goals for the Hospital Program [55].

Examples of errors relating to medication communication include illegible handwritten orders, misheard verbal orders, failure of prescriptions transmitted to the pharmacy, misuse of leading or trailing zeroes, and misunderstood abbreviations [43]. The following reports involving inappropriate abbreviations have been submitted to PA-PSRS [56].

- *An elderly female patient with an INR less than 2.8 received a Coumadin (warfarin) dose that should have been held. The original order stated to give Coumadin if INR < 2.5 (<2.5). However, the "<" (less than) symbol was misinterpreted as "greater than," which led to the administration of Coumadin.*
- *A physician wrote an order to increase Diovan (Valsartan) to 80 mg BID. An up arrow (↑) symbol was used to indicate "increase" in the prescription strength but was read as the numeral 1. The pharmacy interpreted the order to be Diovan 160 mg BID (since no 180 mg form is available), and the patient received one dose of Diovan 160 mg.*
- *A prescriber used an abbreviation for magnesium sulfate and wrote "MgSo$_4$ 2g IV × 1 dose" for a patient. However, the unit clerk and nurse misinterpreted the order as morphine sulfate (MSO4) 2 mg IV × 1 dose, and the patient received a 2 mg dose of morphine sulfate instead of magnesium sulfate.*
- *An elderly patient received an order for Dilaudid (HYDROmorphone) without the use of leading zeroes (0.2–0.4 mg). As a result, the order was misread as 2–4 mg instead of the intended 0.2–0.4 mg.*

The fourth key element in Table 15.5 refers to drug labeling and packaging which constitute a major component of medication error [43]. According to the FDA Fact Sheet, there are over 19,000 prescription medications that are currently on the market [57] which do not include all of the foreign medications that are sometimes imported during drug shortages or utilized by patients who obtain them outside of the country. This raises the problem of numerous look-alike/sound-alike medications which can lead to confused drug names and mix-ups. These can occur between generic names (e.g., acetaminophen and acetazolamide) or brand names (e.g., Celexa and Celebrex), or both (e.g., heparin and Hespan) [58]. Even an entry of the name "aspirin" into the FDA's Phonetic and Orthographic Computer Analysis (POCA) will result in 334 look-alike and sound-alike medication names [59]. ISMP Canada has published the following examples of error reports that involve look-alike sound-alike medication mix-ups [60].

- *A pregnant patient was prescribed Diclectin® (Pyridoxine/Doxylamine), but Dicetel®* (Pinaverium) *was dispensed. She had received Dicetel® many times in the past.*
- *A physician wrote a prescription for Hydrocortisone 1% in Mycostatin®; however, Hydrocortisone 1% in Miconazole (Monistat®) was dispensed instead. The staff member thought Mycostatin® and Miconazole were the same medication.*
- *A patient intended to refill Zopiclone over the phone; however, the technician refilled the existing prescription for Zoloft® (Sertraline).*

In the inpatient settings, providers are at an increased risk of committing an error via mislabeling, missing labels, and lack of standardization when medications are compounded or prepared on patient floors outside of the pharmacy. According to the results of a 2018 ISMP survey of intravenous (IV) push practices in adult care units, more than a quarter (28%) of the respondents reported that they *rarely* or *never* label syringes that are prepared outside the pharmacy and away from the patient's bedside. Rather than labeling the syringes, the respondents claimed to distinguish the medication-containing syringes only by visual appearances, such as the volume of the medication inside, size of the syringe(s), color difference in needle caps or medication, or the location of the syringe in relevance to the practitioner, such as its orientation on a tray or sterile field or placement in different hands or pockets [61]. Therefore, the fifth key element of drug standardization is critical for accurately producing the same IV product every time. Efforts to promote the standardization of IV medications and analyze its impact on safety, effectiveness, and waste reduction have been established through initiatives such as the Standardize 4 Safety initiative, the Indiana Standard Concentrations of Adult Drug Infusions List ("the Indiana List"), and the Vial, Exchange, Rate, and Bag (VERB) analysis [62–64].

As an example of the sixth key element in Table 15.5, compromised medication delivery services can also lead to medication errors. Several wrong-route medication administration errors involving lines and tubing have been documented, such as the inadvertent administration of oral solutions into IV lines and accidental administration of IV contrast media into the external ventricular drain into a patient's brain [65]. Joint Commission Sentinel Event Alert #53 identified that 116 case studies in 34 publications involved misconnections that directed enteral feeding solutions into IV lines [66]. In a *New York Times* article, a 35-week pregnant 24-year-old woman and her unborn child were reported to have died after enteral feeding was inadvertently administered intravenously instead of via nasogastric route [67]. In 2019 the Healthcare Safety Investigation Branch, based in the United Kingdom, completed an investigation on inadvertent administration of an oral liquid into a vein and published several safety findings, including the root causes and safety recommendations to National Health Services (NHS) Improvement and the Royal College of Physicians [68].

Aside from connection mix-ups, additional errors with IV medication administration sets have been reported. Errors involving medications that were trapped inside the IV tubing and later inadvertently administered have been reported to have been caused by an inappropriately setup primary administration set [69]. Insufficient knowledge surrounding the use of smart pumps and medication administration sets is another component of medication error, as, according to a survey performed by nurses and pharmacists, many are unaware of existing guidelines for positioning the primary infusion bag relative to the infusion pump as well as the required head height differentials for secondary infusion [70].

Next, the seventh key element in Table 15.5 describes the environmental factors such as the physical surroundings, organizational unit, ergonomics, workload, staffing patterns, and work schedules [43]. This also includes physical stimulations such as lighting, noise, and foot traffic [43]. When the workspace and schedules do not provide adequate support and may possibly even impede work effort, the practitioners may be left to maneuver important tasks amid distractions and competing priorities that divert from medication safety. The United States Pharmacopeia General Chapter <1066> has official definitions, factors to consider, and guidelines for providing an optimal physical environment for medication safety [71].

The eighth key element in Table 15.5 refers to staff competency and education which are critical in preventing unwanted medication errors. In the case of unsafe IV push practices, ISMP survey results have revealed a wide variability in preparation technique, lack of or unfamiliarity with institutional policies or guidelines, persistence of learned practices without sound scientific evidence, and lack of organized training or competency assessment during formal or professional training [61, 72]. There is further evidence to suggest that providers prepare IV push medications with such variation in technique, not only from practitioner to practitioner but within each individual practitioner from injection to injection [72, 73]. Lack of standardized training and competency assessment can create variable safety risks that can be multifaceted, diverse, and difficult to detect. Purchasing and implementing inventory practices that support safe IV medication use is also essential. Ready-to-administer products are generally preferred whenever possible to help ensure safe IV drug delivery. This underscores the importance of optimizing medication safety at every step of the medication use process [74].

In the ninth key element in Table 15.5, medication errors can also occur at home when patients are not educated, informed, or empowered about their medication therapy. Patients may be reluctant to ask questions about prescription and over-the-counter (OTC) medications that they may not understand due to medical jargon, language barriers, or low health literacy [43]. Approximately 7 out of 10 people have been shown to measure the volume of liquid medication incorrectly by failing to use metric and standardized measurements or inappropriately using the measuring devices [75].

An example of a measuring error is described below [76].

- *A father purchased a store brand diphenhydramine (Benadryl®) per doctor's order to treat his 5-year-old's bad cold. The medication came with a dosing cup and a label that stated 12.5 mg of the medication equals 5 mL. After reading the instruction to give 12.5 mg to 25 mg for a child less than 6 years old, the father filled the dosing cup to 12.5 mL, confusing the dose in mg with the volume in mL. The dose that the father poured into the cup (12.5 mL) was almost three times greater than the amount the child needed (5 mL).*

For patients selecting OTC medications, packaging and brand names also play a role in medication error. A consumer may not be familiar with generic names, brand names, and various combinations of active ingredients that are available in similar packaging. Additionally, poor product container design and labeling can also obscure critical safety information which could lead to dangerous medication errors. An example of an active ingredient packaged in multiple different ways is shown in Fig. 15.4. Lack of patient

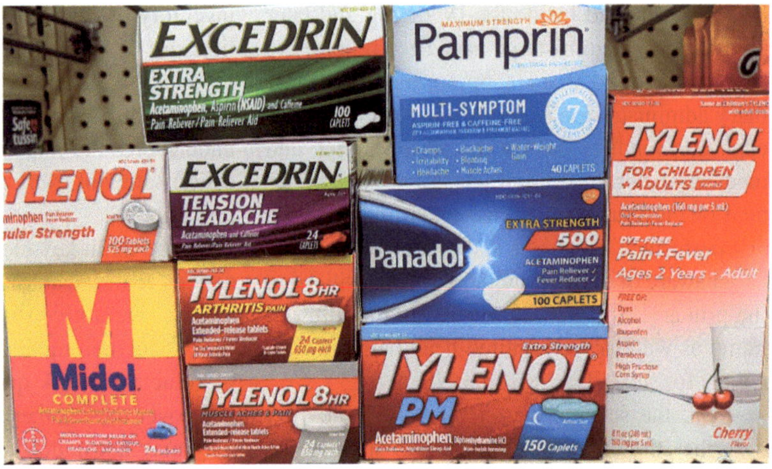

Fig. 15.4 Brand name medications that share the active ingredient acetaminophen at a US pharmacy. These do not include numerous acetaminophen-containing medications that are sold under generic packaging. Note: Acetaminophen is commonly referred to as paracetamol outside of the United States

knowledge and education can result in misuse of medications, missed doses, and failure to promptly respond to warning signs that can lead to serious harm.

Lastly, quality processes and risk management are paramount to ongoing surveillance and quality improvement of safe medication practices. Institutions should strive to create and foster an environment of safety that is perpetuated by encouraging an open and honest culture of reporting and acknowledging each healthcare member as a meaningful contributor to patient and medication safety. Safety goals should be regularly set, benchmarked, reviewed, and monitored for tangible gains in action plans and targeted risk mitigation strategies. When errors do occur, institutions that target individual members or events as standalone deviations, rather than addressing the system as a whole and as lessons in safety, will not learn and grow from their mistakes. A classic non-healthcare example is starting a car in reverse. Rather than isolating the incidents and blaming the individual drivers, the automotive industry created a forcing function from the systems perspective to eliminate the problem altogether [5]. Culture of blame breeds fear, silence, and secrecy, none of which is conducive to collective systems' progress toward safety.

4.2 Human Error, At-risk Behavior, and Reckless Behavior

Human errors can be classified into knowledge-based, rule-based, and skill-based [77]. Knowledge-based human errors occur due to practitioner's deficit in experience or knowledge, rule-based errors occur when practitioners misinterpret or misapply the rules, and skill-based errors occur due to attention and memory failures [77].

The terminology used when describing Just Culture defines human errors as slips of action and lapses of memory that occur when carrying out familiar tasks without giving much conscious attention [78]. Conditions that can prime slips and lapses include familiarity of task, confusion of two similar tasks, convoluted procedures that do not follow naturally, and interruptions or distractions [78].

On the other hand, at-risk behavior is distinguished from human errors by the loss of perception of risk associated with the choice or mistaken belief that the risk is insignificant or justified [79]. David Marx from Just Culture argues that it is natural human tendency to "drift" and engage in at-risk behavior, as over time practitioners become comfortable performing their tasks and habitually engage in shortcuts whose risk they calculate to be present, but low and tolerable [79].

Human errors and at-risk behaviors are distinct from reckless behavior, in which the healthcare practitioner has consciously discarded a known, substantial, and unjustifiable risk of harm [78, 79]. Once a behavior has been found to be reckless following an investigation, it warrants swift and appropriate remediation or disciplinary action as it deliberately violates a healthcare worker's commitment to protect patients from harm [79].

4.3 Technology—Greatest Gift to Medication Safety or Weapon of Mass Destruction?

Health information technology (HIT) has introduced some of the most popular preventative mechanisms against human and medication errors as well as expanded access and availability to medications. BCMA employs barcode scanning that reliably distinguishes the correct medication despite look-alike packaging and confusing labeling. CPOE and EHRs eliminate handwritten prescriptions that are rife with illegible handwriting and misinterpreted abbreviations as well as extend accessibility of patient and medication records to all relevant healthcare practitioners providing care to the patient. ADCs offer a convenient and secure platform to dispense verified and profiled medications directly to the providers on the clinical units. However, the caveat of technology is that its safety profile strictly depends on the user who operates it properly within its safe workflow processes. When it is improperly programmed or utilized, technology and automation have the adverse potential to cause harm on an exaggerated scale until the mistake is detected and corrected.

Such is the case with a former nurse, RaDonda Vaught, who made the fatal error of choosing a wrong medication from the ADC that led to the death of a patient. While attempting to obtain a vial of VERSED (a discontinued brand of midazolam), she typed "VE" into the ADC search field and inadvertently selected vecuronium, a neuromuscular blocker. The death of the patient from a wrong medication administration and the resulting trial and conviction of the former nurse captured the media attention in the United States for several years, prompting discussions on safe medication use, functionalities of ADC, and Just Culture. The case of RaDonda Vaught illustrates that technology, such as the ADC, will only operate safely and effectively as limited by the system rules and designs that outline its optimal use and the individual users who navigate it safely [96, 126, 127].

Additionally, when institutions first acquire new technology or converge their existing technology with another, technology-related adverse events can be created as new demands arise, resources are diverted, current processes are temporarily adjusted or permanently changed, and staff members learn to adapt to new technologies. TJC Sentinel Alert #42 was published in response to technology-related adverse events in healthcare involving CPOE, ADCs, EHRs, clinical decision support (CDS), barcoding or radio frequency identification, and more [128]. Errors can stem from failing to include the frontline practitioners in the planning process, not considering resource and staffing relocations needed for implementation and ongoing maintenance, and rejecting the need to address existing flaws and latent problems prior to installing new technology [128].

Once HIT is implemented, many can offer CDS with warnings to alert the provider from making unsafe practice choices. These can be part of the CPOE, smart infusion pumps, cardiac monitoring devices, automated compounding devices, and more. However, between a staggering number of the various interactive alerts, sounds, and visuals that are constantly triggered during clinical practice, the providers can become overwhelmed and eventually desensitized to safety alerts, leading to ignorance or failure to heed appropriately to such warnings in a phenomenon coined the "alert fatigue" [129]. A 2013 study found that providers selected to "override" important and useful drug–drug interaction alerts that are likely to cause serious patient harm [130].

Alert fatigue from overuse of technology can have the unintended counter-effect of bypassing safety warnings; technology should be supported and monitored comprehensively before, during, and after its implementation for its optimal impact on medication safety.

The advancement of technology continues to widely impact the landscape of healthcare, encouraging a growing number of institutions to adopt new and innovative ways to ensure medication and patient safety. However, technology should not be regarded as a panacea in risk reduction, as it affords safety measures only within the confined limits of safe work processes and adequate user knowledge. Safe use of technology should be deliberated within interdisciplinary teams, assessed in the context of the existing needs and processes at the institution, and continuously monitored for adjustment and improvement.

5 Error Mitigation Strategies

Once the contributing factors or causes for medication error have been identified, the corresponding mitigation strategies need to be implemented in a timely manner and monitored continuously for quality improvement. For an investigation into an unintended medication error or event, the 10 key elements to medication use can be a useful approach to pinpointing various aspects and identifying active and latent failures that contributed to the error.

There are many official and consensus-based error reduction recommendations and resources readily available for practitioners, patients, and industry vendors. The NCC MERP has various recommendations to enhance accuracy of prescription or medication order writing as well as a list of dangerous abbreviations [80, 81]. The ISMP regularly updates its List of Error-Prone Abbreviations, Symbols, and Dose Designations, Look-Alike Drug Names with Recommended Tall Man Letters, High-Alert Medications in various healthcare settings, and Confused Drug Names [46, 58, 82, 83]. ISMP also offers several self-assessments and practice guidelines such as ISMP Targeted Medication Safety Best Practices for Hospitals [84]. Table 15.6 offers a list of some international agencies and organizations offering medication safety-related guidance and updates.

The FDA also has several official guidelines for all users, for example, the Safety

Table 15.6 International regulatory agencies and professional organizations

Name	Country or region	Regulatory, professional, or other
The US Food and Drug Administration (FDA)	United States	Regulatory
The European Medicines Agency (EMA)	Europe	Regulatory
Japan's Pharmaceutical and Medical Devices Agency (PMDA)	Japan	Regulatory
National Agency for the Safety of Medicine and Health Products (ANSM)	France	Regulatory
Medicines and Healthcare products Regulatory Agency (MHRA)	United Kingdom	Regulatory
Health Canada	Canada	Regulatory
Australia's Therapeutic Goods Administration (TGA)	Australia	Regulatory
International Pharmaceutical Federation (FIP)	International	Professional
International Medication Safety Network (IMSN)	International	Professional
International Society of Pharmacovigilance (ISoP)	International	Professional
International Society Pharmacoepidemiology (ISPE)	International	Professional
Patient Safety Authority (PSA)	United States	Other
Institute of Safe Medication Practices (ISMP)	United States	Other
American Society of Health-System Pharmacists (ASHP)	United States	Professional
National Coordinating Council for Medication Error Reporting and Prevention (NCC MERP)	United States, international	Other

These are a few examples of official international organizations that provide useful medication safety-related guidance and announcements

Considerations for Container Labels and Carton Labeling Design to Minimize Medication Errors which has several recommendations for industry to design optimal package labels that minimize confusion and prioritize safety for vendors [85]. Some of these include minimization of corporate trade dress, judicious use of color, display of product strength and concentration, metric measurements, and avoidance of dangerous abbreviations, acronyms, and dose designations [85].

The American Society of Health-System Pharmacists (ASHP) is a professional organization in the United States that represents pharmacists practicing in hospitals, health systems, ambulatory clinics, and other healthcare settings. It offers many resources such as guidelines on preventing medication errors in hospitals [86] and position statement on medication safety [87]. It also provides useful information by clinical specialties, such as the guidelines on medication error prevention in chemotherapy and biotherapy [88].

5.1 Patient and Consumer Education

At the level of patients and consumers, it is of utmost significance that they are educated on the medication they are taking. They should be encouraged to ask questions about their therapy, seek counsel from their pharmacists or prescribing physicians with any questions about medications, and keep a written record of all their prescription and nonprescription, OTC, vitamins, and herbal medications [43]. The FDA recommends that consumers ask questions and seek knowledge surrounding indications for drug therapy, potential adverse effects, risks and causes for medication errors, instructions on appropriate administration, storage, disposal, dangers of drug–drug and drug–food interactions, and submission of medication errors to reporting programs such as FDA's MedWatch [89] and the ISMP Medication Errors Reporting Program (ISMP-MERP).

Patients can use the following list of questions as an example if not already addressed during patient counseling [90]:

1. What is this medication for?
2. What are the brand and generic names of the medication?
3. Can I take the generic version?
4. Should I stop taking any other medications?
5. How much and how often should I take the medication?
6. When should I stop taking the medication?
7. How many and how often are the refills available?
8. How is the medication stored?
9. Does this medication require or recommend any tests?
10. How can I tell if the medication is working?
11. Are there any foods, other medications, or activities that I should avoid while taking this medication?
12. What side effects can I expect?
13. What should I do if I experience a side effect?
14. What should I do if I miss a dose?
15. What other (printed) information is available regarding this medication?

Whenever possible, patients should engage in mutual conversations with their providers in order to continuously learn new information and complement their existing knowledge gaps. When consulting online resources for information, they should seek websites that are supported by the local and federal government, accredited organizations, peer-reviewed journals, and other reputable sources. If healthcare providers cannot be immediately accessed for medication safety inquiries, patients are encouraged to visit their nearby community pharmacies for trusted medication-related information. Furthermore, it is important to note that effective communication requires an understanding between the patient and the prescriber of the perception of the message and the motivations behind the intended alterations in behavior [91].

5.2 Risk Reduction Strategies at Healthcare Settings

At the level of healthcare institutions and facilities, numerous layers of strategies should be

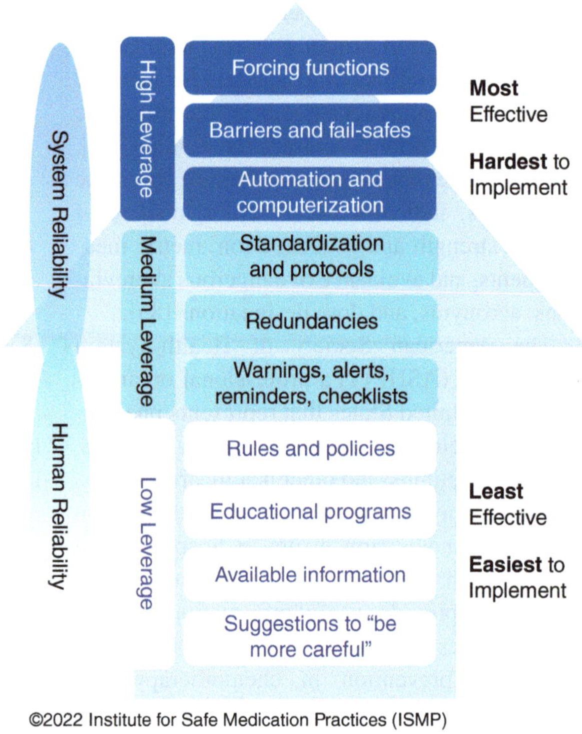

Fig. 15.5 ISMP's hierarchy of effectiveness of **risk reduction strategies.** Some risk mitigation strategies are more effective than others but also more difficult to implement. (c) 2022 Reprinted with permission from ISMP [92]

implemented to prevent the potential for harm from reaching the patient. The spectrum of strategies, ranging from those that are system-based, most difficult to implement, and highly automated to those that are the easiest to implement yet most reliant on human consistency, should be utilized concomitantly to create a robust safety system. ISMP's hierarchy of effectiveness of risk reduction strategies (Fig. 15.5) places the highest priority on forcing functions, barriers and fail-safes, and automation and computerization which are collectively referred to as high leverage, although they can be the most complex, time-consuming, and difficult to implement in practice [93]. These should be mixed with medium- to low-leverage strategies that are easier to implement and less resource-intensive, such as standardization and protocols, warnings and alerts, rules and policies, and educational programs [93]. Also referred to as the hierarchy of hazard control, it is an important concept in human factors engineering as shown in a study involving medication and patient safety in the ICU [94].

For example, in response to the fatal medication error that involved the unintentional retrieval of vecuronium over Versed (midazolam), an institution could implement the following strategies in the order of effectiveness hierarchy. The first is to discontinue using the brand name of midazolam "Versed" which is no longer available on the market [95]. Sequestering high-risk neuromuscular blockers to safe storage inside the pharmacy and limiting them to rapid sequence intubation (RSI) kits are considered high-leverage strategies because they eliminate access to the medications at the systems level. Instituting protocols surrounding ADC overrides and allowing medication searches by both brand and generic names are considered medium- to high-leverage strategies. The easiest to implement but least effective are reminders to healthcare practitioners to double-check their dispensed medications and instructions to search by the first five, not two, letters of the medication name. Combining strategies of various leverage levels helps to create more diverse and robust barriers against potential medication errors [96, 97].

Sequestering physical access to high-alert medications, allowing ADC searches by both brand and generic names as well as multiple letters and implementing forcing functions and barriers in the EHR system are considered high-leverage strategies that utilize principles of human factors engineering.

5.3 Human Factors and System Engineering

Human factors engineering is described as identifying the limitation of human capabilities and designing the system to meet the needs of the workers. It operates on the assumption that [29]:

Fallibility is part of human condition;

We *cannot* change the human condition, however;

We *can* change the conditions under which people work.

In the complex medication use process where humans, technology, and systems processes are inextricably intertwined, there are extensive human factors that play a role in medication errors. The focus is not only on preventing failures but also on controlling or enforcing constraints on system behavior [98]. Similar to the previous descriptions of the systems approach, human factors engineering approaches often add the component of technology into the safety strategies, as viewed from ergonomics perspective that is designed to reduce human error, increase productivity and comfort, and enhance safety.

5.4 Medication Error Classification

When medication errors do occur, there are several ways to classify the error. The NCC MERP Index for Categorizing Medication Errors classifies errors by harm score. They range from Categories A to I, with the least severe Category A having the capacity to cause error and Category B describing an error that did not reach the patient to Category I referring to an error that may have contributed to or resulted in the patient's death [99]. The US Veterans Health Administration uses the Safety Assessment Code Matrix, which adds levels of probability in addition to the harm severity levels [100]. The categories are represented within a 4 × 4 matrix, in which medication errors are scored on a range of 1–3 for probability and severity, with 3 inferring the highest risk and 1 the lowest risk [100].

Another classification and metric system by Healthcare Performance Improvement (HPI) utilizes the safety event classification (SEC) in combination with the serious safety event rate (SSER) [101]. In addition to identifying the harm scores, HPI SEC first distinguishes all events into three initial categories: serious safety event in which the patient was harmed, precursor safety event in which the medication error reached the patient but did not result in serious harm, and near miss safety event which did not reach the patient. Then, based on the SEC information, SSER calculates the number of serious safety events for the previous 12 months per 10,000 adjusted patient days. The combination of SEC and SSER presents a rate trend of the event and aims to reward sustained, over episodic, improvements in preventing serious safety events.

5.5 Risk Analysis Assessments

Regardless of the method used, the purpose of medication event classification is to identify those that have the most potential for patient harm and room for improvement. Typically, the cases that can lead to the biggest impact at the institution, for instance in terms of the biggest harm averted, extensive lessons learned, and creation of robust safety improvement plan, are chosen for further in-depth investigations using techniques such as detailed root cause analysis (RCA).

An RCA is a retrospective risk analysis whose purpose is to determine what happened in an unwanted event, how it happened, and how to prevent it from happening again [102, 103]. A comprehensive RCA assessment is conducted by multidisciplinary frontline workers who are most familiar with the situation and can help delve into the one or few underlying root causes cases of the problem by sequentially asking the "why" questions. Oftentimes, the root causes of a problem may not be readily apparent from the initial error report and may be uncovered by interviewing staff members, connecting the pieces of the timeline, and understanding the processes that occurred versus what should have occurred. Due to its retrospective nature, RCAs should be conducted in a timely manner in order to capture the details of the past event as accurately as possible.

In contrast to its retrospective counterpart, the failure modes and effects analysis (FMEA) is a prospective risk analysis that anticipates all possible failures that may occur in response to the introduction of new or modified processes. Examples may be piloting of new compounding technology, formulary changes amid drug shortages, or changes to the EHR order sets. Like the RCA, the FMEA is performed by an interdisciplinary team that meets regularly to identify failure modes, failure causes, and failure effects [104]. The team then scores the likelihood of occurrence, the likelihood of detection, and the severity of harm for each deviation from the safety processes on a scale of 1–10. The product of the three scores is calculated as the risk profile number (RPN), which is synonymous with risk priority. Failure modes with the highest RPN take precedence over others and demand immediate attention for error reduction strategies. The RPN can also be used as an ongoing benchmarking metric after safety action plans are brainstormed and implemented at the institution.

Another type of a risk analysis model, which is more commonly seen in aviation and petrochemical industries, is the bowtie analysis [105]. With the unintended event in question at the middle of the analysis tree, the diagram is divided on one side as the "fault tree" which probes all potential causes leading to the unintended event and the other side as the "event tree" which identifies the potential downstream consequences of the event [106]. Although there are some published examples of the bowtie analyses used in the investigation of medication safety events [105], more research may be needed to delineate clear applicability and value in healthcare. Some studies indicate that bowtie analysis may be useful in combination with other risk analyses such as the FMEA or the systems-theoretic accident model and processes (STAMP), or as a starting project in a larger safety improvement plan [105–107].

Because error report investigations and formal risk analysis assessments such as an RCA, FMEA, or bowtie analysis can be time- and resource-intensive, institutions must select judiciously which unintended events warrant follow-up attention from the error reports. Furthermore, each risk analysis has its own unique strengths, weaknesses, and applicability to certain situations, and it is recommended that safety experts and leaders are adequately trained and prepared to conduct the risk assessments and relay the findings to the appropriate committees that will help to carry out tangible action plans. In the UK, the nationally funded Healthcare Safety Investigation Branch conducts numerous patient safety investigations through collaborations with diverse stakeholders and healthcare experts [108].

5.6 Error Reporting Culture

Leadership should strive to create a safe culture of error reporting, one that is nonpunitive, open, efficient, and proactive [109]. In this environment, error reporting must be accompanied by tangible and timely system changes that are supported by a multidisciplinary expert body that can affect change from the top administration [110]. Key attributes of an effective event reporting system should have: [111]

- A supportive environment that protects the privacy of staff who report occurrences.
- Participation by a broad range of personnel.
- Dissemination of summarized reports in a timely fashion.
- A structured mechanism for regularly reviewing reports and developing action plans.

An optimal, proactive, and resilient culture of safety is created by incorporating elements of Just Culture, reporting culture, and learning culture in an effort to promote a continuous environment of learning, flexibility, and preparedness [112]. To achieve this purpose, the National Academy of Medicine has recommended two separate national US reporting systems: a mandatory public reporting system that promotes accountability and a voluntary confidential system that encourages learning from errors [113]. However, as previously mentioned, the voluntary reporting systems have historically suffered from severe *under*-utilization; in order to increase the utilization of error reporting and promote a safe reporting culture, ISMP recommends that the reporting systems be confidential, clear, fair, and actionable [109]. Furthermore, ISMP encourages the designation of a medication safety officer (MSO) at each hospital for optimal medication safety culture and practices [114].

5.7 Healthcare Systems Need Medication Safety Officers

An official staff member who champions the priority, integration, and implementation of safe medication practices across a healthcare institution is known as the Medication Safety Officer (MSO) or Medication Safety Leader or Medication Safety Manager or Medication Safety Coordinator. According to the ASHP Statement on the Role of the Medication Safety Leader, MSOs are expected to [115]:

- Serve as the leader in medication safety initiatives and committee meetings for the organization.
- Collect and review data on medication use process, medication errors, drug reactions, and continuous quality improvement (CQI) data.
- Participate in risk analyses and quality improvement efforts.
- Collaborate with interdisciplinary leaders on actively finding solutions to drug shortages, use of replacement drug products, HIT issues, and other medication safety-related problems.

Additionally, ISMP describes an MSO as a diplomat, information steward, proactive strategist, data optimizer, compassionate Just Culture mentor, and agent of change in its article "A Recurring Call to Action: Every Healthcare Organization Needs a Medication Safety Officer!" [114]. Having an MSO to advocate for medication safety within the hospital leadership can positively affect change, ensure continuous learning moments from error reporting, encourage high-leverage strategies to reduce medication errors, and promote Just Culture to achieve better collective safety outcomes. In the United Kingdom, all healthcare trusts are required to appoint an MSO who champions medication error-related learning and reporting and serves as the main contact for National Medication Safety Network, NHS, England, and the Medicines and Healthcare Products Regulatory Agency (MHRA) [116].

Depending on the unique safety needs and delegations of roles at the hospital, the MSO may be expected to oversee several technologies used in medication safety. These may include updating the smart pump library and periodically reviewing the data surrounding the smart pump users and DERS overrides. When change requests for EHR order sets are submitted, the MSO may work in conjunction with informatics and clinical support staff to design and implement appropriate, usable, and up-to-date changes to the system. An MSO may also be expected to review, assess, and oversee sterile compounding technologies such as the IV workflow software, automated compounders, or IV robotics inside the pharmacy clean rooms. Override and other usage data from ADCs, compliance rate of the BCMA, and issues with automated packaging machines may fall within the scope of an MSO's role depending on the specific institution.

In addition, the MSO is expected to complement and collaborate alongside the institution's designated Patient Safety Officer (PSO) to continually identify risk, implement mitigating strategies, monitor for improvement, and lead the multidisciplinary safety efforts among various care groups. TJC standard requires the identification of a clinician or a body of healthcare providers such as, but not limited to, physicians, nurses, pharmacists, or other healthcare providers to complete the tasks of the PSO [117, 118]. In the United States, the local and state legislation requiring the integration of a PSO may vary, such as in the state of Pennsylvania which requires the designation of a PSO and mandatory error reporting according to the Medical Care Availability and Reduction of Error (MCARE) Act [119]. The goal of a PSO and an MSO, in part, is to combine the knowledge and skill sets beyond any one clinical specialization to make medication use and other clinical practices safer for the patient.

An MSO understands that true reform toward medication safety requires a systems approach. For many decades, healthcare has been striving to become high reliability organizations (HROs) such as the nuclear power and commercial aviation industries in which the smallest errors can lead to tragic consequences. HROs adhere to five primary principles: preoccupation with failure, reluctance to accept "simple" explanations, sensitivity to operations, resilience, and deference to expertise [120, 121]. In addition to robust process improvements, HROs harness the predominant safety culture to continuously anticipate emerging threats to safety, proactive detection of risk, and immediate mitigation responses to deter catastrophic events.

5.8 Finding an Improvement Methodology that Works

Generally, improvement in any process requires focus and monitoring over an extended period of time. In healthcare and other industries, improving quality over time requires a functional understanding of the concept of continuous quality improvement (CQI). CQI, as used in healthcare, can be defined as a "structured, organizational process for involving personnel in planning and executing a continuous flow of improvements to provide quality healthcare that meets or exceeds expectations" [122]. Various industries use CQI models and methods; however, the most widely used model is the Plan-Do-Study-Act (PDSA) (sometimes also known as Plan-Do-Check-Act, or PDCA) cycle. The PDSA model is comprised of four steps that can be continuously repeated to: (P) plan a process improvement, (D) implement that improvement, (S) study the results of the process change, and then (A) modify and spread the improvement [123].

When using PDSA, the first action is the development of an action plan for implementation of the change. Often, a test or pilot study is needed to prove the change will have a positive impact. Using small tests of change is especially important for processes involving patient care. Using this approach allows organizations to determine if any modifications to the process will lead to success while at the same time minimizing the potential for patient harm and organizational inefficiency if a project fails. The action plan should include the intended duration of the project, the location of where the project will occur, the measures developed previously, and an operational plan to guide implementation. Scoping the plan correctly is important. During the do phase of PDSA, the action plan is implemented. Successful implementation can depend on many factors. Generally, having the right team members collaborating and communicating effectively is a critical component of success. Any data identified in the action plan should be collected during the study phase of PDSA. The data collected should be easy to retrieve and timely and should be reported regularly to all involved team members. Data collected should be compared to baseline measures and reconciled with what was predicted. Once analyzed, the data will help the team determine whether the study impact was positive, negative, or resulted in no change. Data collection and analysis occurs during the study phase of the PDSA. In the final step in the PDSA cycle, the team uses the information and analysis to make any potential changes to the original intervention. Based on multiple PDSA cycles and the establishment of a reasonable level of success, the change should be adopted and expansion of the changes into the organization should be considered. Ongoing monitoring and data analysis should be included as part of an organization's overall CQI plan.

In addition to PDSA, the *Lean Production System* and *Six Sigma* are improvement methodologies that are also used in CQI activities. Both models migrated to healthcare from other industries. The Lean Management System (Lean) and the Toyota Production System (TPS) are methods that focus on value of a particular process and seek to maximize the uninterrupted flow of that value to the end customer [124]. Unnecessary or wasteful steps that do not add value are removed to make the resulting process "leaner" and more efficient. Six Sigma is a data-driven method that focuses on customer satisfaction and defect (error) reduction. Specifically, Six Sigma refers to six standard deviations from the expected or desired process result (mean) [125]. This translates to reducing the error associated with a specific process to no more than 3.4 defects or errors per million opportunities or activities.

6 Summary and Conclusions

Patients have a right to safe care across the healthcare continuum. Special attention should be given to understanding, practicing, and systematically employing the tools and concepts presented in this chapter. Improving the safe delivery of medication-related care is the responsibility of all healthcare professionals. Although preventing all errors inherent in our systems may not be possible, eliminating preventable patient harm is possible and foundational to the delivery of healthcare. "Primum non nocere" (First, do no harm).

7 Case Studies

7.1 Case Study 1

A patient was admitted to the emergency room with a suspected stroke and administered an overdose of tenecteplase.

The RCA found the following contributing factors:

1. The patient's most recent weight was not recorded. The dose of tenecteplase was calculated using the weight documented from a previous encounter.
2. The prescriber failed to use the designated order set for tenecteplase for the treatment of stroke.
3. The order set for tenecteplase for the treatment of stroke did not have the CDS that would have provided the dosage recommendations.
4. The tenecteplase is excluded from the list of medications approved for the ADC overrides.
5. The dosing instructions inside the tenecteplase medication kit pertained to the dosing of acute myocardial infarction, not stroke.
6. The institution lacked protocol for dispensing and administering high-alert medications, e.g., dual sign-out.

Possible error mitigation strategies include:

1. Obtain the most recent weight of the patient to calculate the accurate dose of tenecteplase.
2. Designated order sets for specific indications should be readily available and easily accessible. The order sets should prominently display the intended indication and the full generic name of the medication.
3. The order set should be equipped with the relevant CDS features to provide additional instructions and guidance for prescribing, dispensing, administration, and monitoring of the medication.
4. Medications that are intended for emergency use need to be on the institution's approved ADC override list for safe and efficient dispensing of the medication.
5. The approved medication kit for tenecteplase for stroke needs to be fully stocked with the relevant supplies (e.g., syringe, needles, and medication) including the accurate dosing instructions.
6. Given their potential for serious harm if used in error, high-alert medications need to be identified and handled accordingly under institutional protocol and guidelines.

Acknowledgments The authors would like to thank Dr. Sarah McDowell for allowing us to reproduce a figure (Fig. 15.1) included in the chapter.

References

1. Flynn E. A brief history of medication errors. American Pharmaceutical Association Published Online; 1999. p. 1–6.
2. Barker KN, McConnell W. The problems of detecting medication errors in hospitals. Am J Hosp Pharm. 1962;19:360–9.
3. http://www.hsph.harvard.edu/lucian-leape/. Accessed 14 Jan 2016.
4. Institute of Medicine. To err is human: building a safer health care system. National Academies Press; 1999.
5. http://aviation-safety.net/airlinesafety/industry/. Accessed 31 Jan 2016.
6. World Health Organization. WHO launches global effort to halve medication-related errors in 5 years. Accessed 8 May 2023. https://www.who.int/news/item/29-03-2017-who-launches-global-effort-to-halve-medication-related-errors-in-5-years.
7. Practices Institute for Safe Medication. A call to action: The case for Medication Safety Officers (MSO). Published online; 2018.
8. American Society of Health-System Pharmacists (ASHP). ASHP statement on the role of the medication safety leader. Am J Health Syst Pharm. 2019;70:448–52.
9. Yu K, Nation R, Dooley M. Multiplicity of medication safety terms, definitions and functional meanings: when is enough enough? Qual Saf Health Care. 2005;14(5):358–63. https://doi.org/10.1136/qshc.2005.014159.
10. Moore S, Jenkins A, Poppe L, Rowe E, Eckel S. Significant publications about the medication use process in 2012. J Pharm Pract. 2015;28(4):387–97. https://doi.org/10.1177/0897190013519821.
11. Leape L, Bates D, Cullen D. Systems analysis of adverse drug events. ADE Prevention Study Group. JAMA. 1995;274(1):35–43.
12. Bates D, Cullen D, Laird N. Incidence of adverse drug events and potential adverse drug events. Implications for prevention. ADE Prevention Study Group. JAMA. 1995;274(1):29–34.
13. al Rowily A, Jalal Z, Price MJ, et al. Prevalence, contributory factors and severity of medication errors associated with direct-acting oral anticoagulants in adult patients: a systematic review and meta-analysis. Eur J Clin Pharmacol. 2022;78(4):623–45. https://doi.org/10.1007/s00228-021-03212-y.
14. Manasse HR. Medication use in an imperfect world: drug misadventuring as an issue of public policy, Part 1. Am J Hosp Pharm. 1989;46(5):929–44.
15. Lisby M. How are medication errors defined? A systematic literature review of definitions and characteristics. Int J Qual Health Care. 2010;22(6):507–18.
16. Lisby M, Nielsen L, Brock B, Mainz J. How should medication errors be defined? Development and test of a definition. Scand J Public Health. 2012;40(2):203–10. https://doi.org/10.1177/1403494811435489.
17. National Coordinating Council for Medication Error Reporting and Prevention (NCC MERP). What is a medication error? Accessed 10 May 2022. https://www.nccmerp.org/about-medication-errors.
18. European Medicines Agency. Medication errors. https://www.ema.europa.eu/en/human-regulatory/post-authorisation/pharmacovigilance/medication-errors.
19. World Health Organization (WHO). International drug monitoring: the role of national centres. Technical Report Series No 498. Published online; 1972.
20. Coleman J, Pontefract S. Adverse drug reactions. Clin Med (Lond). 2016;16(5):481–5. https://doi.org/10.7861/clinmedicine.16-5-481.
21. Aronson J, Ferner R. Clarification of terminology in drug safety. Drug Saf. 2005;28(10):851–70. https://doi.org/10.2165/00002018-200528100-00003.
22. European Medicines Agency. ICH E2A Clinical safety data management: definitions and standards for expedited reporting—Scientific guideline. https://www.ema.europa.eu/en/ich-e2a-clinical-safety-data-management-definitions-standards-expedited-reporting-scientific.
23. Adverse events, near misses, and errors. Accessed May 10, 2022. https://psnet.ahrq.gov/primer/adverse-events-near-misses-and-errors.
24. Glossary | PSNet. Accessed 1 Mar 2022. https://psnet.ahrq.gov/glossary-0.
25. Pintor-Mármol A, Baena M, Fajardo P, et al. Terms used in patient safety related to medication: a literature review. Pharmacoepidemiol Drug Saf. 2012;21:799–809.
26. Manley H, Drayer D, Muther R. Medication-related problem type and appearance rate in ambulatory hemodialysis patients. BMC Nephrol. 2003;4:10.
27. Naseralallah L, Stewart D, Azfar Ali R, Paudyal V. An umbrella review of systematic reviews on contributory factors to medication errors in health-care settings. Expert Opin Drug Saf. 2022;21(11):1379–99. https://doi.org/10.1080/14740338.2022.2147921.
28. Reason J. Human error. Cambridge University Press; UK, 1990.
29. Reason J. Human error: models and management. Br Med J. 2000;320(7237):768. https://doi.org/10.1136/BMJ.320.7237.768.
30. Betsy Lehman's story. https://youtu.be/A44Ipbh71Xk.
31. Lois J. Ayash v. Dana-Farber Cancer Institute & others. Presented at: 2005.
32. The Boston Globe. Dana-Farber tests signaled an overdose, records show.
33. Conway J, Weingart S. Organizational change in the face of highly public errors—I. The Dana-Farber Cancer Institute Experience.
34. Meyer-Massetti C, Cheng C, Schwappach D. Systematic review of medication safety assessment methods. Am J Health-Syst Pharm. 2011;68(3):227–40.
35. Institute of Medicine. Preventing medication errors. The National Academies Press; 2007.

36. Battles J. Disaster prevention: lessons learned from the Titanic. Proc (Bayl Univ Med Cent). 2001;14(2):150–3.
37. Classen D, Pestotnik S, Evans R. Computerized surveillance of adverse drug events in hospital patients. JAMA. 1991;266:2847–51.
38. Rozich J, Haraden C, Resar R. Adverse drug event trigger tool: a practical methodology for measuring medication related harm. Qual Saf Health Care. 2003;12:194–200.
39. Goodwin MA, Stange KC, Zyzanski SJ, Crabtree BF, Borawski EA, Flocke SA. The Hawthorne effect in direct observation research with physicians and patients. J Eval Clin Pract. 2017;23(6):1322–8. https://doi.org/10.1111/jep.12781.
40. Barber N, Cornford T, Klecun E. Qualitative evaluation of an electronic prescribing and administration system. Qual Saf Health Care. 2007;16(4):271–8.
41. Marwitz K. Investigating multiple sources of data for smart infusion pump and electronic health record interoperability. Am J Health-Syst Pharm. 2020;77(17):1417–23.
42. Key Elements of Medication Use | Institute For Safe Medication Practices. Accessed 28 Feb 2022. https://www.ismp.org/key-elements-medication-use.
43. Cohen MR. Causes of medication errors. In: Medication errors. The American Pharmacists Association; 2007. p. 55–66.
44. Haque H, Alrowily A, Jalal Z, et al. Direct oral anticoagulant-related medication incidents and pharmacists' interventions in hospital in-patients: evaluation using reason's accident causation theory. Int J Clin Pharm. 2021;43(6):1693–704. https://doi.org/10.1007/s11096-021-01302-6.
45. Authority PP. Medication errors: significance of accurate patient weights | advisory. PA Patient Saf Advis. 2009;6(1):10–5.
46. High-Alert Medications in Acute Care Settings | Institute For Safe Medication Practices. Accessed 15 Mar 2022. https://www.ismp.org/recommendations/high-alert-medications-acute-list.
47. Neuspiel DR, Taylor MM. Reducing the risk of harm from medication errors in children. Health Serv Insights. 2013;6:47. https://doi.org/10.4137/HSI.S10454.
48. Sentinel Event Alert 39: Preventing pediatric medication errors | The Joint Commission. Accessed 15 Mar 2022. https://www.jointcommission.org/resources/patient-safety-topics/sentinel-event/sentinel-event-alert-newsletters/sentinel-event-alert-issue-39-preventing-pediatric-medication-errors/#.YjDfFHrMI2w.
49. Levine S, Cohen MR. Preventing medication errors in pediatric and neonatal patients. In: Medication errors. 2nd ed. The American Pharmacist Association; 2007. p. 469.
50. Adelman J, Aschner J, Schechter C, et al. Use of temporary names for newborns and associated risks. Pediatrics. 2015;136(2):327–33. https://doi.org/10.1542/PEDS.2015-0007.
51. Medication Safety in Pediatrics. Pharmacy connection Published online 2011, pp. 14–17.
52. Burns AL, Owen JA, Reilly C, Scheckelhoff D. Improving care transitions: optimizing medication reconciliation. J Am Pharm Assoc. 2012;52(4) https://doi.org/10.1331/JAPHA.2012.12527.
53. Amy Harper B, Kukielka E, Jones R. Patient harm resulting from medication reconciliation process failures: a study of serious events reported by Pennsylvania hospitals. Patient Saf. 2021;3(1):10–22. https://doi.org/10.33940/DATA/2021.3.1.
54. Digiantonio N, Lund J, Bastow S. Impact of a pharmacy-led medication reconciliation program. Pharm Ther. 2018;43(2):105.
55. Hospital: 2022 National Patient Safety Goals | The Joint Commission. Accessed 21 Mar 2022. https://www.jointcommission.org/standards/national-patient-safety-goals/hospital-national-patient-safety-goals.
56. Abbreviations: a shortcut to medication errors | Advisory. PA PSRS Patient Saf Advisory. 2005;2(1):19–21.
57. Administration D. FDA at a glance regulated products and facilities. Published online; 2018.
58. List of Confused Drug Names | Institute For Safe Medication Practices. Accessed 23 May 2022. https://www.ismp.org/recommendations/confused-drug-names-list.
59. Phonetic and Orthographic Computer Analysis (POCA) Program | FDA. Accessed 21 Mar 2022. https://www.fda.gov/drugs/information-industry-drugs/phonetic-and-orthographic-computer-analysis-poca-program.
60. ISMP Canada. Preventable medication errors-look-alike/sound-alike drug names. https://www.ismp-canada.org/download/PharmacyConnection/PC2014-02-Spring_LookalikeSoundalike.pdf.
61. Institute for Safe Medication Practices (ISMP). Part I: Survey results show unsafe practices persist with IV push medications. Medication Saf Alert! 2018;23(22)
62. American Society of Health-System Pharmacists. Standardize 4 Safety Initiative. https://www.ashp.org/pharmacy-practice/standardize-4-safety-initiative.
63. Forshay CM, Hansen KN, Eckel SF. Using intravenous pump infusion data to optimize continuous infusion concentrations and reduce drug and fluid waste. Am J Health-Syst Pharm. 2020;77(18):1497–503. https://doi.org/10.1093/ajhp/zxaa199.
64. Walroth TA, Dossett HA, Doolin M, et al. Standardizing concentrations of adult drug infusions in Indiana. Am J Health-Syst Pharm. 2017;74(7):491–7. https://doi.org/10.2146/ajhp151018.
65. Safety Committees Need to Proactively Address the Risk of Accidental Cerebral Injection of Intravenous (IV) Drugs | Institute For Safe Medication Practices. Accessed 21 Mar 2022. https://www.ismp.org/resources/safety-committees-need-proactively-address-risk-accidental-cerebral-injection-intravenous.

66. Sentinel Event Alert 53: Managing risk during transition to new ISO tubing connector standards | The Joint Commission. Accessed 22 Mar 2022. https://www.jointcommission.org/resources/patient-safety-topics/sentinel-event/sentinel-event-alert-newsletters/sentinel-event-alert-53-managing-risk-during-transition-to-new-iso-tubing-connector-standards/#.YjnMXurMI2w.
67. U.S. Inaction Lets Look-Alike Tubes Kill Patients—The New York Times. Accessed 22 Mar 2022. https://www.nytimes.com/2010/08/21/health/policy/21tubes.html.
68. Inadvertent administration of an oral liquid into a vein | HSIB. Accessed 22 Mar 22, 2022. https://www.hsib.org.uk/investigations-and-reports/inadvertent-administration-of-an-oral-liquid-into-a-vein/.
69. Hidden medication loss when using a primary administration set for small-volume intermittent infusions | Institute For Safe Medication Practices. Accessed 12 Jan 2022. https://www.ismp.org/resources/hidden-medication-loss-when-using-primary-administration-set-small-volume-intermittent.
70. Giuliano KK, Blake JWC. Nurse and pharmacist knowledge of intravenous smart pump system setup requirements. Biomed Instrum Technol. 2021;55(1):51–8. https://doi.org/10.2345/0890-8205-55.1.51.
71. General chapter physical environments that promote safe medication use | USP-NF. Accessed 26 June 2022. https://www.uspnf.com/notices/retired-compendial-notices/general-chapter-physical-environments-promote-safe-medication-use.
72. Some IV medications are diluted unnecessarily in patient care areas, creating undue risk | Institute For Safe Medication Practices. Accessed 22 Mar 2022. https://www.ismp.org/resources/some-iv-medications-are-diluted-unnecessarily-patient-care-areas-creating-undue-risk.
73. Muffly MK, Chen MI, Claure RE, et al. Small-volume injections: evaluation of volume administration deviation from intended injection volumes. Anesth Analg. 2017;125(4):1192–9. https://doi.org/10.1213/ANE.0000000000001976.
74. Gabay M, Hertig JB, Degnan D, et al. Third consensus development conference on the safety of intravenous drug delivery systems-2018. Am J Health Syst Pharm. 2020;77(3):215–20. https://doi.org/10.1093/AJHP/ZXZ277.
75. Measuring the dose of liquid medicines—consumer med safety. Accessed 22 Mar 2022. https://consumermed-safety.org/measuring-the-dose-of-liquid-medicines.
76. Example of a measuring error—consumer med safety. Accessed 22 Mar 2022. https://consumermed-safety.org/measuring-the-dose-of-liquid-medicines/measuring-liquid-medicines-safely-2.
77. The Joint Commission. Human factors analysis in patient safety systems. Published online 2015. https://www.jointcommission.org/-/media/deprecated-unorganized/imported-assets/tjc/system-folders/assetmanager/humanfactorsthe_sourcepdf.pdf.
78. Executive S. Leadership and worker involvement toolkit understanding human failure.
79. The differences between human error, at-risk behavior, and reckless behavior are key to a just culture | Institute For Safe Medication Practices. Accessed 13 Apr 2022. https://www.ismp.org/resources/differences-between-human-error-risk-behavior-and-reckless-behavior-are-key-just-culture.
80. Recommendations to enhance accuracy of prescription/medication order writing | NCC MERP. Accessed 21 Mar 2022. https://www.nccmerp.org/recommendations-enhance-accuracy-prescription-writing.
81. Dangerous abbreviations | NCC MERP. Accessed 21 Mar 2022. https://www.nccmerp.org/dangerous-abbreviations.
82. List of error-prone abbreviations | Institute For Safe Medication Practices. Accessed 21 Mar 2022. https://www.ismp.org/recommendations/error-prone-abbreviations-list.
83. Look-alike drug names with recommended tall man letters | Institute For Safe Medication Practices. Accessed 23 May 2022. https://www.ismp.org/recommendations/tall-man-letters-list.
84. Targeted medication safety best practices for hospitals | Institute For Safe Medication Practices. Accessed 1 Mar 2022. https://www.ismp.org/guidelines/best-practices-hospitals.
85. Safety considerations for container labels and carton labeling design to minimize medication errors | FDA. Accessed 21 Mar 2022. https://www.fda.gov/regulatory-information/search-fda-guidance-documents/safety-considerations-container-labels-and-carton-labeling-design-minimize-medication-errors.
86. ASHP. Medication safety-guidelines ASHP guidelines on preventing medication errors in hospitals. https://www.ashp.org/-/media/assets/policy-guidelines/docs/guidelines/preventing-medication-errors-hospitals.ashx.
87. ASHP. Medication safety policy positions. https://www.ashp.org/-/media/assets/policy-guidelines/docs/policy-positions/policy-positions-medication-safety.pdf.
88. ASHP. ASHP Guidelines on preventing medication errors with chemotherapy and biotherapy. https://www.ashp.org/-/media/assets/policy-guidelines/docs/guidelines/preventing-medication-errors-chemotherapy-biotherapy.ashx.
89. Working to reduce medication errors | FDA. Accessed 28 Feb 2022. https://www.fda.gov/drugs/information-consumers-and-patients-drugs/working-reduce-medication-errors.
90. Questions to ask before taking medicine | Agency for Healthcare Research and Quality. Accessed 11 May 2022. https://www.ahrq.gov/questions/resources/your-meds/before-taking.html.
91. Edwards B, Chakraborty S. Risk communication and the pharmaceutical industry. Drug Saf. 2012;35(11):1027–40. https://doi.org/10.1007/BF03261989.

92. Institute for Safe Medication Practices. Education is "predictably disappointing" and should never be relied upon alone to improve safety. https://www.ismp.org/resources/education-predictably-disappointing-and-should-never-be-relied-upon-alone-improve-safety. Published online June 4, 2020.
93. Education is "predictably disappointing" and should never be relied upon alone to improve safety | Institute For Safe Medication Practices. Accessed 11 May 2022. https://www.ismp.org/resources/education-predictably-disappointing-and-should-never-be-relied-upon-alone-improve-safety.
94. Scanlon MC, Karsh BT. Value of human factors to medication and patient safety in the intensive care unit. Crit Care Med. 2010;38:S90–6. https://doi.org/10.1097/CCM.0b013e3181dd8de2.
95. US Food & Drug Administration (FDA). Drugs@FDA: FDA-Approved Drugs. https://www.accessdata.fda.gov/.
96. Ro M, Holcomb E. More lessons learned from RaDonda Vaught case. Pharmacy Practice News—June 2022. 2022:21–23.
97. Institute for Safe Medication Practices. Safety enhancements every hospital must consider in wake of another tragic neuromuscular blocker event. https://www.ismp.org/resources/safety-enhancements-every-hospital-must-consider-wake-another-tragic-neuromuscular.
98. Leveson N, Couturier M, Thomas J, et al. Applying system engineering to pharmaceutical safety. J Healthc Eng. 2012;3(3):391–414. https://doi.org/10.1260/2040-2295.3.3.391.
99. Types of medication errors | NCC MERP. Accessed 1 Mar 2022. https://www.nccmerp.org/types-medication-errors.
100. Safety Assessment Code (SAC) Matrix—VHA National Center for Patient Safety. Accessed 1 Mar 2022. https://www.patientsafety.va.gov/professionals/publications/matrix.asp.
101. Health Performance Improvement. The HPI SEC & SSER Patient Safety Measurement System for Healthcare; 2020.
102. Root cause analysis—VHA National Center for Patient Safety. Accessed 1 Mar 2022. https://www.patientsafety.va.gov/professionals/onthejob/rca.asp.
103. Getting the most out of root-cause analyses. Accessed 1 Mar 2022. https://www.ecri.org/components/HRC/Pages/RiskQual23.aspx?tab=2.
104. Failure Modes and Effects Analysis (FMEA) Tool | IHI—Institute for Healthcare Improvement. Accessed 11 May 2022. http://www.ihi.org/resources/Pages/Tools/FailureModesandEffectsAnalysisTool.aspx?PostAuthRed=/resources/_layouts/download.aspx?SourceURL=/resources/Knowledge Center Assets/Tools-FailureModesandEffectsAnalysisFMEATool_3fd4e6fd-b819-4f14-89ba-fb3563dd4e2d.
105. Wierenga PC, Lie-A-Huen L, De Rooij SE, Klazinga NS, Guchelaar HJ, Smorenburg SM. Application of the Bow-Tie model in medication safety risk analysis: consecutive experience in two hospitals in the Netherlands. Drug Saf. 2009;32(8):663–73. https://doi.org/10.2165/00002018-200932080-00005.
106. Afefy IH. Hazard analysis and risk assessments for industrial processes using FMEA and bow-tie methodologies. Indust Eng Manage Syst. 2015;14(4):379–91. https://doi.org/10.7232/IEMS.2015.14.4.379.
107. Chatzimichailidou MM, Ward J, Horberry T, Clarkson PJ. A comparison of the Bow-Tie and STAMP approaches to reduce the risk of surgical instrument retention. Risk Anal. 2018;38(5):978–90. https://doi.org/10.1111/RISA.12897.
108. Healthcare Safety Investigation Branch. Investigations and reports. https://www.hsib.org.uk/investigations-and-reports/.
109. Pump up the volume: tips for increasing error reporting and decreasing patient harm | Institute For Safe Medication Practices. Accessed 22 Mar 2022. https://www.ismp.org/resources/pump-volume-tips-increasing-error-reporting-and-decreasing-patient-harm.
110. Cohen MR. Why error reporting systems should be voluntary: they provide better information for reducing errors. BMJ: Br Med J. 2000;320(7237):728. https://doi.org/10.1136/BMJ.320.7237.728.
111. Reporting Patient Safety Events | PSNet. Accessed 22 Mar 2022. https://psnet.ahrq.gov/primer/reporting-patient-safety-events.
112. Seal C, Edwards B, Morrisroe J, Harden S, Krokstad TH, Powell S. We should move from a culture of blame to a culture of fairness. Pharm J. 2009;282:743.
113. Kohn LT, Corrigan JM, Donaldson MS. To err is human: building a safer health system. Washington, DC: the National Academies Press; 2000. https://doi.org/10.17226/9728.
114. A Recurring Call to Action: Every Healthcare Organization Needs a Medication Safety Officer! | Institute For Safe Medication Practices. Accessed 11 May 2022. https://www.ismp.org/resources/recurring-call-action-every-healthcare-organization-needs-medication-safety-officer.
115. ASHP. Medication safety-statements ASHP statement on the role of the medication safety leader position.
116. Jethwa R. A day in the life of a medication safety officer. Pharm J. 2019; https://doi.org/10.1211/PJ.2019.20206032.
117. The Joint Commission. Is there a requirement to specify or identify a safety officer? https://www.jointcommission.org/standards/standard-faqs/critical-access-hospital/environment-of-care-ec/000001217/.
118. Institute for Healthcare Improvement. Designate a Patient Safety Officer. Accessed 8 May 2023. https://www.ihi.org/resources/Pages/Changes/DesignateaPatientSafetyOfficer.aspx.
119. Pennsylvania General Assembly. Medical Care Availability and Reduction of Error (MCARE) Act.

https://www.legis.state.pa.us/cfdocs/legis/li/uconsCheck.cfm?yr=2002&sessInd=0&act=13. Published online 2002.
120. Veazie S, Peterson K, Bourne D. Evidence brief: implementation of high reliability organization principles. Evidence brief: implementation of high reliability organization principles. Washington, DC: Department of Veterans Affairs (US); 2019. p. 1–84.
121. High Reliability | PSNet. Accessed 11 May 2022. https://psnet.ahrq.gov/primer/high-reliability.
122. Johnson J, Sollecito W. McLaughlin and Kalazny's continuous quality improvement in healthcare. 5th ed. Jones and Bartlett Learning; 2019.
123. Langley G. The improvement guide: a practical approach to enhancing organizational performance. 1st ed. Jossey-Bass Publishers; 1996.
124. The Toyota production system: what does it mean, and what does it mean for health care? Health Affairs.
125. Arthur J. Arthur J. Lean Six Sigma for hospitals: simple steps to fast, affordable, and flawless healthcare.
126. TN Board of Nursing's Unjust Decision to Revoke Nurse's License: Travesty on Top of Tragedy! | Institute For Safe Medication Practices. Accessed 26 June 2022. https://www.ismp.org/resources/tn-board-nursings-unjust-decision-revoke-nurses-license-travesty-top-tragedy.
127. More lessons learned from RaDonda Vaught case—Pharmacy Practice News. Accessed 28 June 2022. https://www.pharmacypracticenews.com/Operations-and-Management/Article/06-22/More-Lessons-Learned-From-RaDonda-Vaught-Case/67213.
128. Sentinel Event Alert 42: Safely implementing health information and converging technologies | The Joint Commission. Accessed 1 Mar 2022. https://www.jointcommission.org/resources/patient-safety-topics/sentinel-event/sentinel-event-alert-newsletters/sentinel-event-alert-issue-42-safely-implementing-health-information-and-converging-technologies/.
129. Alert Fatigue | PSNet. Accessed 11 May 2022. https://psnet.ahrq.gov/primer/alert-fatigue.
130. Slight SP, Seger DL, Nanji KC, et al. Are we heeding the warning signs? Examining providers' overrides of computerized drug-drug interaction alerts in primary care. PLoS One. 2013;8(12) https://doi.org/10.1371/JOURNAL.PONE.0085071.

Methods to Detect, Predict, and Prevent Adverse Drug Reactions in Pharmacovigilance and Clinical Practice

16

Jeffrey Pradeep Raj, Nithya J. Gogtay, and Suparna Chatterjee

Abstract

The fundamental principle in any drug approval process is that the drug's perceived benefits outweigh the risks at the population level. However, post-marketing authorization, adverse drug reactions (ADRs) abound in clinical practice as individual-level factors vary. Further, the number of subjects on whom a drug is tested during the process of drug development is relatively small and thus continuous monitoring is warranted. This is undertaken through the process of pharmacovigilance, which is defined by the World Health Organization as the science and activities related to detecting, assessing, understanding, and preventing adverse effects and other medicine/vaccine-related problems. This chapter outlines the various study designs of post-authorization safety studies used to identify ADRs and the various challenges in detecting ADRs. This chapter also summarizes the various strategies to predict and prevent ADRs in clinical practice and by other means such as pharmacogenetics, use of omics, and in silico approaches including artificial intelligence.

Keywords

Adverse drug reactions · Post-authorization safety studies · Pharmacovigilance study methods · Risk factors · Pharmacogenetics · Omics · Artificial intelligence · Preventability · Predictability

J. P. Raj (✉)
Division of Clinical Pharmacology, Department of Pharmacology, Kasturba Medical College, Manipal, Karnataka, India

Manipal Academy of Higher Education, Manipal, Karnataka, India
e-mail: jpraj.m07@gmail.com

N. J. Gogtay
Department of Clinical Pharmacology, Seth GS Medical College and King Edward Memorial Hospital, Mumbai, India

S. Chatterjee
Department of Pharmacology, Institute of Postgraduate Medical Education & Research, Kolkata, India

Learning Objectives

- To understand the various methods used in pharmacovigilance for detecting adverse drug reactions (ADRs)/pharmacovigilance study methods.
- To list the challenges in identifying/diagnosing ADRs.
- To describe various methods and strategies to predict, prevent, and manage ADRs.

J. Jose et al. (eds.), *Principles and Practice of Pharmacovigilance and Drug Safety*,
https://doi.org/10.1007/978-3-031-51089-2_16

Key Points

- ADR is any response that is noxious, unintended, and which occurs at doses normally used in humans for prophylaxis, diagnosis, or therapy of disease or for the modification of a physiological function.
- Before the drug is approved, it is exposed only to a few patients in a controlled research setting and a drug is approved based on its perceived benefits over the risks at a population level rather than at an individual level. On the other hand, ADRs abound in routine clinical practice and post-authorization safety studies help identify ADRs in real-world setting.
- The strategies for the prediction and prevention of ADRs include genomics, metabolomics, proteomics, transcriptomics, epigenomics, and in silico approaches including artificial intelligence.
- Management of ADRs includes early detection, symptomatic and/or specific management, documentation, follow-up, and monitoring.

1 Introduction

Benefits and risks are two sides of the same coin, and there really is no medication that can be claimed to be devoid of adverse effects. The fundamental principle in a drug approval process is that the drug's perceived benefits outweigh the risks at the population level, and this permits the marketing of the drug. However, in clinical practice, routine monitoring for adverse effects at an individual level is warranted as safety data generated in pre-approval phases are insufficient and need to be constantly updated with real-world safety data for estimating risks associated with drug usage. The process of continuous monitoring of a drug for its safety is called pharmacovigilance which is derived from the words *pharmakon* (Greek word for drug) and *vigiliare* (Latin word to keep watch) [1].

Monitoring of adverse drug reactions (ADRs) has become more important than ever before, given the rapidly growing complexity of therapeutics (biologics, biosimilars, and novel vaccines to name a few), an aging population, and the presence of comorbidities leading to polypharmacy. What once started off as a branch of science that deals with the safety of a small number of drugs has now widened its scope to include herbals, traditional and complementary medicines, biologics, vaccines, and even medical devices [2, 3]. Of late, specialized branches of pharmacovigilance programs such as hemovigilance that deals with the surveillance of blood and blood products [4] and materiovigilance that deals with medical devices have gained importance globally [5].

ADRs abound in routine clinical practice and can be something as simple as nausea, vomiting, or gastritis associated with antimalarials that can be easily treated to something more sinister such as warfarin-induced bleeding leading to intracranial hemorrhage and even death. While mortality and morbidity can be appreciated by the patient and prescriber alike, there are significant financial costs associated with ADRs that impact the patient, hospital, insurer, or society and also impact the physician–patient relationship [6]. A successful pharmacovigilance program is one that can predict, minimize, and mitigate mortality and morbidity. The withdrawal of drugs such as pergolide (for Parkinson's disease) due to increased risk of cardiac valvulopathy and pemoline (for attention-deficit hyperactivity disease) due to hepatotoxicity are some examples of a successful pharmacovigilance program. Had it not been for the continued monitoring for safety after its marketing, these important adverse events may not have been picked up [7].

Hence, this chapter aims to outline the various study designs of post-authorization safety studies (PASS) used to identify ADRs and the various challenges in diagnosing ADRs. This chapter also aims to summarize the various strategies to predict and prevent ADRs such as pharmacogenetics, use of omics, and in silico approaches including artificial intelligence (AI).

2 Detecting Adverse Drug Reactions/ Pharmacovigilance Study Methods

ADRs can be detected at various levels. Since most of the adverse reactions are likely to be detected after the drug is marketed, PASS becomes very important and forms a significant part of a drug's pharmacovigilance life cycle. These can be defined as "any study relating to an authorized medicinal product conducted with the aim of identifying, characterizing, or quantifying a safety hazard, confirming the safety profile of the medicinal product, or of measuring the effectiveness of risk management measures". These are noninterventional with the primary objective of collecting safety information beyond clinical trials and can also be used to assess drug utilization [8].

The following are the various pharmacovigilance methods employed to evaluate drug safety [9, 10]:

1. Passive surveillance

   (a) Spontaneous reports/spontaneous reporting

   The International Council for Harmonisation of Technical Requirements for Pharmaceuticals for Human Use (ICH) has defined spontaneous reporting as "an unsolicited communication by a healthcare professional or consumer to a company, regulatory authority, or other organization (e.g., a national pharmacovigilance center) that describes one or more adverse drug reactions in a patient who was given one or more medicinal products and that does not derive from a study or any organized data collection scheme" [11]. This form of reporting to detect ADRs forms the cornerstone of many national pharmacovigilance systems worldwide and can be both paper-based or electronic. Though the modality is passive, it is a low-maintenance, cost-effective approach that has picked up several ADRs of consequence. Reports from individual patients are called as Individual Case Safety Reports (ICSRs) and help identify early warning signals, especially to newly introduced medicinal products [12]. An example of a well-known spontaneous reporting system is the "Yellow Card" reporting system from the UK regulator that collects information not just about medicinal products but also about devices. This is available in both paper and electronic versions including a Yellow Card app. The system was established in 1964, and patients are also able to report ADRs effective from 2005 [13]. Cough induced by the angiotensin inhibitors captopril and enalapril is an example of an adverse event picked up through analysis of spontaneous reports [14].

   (b) Case series

   It is a series of case reports reporting the same event spontaneously in at least two or more patients. They are useful in generating hypotheses rather than for testing association or causation of the event with the medicinal agent.

2. Stimulated reporting/targeted spontaneous reporting

   This system of stimulated reporting is identical to the spontaneous reporting system except this is drug-specific or with a focus on drugs for a certain disease condition (e.g., antiretroviral therapy) and is also at times called targeted spontaneous reporting [15]. Targeted spontaneous reporting was introduced by the World Health Organization (WHO) in 2010 and uses the same principles and methodology as spontaneous reporting except the specific focus of the former. Although this method increases the rate of ADR reporting, it is not devoid of the usual drawbacks of passive surveillance such as underreporting and incomplete information. An example of this method is the identification of nephrotoxicity in patients receiving antiretroviral therapy, specifically tenofovir in Uganda [16]. This methodology led to both a fivefold increase in overall reporting of ADRs for all antiretrovirals and identification of one suspected case of nephrotoxicity per 200 patients treated with tenofovir.

3. Active surveillance

   In an active surveillance system, a continuous pre-organized process is established as an attempt to ascertain the total number of adverse events. For instance, patients prescribed a specific drug may be followed up using a risk management program wherein they may be asked to complete a brief survey and sought permission to be contacted at a later time as well. For instance, brexanolone (Zulresso) has a risk evaluation and mitigation strategy program as this drug when given as per its approved mode of administration of continuous IV infusion over 60 h for postpartum depression can cause some people to faint or even lose consciousness. The regulators too, many a times, recommend the innovators to propose a risk management plan (RMP) detailing the commitments of post-marketing pharmacovigilance with an aim to identify safety signals that continue to emerge early in the post-approval phase [17]—e.g., bedaquiline (antituberculosis drug) RMP.

   (a) Sentinel sites/sentinel surveillance

      Here, a sample of sentinel sites are selected, and active surveillance is achieved by thoroughly interviewing patients and/or pharmacists/physicians or by reviewing medical records in order to ensure accurate and complete reporting of ADRs. The advantages are that the data from specific patient subgroup may be collected and information on the use of certain medicinal products with a potential for abuse could also be targeted. However, the disadvantages are the small number of patients, selection bias, and increased cost. Therefore, this type of active surveillance with sentinel sites works efficiently in an institutional setup where certain drug products are used in higher frequency, for example, drugs used in ICU such as colistin.

   (b) Cohort event monitoring and prescription event monitoring [9, 18]

      Cohort event monitoring (CEM) is a system of pharmacovigilance which is often used following the approval of a new drug or vaccine to identify signals or adverse events not picked up during the clinical trials due to a limited sample size. Essentially, CEM studies select a defined group of individuals (e.g., those who have received a COVID-19 vaccine) or a drug and prospectively monitor them after defining a specified time interval for follow-up. The initial visit captures demographic data and relevant medical information—for example, medication history, comorbidities, past history of drug allergy, and the like. The studies are observational (noninterventional) and form safety assessments in the early period after marketing. Participants in these studies are followed up at predefined intervals. Adverse events that occur are collated regardless of causality. The method is based on prescription event monitoring (PEM) that originated in the 1970s, but the only difference between the two is that the enrollment into the CEM is done by the physician directly, whereas in the PEM it is through the prescription details provided by the pharmacists/pharmacies. Here, patients are identified via electronic prescriptions or health insurance claims. A predefined questionnaire is sent to patients and/or the prescribing physicians at prespecified time intervals to obtain outcome information such as clinical events, reason for discontinuation, ADRs, and likewise. The disadvantages are the unfocussed nature of data collection that can obscure important signals, difficulty in maintaining patient confidentiality, and poor response rates to the questionnaires sent. However, the main advantage is that more detailed information on adverse events may be collected from a large number of patients and physicians. The methodology is also used by the WHO for safety monitoring for drugs used in public health programs. The WHO has published handbooks for the conduct of these studies in the fields of HIV/AIDS, malaria, tuberculosis, and even for COVID-19 vaccines. Studies of this nature have the advantage of both a numerator and a denominator and thus give us incidence rates of adverse events. Multiple adverse events can also be picked up during the course of the monitoring. However, these studies can become difficult if the drug of interest is an orphan drug, as an adequate sample may be difficult to come by. Similarly, rare outcomes may still be missed if the cohort is not sufficiently large.

(c) Specialist cohort event monitoring studies [19]

Specialist cohort event monitoring (SCEM) studies involves a cohort of patients from the hospital and secondary care settings who have been prescribed a particular medicinal agent to be monitored for ADRs. It also allows concurrent monitoring of a comparator cohort of patients on standard of care or another counterfactual comparator group depending on the research question. These studies are proposed with a preamble that the study population is usually under the care of specialists due to their complex health situation in terms of comorbidities, underlying disease severity, and concurrent medications when compared to a general population that gets treated in primary care. An example of an SCEM study is the ROSE study—Rivaroxaban Observational Safety Evaluation, where specialist healthcare professionals from the Cardiovascular Specialty Group, Non-Malignant Haematology Speciality Group, and Stroke Research Network were invited to participate.

(d) Registries [10]

There are two types of registries that collect data on patients; product registries that focus on a specific product or drug and disease registries that focus on a specific disease—for example, aplastic anemia or glomerulonephritis. Both these registries are extremely useful sources for drug safety for the simple reason that the population enrolled is far more heterogenous than the homogenous population that is enrolled in regular clinical trials. Information in product-specific registries should record the maximum amount of variables for suitable inferences to be made. These could be apart from dose, duration, and start and stop date information on whether a branded or generic product was used or the nature of the excipient which would make it product-specific. For example, the adjuvants of interest in COVID-19 vaccines are polyethylene glycol (PEG found in mRNA vaccines) and polysorbate 80 (present in the AstraZeneca COVID-19 vaccine). This will give an indication of the diversity of adverse events with the two vaccines and also help make comparisons. If details of unvaccinated patients who are similar in characteristics are available in such registries or other nation-wide large databases, then it would help by giving an indication of the baseline/background risk of a certain condition, for example, Guillain–Barre syndrome [20]. This also enables the calculations of the "odds" of these specific adverse events. These registries thus provide real-world data on a wider population by keeping the selection criteria broad and inclusive. Registries can similarly be established for biologics, biosimilars, and devices. The variables of interest here would be different, for example, production batch, device identifier, the company making the biosimilar, and so forth. Proportions of both total adverse events and specific adverse events seen would help sample size calculation for future epidemiological studies as well as for similar products.

4. Comparative observational studies [10]

These are the traditional epidemiological study designs centered around the time of exposure and occurrence of the outcome/event, namely, cross-sectional, case–control, and cohort studies, which are discussed in detail in Chap. 9.

5. Targeted clinical investigations

   At times, after the marketing approval has been obtained, further clinical studies may be planned to delineate the mechanism of action of an ADR, especially when significant risks are identified in the pre-approval clinical trials. These studies may include pharmacokinetic, pharmacodynamic, or pharmacogenetic studies. With the growing emphasis on personalized medicine and dose individualization, these clinical investigations are gaining importance and are utilized in modeling studies such as the population pharmacokinetics or physiology-based pharmacokinetics studies with the main goal of maximizing therapeutic benefit and at the same time minimizing safety concerns. These studies are more useful in establishing potential risks or unforeseen benefits in special populations such as children, the elderly, or those with renal or hepatic impairment who usually get excluded from the traditional clinical trials. This category of studies also includes the drug–drug interaction studies as well as the food–drug interaction studies that are also conducted with an aim to minimize ADRs due to concomitant drugs or specific food intake.

6. Descriptive studies

   These studies are used to estimate the background rate of ADRs that occur in a specified population that uses a specific drug.

   (a) Natural history of disease

   This includes the study of the natural course of the disease such as the distribution of the disease in the said population, characteristics of a diseased patient, treatments used, and the adverse events or favorable outcomes encountered. For example, a natural history of disease study could be conducted in a certain disease registry in a specific sub-population of patients such as those with comorbid illnesses like cardiovascular diseases and estimate the background incidence rate of ADRs. Similarly, in the pharmacovigilance of vaccines, knowing the background rates allows to perform observed (adverse events reported) *versus* expected analysis, as a method to continuous and proactive surveillance [20].

   (b) Drug utilization studies

   The WHO defines drug utilization studies (DUS) as *"studying the marketing, distribution, prescription, and use of medicinal products in a society, with special emphasis on the resulting medical and socioeconomic consequences"* [19]. Thus, DUS can be used to determine if a medicinal product is being used in a specific sub-population or a special population and, if used, what are the ADRs encountered in that population.

3 Identifying Adverse Drug Reactions in Clinical Practice

Many a times, patients themselves can pick up early warning signs of ADRs and report them to their treating physicians, provided the physicians adequately communicate with their patients on what to expect and bring it to their attention. In addition, any new complaint that the patient reports must be considered as a potential ADR. Practical methods of identification of ADRs in clinical practice to facilitate their early identification are to identify and monitor patients at high risk of ADRs, monitor for clinical signs and laboratory parameters, keep a high level of suspicion, and consider ADRs as a differential diagnosis. This would be aided by a thorough review of the patients' medical and medication history, ordering necessary laboratory investigations and, wherever appropriate, subjecting the patients to drug dechallenge and/or rechallenge. However, the responsibility of identifying an ADR is not merely confined to the treating physician and the patient, but to the wider care team including pharmacists, staff nurses, and caregivers. With advances in science and technology, the identification of ADRs also includes various advanced methods such as the use of trigger tools, tracer drugs, and coding of diseases/events that flag potential ADRs [21, 22].

4 Challenges in Diagnosing Adverse Drug Reactions

In clinical practice, prescribers tend to remain better informed about the perceived benefits of prescribed drugs rather than their risks, especially if such ADRs are rare and not likely to be serious. ADRs are classically described as "Type A" reactions called augmented reactions and can be predicted based on the drug's pharmacology. These can be prevented or at the least mitigated by identifying a susceptible cohort of individuals (e.g., patients at extremes of age) and tailoring an appropriate treatment plan along with effective communication. The "Type B" or the bizarre reactions are the ones like anaphylaxis that are unpredictable and potentially cannot be prevented [23]. Type A ADRs are akin to the pharmacological effects of the drug and may pose diagnostic difficulties when they resemble the disease for which it is indicated [23]. For example, arrhythmias occurring in patients on digoxin may be either drug-induced or due to the underlying disease, i.e., heart failure for which digoxin was prescribed. Similarly, many a times, patients do not report the common, mild, or nonserious ADRs to their prescribing physicians [24]. This is more so with Type A ADRs which are merely an extension of the pharmacological activity of the drug prescribed, for example, constipation following opioid use and dry mouth following the use of anticholinergics.

On the contrary, for Type B reactions, which are bizarre or unpredictable reactions, a strong clinical suspicion is the basic tenet in the detection of ADR, for instance, the recent identification of adenovirus vector-based COVID-19 vaccine-induced thrombosis with thrombocytopenia syndrome [25]. Furthermore, the diagnoses of immunological ADRs like acute exanthematous generalized pustulosis which is reported to occur rarely with some antimicrobial drugs like beta-lactam antibiotics and macrolides are often indistinguishable from the indication for their use [26]. Similarly, some neurological adverse effects seen with high doses of antiseizure medications like phenytoin may be indistinguishable from the disease for which it is being prescribed [27]. Thus, a thorough knowledge of the safety profile of drugs is important for all the stakeholders involved in patient care, especially in the diagnosis of idiosyncratic and immune-mediated ADRs. With the advent of several biologics and small molecules with complex therapeutics, establishing a causal association needs consideration of several additional issues.

Though infrequent, we also encounter situations where multiple drugs can cause similar ADRs. A common example is when a patient on antituberculosis drugs develops hepatotoxicity. The suspect drugs can be isoniazid, rifampicin, and pyrazinamide singly or in combination. It is well known that theoretically all these drugs can cause liver injury, but all of them may not be the suspect drug(s) in a given patient [28]. Establishing causality in such scenarios is often challenging mainly because withholding drugs which may not be causally related is indeed undesirable.

Similarly, diagnosis of ADRs in special populations and settings also needs careful consideration. For example, it is often difficult to diagnose ADR in neonates and infants or critically ill patients with altered consciousness. Such patients (neonates and unconscious patients) are unable to communicate, and it is likely that diagnosis of an ADR may be delayed or missed unless there is a strong clinical suspicion. This is because most ADRs detected in such settings need to manifest as abnormalities in investigational parameters or present as overt clinical signs.

5 Predicting and Preventing Adverse Drug Reactions

It is estimated in several studies that the median proportion of preventable ADRs-related admissions to hospital was 3.7% (range 1.4–15.4). The drugs commonly implicated in these hospital admissions include diuretics, nonsteroidal anti-inflammatory drugs, antiplatelets, and anticoagulants. These four groups of drugs account for a little more than 50% of all the drug groups that are associated with preventable drug-related hospital admissions [29].

The nature, frequency, and severity of ADRs can be diverse, ranging from innocuous, frequently occurring ones like skin rash, nausea, and vomiting to life-threatening or fatal rare events like ventricular arrhythmias or Stevens–Johnson syndrome. Since any organ or biological system can be the target of adverse effects of drugs, the act of identifying and predicting such risks is one of the most challenging tasks. Though complex, efforts to identify ADR and its predictors are initiated in the early phases of drug development and continue well beyond approval stage. The strategies to identify predictive factors include in vitro and in vivo nonclinical studies such as computational tools of simulation and modeling, AI-based approach in the early stages of new drug development [30], and active and passive safety surveillance in the post-marketing phase. Complex predictive models and algorithms are often formulated, but often their clinical applicability becomes limited as the extent of contribution of a predictive factor for a drug of interest is not uniform and may demonstrate significant interindividual variability. Additionally, assessment of any risk associated with drugs entails identification as well as quantification of risk compared to the background rates of such events. Unless comprehensive information is available about background rates, quantifying the risk attributable to a drug is not feasible or scientifically sound. A thorough understanding and consideration of risk factors for ADRs is very essential in preventing ADRs to the best way possible. The same should be considered while prescribing medications, dispensing, administering, patient education, and monitoring of patients. A detailed discussion on predisposing factors for ADRs is included in Chap. 3.

5.1 Methods to Predict Adverse Drug Reactions

1. Pharmacogenomics to predict ADRs.
2. Omics approaches to predict ADRs in drug development practice.
   (a) Metabolomics
   (b) Proteomics
   (c) Transcriptomics
   (d) Epigenomics
3. In silico approaches and use of artificial intelligence to predict ADRs in silico techniques in drug safety assessments are as follows:
   (a) Structure-related data
   (b) Drug target and pathways
   (c) Drug-induced gene expression profiles
   (d) Phenotypic features from primary cell cultures

1. Pharmacogenomics to predict and prevent ADRs

   Several ADRs that occur in clinical practice can be anticipated and prevented or at least their impact mitigated. The role of pharmacogenetics/pharmacogenomics in predicting drug response has transformed from being a mere research tool to one that guides and shapes clinical practice. Pharmacogenetics is the study of how individual genetic variations impact the drug response whereas pharmacogenomics deals with how the genome as a whole with simultaneous multiple mutations may determine a patient's response to drug therapy [54]. Despite the restricted availability of such testing in resource-limited settings, their utility in predicting some ADR risks has been well documented. In countries where such screening facilities are readily available, the Clinical Pharmacogenetics Implementation Consortium (CPIC) guidelines-based prescribing has reduced the occurrence of these ADRs [55].

   Specific examples of the use of pharmacogenetics to predict and therefore prevent ADRs are discussed as part of Chap. 23.

2. Omics approaches to predict ADRs in drug development

   Omics refers to the study of the sum of specific constituents in the cell. These constituents could be proteins, metabolites, or genetic material. It is a scientific discipline that aims to understand biological systems at a molecular level [31]. Omics technologies provide a comprehensive view of the biological effects of drugs on different biological systems and therefore have the potential to significantly improve our understanding of drug safety both in the drug development stage and in the post-marketing phase [31]. Although these omics technologies offer a great potential to understand drug safety, they are not yet extensively applied in routine clinical practice. Some important types of omics are described below.

   (a) Metabolomics

      It is the study of small molecules called metabolites such as the carbohydrates, amino acids, fatty acids, or other by-products of metabolic function found within the cells, biofluids, tissues, or organisms [32].

Metabolomics helps to investigate toxicities due to drugs and xenobiotics. As a result of drug metabolism, three types of metabolites, namely, active, inactive, and reactive metabolites, are produced. These reactive metabolites can bind to normal cellular macromolecules such as the DNA or cellular proteins and disrupt the homeostasis. These reactive metabolites are also unstable, unpredictable, and thus are sometimes difficult to be detected using regular technology if not for metabolomics [33]. Thus, metabolomics can be used to predict ADRs in the early phases of drug development as well as to predict etiopathogenesis of ADRs of old drugs and their likelihood to cause the ADR in a patient. One such example is the use of liquid chromatography and mass spectrometry-based metabolomics approach in screening the bioactivation pathways of ritonavir, a protease inhibitor used in the management of HIV infection. Ritonavir frequently causes hepatoxicity and metabolomics helped to identify 26 metabolites of which 5 were reactive [33].

(b) Proteomics

It refers to the large-scale study of genome-wide proteomes. Proteome is a complete set of proteins produced by the organism post-translation based on the genetic makeup [32]. The subspecialty of proteomics that deals with toxicity due to drugs and xenobiotics is called as toxicoproteomics. The principle is that a specific group of xenobiotic will bring about a specific pattern of protein expression that would aid in predicting the ADR/toxicity [34]. An example of the successful utilization of proteomics in ADR prediction was that of a novel lipid-lowering agent, torcetrapib, a cholesteryl-ester transfer protein inhibitor used in the ILLUMINATE trial conducted among 15,000 patients at high risk for coronary heart disease. The study was abruptly stopped after a median follow-up of 550 days due to reports of an increased cardiovascular event in the intervention arm. A subsequent retrospective study by Williams et al. analyzed paired plasma samples (baseline and 3-month post-intervention) using aptamer-based arrays and identified a significant increase within group, in nearly 200 proteins, including proteins functioning in the aldosterone pathways, inflammation, and immunity pathways post-intervention in the torcetrapib group when compared to the control group. Thus, the authors were able to identify the likely deleterious plasma proteins that were responsible for torcetrapib-associated increased cardiovascular events [35].

(c) Transcriptomics

A transcriptome is a complete set of RNA transcripts that are produced by a genome. As per the central dogma of biology, the process of transcription produces the RNA from the DNA followed by the process of translation which produces the required proteins necessary for biological action from the RNA. Thus, transcriptomics is the study of transcriptome both qualitatively (the types of RNA present, RNA editing sites, identification of novel splicing sites, etc.) and quantitatively (the number of each transcript that is present) using high throughput methods [32]. ADRs are often related to immunological features, as many drugs or metabolites can interact with major histocompatibility molecules, and these associations have been detected in the early genome-wide association studies of ADRs. An example of the use of transcriptomics in pharmacovigilance was in the understanding of the mechanism of peroxisome proliferators clofibrate and gemfibrozil causing hepatotoxicity in rat liver cells in comparison with an enzyme-inducer phenobarbital, and there were striking differences in the RNA transcripts suggesting novel mechanisms of hepatotoxicity [31, 36].

(d) Epigenomics

It is the study of the genome-wide epigenetic modifications found on the genetic material of the cell. These are reversible modifications of the DNA or the DNA-associated proteins such as histone acetylation, histone deacetylation, DNA methylation, DNA demethylation, and likewise [35]. Although currently there is much evidence that suggests differential response of certain diseases to drug therapies based on epigenetic changes, none have yet obtained a regulatory approval to be incorporated in routine practice. Some examples include hypomethylation of the CYP2E1 gene promoter in the CNS being associated with Parkinson's disease, prostate cancer with methylation levels at CYP1A1 and CYP1B1, and colon cancer with CYP2W1 [37]. It is further hypothesized that some iatrogenic ADRs such as drug-induced lupus and tardive dyskinesia are epigenetic in nature [38]. For instance, hydralazine is known to inhibit DNA methylation which is believed to cause the drug-induced lupus-like syndrome [39].

3. In silico approaches and use of AI to predict ADRs [40–42]

   Traditional clinical trials cannot identify all serious ADRs because of genetic factors, nongenetic factors, and ethnic diversity of patients who are enrolled in clinical trials. In contrast to traditional toxicological studies, the in silico method is an innovative and highly efficient technique to evaluate the toxicity and hazards of drugs. In silico modeling is an organ-on-a-chip technology that employs applied computer, omics, and mathematical biology, which can provide complementary knowledge of specific biological interactions and pathway analysis of the potential response of an organism to a chemical stressor [42]. In silico approaches have become a part of the drug discovery pathway that includes target protein identification, chemical library screening, and toxicity assessments using machine learning approaches. The in silico technique and computational pharmacology can be used to repurpose existing drugs to understand their pharmacological effect. They may be useful in improving clinical use and preventing potential ADRs [42].

   In silico approaches often use principles of AI wherein a machine simulates human intelligence processes like learning, reasoning, and decision-making. Some commonly used types of AI in predicting ADRs are machine learning and deep learning. Machine learning is the science and study of algorithms that depict mathematical models derived from available sample data to make predictions or decisions, but the machine itself is not programmed to perform that task directly. Deep learning is a subset of machine learning where there is a neural network across multiple layers of transformed data to extract higher-level information/features from raw data. Deep learning simulates the function of the human brain [43].

   Some approaches and applications of in silico techniques in drug safety assessments are as follows:

   (a) Structure-related data

      In-silico technique is an overriding approach involved in the assessment of drug toxicity based on their quantitative structure–activity relationships [44]. In silico modeling can be used in predicting severe cutaneous adverse reactions (SCARs) by deep learning. It is considered a useful technique to assess the association between the chemical substances and SCARs [45].

   (b) Drug target and pathways

      The technique includes the identification of ADR-related proteins that are used to predict ADRs based on existing literature on known drugs and their ADR profile. The known information regarding ADR-related proteins is compiled in databases such as the Drug-Induced Toxicity Related Protein Database (DITOP) and the Drug Adverse Reaction Target Database (DART) which are in the public domain. In silico drug target search approach (INVDOCK) was a helpful technique for predicting ADRs of 11 marketed anti-HIV drug interactions with related proteins. INVDOCK-predicted ADRs of these drugs were consistent with the literature-reported ADRs. This method proved that 86–89% of all predicted ADRs were consistent with known anti-HIV drug ADRs.

(c) Drug-induced gene expression profiles

This is a novel genomic prediction technique that compares drug-induced gene expression (DIGE) profiles after in vitro incubation of a drug with a culture of tumor cells or primary cell line with that of a normal condition. DIGE profiles can be obtained from three major public sources: Gene Expression Omnibus, Comparative Toxicogenomics Database, and Connectivity Map.

(d) Phenotypic features from primary cell cultures

The predefined set of phenotypic features relevant to toxic pathways can be used to predict ADR mechanisms. For instance, in silico validated hybrid models were developed based on a set of 156 drug-induced liver injury (DILI)-positive and 136 DILI-negative compounds screening to predict hepatotoxicity [46].

5.2 Preventability and Predictability of Adverse Drug Reactions in Clinical Practice

In clinical practice, ADRs could be prevented by ensuring rational medication use (the right patient, the right drug, the right time, the right dose, and the right route), evaluating for the risk factors, availability of alternative safer options, taking a thorough concomitant medication history and history of allergies, allergy testing, deprescribing, giving preventive medications, and likewise [47]. Inappropriate prescription is considered as one of the most important risk factors for ADRs, especially in the elderly. It includes a wide spectrum ranging from potentially inappropriate medications (PIMs) to potential prescribing omissions (PPOs). To tackle this, the screening tool of older people's prescriptions (STOPP) and screening tool to alert to right treatment (START) criteria have been developed to address PIMs and PPOs, respectively [48]. It is to be noted that the STOPP/START criteria, when applied as an intervention within 72 h of hospital admission, significantly reduced ADRs (absolute risk reduction = 9.3%; number needed to treat = 11) and the average length of stay by 3 days in elderly who were admitted with any acute illness [49]. Preventability of an ADR from already reported individual ADR reports could also be assessed using validated scales such as the Schumock and Thornton preventability scale [50]. Details of the mentioned scale is provided in Case 2 of the chapter.

Predictability, on the other hand, refers to the ability to forecast the likelihood of occurrence of an ADR based on certain factors or indicators. Type A ADRs are more predictable, and a good knowledge of the drug with a good medical history elicited from the patient would help predict ADRs better. Further, the Council for International Organizations of Medical Sciences (CIOMS) scale can also be used to assess the frequency of ADRs and help predict and categorize ADRs based on their frequency of occurrence. The following are the categories of CIOMS scale: (a) very rare: < 1 in 10,000 patients, (b) rare: ≥1 in 10,000 to <1 in 1000 patients, (c) uncommon: ≥1 in 1000 to <1 in 100 patients, (d) common: ≥1 in 100 to <1 in 10 patients, and (e) very common: ≥ 1 in 10 patients. The frequency of ADRs is usually identified through clinical trials, post-marketing surveillance, and other pharmacovigilance methods described previously in this chapter. By using the CIOMS scale for frequency of ADRs, healthcare professionals can better understand the likelihood and potential impact of ADRs associated with a particular drug. However, the downside is that the frequency of ADRs can vary depending on the patient population, dose, and duration of treatment, among many other factors [51].

6 Seriousness and Severity of Adverse Drug Reactions

As per the ICH, a serious adverse event (SAE) is defined as *"any untoward medical occurrence that at any dose results in death; or is life threatening or requires inpatient hospitalisation or*

Table 16.1 Modified version of Hartwig et al.'s severity assessment scale

Level	Description
1	An ADR occurred but required no change in treatment with the suspected drug
2	The ADR required that treatment with the suspected drug be held, discontinued, or otherwise changed. No antidote or other treatment requirement was required. No increase in length of stay (LOS)
3	The ADR required that treatment with the suspected drug be held, discontinued, or otherwise changed. AND/OR an antidote or other treatment was required. NO increase in LOS
4	(A) Any level 3 ADR which increases LOS by at least 1 day OR: (B) The ADR was the reason for admission
5	Any level 4 ADR which requires intensive medical care
6	The adverse reaction caused permanent harm to the patient
7	The adverse reaction either directly or indirectly led to the death of the patient

Mild = levels 1 and 2, moderate = levels 3 and 4, severe = 5, 6, and 7 as represented in the second table of Q 3 of Case 2. Thus, not all SAEs are severe in grade. For instance, let us consider a patient on a new drug who develops a rash, and he/she gets admitted to the hospital for observation or treatment for just 1 day and gets discharged. This would qualify as an SAE due to hospitalization but will not qualify as a severe grade SAE as ascertained by the modified version of Hartwig et al.'s severity assessment scale. The SAE will be considered as a moderate-grade ADR

prolongation of existing hospitalisation; or results in persistent or significant disability/ incapacity or is a congenital anomaly/birth defect." Severity, on the other hand, is graded using the Hartwig et al. severity assessment scale which categorizes ADRs into seven levels. The modified version of the scale available in literature further combines these levels into three grades of severity: mild, moderate, and severe. Mild = Levels 1 and 2; Moderate = Levels 3 and 4; Severe = Levels 5, 6, and 7 [47] (Table 16.1). On a little different note, the "severity" of an ADR also represents a measure of the "extent" to which the adverse effect develops and the same concept is discussed in Chap. 1.

7 Broad Principles Regarding Management of Adverse Drug Reactions

Although the best way to manage ADRs is to prevent them from occurring, patients do suffer from ADRs due to myriad reasons. The main aim of ADR management is therefore to mitigate harm to the patient through various strategies. These include the following:

(a) Early detection: Close monitoring and increasing the awareness of patients to watch out for known ADRs would help identify ADRs early, thereby prompting appropriate medical attention and preventing it from becoming severe.
(b) Documentation: Documentation of ADRs in patient files and providing alert cards is critical for tracking and monitoring adverse events and informing clinical decision-making.
(c) Treatment: Treating the presenting clinical symptoms is key to keeping the patient comfortable and minimizing the impact on the patient's quality of life. This may involve providing an antidote, providing supportive care, or using other therapies to manage specific symptoms.
(d) Discontinuation or switching medications: In some cases, ADRs may require discontinuation of the offending medication, reducing the dose, or switching to an alternative therapy.
(e) Follow-up and monitoring: This is the final step in the management wherein patients who had experienced an ADR are closely monitored and followed up for any further symptoms or complications that may require ongoing care to manage/prevent any long-term effects or complications associated with the ADR.

8 Summary and Conclusions

While detecting ADRs is relatively easy, predicting and preventing them is more challenging. Over the years, a lot of thrust has been given to the prevention approaches and some of this has found its way into patient care and mitigated and minimized ADR burden. As the knowledge base evolves, it is hoped that as more and more predictive and preventative tools become available that are not too expensive, the clinician will be able to deliver better quality patient care. This will be particularly impactful for developing countries.

9 Case Studies

9.1 Case Study 1

A 79-year-old male patient who is a known case of cerebral amyloid angiopathy developed headache and seizures. He was diagnosed to have subarachnoid hemorrhage. He was started on Tab. Phenytoin 100 mg twice daily. However, he had an episode of seizure 2 weeks later, and hence the evening dose of phenytoin was increased to 150 mg. He continued to have seizures and within 2 days of the dose hike, he developed altered sensorium and was admitted to the hospital. At admission, his plasma phenytoin level was 30.8 μg/ml (normal range: 10–20 μg/ml). Pharmacogenetic testing for CYP2C9 polymorphism revealed a diplotype of *2/*3. Tab. Phenytoin was thus replaced with Tab. Clobazam 10 mg twice daily and the plasma phenytoin levels normalized within 4 days and the patient was relieved of his symptoms.

1. *What is the interpretation of the pharmacogenetic test in this patient?*

   *3 is a no function allele and *2 is a decreased function allele. Therefore, this patient's phenotype may be considered as poor metabolizer [49].
2. *Name the other pharmacogenetic test that is recommended to be done along with CYP2C9 in patients prescribed with phenytoin.*

   HLA-B *15:02
3. *Describe the clinical application of these pharmacogenetic tests while prescribing phenytoin.*

The following are excerpts from the Clinical Pharmacogenetics Implementation Consortium (CPIC) guidelines for phenytoin [49].

(a) Assignment of HLA-B phenotypes based on genotypes

HLA phenotype	Genotype	Examples of diplotypes
HLA-B*15:02 negative	Homozygous for an allele other than HLA-B*15:02	*X/*X Where *X = any HLA-B allele other than HLA-B*15:02
HLA-B*15:02 positive	Heterozygous or homozygous variant	*15:02/*X, *15:02/*15:02 Where *X = any HLA-B allele other than HLA-B*15:02

(b) Assignment of CYP2C9 phenotypes based on genotypes

CYP2C9 phenotype	Activity score	Genotypes	Examples of diplotypes
Normal metabolizer	2	An individual carrying two normal function alleles	*1/*1
Intermediate metabolizer	1.5	An individual carrying one normal function allele and one decreased function allele OR	*1/*2
	1	One normal function allele plus one no function allele OR two decreased function alleles	*1/*3, *2/*2
Poor metabolizer	0.5	An individual carrying one no function allele and one decreased function allele OR	*2/*3
	0	Two no function alleles	*3/*3

(c) Algorithm for phenytoin prescription

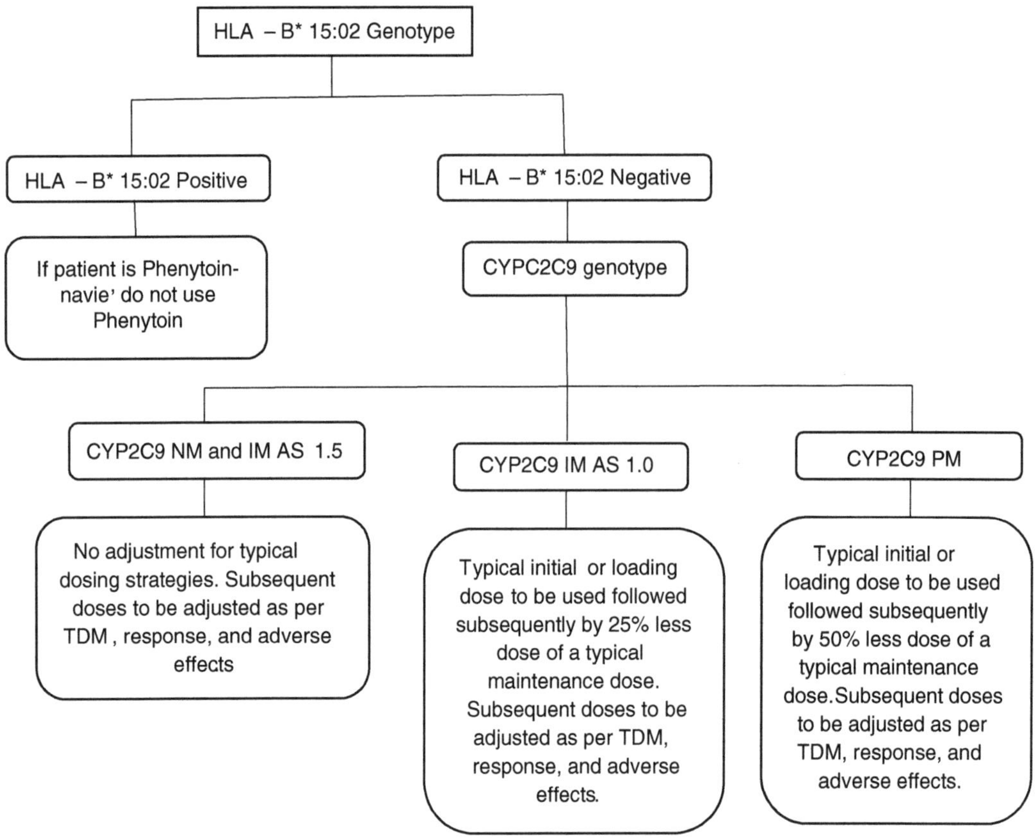

HLA human leukocyte antigen, *NM* normal metabolizer, *IM* intermediate metabolizer, *PM* poor metabolizer, *AS* activity score, *TDM* therapeutic drug monitoring

9.2 Case Study 2

A 54-year-old male patient who is a known person living with HIV infection was started on antiretroviral treatment (ART) regimen containing tenofovir, lamivudine, atazanavir, and ritonavir. Within 6 months of starting the ART, the patient developed puffiness of the face and pitting pedal edema during his routine follow-up. There was no change in the ART regimen recommended then, and in the subsequent 1 month, he was diagnosed to have high blood pressure and severe pitting pedal edema, new onset pleural effusion requiring intensive care unit admission.

1. *Identify the ADR and name the drug that is likely to have caused this. What is the possible mechanism of this ADR?*

   Tenofovir-induced nephrotoxicity [56]. The major pathway of renal elimination of tenofovir is glomerular filtration. However, approximately 20–30% gets eliminated by tubular secretion through the human organic anion transporter-1 (hOAT-1) transporter. But cellular accumulation through increased entry from the OAT and decreased efflux into tubular lumen results in cytotoxicity secondary to mitochondrial dysfunction of the proximal tubular cells [56].

2. *Name the other drugs that interfere with the renal tubular function similar to the offending drug?*

Transporter	Drug interaction	Effect [56]
hOAT-1	Probenecid inhibits hOAT-1 acyclovir and didanosine compete with tenofovir	Probenecid may decrease the incidence of nephrotoxicity by tenofovir. Acyclovir increases serum tenofovir concentrations, while tenofovir increases didanosine concentrations
MRP-4	NSAIDs and acyclovir group of drugs inhibit MRP-4	Increased risk of tenofovir associated nephrotoxicity
MRP-2	Ritonavir gets transported by MRP-2	Ritonavir increases tenofovir concentration and thereby increases the risk of nephrotoxicity

hOAT-1 human organic anion transporter-1, MRP multidrug resistance protein

3. *Could this ADR have been prevented? Assess using the Schumock and Thornton criteria and also grade the severity using the modified version of Hartwig et al.'s severity assessment scale.*

Preventable ADR of severe grade. There is a reported interaction between tenofovir and ritonavir which increases the risk of nephrotoxicity with tenofovir.

Sr. no.	Schumock and Thornton criteria [54]	Yes	No
1.	Was the drug involved in the ADR *not* considered appropriate for the patient's clinical condition?		
2.	Was the dose, route, and frequency of administration *not* appropriate for the patient's age, weight and disease state?		
3.	Was therapeutic drug monitoring or other necessary laboratory test *not* performed?		
4.	Was there a history of allergy or previous reactions to the drug?		
5.	Was a drug interaction involved in the reaction?	✓	
6.	Was a toxic serum drug level documented?		
7.	Was poor compliance involved in the reaction?		

Answering "yes" to one or more of the above questions suggests that the ADR in question may indeed have been preventable

Level	Modified version of Hartwig et al.'s severity assessment scale	Choose the right level
1	An ADR occurred but required no change in treatment with the suspected drug	
2	The ADR required that treatment with the suspected drug be held, discontinued, or otherwise changed. No antidote or other treatment requirement was required. No increase in length of stay (LOS)	
3	The ADR required that treatment with the suspected drug be held, discontinued, or otherwise changed. AND/OR An Antidote or other treatment was required. NO increase in LOS	
4	(A) Any level 3 ADR which increases LOS by at least 1 day OR: (B) The ADR was the reason for admission	
5	Any level 4 ADR which requires intensive medical care	✓
6	The adverse reaction caused permanent harm to the patient	
7	The adverse reaction either directly or indirectly led to the death of the patient	

Mild = levels 1 and 2, moderate = levels 3 and 4, severe = 5, 6, and 7

Acknowledgments Both the case studies were reported to an ADR monitoring center (AMC), West Zone, established under the aegis of the Pharmacovigilance Program of India and were also discussed in the monthly causality assessment meeting held at this AMC.

References

1. Fornasier G, Francescon S, Leone R, Baldo P. An historical overview over pharmacovigilance. Int J Clin Pharm. 2018;40(4):744–7.
2. World Health Organization. WHO Collaborating Centre for International Drug Monitoring. The importance of pharmacovigilance: safety Monitoring of medicinal products. World Health Organization; 2002. 48 p.
3. Alomar MJ. Factors affecting the development of adverse drug reactions (review article). Saudi Pharm J. 2014;22(2):83–94.
4. Mukherjee S, Maiti R. Haemovigilance: a current update in Indian perspective. J Clin Diagn Res. 2016;10(11):EE05–9.
5. Joshi D, Sharma I, Gupta S, Singh TG, Dhiman S, Prashar A, et al. A global comparison of implementation and effectiveness of materiovigilance program: overview of regulations. Environ Sci Pollut Res. 2021;28(42):59608–29.
6. Suh DC, Woodall BS, Shin SK, De Santis ERH. Clinical and economic impact of adverse drug reactions in hospitalized patients. Ann Pharmacother. 2000;34(12):1373–9.
7. Alomar M, Palaian S, Al-tabakha MM. Pharmacovigilance in perspective: drug withdrawals, data mining and policy implications. F1000Res. 2019;8:2109.
8. Engel P, Almas MF, De Bruin ML, Starzyk K, Blackburn S, Dreyer NA. Lessons learned on the design and the conduct of post-authorization safety studies: review of 3 years of PRAC oversight. Br J Clin Pharmacol. 2017;83(4):884–93.
9. ICH. ICH harmonised tripartite guideline E2E pharmacovigilance planning. ICH Guidelines. Curr Step. 2004;4:1–20.
10. ECA Academy. Eudralex Volume 9 Volume 9a—Guidelines on pharmacovigilance for medicinal products for human use. EudraLex; 2008. Available from: https://www.gmp-compliance.org/files/guidemgr/vol9a_09-2008_en.pdf
11. International Conference on Harmonisation of Technical Requirements for Registration of Pharmaceuticals for Human Use. Harmonised tripartite guideline: clinical safety data management: definitions and standards for expedited reporting E2A. ICH. 1994. p. 1–12.
12. Streefland MB. Why are we still creating individual case safety reports? Clin Ther. 2018;40(12):1973–80.
13. Anderson C, Gifford A, Avery A, Fortnum H, Murphy E, Krska J, et al. Assessing the usability of methods of public reporting of adverse drug reactions to the UK Yellow Card Scheme. Health Expect. 2012;15(4):433–40.
14. Capellà D, Torres F, Avila P, Moreno V, Laporte JR. Cough caused by angiotensin-converting enzyme inhibitors. A series of cases collected by spontaneous notification of adverse reactions. Med Clín. 1991;96(4):126–8.
15. Rachlis B, Karwa R, Chema C, Pastakia S, Olsson S, Wools-Kaloustian K, et al. Targeted spontaneous reporting: assessing opportunities to conduct routine pharmacovigilance for antiretroviral treatment on an international scale. Drug Saf. 2016;39(10):959–76.
16. Ndagije H, Nambasa V, Namagala E, Nassali H, Kajungu D, Sematiko G, et al. Targeted spontaneous reporting of suspected renal toxicity in patients undergoing highly active anti-retroviral therapy in two public health facilities in Uganda. Drug Saf. 2015;38(4):395–408.
17. Frau S, Font Pous M, Luppino MR, Conforti A. Risk management plans: are they a tool for improving drug safety? Eur J Clin Pharmacol. 2010;66(8):785–90.
18. Suku CK, Hill G, Sabblah G, Darko M, Muthuri G, Abwao E, et al. Experiences and lessons from implementing cohort event monitoring programmes for antimalarials in four African countries: results of a questionnaire-based survey. Drug Saf. 2015;38(11):1115–26.
19. Layton D, Shakir SAW. Specialist cohort event monitoring studies: a new study method for risk management in pharmacovigilance. Drug Saf. 2015;38:153–63.
20. Willame C, Dodd C, Durán CE, Elbers RJHJ, Gini R, Bartolini C, et al. Background rates of 41 adverse events of special interest for COVID-19 vaccines in 10 European healthcare databases—an ACCESS cohort study. Vaccine. 2023;41(1):251–62.
21. Gohil J, Desai C, Panchal J, Patel R, Rathod G. An evaluation of trigger tool method for adverse drug reaction monitoring at a tertiary care teaching hospital. Indian J Pharmacol. 2022;54(1):19–23.
22. Bates DW, Evans RS, Murff H, Stetson PD, Pizziferri L, Hripcsak G. Detecting adverse events using information technology. J Am Med Inform Assoc. 2003;10(2):115–28.
23. Kant A, Bilmen J, Hopkins PM. Adverse drug reactions. In: Pharmacology and physiology for anesthesia: foundations and clinical application, vol. 16(5). Elsevier; 2018. p. 130–43.
24. Jarernsiripornkul N, Krska J, Richards RME, Capps PAG. Patient reporting of adverse drug reactions: useful information for pain management? Eur J Pain. 2003;7(3):219–24.
25. Islam A, Bashir MS, Joyce K, Rashid H, Laher I, Elshazly S. An update on covid-19 vaccine induced thrombotic thrombocytopenia syndrome and some management recommendations. Molecules. 2021;26(16):5004.
26. Beylot C, Doutre MS, Beylot-Barry M. Acute generalized exanthematous pustulosis. Semin Cutan Med Surg. 1996;15(4):244–9.

27. Reynolds EH, Trimble MR. Adverse neuropsychiatric effects of anticonvulsant drugs. Drugs. 1985;29:570–81.
28. Molla Y, Wubetu M, Dessie B. Anti-tuberculosis drug induced hepatotoxicity and associated factors among tuberculosis patients at selected hospitals, Ethiopia. Hepatic Med: Evid Res. 2021;13:1–8.
29. Howard RL, Avery AJ, Slavenburg S, Royal S, Pipe G, Lucassen P, et al. Which drugs cause preventable admissions to hospital? A systematic review. Br J Clin Pharmacol. 2007;63(2):136–47.
30. Jamal S, Goyal S, Shanker A, Grover A. Predicting neurological Adverse Drug Reactions based on biological, chemical and phenotypic properties of drugs using machine learning models. Sci Rep. 2017;7(1):1–12.
31. Nguyen N, Jennen D, Kleinjans J. Omics technologies to understand drug toxicity mechanisms. Drug Discov Today. 2022;27(11):103348.
32. Hasin Y, Seldin M, Lusis A. Multi-omics approaches to disease. Genome Biol. 2017;18(1):1–15.
33. Wang P, Shehu AI, Ma X. The opportunities of metabolomics in drug safety evaluation. Curr Pharmacol Rep. 2017;3(1):10–5.
34. Ge F, He QY. Genomic and proteomic approaches for predicting toxicity and adverse drug reactions. Expert Opin Drug Metab Toxicol. 2009;5(1):29–37.
35. Williams SA, Murthy AC, DeLisle RK, Hyde C, Malarstig A, Ostroff R, Weiss SJ, Segal MR, Ganz P. Improving Assessment of Drug Safety Through Proteomics: Early Detection and Mechanistic Characterization of the Unforeseen Harmful Effects of Torcetrapib. Circulation. 2018;137(10):999–1010. https://doi.org/10.1161/CIRCULATIONAHA.117.028213. Epub 2017 Oct 3. PMID: 28974520; PMCID: PMC5839936.
36. Zhu XW, Sedykh A, Liu SS. Hybrid in silico models for drug-induced liver injury using chemical descriptors and in vitro cell-imaging information. J Appl Toxicol. 2014;34(3):281–8.
37. Kronfol MM, Dozmorov MG, Huang R, Slattum PW, Mcclay JL, Science O. The role of epigenomics in personalized medicine Mohamad. Expert Rev Precis Med Drug Dev. 2017;2(1):33–45.
38. Csoka AB, Szyf M. Epigenetic side-effects of common pharmaceuticals: a potential new field in medicine and pharmacology. Med Hypotheses. 2009;73(5):770–80.
39. Arce C, Segura-Pacheco B, Perez-Cardenas E, Taja-Chayeb L, Candelaria M, Dueñnas-Gonzalez A. Hydralazine target: from blood vessels to the epigenome. J Transl Med. 2006;4:1–16.
40. Ivanov SM, Lagunin AA, Poroikov VV. In silico assessment of adverse drug reactions and associated mechanisms. Drug Discov Today. 2016;21(1):58–71. DRUDIS 1663
41. Madden JC, Enoch SJ, Paini A, Cronin MTD. A review of in silico tools as alternatives to animal testing: principles, resources and applications. Altern Lab Anim. 2020;48(4):146–72.
42. Hodos RA, Kidd BA, Shameer K, Readhead BP, Dudley JT. In silico methods for drug repurposing and pharmacology. WIREs Syst Biol Med. 2016;8(8):186–210.
43. Golan D, Hanna SA, Ramachandran M. Artificial intelligence, machine learning and the evolution of healthcare. Bone Joint Res. 2018;7(3):223–5.
44. Myshkin E, Brennan R, Sitnik T, Litvinova E, Nikolsky Y. Prediction of organ toxicity endpoints by QSAR modeling based on precise chemical-histopathology annotations. Chem Bio Drug Des. 2012;80(13):406–16.
45. Ambe K, Ohya K, Takada W, Suzuki M, Tohkin M. In silico approach to predict severe cutaneous adverse reactions using the Japanese Adverse Drug Event Report Database. Clin Transl Sci. 2021;14:756–63.
46. Church RJ, Watkins PB. In silico modeling to optimize interpretation of liver safety biomarkers in clinical trials. Exp Biol Med. 2018;243:300–7.
47. Hartwig SC, Siegel J, Schneider PJ. Preventability and severity assessment in reporting adverse drug reactions. Am J Hosp Pharm. 1992;49(9):2229–32.
48. O'Mahony D, O'Sullivan D, Byrne S, O'Connor MN, Ryan C, Gallagher P. STOPP/START criteria for potentially inappropriate prescribing in older people: version 2. Age Ageing. 2015;44(2):213–8.
49. Karnes JH, Rettie AE, Somogyi AA, Huddart R, Fohner AE, Formea CM, et al. Clinical Pharmacogenetics Implementation Consortium (CPIC) guideline for CYP2C9 and HLA-B genotypes and phenytoin dosing: 2020 update. Clin Pharmacol Ther. 2021;109(2):302–9.
50. Schumock GT, Thornton JP. Focusing on the preventability of adverse drug reactions. Hosp Pharm. 1992;27(6):538.
51. CIOMS. CIOMS 7—DSUR harmonizing the format and content for periodic safety report during CTs. Guideline; 2006.
52. Leena LM. Neuroinformatics and computational modelling as complementary tools for neurotoxicology studies. Basic Clin Pharmacol Toxicol. 2018;123:56–61.
53. Cai C, Fang J, Guo P, Wang Q, Hong H, Moslehi J, et al. In silico pharmacoepidemiologic evaluation of drug-induced cardiovascular complications using combined classifiers. J Chem Inf Model. 2018;58(5):943–56.
54. Dere WH, Suto TS. The role of pharmacogenetics and pharmacogenomics in improving translational medicine. Clin Cases Mineral Bone Metab. 2009;6(1):13–6.
55. Turongkaravee S, Jittikoon J, Rochanathimoke O, Boyd K, Wu O, Chaikledkaew U. Pharmacogenetic testing for adverse drug reaction prevention: systematic review of economic evaluations and the appraisal of quality matters for clinical practice and implementation. BMC Health Serv Res. 2021;21(1):1–23.
56. Fernandez-Fernandez B, Montoya-Ferrer A, Sanz AB, Sanchez-Niño MD, Izquierdo MC, Poveda J, et al. Tenofovir nephrotoxicity: 2011 update. AIDS Res Treat. 2011;2011:354908.

Information Sources for Drug Safety and Communicating Risks in Practice

17

Vivien Tong, Mathias Møllebæk, and Parisa Aslani

Abstract

Drug safety is an important goal of clinical practice, where healthcare professionals must balance the benefits versus harms of medication use to optimize treatment outcomes. To facilitate this decision-making process and subsequent communication of drug safety issues to patients and their families, identifying and utilizing appropriate health and medicines information sources are critical. Drug safety-related information can be obtained from numerous sources, including government/regulatory bodies, non-government sources such as drug sponsors and other academic, commercial, and patient/healthcare professional organizations. These sources contribute toward the publication of different information types, including research studies, product information, clinical guidelines, safety advisories, and patient information leaflets, intended for healthcare professionals and/or patients/consumers. Healthcare professionals should source high-quality drug safety information. Assessing risk of bias, currency of information, and the reliability and trustworthiness of information are practical ways to help evaluate information quality. Harms and benefits information is important for safe and effective use of medicines by patients. They can be expressed in several ways, and risk information should be carefully appraised, considering the context in which the data were derived and communicated, when applying it in clinical practice and communicating to patients.

Keywords
Drug information · Drug safety · Patient information · Safety advisories · Risk of bias · Trustworthiness of information · Side effect risk · Risk communication · Medication harms · Medication benefits · Information sources

Learning Objectives

- Describe the range of sources that are available through which healthcare professionals can obtain accurate and up-to-date information about the safety of medicines
- Identify the approaches and methods used to assess the quality, bias, accuracy, and reliability of drug safety-related information across the range of information sources

V. Tong (✉) · P. Aslani
The University of Sydney School of Pharmacy, Faculty of Medicine and Health, The University of Sydney, Camperdown, NSW, Australia
e-mail: vivien.tong@sydney.edu.au

M. Møllebæk
Copenhagen Centre for Regulatory Science, Department of Pharmacy, University of Copenhagen, Copenhagen, Denmark

J. Jose et al. (eds.), *Principles and Practice of Pharmacovigilance and Drug Safety*,
https://doi.org/10.1007/978-3-031-51089-2_17

- Describe the types of risk of harms and benefits information that are available for medicines, and various sources of such information
- Utilize the sourced information on risk of harms and benefits to communicate to healthcare professionals and patients/the public

Key Points

- Drug safety-related information can be obtained from numerous sources, including government/regulatory bodies, non-government sources such as drug sponsors and other academic, commercial, and patient/healthcare professional (HCP) organizations
- These sources contribute toward the publication of different information types, including research studies, product information, clinical guidelines, safety advisories, and patient information leaflets, intended for HCPs and/or patients/consumers
- High-quality drug safety information should be sourced by HCPs for use. Assessing for risk of bias, recency of information, and the reliability and trustworthiness of information are practical ways to help evaluate information quality
- Harms and benefits information can be expressed in several ways via framing of information and the use of qualifiers versus numbers. Numerical risk information should be carefully appraised, considering the context in which the data was derived and how it has been communicated, when applying it in clinical practice

1 Introduction

Drug safety is an important goal of clinical practice, where healthcare professionals (HCPs) who prescribe and/or oversee the use of medicines must balance the benefits versus harms of medication use to optimize treatment outcomes. To facilitate this decision-making process and subsequent communication of drug safety issues to patients and their families, identifying and utilizing appropriate health and medicines information sources are critical.

The overall goals of the chapter are to:

- Provide a broad outlook on the range of information sources that are available to clinicians, pharmacists, and other HCPs on medicines and, specifically, on the safety aspects of medicines
- Outline practical approaches to assess the quality and reliability of information sources on risk of harms and benefits
- Demonstrate how information on risk of harms and benefits obtained from the sources can be best utilized for communicating to other HCPs and patients/the public

2 Sources of Drug Safety-Related Information

Drug safety information can be communicated via several means, including spoken, written, multimedia, and other hybrid communication formats. HCPs should be aware of the breadth of information sources that are available that tailor information intended for their use, as well as common information sources that patients or consumers are exposed to. From a safety perspective, optimal drug safety information can support medication literacy for both HCPs and consumers, as well as drug safety. Medication literacy can be defined as:

> *The degree to which individuals can obtain, comprehend, communicate, calculate and process patient-specific information about their medications to make informed medication and health decisions in order to safely and effectively use their medications, regardless of the mode by which the content is delivered (e.g. written, oral and visual).* (p.801) [1]

Effective understanding of drug safety-related information underpins effective communication within multidisciplinary healthcare teams about drug safety. Broadly, from a user perspective, information sources can be consumer-focused or targeted toward HCPs. HCPs can acquire information about drugs and drug safety from a wide range of sources which may differ in multiple ways with respect to their content and communication style. The information may be communicated with different intended uses; that is, clinical treatment guidelines, news bulletins, or safety advisories. Due consideration should also be given to the provider of the information. For example, organizations that provide information may have financial or other interests in the drugs they inform about, or the provision of information may be a result of regulatory requirement or may be integrated in an electronic system or software, such as prescribing and dispensing software and processes. The following sections go into more detail about potential information sources relevant to drug safety.

2.1 Government and Regulatory Agencies

Government agencies and public bodies, such as drug regulators or health technology assessment (HTA) bodies (e.g., the National Institute for Health and Care Excellence (NICE), Finnish Coordinating Center for Health Technology Assessment (FinCCHTA)), provide information about drugs and drug safety as part of their remit to protect public health and individual consumers from harm. Importantly, regulators and HTA bodies have different functions in the regulation and assessment of drugs, and the information they provide may differ accordingly. Whereas HTA bodies provide recommendations on the value of new health technologies in the context of existing therapeutic options and healthcare provision more generally, regulators are mandated to ensure the safety, efficacy, and quality of health products upon market entry and monitor them after marketing. While recommendations by HTA bodies include the harms and benefits of drugs, they typically do not aim to provide a comprehensive picture of potential safety issues in clinical practice to the same extent as information from regulators.

Regulators oversee the information provided by medicine sponsors and available pharmacovigilance data and issue postapproval safety advisories if new safety concerns have emerged and need to be communicated to HCPs and/or the public, as appropriate. Regulatory safety advisories may come in the form of information letters to HCPs, drug safety bulletins, media alerts, and public website announcements, with different examples available from regulatory bodies [2]. HTA bodies may include emergent safety concerns in their guidelines, although the degree of coordination and harmonization between information material from regulatory authorities and HTA bodies is currently unknown. The adverse event reporting databases in some countries may also be accessible by users to see the reporting that has been received for medicines. Examples include:

- United States of America: Food and Drug Administration (FDA) Adverse Event Reporting System (FAERS) Public Dashboard [3]
- European Union: EudraVigilance—European database of suspected adverse drug reaction reports [4]
- Australia: Database of Adverse Event Notifications (DAEN) for medicines and medical devices [5]

2.2 Professional Organizations

Professional organizations have considerable influence in the provision of drug information to HCPs. Professional organizations typically produce publicly available medical information for their membership, which may include different types of healthcare professionals (e.g., physicians, pharmacists, nurses) at varying levels of speciality (e.g., endocrinologists, diabetes education nurses, diabetes educators). Drug safety information may be delivered as part of continuing professional development activities spearheaded by the organizations such as presentations, articles, newsletters, and online publications, to name a few. Notably, as HCP organizations are key stakeholders when representing their profession, a key information product is clinical practice guidelines which would be relevant for their membership and other HCPs working in collaboration.

2.3 Independent Academic Institutions/ Research Groups/ Organizations

Research centers and drug information initiatives have been established with the primary aim of providing information independent from commercial and policy interests. An important driver for such activities is the perceived risk of bias in information about drugs and drug safety. Therefore, independent organizations employ editorial policies that emphasize transparency, rigorous peer review, and requirement for declarations of potential conflict of interests. The International Society of Drug Bulletins is an international network of such drug information initiatives that are independent of the pharmaceutical industry both financially and intellectually [6]. The Therapeutics Initiative based at the University of British Columbia is another example [7]. The primary information outlet is the *Therapeutics Letter*, a bimonthly newsletter that aims to provide physicians and pharmacists with up-to-date, evidence-based, practical information on prescription drug therapy. The publication process typically involves systematic literature reviews by different working groups and peer review conducted by national and international specialists.

A range of academic journals about drug safety and pharmacovigilance are also available. These include *Drug Safety* (Electronic ISSN 1179-1942), *Pharmacoepidemiology and Drug Safety* (ISSN:1099-1557), *Therapeutic Advances in Drug Safety* (ISSN: 2042-0994), and *Expert Opinion on Drug Safety* (ISSN: 1744-764X). They are all international peer-reviewed academic journals that publish review articles and research articles on all aspects of drug treatment safety issues, including clinical implications of drug safety issues.

2.4 Commercial Organizations

HCPs also search and retrieve drug safety information from a range of for-profit sources. WebMD.com and drugs.com are two US-based examples. While the for-profit information sources differ from not-for-profit sources in important ways, the dividing line is not always clear. For example, in Denmark, the online medical compendium, which is widely used by HCPs and integrated in various ways in informational platforms, is privately owned by the federation of the Danish pharmaceutical companies and operates on a for-profit basis of fees from drug companies per drug. However, in order to reduce risk of commercial bias, the articles in the compendium are authored by independent experts who are compensated, reviewed by independent reviewers, and overseen by an editorial board [8].

2.5 Patient Groups/Organizations

Patient groups or organizations exist to provide appropriate and relevant information and empower patients in their own healthcare journey or the journey of those they care for. They may also provide information about drug safety to HCPs, in addition to information to patients. Such information can emphasize patients' perspectives in pharmaceutical care in ways that other sources cannot. In general, however, while some patient organizations have well-established and longstanding relations with medical professions and other healthcare communities, it is important to note that patient organizations may receive various forms of funding from industry [9]. HCPs should therefore consider the potential biases of information in relation to the financial interests held by those who sponsor these organizations.

Medical condition-specific organizations may focus on specific conditions, the medicines used to treat those conditions, and the subsequent benefits and harms, e.g., Arthritis Australia and the rheumatological drug fact sheets available [10]. Videos, interactive media, and other print resources may also be available. Other organizations offer a platform to facilitate patient-specific information and engagement to improve drug safety, for example, the former organization NPS Medicinewise in Australia [11] and the National Council on Patient Information (NCPIE)/NeedyMeds and the BeMedWise program in the United States [12].

The benefits of information sources that have been endorsed and published by patient organizations (or organizations with a patient-centered arm) are that information would be more likely to be fit for purpose for the target audience and worded using consumer-friendly language. The transformation of more complex data into easy-to-understand information that reflect the interests of the patient groups/patient organizations is beneficial as these resources can then be used as patient education and counseling tools to supplement spoken information provided in consultations.

2.6 Social Networking Sites

Online communities have been conceptualized and are commonplace within social networking sites, which contribute toward user-created sources of information by both consumers and HCPs. Social networking sites provide an important forum for users to exchange and mutually learn from insights and experiences about medical conditions and subsequent treatment(s). From a user perspective, side effects are a key driver prompting online information searching [13]. Interestingly, information derived from the personal experiences of others when using medicines was valued and seen as less generic in comparison to information provided by medicine sponsors [13]. Perceived advantages of user-created content include the personal nature of the information, with documented experiences from actual reported medicine users that then resonate with potential medicine users, which can in turn impact treatment decision-making and adherence [13].

Social media use among online communities of fellow HCPs, medicine users, or parents/carers of children or older persons who may also be living with similar medical conditions or have similar medication use provide opportunities to create online conversation about experienced side effects. This may be a data source for signal detection, monitoring of side effects, and additional adverse drug reaction (ADR) reporting, where individuals collectively create insight into real-world drug safety data via discussing their experiences [14]. However, with this opportunity to leverage this type of data in drug safety monitoring initiatives alongside more "traditional" ADR reporting avenues, variation in how online discussions ensue needs to be considered [14].

3 Types of Information on Drug Safety

Given the wealth of information sources, both patient and HCP-centered, that provide information to end users, there are several different information types that are relevant to refer to and help communicate risks in clinical practice. This section details some of the types of information sources available to HCPs, depending on their drug safety information needs.

3.1 Research Studies

Research informs the available evidence base for drug safety. Clinical guidelines should be evidence-based and rely on high-quality research studies to inform them. Given the emergence of new medicines and health technologies over time and their implications on guidelines, keeping abreast of empirical research such as high-quality clinical trials in the clinical area(s) specific to one's clinical practice will help HCPs establish an understanding of the specific evidence that informs clinical guidelines and practice.

Drug safety evidence can be derived from multiple research study types and available data such as case reports, randomized clinical trials, non-randomized studies such as cohort and case-control studies, and meta-analysis of controlled observational studies and/or trials [15]. The resulting drug safety data are therefore influenced by the study design and how it was obtained [15]. One notable example is that the shorter duration of clinical trials may mean that long-term drug safety issues may not be detected [15].

Literature reviews collate and critique available evidence. They are designed to address specific research aim(s) and objective(s) and are useful if wanting to access a summary of existing drug safety evidence within certain parameters. There are several review types that are commonly seen in the context of healthcare, such as systematic reviews with or without meta-analyses, scoping reviews, rapid reviews/rapid evidence assessments, and narrative reviews, to name a few, each with their pros and cons [16]. Systematic reviews are regarded as the gold standard of the review types, seeking to answer a focused clinical question through the utilization of well-documented, reproducible methods of literature searching, appraisal, and reporting [16].

Database searches yield relevant peer-reviewed research publications. Common databases that are available to use when searching the literature include MEDLINE, Embase, PubMed, CINAHL, and Cochrane Library, among others. Other search platforms are also available such as Scopus and Web of Science.

3.2 Product Information/Summary of Product Characteristics

As part of their market approval, drugs are also accompanied by a comprehensive document that describes the approved uses and characteristics of the drug, for example, the Summary of Product Characteristics (SPC; sometimes abbreviated as SmPC, and also known as the Product Information (PI) in Australia). In a review conducted on the regulations for written medicine information across Australia, the United States, and Europe, regulatory similarities were seen between the regions with respect to PI/SPC (and the package insert, as it is known in the United States) [17]. The SPC is generally considered the definitive source of drug information [17, 18]. This information is generally written for HCPs, where clinical trials data and adverse effects information are included alongside other product-specific information such as contraindications and precautions, directions for use, and product details [17]. The incorporation of data derived from research in PI/SPC emphasizes the important role that research plays in informing these sources of drug safety information.

3.3 Patient Information Leaflets/Consumer Medicines Information

Alongside the PI or SPC, which are designed with HCPs in mind, written medicine information leaflets are produced for consumers to communicate medicine-specific information. The content of these leaflets is based on the respective PI/SPC [17]. A core section included in this information is that on adverse effects, where known side effects for a medication are communicated together with an indication of the likelihood of experiencing the side effect(s) and/or relevant action(s) to be taken by the patient, if experienced. While in many countries, this information is produced by the medicine sponsor, in the United States, for instance, depending on the medicine and legislative requirements, some information may be produced by the sponsor and others by varying organizations/companies which may lead to variation in content [17]. HCPs should be aware of these information sources as they can be used to help communicate benefit and harm information to consumers/patients in clinical practice.

3.4 Other Drug Information Sources

3.4.1 Clinical Guidelines

Clinical guidelines summarize current medical knowledge and provide evidence-based treatment recommendations for specific therapeutic areas. They play an important role in assisting clinicians in their healthcare decisions and synthesizing input from a range of different stakeholders in healthcare practices. While research has shown that clinical guidelines are important for drug safety, there is a lack of knowledge on how postmarketing safety advisories are integrated into clinical practice guidelines, and particularly how quickly clinical guidelines are updated to include new safety concerns [8]. Specifically, detailed information on drug safety may not be fully encapsulated in clinical guidelines, highlighting the role of other complementary drug information sources to gain a comprehensive understanding of the individual drug safety profile(s).

Clinical guidelines are available on a local (institutional, e.g., hospital-based), national, and international basis. Leading national organizations may publish guidelines relevant to their remit, e.g., the National Heart Foundation of Australia and guidelines on the management of cardiovascular diseases [19]. Prominent guidelines that are well-known internationally may be published by consortia or bodies such as The National Institute for Health and Care Excellence (NICE) in the United Kingdom. As detailed in "Developing NICE guidelines: the manual—Process and methods [PMG20]," a systematic review of the available evidence is a critical component of the guideline development process [20]. This reiterates that research studies and rigorous literature reviews form the evidence base on which evidence-based clinical guidelines are formulated.

3.4.2 Drug Compendiums

In many countries, online drug compendiums (also known as drug monographs or pharmacopoeia) source government-approved information typically based on the SPC. However, information included in compendium monographs can differ due to how quickly and frequently the information is revised, and emergent safety concerns added in. Notwithstanding, due to their ease of search and retrieval, medical compendia are widely used by both HCPs and the public. For example, the Electronic Medicines Compendium (EMC) provides information about drugs licensed for use in the United Kingdom [21]. EMC has more than 14,000 documents on medicines sourced from or approved by either the UK or European government agencies that license drugs [21]. Monthly Index of Medical Specialties (MIMS) is a prominent source of medicines information especially within the Asia-Pacific region, offering medicines information references, as well as specialty resources and clinical decision support [22].

3.4.3 Safety Advisories

Safety advisories are notifications from regulators that inform HCPs, patients, and/or the public about a potential or confirmed safety risk that is inherent to a drug and not due to manufacturing problems or improper use [23]. The identification and confirmation of safety risk is based on regulatory surveillance and assessment of postmarketing data. A range of communication modalities can be used to inform HCPs about newly identified safety risks in prescription drugs [2]. They vary depending on how acute their message is (e.g., acute risk or notification on ongoing drug safety review), what their objective is (e.g., share information, change beliefs, change behavior), who the intended recipients are (e.g., various groups of HCPs), and what the channel of communication is (e.g., hardcopy letter, website posting, newsletter article).

4 Quality and Reliability of Drug Safety Information

As HCPs rely on up-to-date, clear, and evidence-based information for their decisions, it is important to assess the independence, usability, and evidential strength of the information when choosing which sources to rely on. When assessing the quality and reliability of information, there are several factors that must be considered, which would also be dependent on the type of information source being evaluated. Overall, information should be assessed for risk of bias, currency, and reliability and trustworthiness.

4.1 Risk of Bias

In a clinical context, HCPs should continually strive to source and utilize information of the highest available quality. However, given the sheer amount of information available via several sources, as outlined earlier in the chapter, HCPs need to be cognizant of the information they are sourcing and utilizing to inform their practice.

Assessing the risk of bias for drug benefit and safety-related information (e.g., clinical trials) and other relevant information to inform clinical decision-making guidelines is an imperative step. Established tools are available to assess the risk of bias, which essentially helps the user determine the strengths and limitations of the research that was conducted and reported, and potential factors that can contribute toward interpretation of study results [24]. For example, non-randomized interventional studies can be assessed for the risk of bias using tools such as the ROBINS-I or SIGN checklist (case-control and cohort studies) [24]. For randomized trials, the Cochrane RoB 2.0 Tool or SIGN checklist for randomized controlled trials can be used [24]. A review conducted by Ma et al. in 2020 provides an overview of the risk of bias assessment tools that are available for use when examining medical research [25]. Risk of bias assessment is also reiterated in guidelines developed to support guidelines development [24]. Through understanding the risk of bias, conclusions based on the available body of research can be contextualized within the parameters of the studies that were conducted. This will facilitate a grounded approach to evidence-based practice.

4.2 Currency of Information

Currency of information is informed by the date of availability of the risk information, when the risk data were obtained or made available, e.g., when a clinical trial was conducted in which side effects risk information was obtained, and when the information was last reviewed and/or updated. Currency of information for well-established, longstanding medicines with largely unchanged safety profiles may not lead to significant fluctuations of information over time. Novel medicines, where postmarketing surveillance is helping to inform understanding of risks that become clearer once medicines are taken by a broader population, may see a substantial difference in data when stratified by currency. A recent global example would be the COVID-19 vaccine roll-out and the ensuing changes to COVID-19 vaccination guidelines due to the emergent adverse effects and safety profile aspects—one notable example was observed with the AstraZeneca COVID-19 vaccine and age-related guidelines for use [26].

When retrieving drug safety information from the available literature, it is important to consider:

- When the research was conducted, if referring to empirical research papers
- When the systematic review or meta-analysis was conducted and the years of published literature that was captured and critically reviewed as part of the review; for instance, consider whether known recent seminal research has been captured
- Whether there have been any review updates subsequently conducted since the initial review to provide further information about evolving safety information drawn from pharmacovigilance efforts—search strategies may be repeated in review updates, which may contribute to slight differences in interpretation of all available data
- The currency of evidence utilized to inform clinical guidelines in comparison to available literature. Guidelines may not be updated as quickly as evidence emerges; therefore, clinical practice may rely on other update avenues

4.3 Reliability and Trustworthiness of Information

Reliability of information can refer to the level of trust in the information source as well as its "repeatability" or consistency of information being delivered about the medicine. Mandatory safety information that is required to be reported by medicine sponsors helps to ensure reliable and consistent safety information for a specific medicinal product. Sourcing information directly from the sponsor, regulator repository, or well-known, trusted drug compendiums/pharmacopoeias will help to ensure that the correct information about the product is being accessed.

For proprietary medicines that go off patent, information provided by generic medicine manufacturers should largely be consistent with the safety profile information reported for the proprietary product. Any further changes in the safety profile between marketed products should be detected via pharmacovigilance systems overseen by the relevant regulatory bodies. This can possibly lead to updated information about the medicine itself. In these instances, with multiple medicines on the market with the same active ingredient, the reliability of information available on the safety profile is improved if appropriate documentation, reporting, and monitoring systems are in place from a regulatory and reporting perspective.

With respect to online resources, mechanisms to help verify whether the drug safety-related information is from a reputable source should be checked. For example, looking to see whether the website/online resource had been Health On the Net (HON) code certified was one way. Health On the Net *"promotes transparent and reliable health information online"* [27]; however, HON was discontinued in December 2022. Previously, HONcode certification could also be sought for social networking sites [28].

5 Information on Risk of Harms, and Benefits: How to Frame the Information

While it is important to know the types of harms and benefits that can be experienced when using a medicine, it is important for the user to understand the proportion of people that experience these benefits versus harms so that the benefits of treatment can be appropriately weighed up at timely points during the treatment continuum. Appropriately conveying benefit and harm information to the user and engaging in discussions between users and their treating HCP(s) can help facilitate informed treatment decision-making.

5.1 How to Frame the Information: Loss (Harm) vs. Gain (Benefit)

Benefits are intrinsically tied in with the medicine's indication or purpose and the harms with potential side effects that can be experienced. Framing of information can therefore have an important impact upon people's perception and understanding of harms and benefits of a medicine. For example, side effects information is typically conveyed using negative framing, i.e., the proportion of people who will experience the side effect. However, there is also the possibility of positively framing information, e.g., conveying the proportion of people who will **not** experience a particular side effect [29]. However, given the nature of medicine sponsor drafted information about their products, there may be reluctance to positively frame harm information or convey benefit information upfront as it may be perceived as promotional in nature. In many ways, information that medicine users receive, such as patient information leaflets, convey long lists of side effects information and less benefit information. This may lead to incomplete understanding of the benefits for starting and adhering to the medicine and altered perceived safety of medication use due to this "imbalance" of information presented before them.

5.2 Qualifiers Versus Numbers

Empirical research has shown that people's judgments about health risks may not only be influenced by their individual risk tolerance and how well they understand the health risk but also by the ways in which risk information is presented. For example, researchers presented a sample of individuals with two different statements about a cancer mortality risk and asked them which they considered to present the highest risk: A cancer that kills 1286 out of 10,000 people, or a cancer that kills 24.14 out of 100 people? The first statement was judged as being a much higher risk even though the risk described in the second is, in fact, twice as high [30].

Generally, research has shown that for both written and oral information, patients gain a more accurate perception of risk if probabilistic information is relayed in numbers rather than words [31]. But there are multiple ways to numerically present risk information to patients. Therefore, it is important that HCPs understand what the different formats of risk information express and when to use them most appropriately [32].

With respect to the likelihood of experiencing side effects for a medicine, in order to simplify messaging, patients have been exposed to verbal descriptors for risk information. These verbal descriptors have been mapped to specific numerical ranges, which can then in turn be expressed as either percentages or frequencies, as detailed in an earlier version of the European Commission guidelines for readability of medicine labels and leaflets [33]. Similarly, for example, the New Zealand Medicines and Medical Devices Safety Authority have published on their website the numerical descriptors mapped to each of the verbal descriptors very common, common, uncommon, rare, and very rare [34]. A very common side effect equates to 1 in 10 (or 10%) of those taking the medicine experiencing the side effect in comparison to a very rare side effect being less than 1 in 10,000 medicine users likely to experience that particular side effect [34]. These numerical frequency ranges may or may not be explicitly stated in the information received by patients, which can lead to misunderstanding of what the likelihood of a "common" side effect is. Research studying verbal descriptors advocated for use by the European Commission has shown that people misunderstand verbal descriptors used to communicate side effect risk in patient information leaflets [35]. A systematic review demonstrated that verbal descriptors contribute to risk overestimation in comparison to numerical descriptors [36]. The authors concluded that numerical risk information would be preferred for communication in consumer-oriented information where possible [36].

However, HCPs should be educating patients on what verbal descriptors for side effect risk mean to avoid misunderstanding. Furthermore, it is imperative that HCPs communicate to their patients the relevant action to be taken if side effects are experienced—while it may be of interest to understand the population statistics, patients need to understand the relative severity of the side effects/adverse events if experienced and what to do. Seeking medical attention in a timely manner could affect prognosis.

5.3 Understanding Numerical Drug Safety-Related Data

There are several ways in which drug safety data derived from clinical studies can be communicated. When reading clinical research data, alongside frequencies and percentages, drug safety studies may also report other numerical data measures. While not exhaustive, below are some relevant numerical data examples that HCPs should be able to understand within the context of drug harm and benefit.

5.3.1 Absolute and Relative Risk Reduction

Absolute risk refers to the number of harmful events (e.g., ADRs) that occur in a group, divided by the number of people in that group. The reduction of risk in absolute terms (absolute risk reduction or risk difference) is the difference between risk of a harmful event in a control group and the risk of an event in a treatment group.

In contrast to absolute risk, relative risk is the ratio of risks of the treatment group and control group. The reduction of risk in relative terms (relative risk reduction) is the difference in the rate of events between the control and treatment group. For example, if 20% of patients experience ADRs *before* exposure to risk minimization measures and 15% of patients experience ADRs *after* exposure to a risk minimization measure, the relative risk would be 15%/20% = 0.75. The relative risk reduction of the risk minimization measure is therefore 25%. But to HCPs and lay audiences, the magnitude of risk may be difficult to interpret in light of relative risk measures and related odds ratio reporting from a clinical perspective [37]. HCP and lay audiences can also falsely conclude that strong statistical associations or statistical significance imply high clinical importance [38].

The potential problem with explaining risk in absolute and relative terms is the risk of bias. Health researchers such as Leung [39] have argued for providing a baseline level of risk for consideration as well as the relative risk reduction. For example, when referring to the data published as part of an older prescriber update released several years ago [40], patients using a third-generation oral contraceptive should not only be told that the risk of venous thromboembolism is about twice that of alternative contraceptives containing levonorgestrel, but also be informed about the absolute risk for venous thromboembolism for these contraceptives to provide further context for interpretation; for example, observed to be about 10 per 100,000 women/years for second-generation contraceptives compared to about 21 for third generation [40]. Experimental evidence about effectiveness and safety information about vaccines suggest that the inclusion of baseline levels of risk is a key factor in people's perception of risk and that it may lead to increased levels of perceived effectiveness of vaccination and intention to be vaccinated [41]. Communicating baseline level of risk information to patients is useful to support understanding of flu risk whether it is presented in absolute or relative risk formats [41].

5.3.2 Odds Ratio

The odds ratio refers to the odds of an event occurring versus the odds of it not occurring. In the context of pharmacovigilance, the odds ratio may be used to express the odds of an ADR occurring. So, an odds ratio of 3 in this case means that a patient taking a specific treatment is three times more likely to experience an ADR than the patient who takes a placebo treatment. Odds ratios are typically used in case-control studies where the relative risk cannot be estimated. It can also be used in retrospective and cross-sectional studies with the aim of examining associations rather than differences [42].

5.3.3 Number Needed to Treat

To communicate the benefits of a therapeutic intervention, HCPs often use the "number needed to treat" (NNT) format. In practice, NNT expresses "the number of patients you need to treat to prevent one additional bad outcome (death, stroke, etc.)" [43]. NNT is the inverse of absolute risk reduction (ARR; see Sect. 5.3.1), i.e. NNT=1/ARR. It provides quantitative basis for making decisions about therapies that align better with patient perspectives, and it is often preferred by patients and clinicians because it is more intuitively understandable than other formats [44]. However, this is not always the case. In a study conducted by Hamrosi et al. [45], when the benefit information in the form of NNT was included in revised information leaflets, some had difficulty understanding the NNT data presented. Additionally, people were surprised that more people did not benefit from taking the medicine [45].

However, there are notable limitations to NNT. It is more difficult to compare different NNTs than formats that use natural frequencies (e.g., benefit per hundred patients) because NNTs are expressed as fractions with different denominators. Moreover, NNT reflects the number but not the importance of events. As different outcomes of a treatment are reflected in separate NNT values, using the NNT format may lead to emphasizing less important outcomes [44].

NNT can also be calculated for harmful events: "number needed to treat for an additional harmful outcome" (NNTH). It has been used to describe harmful drug effects in randomized clinical trials [46] and in observational studies [47]. Researchers argue that NNTH is a more intuitively understandable measure of risk than the odds ratio and that it contains more information than the odds ratio alone. However, while the NNTH has been deemed a useful risk measure in clinical practice and regulatory evaluation, a consensus on how to calculate NNTH in clinical practice outside the randomized controlled trial remains to be achieved [48].

6 Summary and Conclusions

There are a multitude of information sources that are relevant to drug safety. Government and non-government sources play an important role in disseminating safety-related information in a timely and appropriate manner to both HCPs and the public. Several organizational and systems-related factors, such as research, pharmacovigilance, and postmarketing surveillance communication efforts, support the development and quality assurance of different types of information sources communicating harms and benefits information to end users. The information "pipeline", where drug research and development proceeds to inform sources of information provided by drug sponsors and eventual postmarketing surveillance, has implications for clinical practice via information inclusion and application in drug compendiums and clinical guidelines. A multidisciplinary approach to the development and availability of information sources can therefore help provide a more complete drug safety picture for all. Importantly, patient/consumer information needs should be taken into consideration when developing and communicating drug safety information.

HCPs should have a strong understanding of drug safety information in order to engage in evidence-based practice. The quality of drug safety information can be assessed by considering the risk of bias, currency, and reliability and trustworthiness of the information at hand. When appraising drug safety-related information, risk information can be conveyed verbally using descriptors, and numerically in various ways, such as through absolute risk, relative risk, and NNT. Understanding and communicating this risk to others also relies on interpreting and communicating adequate context such as the baseline level of risk and addressing common misunderstandings that are identified.

7 Case Studies

7.1 Case Study 1

A patient of yours comes to see you at the community pharmacy in which you work, expressing concern about media reports regarding the risk of myocarditis and pericarditis after receiving the COVID-19 vaccination. He is a 51-year-old male with a history of coronary artery disease. He has already had his first dose and wants to know whether it would be safe for him to receive the second dose of the mRNA vaccine.

Before coming to see you, he checked the Consumer Medicine Information (CMI) leaflet for Comirnaty™ COVID-19 vaccine, and from what he could see, it did not contain the detailed information he was seeking. He would like to know more about the harms and benefits and specifically, to have a stronger understanding of the risks involved. He tried to look up information on the Internet but was not sure if he was understanding the "numbers" correctly.

1. *What would be the best approach to address the patient's concern?*

Step 1: Familiarize yourself with the information cited by the patient

- It is important, as a first step, to familiarize yourself with the information available in the CMI leaflet that the patient is referring to, so that you have a baseline of the information presented and the gaps in safety information that need to be addressed based on the patient's enquiry.
- You check the latest CMI available for Comirnaty™ Covid-19 Vaccine (prepared in April 2022 for the Australian market), and it lists myocarditis and pericarditis under the heading and table "Other side effects (frequency unknown)" [49]. This was sourced from the Australian Therapeutic Goods Regulation repository of PI and CMI products—the regulator for a particular country may have a similar one for approved informa-

tion in their jurisdiction. Alternatively, a drug compendium such as MIMS will also be another suitable repository to source PI and CMI within clinical practice settings.

- It should be noted that previous research has shown that people are strongly against stating that the frequency or likelihood of side effects is unknown [29]—later on when thinking about how you will communicate what you have found to the patient, consider explaining the reason why this is stated as such here.
- Upon a quick Internet search, you also find an older CMI version that was drafted in January 2021 [50] which does not mention myocarditis or pericarditis as known side effects. This is one example where currency of information must be considered when evaluating drug safety information as well as where it was sourced from, given the emergent safety data from postmarketing surveillance. If referring to an older document version, this may lead to further misunderstanding and the patient being misinformed based on outdated information. Some online repositories may update their hosted information more frequently than others—it is important that HCPs and patients/consumers are aware of this.

Step 2: Refer to the PI and relevant clinical guidelines for further information

- Now that you have an understanding of the information that the patient has read, it is important to consult the PI and source relevant clinical guidelines that are relevant to the context in which you practice—in this case, evidence-based vaccination guidelines and recommendations will be useful to seek out as it will be helpful to understand the prevalence of observed myocarditis and pericarditis, the implications on vaccine recommendations, and diagnosis and management pathways where applicable.
- For example, if you were practicing in the Australian context, you identify a clinical guidance document entitled "Guidance on myocarditis and pericarditis after mRNA COVID-19 vaccines" which was first published in July 2021 and updated in April 2022 [51]—this is a government publication that has been developed and endorsed by reputable groups, which provide reassurance on the currency and quality of drug safety information provided specifically around myocarditis and pericarditis.
- When accessing the Comirnaty® PI [52], you find that myocarditis and pericarditis are reported adverse effects from postmarketing surveillance, with cases reported as very rare. There is a cross-reference to refer to further information found in clinical guidelines published by the Australian Technical Advisory Group on Immunisation (ATAGI)—this triangulation of information and relevant references is also a point of assurance that you have sourced the appropriate information source and guidance.

Step 3: Identify and source further information if required, e.g., from published research studies or other empirical data

- While clinical guidelines provide an evidence-based summary, if you would like further details, refer to the literature that has been cited in clinical guidelines where applicable—published research may be cited and included as part of the references.
- Conduct a literature search for additional research, such as reviews and highly cited quality research published in high-impact, reputable, international, peer-reviewed journals. They may help provide further insight into real-world data research and statistics on the observed rates of myocarditis/pericarditis. Some papers that you may come across may include:
  - Risks of myocarditis, pericarditis and cardiac arrhythmias associated with COVID-19 vaccination or SARS-CoV-2 infection [53]
  - Myocarditis with COVID-19 mRNA vaccines [54]

Step 4: Consolidate gained knowledge on pericarditis and myocarditis and relate it back to the patient

Step 5: Communicate this data on the adverse effects of pericarditis and myocarditis to the patient to address his query

Consider the following when communicating the information you have found to the patient:

- Acknowledge that the CMI does not contain detailed information about the incidence of myocarditis and pericarditis for this vaccine.
- Explain why there is limited information—i.e., given that the vaccine has been recently rolled out, the postmarketing surveillance (with real-world data) is ongoing, and as updates are available, the CMI will be updated in due course where appropriate. Emphasize that at present, myocarditis and pericarditis cases do not appear to be common, based on reports received, though this could change as more vaccines are used and data is collated.
- Relate the "statistics" to the patient's own situation to tailor the risk information being communicated, e.g., noting that although the patient is male, cases tend to be observed more so in males below the age of 40 and after receiving the second dose of the vaccine [51].
- Communicate the benefits versus harms of COVID-19 vaccination with the possibility of developing myocarditis and pericarditis, and compare and contrast against not being vaccinated.
- State the current clinical guidelines and recommendations—by consensus, guidelines still reinforce that the benefits of COVID-19 vaccination greatly outweigh the risks of potential myocarditis and pericarditis [51].

7.2 Case Study 2

You are currently working as one of the diabetes educator nurses in a large hospital. A junior colleague at the hospital approaches you with a query. Your colleague is currently completing a rotation with the endocrinology team based in the diabetes outpatient clinic. They have recently heard about the Ozempic® shortage in the community due to it being increasingly prescribed for the management of obesity. They ask you to recommend a research paper that outlines the harms and benefits of semaglutide use in the context of obesity and provide details on its place in current local clinical guidelines, as they are unfamiliar with the evidence supporting this "indication."

1. *How will you respond to this request?*

Step 1: Refer to the Ozempic® PI/SPC to verify the approved indications and available clinical trial data from the medicine sponsor for your specific country/region

- Not all proprietary products containing semaglutide are approved for use for weight loss specifically. In Australia, for example, Ozempic® use in weight management is considered "off-label" as the proprietary product Ozempic® is only indicated for use in diabetes management. The PI/SPC provides information on the indication for a specific medicinal product, as approved by the regulator based on the data submitted by the sponsor for evaluation. Refer to the Ozempic® PI for clinical trial data regarding adverse effects. It should also be noted that weight loss is consistently statistically significant across various clinical trials reported as part of the PI [55].

Step 2: Search for clinical updates and seminal papers to understand the available data supporting the use of semaglutide for weight management

- Look for primary research where possible, published in reputable journals with a high-quality study design, e.g., a well-conducted randomized controlled trial.
- After conducting a literature search, you find a paper published in the *New England Journal of Medicine* by Wilding et al. entitled "Once-weekly semaglutide in adults with overweight or obesity" [56]—this trial is known as the STEP 1 trial, funded by Novo Nordisk.

Step 3: Extract benefit and harm information for semaglutide from the trial data

- When evaluating the data published by Wilding et al., you note the following:
  - When comparing the group treated with semaglutide versus the placebo group, there was a difference of −12.44% (95% CI, −13.37 to −11.51) body weight change between baseline weight and after 68 weeks, that was statistically significant ($P < 0.001$) [56].
  - There was an odds ratio of 11.2 (95% CI 8.9–14.2) reported in relation to those who were able to lose 5% or more of their body weight ($P < 0.001$) as measured at 68 weeks when comparing between the groups [56]—this means that those who utilized semaglutide were about 11 times more likely than those who were using the placebo to exhibit weight loss of 5% or more of their body weight at this time point.
  - Wilding et al. present a comprehensive profile of side effects experienced, with more common side effects being gastrointestinal-related [56]—see the full publication for further information that can be presented alongside the benefits of semaglutide treatment.

Step 4: Consult local and international clinical guidelines

- Internationally, there may be provisional guidance to recommend its use, such as that from the National Institute for Health and Care Excellence [57].
- Regulators may have also approved a product containing semaglutide for use in managing overweight/obesity in your jurisdiction, as seen in the United States [58] and more recently, Australia. Wegovy®, a proprietary product containing semaglutide that is specifically indicated for use in chronic weight management, has recently been approved to be included in the Australian Therapeutic Goods Register as of 1 September 2022 [59]. However, it is currently not supplied in Australia as of yet by the medicine sponsor, and a clear statement was made in that Ozempic® and Wegovy® cannot be substituted for one another given their different approved indications [59].
- If a medicinal product has not been approved for managing a specific condition or is not currently being supplied yet, this may limit its integration into local treatment protocols and clinical guidelines for that country or region.
- Clinical guidelines may be updated in the future, given the recent trend in approvals and clinical direction. Therefore, it is important to keep up to date with emerging evidence, approvals, and clinical guideline updates.

Step 5: Communicate your findings from the previous steps and explain the benefit and harm information for semaglutide

7.3 Case Study 3

You are a clinician working in a cardiology clinic. You receive a safety advisory from the regulatory authority in your jurisdiction about an increased risk of bleeding with direct oral anticoagulants (DOACs). DOACs have been authorized for indications where Vitamin K antagonists were previously used. An important clinical benefit of DOACs is that there is less need for routine monitoring of anticoagulant activity. The safety advisory states that although DOACs were expected to be significantly safer than previous treatments, major bleeding events, including events leading to death, also constitute a significant risk with DOACs, as with Vitamin K antagonists.

Every couple of weeks you see patients who use these medicines, but they differ widely in age, overall health, concomitant medicines, and adherence. You are concerned about the information received and patients being treated.

1. *Suggest the best way to introduce this safety advisory in your practice.*

Step 1. Consider the extent to which you are already aware of the risks outlined in the letter

- Ask yourself whether you were already aware of the risks outlined in the letter and whether you are taking them into account in your prescribing and counseling. In some cases, the emergent safety concerns described in regulatory warnings have already been established in clinical communities as precautions or they have been discussed prior to the emergence of the evidence that would trigger a regulatory warning. In any case, the warning may include important new information to update you.

Step 2. Search for additional information on the emergent risks

- Drug safety advisories and news bulletins about drug safety are typically short-format notifications that do not allow much background information or information on recommendations. Therefore, detailed information about the basis for the emergent concerns and the clinical measures to be taken will most often be found in the material referred to in the safety advisory.
- Consult clinical practice guidelines on the use of DOACs for further recommendations.

Step 3. Consider whether you have patients for whom this would be a concern

- Go through your list of patients and identify patients for whom the new contraindications in the drug safety advisory warning are relevant.

Step 4. For patients of concern, reconsider treatment and explain any changes to them.

References

1. Pouliot A, Vaillancourt R, Stacey D, Suter P. Defining and identifying concepts of medication literacy: an international perspective. Res Soc Adm Pharm. 2018;14(9):797–804. https://doi.org/10.1016/j.sapharm.2017.11.005.
2. Puil L, Lexchin J, Bero L, Mangin D, Hallgreen CE, Wong GWK, Mintzes B. The impact of post-market regulatory safety advisories on patients, prescribers, and the healthcare system. Cochrane Database Syst Rev. 2019;(12) https://doi.org/10.1002/14651858.CD013510.
3. U.S. Food and Drug Administration. FDA Adverse Event Reporting System (FAERS) Public Dashboard; 2021. https://www.fda.gov/drugs/questions-and-answers-fdas-adverse-event-reporting-system-faers/fda-adverse-event-reporting-system-faers-public-dashboard. Accessed 03 April 2023.
4. European Medicines Agency. Online access to suspected side-effect reports; n.d.. https://www.adrreports.eu/en/. Accessed 03 April 2023.
5. Australian Government Department of Health and Aged Care Therapeutic Goods Administration. Database of Adverse Event Notifications (DAEN); 2023. https://www.tga.gov.au/safety/safety/safety-monitoring-daen-database-adverse-event-notifications/database-adverse-event-notifications-daen. Accessed 16 Feb 2023.
6. International Society of Drug Bulletins. About the International Society of Drug Bulletins (ISDB); n.d.. https://www.isdbweb.org/what-is-isdb. Accessed 03 April 2023.
7. Therapeutics Initiative. Therapeutics Initiative; n.d.. https://www.ti.ubc.ca/. Accessed 03 April 2023.
8. Møllebæk M, Kaae S. Are drug safety advisories compatible with physicians' information behaviour? Semi-structured interviews with general practitioners about direct to healthcare professional communication. Eur J Health Commun. 2022;3(3):1–17. https://doi.org/10.47368/ejhc.2022.301.
9. Fabbri A, Parker L, Colombo C, Mosconi P, Barbara G, Frattaruolo MP, et al. Industry funding of patient and health consumer organisations: systematic review with meta-analysis. BMJ. 2020;368:l6925. https://doi.org/10.1136/bmj.l6925.
10. Arthritis Australia. Medication Search; 2017. https://arthritisaustralia.com.au/managing-arthritis/medical-management/medication-search/. Accessed 06 Sep 2022.
11. NPS MedicineWise. NPS MedicineWise; n.d.. https://www.nps.org.au/. Accessed 03 April 2023.

12. Needy Meds. Needy Meds Be MedWise Patient Information and Education; n.d.. https://www.bemedwise.org/. Accessed 03 April 2023.
13. Benetoli A, Chen TF, Aslani P. Consumer health-related activities on social media: exploratory study. J Med Internet Res. 2017;19(10):e352. https://doi.org/10.2196/jmir.7656.
14. Sloane R, Osanlou O, Lewis D, Bollegala D, Maskell S, Pirmohamed M. Social media and pharmacovigilance: a review of the opportunities and challenges. Br J Clin Pharmacol. 2015;80(4):910–20. https://doi.org/10.1111/bcp.12717.
15. Singh S, Loke YK. Drug safety assessment in clinical trials: methodological challenges and opportunities. Trials. 2012;13:138. https://doi.org/10.1186/1745-6215-13-138.
16. Noble H, Smith J. Reviewing the literature: choosing a review design. Evid Based Nurs. 2018;21(2):39. https://doi.org/10.1136/eb-2018-102895.
17. Yuan H-CT, Raynor DK, Aslani P. Comparison of international regulations for written medicine information (WMI) on prescription medicines. Ther Innov Regul Sci. 2018;53(2):215–26. https://doi.org/10.1177/2168479018776949.
18. Anonymous. Why look at an SPC? Drug Ther Bull. 2009;47(5):56–8. https://doi.org/10.1136/dtb.2009.04.0016.
19. Heart Foundation. Clinical guidelines and position statements; 2021. https://www.heartfoundation.org.au/Bundles/For-Professionals/Clinical-guidelines-position-statements. Accessed 06 Sep 2022.
20. National Institute for Health and Care Excellence. (18 Jan 2022). Developing NICE guidelines: the manual—process and methods [PMG20]; 2014. https://www.nice.org.uk/process/pmg20/chapter/introduction. Accessed 03 April 2023.
21. Datapharm. About emc; n.d.. https://www.medicines.org.uk/emc/about-the-emc. Accessed 03 April 2023.
22. MIMS. Products and services; n.d.. https://corporate.mims.com/healthcare-professional/. Accessed 03 April 2023.
23. Perry LT, Bhasale A, Fabbri A, Lexchin J, Puil L, Joarder M, Mintzes B. A descriptive analysis of medicines safety advisories issued by national medicines regulators in Australia, Canada, the United Kingdom and the United States - 2007 to 2016. Pharmacoepidemiol Drug Saf. 2020;29(9):1054–63. https://doi.org/10.1002/pds.5072.
24. NHMRC. Guidelines for guidelines: assessing risk of bias; 2019. https://www.nhmrc.gov.au/guidelinesforguidelines/develop/assessing-risk-bias. Accessed 22 Aug 2022.
25. Ma L-L, Wang Y-Y, Yang Z-H, Huang D, Weng H, Zeng X-T. Methodological quality (risk of bias) assessment tools for primary and secondary medical studies: what are they and which is better? Mil Med Res. 2020;7(1):7. https://doi.org/10.1186/s40779-020-00238-8.
26. Wong, A. AstraZeneca COVID-19 vaccine FAQ: Why do the age recommendations keep changing? Does it cause VIPIT blood clots? Is it effective against variants? 2021. https://theconversation.com/astrazeneca-covid-19-vaccine-faq-why-do-the-age-recommendations--keep-changing-does-it-cause-vipit-blood-clots-is-it-effective-against-variants-158302. Accessed 06 Sep 2022.
27. Health On the Net. Health On the Net; 2020. https://www.hon.ch/en/. Accessed 21 April 2023.
28. Health On the Net. HONcode Certification; 2020. https://www.hon.ch/en/certification.html. Accessed 23 Aug 2022.
29. Tong V, Raynor DK, Blalock SJ, Aslani P. Exploring consumer opinions on the presentation of side-effects information in Australian Consumer Medicine Information leaflets. Health Expect. 2016;19(3):543–56. https://doi.org/10.1111/hex.12215.
30. Yamagishi K. When a 12.86% mortality is more dangerous than 24.14%: implications for risk communication. Appl Cogn Psychol. 1997;11(6):495–506. https://doi.org/10.1002/(SICI)1099-0720(199712)11:6<495::AID-ACP481>3.0.CO;2-J.
31. Trevena LJ, Davey HM, Barratt A, Butow P, Caldwell P. A systematic review on communicating with patients about evidence. J Eval Clin Pract. 2006;12(1):13–23. https://doi.org/10.1111/j.1365-2753.2005.00596.x.
32. Schechtman E. Odds ratio, relative risk, absolute risk reduction, and the number needed to treat—which of these should we use? Value Health. 2002;5(5):431–6. https://doi.org/10.1046/J.1524-4733.2002.55150.x.
33. European Commission. A guideline on the readability of the label and package leaflet of medicinal products for human use; 1998. http://www.pharma-eu.com/pdfs/Guideline%20on%20Readbaility%20EMEA.pdf. Accessed 06 Sep 2022.
34. New Zealand Medicines and Medical Devices Safety Authority. Safety information: adverse reactions to medicines; 2019. https://www.medsafe.govt.nz/consumers/Safety-of-Medicines/Medicine-safety.asp#:~:text=common%20%E2%80%93%20this%20means%20that%20between,10%2C000%20people%20may%20be%20affected. Accessed 22 Aug 2022.
35. Webster RK, Weinman J, Rubin GJ. People's understanding of verbal risk descriptors in patient information leaflets: a cross-sectional national survey of 18- to 65-year-olds in England. Drug Saf. 2017;40(8):743–54. https://doi.org/10.1007/s40264-017-0542-1.

36. Büchter RB, Fechtelpeter D, Knelangen M, Ehrlich M, Waltering A. Words or numbers? Communicating risk of adverse effects in written consumer health information: a systematic review and meta-analysis. BMC Med Inform Decis Mak. 2014;14(1):76. https://doi.org/10.1186/1472-6947-14-76.
37. Sackett DL, Deeks JJ, Altman DG. Down with odds ratios! Evid Based Med. 1996;1(6):164. https://doi.org/10.1136/ebm.1996.1.164.
38. Gigerenzer G, Gaissmaier W, Kurz-Milcke E, Schwartz LM, Woloshin S. Helping doctors and patients make sense of health statistics. Psychol Sci Public Interest. 2007;8(2):53–96. https://doi.org/10.1111/j.1539-6053.2008.00033.x.
39. Leung WC. Risk information study was marred by poor questionnaire design. Br J Gen Pract. 2001;51(467):493.
40. Medsafe Editorial Team. The risk of thromboembolism with third generation oral contraceptives; 1998. https://www.medsafe.govt.nz/profs/PUarticles/contraceptivesFeb96.htm. Accessed 06 Sep 2022.
41. Natter HM, Berry DC. Effects of presenting the baseline risk when communicating absolute and relative risk reductions. Psychol Health Med. 2005;10(4):326–34. https://doi.org/10.1080/13548500500093407.
42. Berry D. Risk, communication and health psychology. Maidenhead: McGraw-Hill Education; 2004.
43. Centre for Evidence-Based Medicine. Number Needed to Treat (NNT); n.d.. https://www.cebm.ox.ac.uk/resources/ebm-tools/number-needed-to-treat-nnt. Accessed 03 April 2023.
44. Saver JL, Lewis RJ. Number needed to treat: conveying the likelihood of a therapeutic effect. JAMA. 2019;321(8):798–9. https://doi.org/10.1001/jama.2018.21971.
45. Hamrosi K, Dickinson R, Knapp P, Raynor DK, Krass I, Sowter J, Aslani P. It's for your benefit: exploring patients' opinions about the inclusion of textual and numerical benefit information in medicine leaflets. Int J Pharm Pract. 2013;21(4):216–25. https://doi.org/10.1111/j.2042-7174.2012.00253.x.
46. Altman DG. Confidence intervals for the number needed to treat. BMJ. 1998;317(7168):1309–12. https://doi.org/10.1136/bmj.317.7168.1309.
47. Bjerre LM, LeLorier J. Expressing the magnitude of adverse effects in case-control studies: "the number of patients needed to be treated for one additional patient to be harmed". BMJ. 2000;320(7233):503. https://doi.org/10.1136/bmj.320.7233.503.
48. Hallas J, Christensen RD, Stürmer T, Pottegård A. Measures of 'exposure needed for one additional patient to be harmed' in population-based case-control studies. Pharmacoepidemiol Drug Saf. 2014;23(8):868–74. https://doi.org/10.1002/pds.3635.
49. Pfizer Australia Pty Ltd. (April 2022). Comirnaty(TM) Covid-19 Vaccine Consumer Medicine Information; 2022. https://www.ebs.tga.gov.au/ebs/picmi/picmirepository.nsf/pdf?OpenAgent&id=CP-2021-CMI-01093-1&d=20220821172310101. Accessed 21 Aug 2022.
50. Pfizer Australia Pty Ltd. Comirnaty(TM) Covid-19 Vaccine Consumer Medicine Information; 2021. https://www.nps.org.au/assets/medicines/85567460-870f-4f5c-8300-accb00f51f39-reduced.pdf. Accessed 21 Aug 2022.
51. Australian Technical Advisory Group on Immunisation (ATAGI), Cardiac Society of Australia and New Zealand (CSANZ), Royal Australian College of General Practitioners (RACGP), Australian College of Rural and Remote Medicine (ACRRM), Australasian College for Emergency Medicine (ACEM), Paediatric Research in Emergency Departments International Collaborative (PREDICT). Guidance on Myocarditis and Pericarditis after mRNA COVID-19 Vaccines; 2022. https://www.health.gov.au/sites/default/files/documents/2022/05/covid-19-vaccination-guidance-on-myocarditis-and-pericarditis-after-mrna-covid-19-vaccines.pdf. Accessed 22 Aug 2022.
52. Pfizer Australia Pty Ltd. (11 May 2022). Australian Product Information—Comirnaty® (tozinameran) COVID-19 Vaccine; 2022. https://www.ebs.tga.gov.au/ebs/picmi/picmirepository.nsf/pdf?OpenAgent&id=CP-2021-PI-01092-1. Accessed 22 Aug 2022.
53. Patone M, Mei XW, Handunnetthi L, Dixon S, Zaccardi F, Shankar-Hari M, et al. Risks of myocarditis, pericarditis, and cardiac arrhythmias associated with COVID-19 vaccination or SARS-CoV-2 infection. Nat Med. 2022;28(2):410–22. https://doi.org/10.1038/s41591-021-01630-0.
54. Bozkurt B, Kamat I, Hotez PJ. Myocarditis with COVID-19 mRNA vaccines. Circulation. 2021;144(6):471–84. https://doi.org/10.1161/CIRCULATIONAHA.121.056135.
55. Novo Nordisk Pharmaceuticals Pty Limited. Australian Product Information—Ozempic® (semaglutide) solution for injection; 2022. https://www.ebs.tga.gov.au/ebs/picmi/picmirepository.nsf/pdf?OpenAgent&id=CP-2019-PI-01881-1&d=20220906172310101. Accessed 06 Sep 2022.
56. Wilding JPH, Batterham RL, Calanna S, Davies M, Van Gaal LF, Lingvay I, et al. Once-weekly semaglutide in adults with overweight or obesity. N Engl J Med. 2021;384(11):989–1002. https://doi.org/10.1056/NEJMoa2032183.
57. National Institute for Health and Care Excellence. Final appraisal document: semaglutide for managing overweight and obesity; 2022. https://www.nice.org.uk/guidance/gid-ta10765/documents/final-appraisal-determination-document. Accessed 22 Aug 2022.
58. U.S. Food and Drug Administration. FDA approves new drug treatment for chronic weight management, first since 2014; 2021. https://www.fda.gov/news-events/press-announcements/fda-approves-new-drug-treatment-chronic-weight-management-first-2014. Accessed 22 Aug 2022.
59. Australian Government Department of Health and Aged Care Therapeutic Goods Administration. Update: Limited semaglutide (Ozempic) supply; 2022. https://www.tga.gov.au/safety/shortages/medicine-shortage-alerts/update-limited-semaglutide-ozempic-supply. Accessed 06 Sep 2022.

Polypharmacy and Deprescribing

18

Alpana Rajesh Mair, Margaret Jordan, and Judy Mullan

Abstract

Polypharmacy contributes to medication-related harm. Medication-related harm accounts for approximately 9% of hospital admissions worldwide, and it is estimated that many of these hospitalisations are preventable. It is therefore important to consider significant opportunities which can be used to reduce the burden of medication-related harm. These opportunities could involve the provision of timely and effective interventions, which include shared decision-making and a person-centred approach when undertaking reviews, where deprescribing may be an outcome as well as starting medications, to ensure optimised treatment. Strategies to avoid inappropriate polypharmacy, as a whole system and integrated approach by various members of the healthcare team, could also be considered as important interventions to reduce medication-related harm.

This chapter will discuss why polypharmacy is on the increase and why it is important to consider appropriate and inappropriate polypharmacy as well as the significance of deprescribing. It will describe why a person-centred prescribing and management of multimorbidity approach are important to consider during all stages of the medication management process.

Keywords

Polypharmacy · Deprescribing · Medication-related harm · Person-centred approach Appropriate polypharmacy · Inappropriate polypharmacy

Learning Objectives

- Understand why prevalence of polypharmacy is increasing and understand when polypharmacy can be appropriate and when it is inappropriate.
- List the medicines that have been identified to cause most harm and how to prioritise patients for review.

A. R. Mair (✉)
Effective Prescribing & Therapeutics Division, Scottish Government, Edinburgh, UK

Edinburgh Napier University, Edinburgh, UK
e-mail: alpana.mair@gov.scot

M. Jordan
School of Pharmacy, Faculty of Science, Medicine and Health, University of Sydney, Sydney, Australia

Faculty of Science, Medicine and Health Faculty, Graduate School of Medicine, University of Wollongong, Wollongong, Australia

J. Mullan
Faculty of Science, Medicine and Health Faculty, Graduate School of Medicine, University of Wollongong, Wollongong, Australia

J. Jose et al. (eds.), *Principles and Practice of Pharmacovigilance and Drug Safety*,
https://doi.org/10.1007/978-3-031-51089-2_18

- Understand how to involve patients in discussions about their medicines and take a person-centred approach to medication review.
- Identify the barriers and enablers that need to be considered when implementing polypharmacy reviews and supporting resulting deprescribing.
- Describe the economic benefits of undertaking the review of patients to ensure appropriate polypharmacy and deprescribing.

Key Points

- Polypharmacy (use of multiple medications) can cause medication-related harm. However, it is important to consider not only the number of medicines an individual is taking but also if polypharmacy is appropriate or inappropriate. Therefore, considering if the therapeutic objectives are being achieved as well as the benefits, harms and applicability of numbers needed to treat are important.
- Causes of polypharmacy include increase in multimorbidity, receiving care from multiple prescribers without adequate integration and the prescribing cascade, where an adverse event is misinterpreted as a new medical condition and subsequently prescribed treatment for it.
- There are some medicines that are regarded as high-risk medications, that is, they have an increased risk of causing harm or death when used in error, e.g. non-steroidal anti-inflammatory drugs. People using these medications with additional risk factors such as age and impaired kidney function should be prioritised for review.
- There are many tools to help identify patients at risk of inappropriate polypharmacy. Healthcare professionals involved should take a person-centred approach to prioritise patients for review, e.g. people on high-risk medications together with other factors that would predispose the patient to risk, e.g. frailty.
- People from deprived communities often present with polypharmacy at a younger age as they have multi-morbidities at an earlier age and hence more likely to be needing medication review.
- The '7-steps' approach not only takes a person-centred approach to review appropriate polypharmacy, asking 'what matters to the person', but also considers numbers needed to treat and whether the person is likely to benefit from the treatment considering individual circumstances. Deprescribing should be taken in this context once the medications are reviewed.
- As part of a person-centred approach, shared decision-making tools should be used to support the person make decisions about their medication.
- Medication safety indicators are available in many countries and can be used not only to prioritise patients for review but also to support improvement.
- Implementing programmes to address inappropriate polypharmacy and resulting deprescribing should take a systems approach that has a multidisciplinary approach with clinical and policy leadership, and patient and public involvement. It needs to address medication safety culture, using change management tools and data to drive change.

1 Introduction

This chapter will consider why polypharmacy is increasing and the need to focus on appropriate and inappropriate polypharmacy and causes of medication-related harm. It will explain why person-centred prescribing and management of multimorbidity are important to consider at initiation of prescribing and as part of regular medication reviews and in all stages of medication management. The role of shared decision-making tools will be considered to support patients and prescribers to make decisions about the benefits and potential harms of medicines.

Medication-related harm accounts for approximately 11% of unplanned hospital admissions in the UK, of which 50% are avoidable and with the majority occurring in older patients with polypharmacy, use of multiple medicines [1]. If this was extrapolated across the EU, it would result in 8.6 M admissions each year. There are, therefore, significant opportunities to reduce this burden by timely and effective interventions. Strategies used to address medication-related harm that include a person-centred approach will be considered as these have been shown to address up to 15% of harm [2].

Actions that can be taken by various members of the healthcare team, as well as mechanisms and strategies to avoid inappropriate polypharmacy, will be discussed in this chapter. Various tools to assess potentially inappropriate medication (PIM) use, approaches and steps, and challenges for deprescribing will be covered.

The importance of a whole system and integrated approach will be considered to ensure that inappropriate polypharmacy is addressed as patients access care in all care settings. This is highlighted by WHO in their Global Patient Safety technical report, Medication Safety in Polypharmacy [3].

2 Polypharmacy, Multimorbidity, Adherence and the Scale of Medication-Related Harm

It has been estimated that the global population aged over 65 years will double from 8% in 2010 to 16% in 2050 due to advances in disease prevention, healthcare, education and socio-economic circumstances [4]. Along with this, there is an increase in multimorbidity, which is defined by the World Health Organization as the 'co-occurrence of two or more chronic medical conditions in one person' [5]. Patients with multimorbidity may require medicines to treat each condition, which can lead to polypharmacy. Also, for some conditions, several medicines are routinely prescribed, for instance after an acute myocardial infarction. Polypharmacy is the concurrent use of multiple medications, and while polypharmacy is often defined as routinely taking a minimum of five medicines [6], it is being more frequently suggested that the emphasis should be on evidence-based and appropriateness of the prescription rather than the number [3, 7]. All medications that a patient is using should be considered when reviewing polypharmacy for its appropriateness, including traditional medications, complementary preparations as well as those purchased by the patient over the counter. Despite increasing multimorbidity, most medical research, clinical guidelines and contractual agreements (such as pay-for-performance initiatives such as the General Medical Contract (GMS) that sets out what GPs are tasked and paid to deliver on for reimbursement) are focused on the management of single disease states [8]. In these multimorbid patients, referrals to specialists and individually treating each condition inevitably lead to the use of multiple medications, that is, polypharmacy [9]; the risks and benefits of which are largely unproven and often unpredictable.

It is important to note that all polypharmacy is not inappropriate per se (see below), and it is often beneficial. See Boxes 18.1 and 18.2 [7].

Box 18.1 Appropriate Polypharmacy

Appropriate polypharmacy is present, when:

(a) all drugs are prescribed for the purpose of achieving specific therapeutic objectives that have been agreed with the patient,
(b) therapeutic objectives are actually being achieved or there is a reasonable chance they will be achieved in the future,
(c) drug therapy has been optimised to minimise the risk of adverse drug reactions and,
(d) the patient is motivated and able to use all medicines as intended.

From: Polypharmacy Guidance, Realistic Prescribing Third Edition [7].

An example of appropriate polypharmacy is for a 65-year-old male patient who has developed atrial fibrillation on the background of cardiac disease and type 2 diabetes, for which he is prescribed lipid-lowering therapy, an angiotensin II receptor blocker (ARB), an antiplatelet agent and two oral hypoglycaemic medicines, to reduce the further risk of cardiovascular events and manage blood glucose. With the additional diagnosis, rate control is commenced, and after considering the potential benefits and risks of anticoagulant therapy, the patient commences apixaban and ceases aspirin. Blood pressure, kidney function and blood glucose are monitored regularly. The patient understands the purpose of the medicines and the degree of monitoring required.

Polypharmacy, however, becomes inappropriate when the risks of multiple medications begin to outweigh their potential benefits for an individual patient, especially as the person ages [7].

Box 18.2 Inappropriate Polypharmacy

Inappropriate polypharmacy is present, when one or more drugs are prescribed that are not or no longer needed, either because

(a) there is no evidence-based indication, the indication has expired, or the dose is unnecessarily high,

(b) one or more medicines fail to achieve the therapeutic objectives they are intended to achieve,

(c) one or the combination of several drugs cause unacceptable adverse drug reactions (ADRs), or put the patient at an unacceptably high risk of such ADRs,

or because

(d) the patient is not willing or able to use one or more medicines as intended.

Inappropriate polypharmacy is also referred to as 'problematic' or 'unacceptable'.

From: Polypharmacy Guidance, Realistic Prescribing Third Edition [7].

The appropriateness of polypharmacy should be considered at every point of initiation of a new treatment for the patient and when the patient moves across different healthcare settings, that is, through transitions of care. The increased risk of harm is not always offset by increased benefits, and for many preventive medicines, such benefits may never be realised due to a shortened life expectancy. The risk of harm is generally higher in older people with multimorbidity than in younger patients due to pharmacokinetic factors, such as reduced ability to clear drugs (e.g., due to kidney and/or liver impairment) and pharmacodynamic factors such as increased vulnerability to drugs' adverse effects (due to general frailty, and drug–drug and drug–disease interactions) and medication burden [8, 10, 11].

2.1 Causes of Inappropriate Polypharmacy

Poor coordination of care increases the likelihood of polypharmacy and medication-related harm. For instance, patients with multimorbidity often receive care from multiple prescribers and have complex medication regimen [12]. This can result in communication breakdowns and fragmentation of care [9, 12]. There is also at times a reluctance by primary care prescribers to alter their patients' medicine prescribed during a hospital admission or by a medical specialist [13], which highlights a need to change the medical culture and to improve the communication between all levels of care [13]. However, care transitions can also present an opportunity to identify inappropriate polypharmacy and potentially deprescribe [14, 15].

A case to illustrate how a person-centred approach could be taken to consider appropriate polypharmacy is discussed as Case 1 in Sect. 9.

2.2 Prescribing Cascade

A 'prescribing cascade' arises when an adverse drug event occurs that is misinterpreted as a new medical condition, and a subsequent therapy prescribed for treatment [16]. If a medicine is used, it may contribute to additional adverse effects, for instance, initiating a diuretic for oedema associated with a dihydropyridines may put the patient at risk of fluid depletion. Some examples of prescribing cascades are illustrated in Box 18.3.

To have a better understanding of the impact of prescribing cascade, please refer to Case 2 in Sect. 9.

Box 18.3 Examples of Prescribing Cascades

Initial medicine	Adverse effect/s	Subsequent medicine/s or device
Cholinesterase inhibitor	Nausea, vomiting, abdominal pain, dyspepsia	Proton pump inhibitor; antacid
Cholinesterase inhibitor	Bradycardia, heart block	Pacemaker insertion
Non-steroidal anti-inflammatory drug	Hypertension	Antihypertensive
Dihydropyridine calcium channel blocker	Ankle oedema	Diuretic
Gabapentinoid	Peripheral oedema, heart failure	Diuretic; angiotensin receptor blockers

3 Medicines Implicated in Causing Harm: 'High-Risk' Medicines

High-risk medicines are those that have an increased risk of causing significant patient harm or death if they are misused or used in error [17, 18]. Errors with these medicines are not necessarily more common than with other medicines, but the consequences of any misadventure can be more devastating [17, 18]. Medicines considered 'high-risk' vary between hospitals and other healthcare settings, such as primary and aged care, and depend on the context and the clinical conditions treated [17, 18].

An Australian mnemonic which has been widely used to raise awareness of medicines identified as high risk in acute care is 'A-PINCH', based on analyses of incident data and literature [18]. See Box 18.4. 'O' may be added to A-PINCH to consider any other medications that have been identified as being relevant for the organisation or setting.

Box 18.4 A-PINCH—Medicines Identified as High Risk in Acute Care

A **Anti-infectives**
P **Potassium** and other electrolytes
I **Insulin** and other hypoglycaemic agents
N **Narcotics** and other sedatives
C **Chemotherapeutic** agents
H **Heparin** and anticoagulants

N = narcotic, used for the purpose of the pneumonic. This refers to opioid medicines.

Although some medicines are recognised as 'high risk' regardless of context, such as anticoagulants and opioid agents, there are many others in common usage that are responsible for potential adverse events due to the changing clinical condition of the patients for whom they are prescribed, concomitant medicines and deficiencies in the medication management pathway. Empirical research has identified medications commonly associated with adverse drug reactions (ADRs) and medication-related harm [19–21]. Some of these can be found in Table 18.1. Note that this list is not exhaustive. Please refer to Case 1 and 2 in Sect. 9 to note the use of high-risk medications.

If we consider the high-risk medications in the cases of Ms AK and Mr PC discussed in Sect. 9

In Case 1, Ms AK is taking aspirin, beta blockers, ramipril and zopiclone.

In Case 2, Mr PC is taking diclofenac, ramipril, bendroflumethiazide and glibenclamide

Table 18.1 Medications commonly associated with adverse drug reactions and medication-related harm in inappropriate polypharmacy[a]

Medication group/ medication	Examples of individual medications	Issues/important areas to consider [7, 22]
Angiotensin-converting enzyme inhibitors (ACEIs)/ Angiotensin receptor blockers (ARBs)	Ramipril, enalapril, captopril, lisinopril, perindopril, irbesartan, losartan	• The indication for ACEIs and ARBs and the evidence base for their use is the indication for symptomatic management for heart failure or for secondary prevention after myocardial infarction. • Kidney function before starting and while titrating the dosage. • Can also cause a drop in BP and cause dizziness and falls.
Antibiotics	Cephalosporins (e.g. cefalexin), penicillin (e.g. amoxicillin), quinolones (e.g. ciprofloxacin), macrolides (e.g. azithromycin)	• Use antibiotics only when indicated and avoid prophylactic use in care homes. • Commonly used antibiotics, such as cephalosporins, fluoroquinolones and amoxicillin with clavulanic acid increase the risk of *C. difficile* and antimicrobial resistance.
Antidepressants	Fluoxetine, paroxetine, amitriptyline, citalopram, venlafaxine, dosulepin	• Antidepressants have been implicated in causing falls. • Tricyclic antidepressants have more anticholinergic and cardiotoxic effects than other antidepressants and should be used with caution in patients with cardiovascular or cognitive comorbidities.
Anti-thrombotics	Antiplatelet agents (e.g. aspirin, clopidogrel) Oral anticoagulants (warfarin and direct Oral anticoagulants [DOACs], e.g. dabigatran, edoxaban, rivaroxaban, apixaban)	• Kidney function declines as people age, which has an impact on the dose and suitability of DOACs • Patent factors can contribute to increased risk of bleeding, such as age, previous bleeding or stroke, raised blood pressure, reduced kidney/liver function and drug–drug interactions. • Review dual antiplatelet therapy and its intended duration, due to the risk of gastrointestinal haemorrhage.
Beta blockers	Atenolol, propranolol, sotalol, bisoprolol, metoprolol, carvedilol	• Adverse effects such as bradycardia and fatigue can be exacerbated with age and by drug–drug interactions
Digoxin		• Kidney function, electrolytes and digoxin serum concentration require monitoring. • Drug–drug interactions can impact on digoxin clearance and increase toxicity.
Diuretics	Furosemide, bendroflumethiazide, bumetanide, spironolactone	• Potent diuretics, useful for symptomatic management (e.g. of heart failure), require regular review due to risk of hypotension and electrolyte disturbances.
Hypoglycaemic agents	Insulin, sulfonylureas (e.g. glibenclamide, glipizide)	• Intensive glycaemic control strategies markedly increase the risk of hypoglycaemia, associated with increased mortality, cardiovascular events, falls and accidents [23], especially sulfonylureas in over 75-year-old persons.
Mood stabilisers	Lithium	• Lithium concentrations require regular monitoring, especially when other medicines are added or withdrawn, or with changes to the patient's clinical conditions (e.g. kidney impairment, dehydration) • Adverse effects that can develop over time and require dosage adjustment

Table 18.1 (continued)

Medication group/ medication	Examples of individual medications	Issues/important areas to consider [7, 22]
Non-steroidal Anti-Inflammatory Drugs (NSAIDs)	Diclofenac, ibuprofen, celecoxib, ketoprofen, naproxen	• In a landmark UK study, gastrointestinal bleeding due to NSAIDs and antiplatelet agents was the leading cause of drug-related hospital admissions, accounting for approximately a third of all drug-related admissions and half of drug-related deaths [21]. This is exacerbated with a history of peptic ulcer disease and the use of several medicines, including antiplatelets, anticoagulants, corticosteroids and selective serotonin reuptake inhibitors. • Consider, gastroprotection (usually with a proton pump inhibitor if unavoidable, which approximately halves the risk of gastrointestinal bleeding) in those at highest risk • Cardiovascular risk associated with many of the NSAIDs
Opioids	Morphine, dihydrocodeine, codeine (± paracetamol) tramadol, fentanyl	• Opioids are rarely indicated for long-term use for chronic, noncancer pain • Adverse effects such as respiratory and cognitive dysfunction are exacerbated with drug–drug interactions and altered pharmacodynamics in older persons.
Psychotropic agents	Benzodiazepines and hypnotics (e.g. diazepam, nitrazepam, temazepam)	• Long-term use of hypnotics and anxiolytics in general practice is not appropriate, maximum duration for most patients is three to four weeks [24]. • Long-term use is associated with numerous risks, including drowsiness and falls, forgetfulness, confusion, depression, irritability, aggression, impulsivity, digestive problems and dependence.
	Antipsychotics (e.g. olanzapine, clozapine, quetiapine)	• Antipsychotics are frequently prescribed to reduce symptoms of stress and distress in people with dementia. However, these drugs have (time) limited benefits, and older patients are particularly vulnerable to their adverse effects [25]. They should therefore be used as the last resource. • Long-term use is associated with cerebrovascular events and death in people with dementia [26].
Systemic corticosteroids	Prednisolone	• Require ongoing review to wean or use the lowest, effective dose • Adverse effects with long-term use necessitate management, such as osteoporosis and glaucoma.

[a]Adapted from [19–21]

3.1 Anticholinergic Burden

It is also important to consider the anticholinergic symptoms that are caused by multiple medications that have anticholinergic side effects. These include impaired cognition, increased risk of falls, functional decline, cardiovascular events and mortality. Sensitivity varies across individuals and are dose-dependent [27–31]. This is why it is essential to take a person-centred approach when reviewing medications with anticholinergic side effects, as the impact will vary depending on individual sensitivity, although at the time of writing this chapter, there is currently not a commonly accepted measure of cumulative anticholinergic burden [32]. However, several tools have been developed to estimate the anticholinergic load of an individual's medicine regimen, including the Drug Burden Index (DBI) [33] and the Anticholinergic Risk Score (ARS) [34].

4 People Most Affected by Polypharmacy

People prescribed multiple concurrent medicines are at risk of medication-related harm, as polypharmacy increases the chances of experiencing ADRs, poor medication adherence and drug–drug interactions [35]. The major risk factors for medication-related harm include old age, polypharmacy, comorbidities, those visiting multiple prescribers [36, 37] and those living with cognitive impairment, including Alzheimer's and related dementias [38]. One study found that for those people admitted to hospital with a PIM, there was at least three further readmissions [39].

Deprivation can have an impact on the numbers of medicines that people take, as multimorbidity occurs earlier for those in more deprived communities [40]. Figure 18.1 illustrates this for the Scottish population, where the Scottish Index of multiple deprivation (SIMD) shows that those from more deprived communities will take medications at an earlier age and may need more support to manage their medication and medication review to prevent harm [41].

The figure supports that people from more deprived populations are taking more medications in each age group. This is in line with multimorbidity also presenting earlier in life in those from more deprived communities, so that people from more deprived backgrounds experience polypharmacy at an earlier age and are potentially at increased risk of medication-related harm.

4.1 Tools to Identify People at Risk of Potentially Inappropriate Polypharmacy

Inappropriate prescribing is also a major risk factor for medication-related harm [42]. There are several screening tools that have been developed to help identify PIMs and appropriate prescribing, in an effort to improve medication prescribing practices. Some examples of these screening tools, typically used to assess older adults, are presented in Table 18.2.

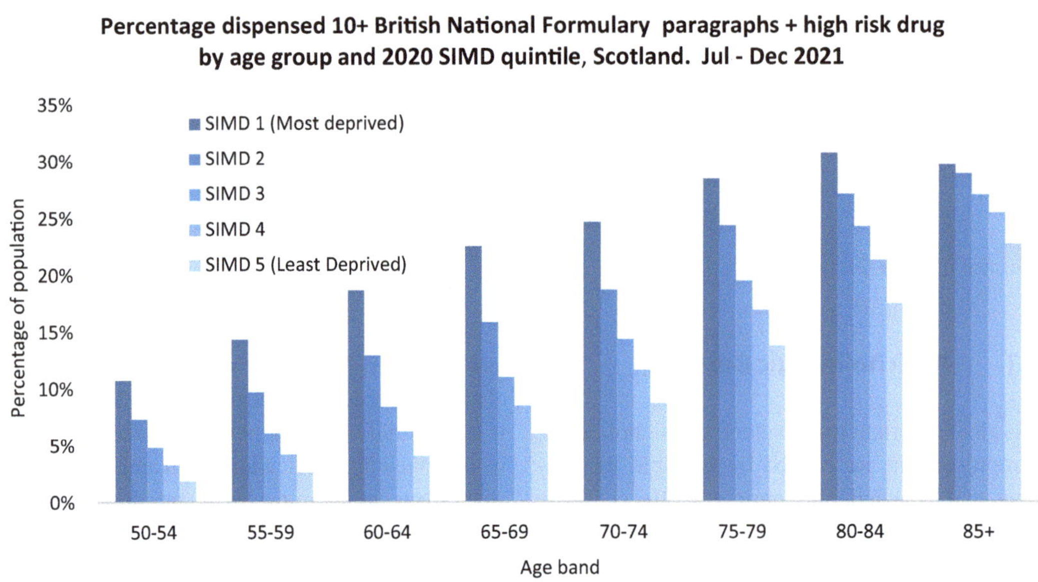

Fig. 18.1 The number of people taking multiple medications by age and deprivation

Table 18.2 Examples of screening tools developed to help identify potentially inappropriate medications and inappropriate prescribing

Name of tool/instrument	Contents of tool/instrument	Where has the tool/instrument been used?
Tools used in community settings		
Beers Updated Criteria for Potentially Inappropriate Medication (PIMs) use in Older Adults [43]	An explicit list of PIMs to avoid in older adults or in certain circumstances	In acute and community settings
STOPP/START criteria [44]	Screening Tool for Older People's Potentially Inappropriate Prescriptions (STOPP) Screening Tool to Alert Doctors to the Right Treatment (START)	These tools/instruments have been used in a variety of settings and to identify potentially inappropriate prescribing in older adults (≥65 years).
FORTA (Fit fOR The Aged) tool [45]	FORTA is a validated tool based on a drug list approach	
Medication Appropriateness Index (MAI) [46]	MAI is a valid and reliable measure of potentially inappropriate prescribing based on the following 10 criteria: (i) indication, (ii) effectiveness, (iii) dosage, (iv) correct directions, (v) practical directions, (vi) drug–drug interactions, (vii) drug–disease interactions, (viii) duplication, (ix) duration and (x) expense.	
PRIME (Prospective study to develop a model to stratify the RIsk of Medication-related harm in hospitalised Elderly patients) tool [47]	The PRIME tool includes a combination of demographic (age, female gender), medication-specific (number of medicines, antiplatelet drug, antidiabetic drug, past ADR), biochemical (sodium level) and social predictors (living alone)	PRIME is a prediction tool used to identify high-risk medication-related harm requiring healthcare within 8 weeks post discharge from hospital.
Scottish Polypharmacy Case finding indicators [7]	This is a suite of 68 case finding indicators that prioritise patients using diagnosis, examination signs and laboratory data. Composite indicators will prioritise on, for example, falls risk, bleeding risk as well as age and frailty	Patients taking 10 or more medicines are prioritised where there are limited resources considering: 1. Age >75 years 2. Frailty 3. High-risk medication Tool is used across Scotland and has also been piloted in the Republic of Ireland
Goal-directed Medication review Electronic Decision Support System (G-MEDSS) [48]	This provides clinical decision support for healthcare practitioners conducting medication reviews for older people with and without dementia, to tailor care to meet the person's goals and preferences.	In clinical practice, mainly by pharmacists, during medication reviews in their homes and aged care residences [49].
Tools used for frail older persons		
Screening Tool of Older Persons Prescriptions in Frail adults with limited life expectancy (STOPPFrail_v2) [50]	Emphasises the importance of shared decision-making in deprescribing medicines for older persons approaching end-of-life.	Used also to identify older people approaching the end-of-life, e.g. in residential aged care, and the deprescribing criteria for antihypertensive agents, anti-anginal medicines and vitamin D.
Norwegian General Practice Nursing Home (NORGEP-NH) [51]	A list of 34 explicit criteria for PIM use.	Suitable for use in aged care residents to reduce concomitant PIMs, risk of falls, acute infection, dehydration.

(continued)

Table 18.2 (continued)

Name of tool/instrument	Contents of tool/instrument	Where has the tool/instrument been used?
Tools used in hospital settings		
Shed-MEDS [52]	Shed-Meds considers patient and disease-related factors, life expectancy, goals of care, appropriate treatment targets and the duration of treatment required.	Shed-Meds is a person-centred deprescribing tool initiated in hospital and continued in post-acute care facilities
MedSafer [53]	MedSafer is an electronic decision support tool for deprescribing, based on the Beers Screening Tool for Older People's Potentially Inappropriate Prescriptions (STOPP) [44] and the 'Choosing Wisely' lists from Canada [54–56].	MedSafer is especially useful in deprescribing antipsychotics and high dose iron salt medications in an acute care setting.
PADR-EC (Prediction of Hospitalization due to Adverse Drug Reactions in Elderly Community-Dwelling Patients) score [57, 58]	Variables included in the PADR-EC are: ≥4 comorbid conditions, heart failure, liver disease, number of medications (≤5, 5–7, ≥8), previous ADR, renal failure.	PADR-EC is used to help identify older adults at increased risk of adverse drug reactions (ADRs) in hospital and among community-dwelling older adults at risk of hospitalisation due to ADRs, which include inappropriate medications, anticholinergic medications and antihypertensive medications
Brighton Adverse Reactions Risk (BADRI) score which has been used to assess the risk of older adults experiencing an ADR while in hospital [59].	The BADRI score is based on the following five clinical variables: (i) taking eight or more medications, (ii) hyperlipidaemia, (iii) raised white cell count, (iv) taking antidiabetic medications and (v) length of stay ≥12 days.	BADRI is used to assess the risk of older adults experiencing an ADR while in hospital
Prediction of Adverse Drug Reactions in Older Inpatients (PADROI) Risk Assessment Tool [60]	The PADROI risk assessment tool is based on the following eight predictors: (i) age 60–75 years, (ii) ADR in the previous 12 months, (iii) PIMs, (iv) polypharmacy (≥5 medications), (v) Charlson Comorbidity Index Score ≥6, (vi) heart failure, (vii) kidney disease and (viii) hospital stay ≥11 days	PADROI is used to assess older adults experiencing ADRs while in hospital

These screening tools are recommended to identify those high-risk medicines (as shown in Table 18.1) which require monitoring to reduce the risk of adverse events, as well as high-risk situations that place patients at greater risk of harm. However, using screening tools may generate many more patients than can practically be reviewed, and in these cases, organisations may use additional criteria to prioritise those eligible for a comprehensive medication review [7, 61].

Once people are prioritised, it is then important to use a process of review using a person-centred approach, which the next section will consider. This process should be one that can be used by all healthcare professionals and involve shared decision-making with the patient.

5 A Person-Centred Approach to Address Polypharmacy

Strategies used to address medication-related harm that include a person-centred approach to address polypharmacy will be considered as these have been shown to reduce harm by up to 15% [2].

5.1 7-Step Approach to Appropriate Polypharmacy

One method to apply a person-centred attitude to review polypharmacy is the '7-step approach', which starts by matching therapeutic objectives to current life priorities with the patient. This is illustrated in Fig. 18.2. This initial discussion guides decision-making in subsequent steps that consider medication need, effectiveness and safety before a therapeutic plan and follow-up strategy are agreed upon. Applying the seven steps as part of a holistic medication review has the potential to address all six dimensions of quality in healthcare: efficacy, safety, efficiency, timeliness, equity and acceptability [7]. Although the seven-step approach was primarily designed to be applied at the point of medication review to *correct* inappropriate prescribing, its principles may equally be applied when initiating new medicines, to *prevent* inappropriate prescribing or when a patient moves across transitions of care. This may result in reducing the dose or stopping a medication completely, although this should not be the primary objective of a medication review. Addressing unmet needs may include starting new medications.

The actions undertaken in each step are summarised and begin with asking 'what matters to the patient?'

- Step 1: sets the context within which all further decisions are made, namely establishing what matters to the patient
- Step 2: identify essential treatment
- Step 3: determine if the patient is taking unnecessary treatment
- Step 4: identify whether therapeutic objectives that matter to the patient are achieved
- Step 5: assess if any medicines are too risky or cause unacceptable adverse effects
- Step 6: consider which medicines are cost-effective and environmentally sustainable
- Step 7: determine whether the patient is willing and able to manage their medicines in a way that avoids harm and maximises benefit.

Please refer to Case 1 and Case 2 in Sect. 9 to better understand the use of the 7-step approach to appropriate polypharmacy.

5.2 Sick Day Guidance

Dehydration can be a significant risk for people taking certain medicines. 'Medicine Sick Day guidance' provides information on medicines that should be temporarily stopped during illness that can result in dehydration (vomiting, diarrhoea and fever). This advice does not apply to minor sickness or diarrhoea, which is defined as a single episode.

Some key medicines and contexts are:

- Diuretics can cause dehydration or make dehydration more likely in an ill patient.
- In a dehydrated patient, ACE inhibitors, ARBs and non-steroidal anti-inflammatory drugs (NSAIDs) may impair kidney function which can reduce elimination of other medicines such as DOACs or could lead to kidney failure
- Dehydration increases the risk of lactic acidosis, a serious and potentially life-threatening side effect of metformin.

Prescribers should discuss with the patient which of their medicines might cause harm if they are dehydrated and provide appropriate guidance. An example of 'sick day guidance' is for people with diabetes and the changes required to medicines during a bout of illness [62].

5.3 Numbers Needed to Treat (NNT)

In the context of multimorbidity and assessing if therapeutic objectives are likely to be achieved, the numbers needed to treat (NNT) can be used as an aid to assess medication benefit in assessing

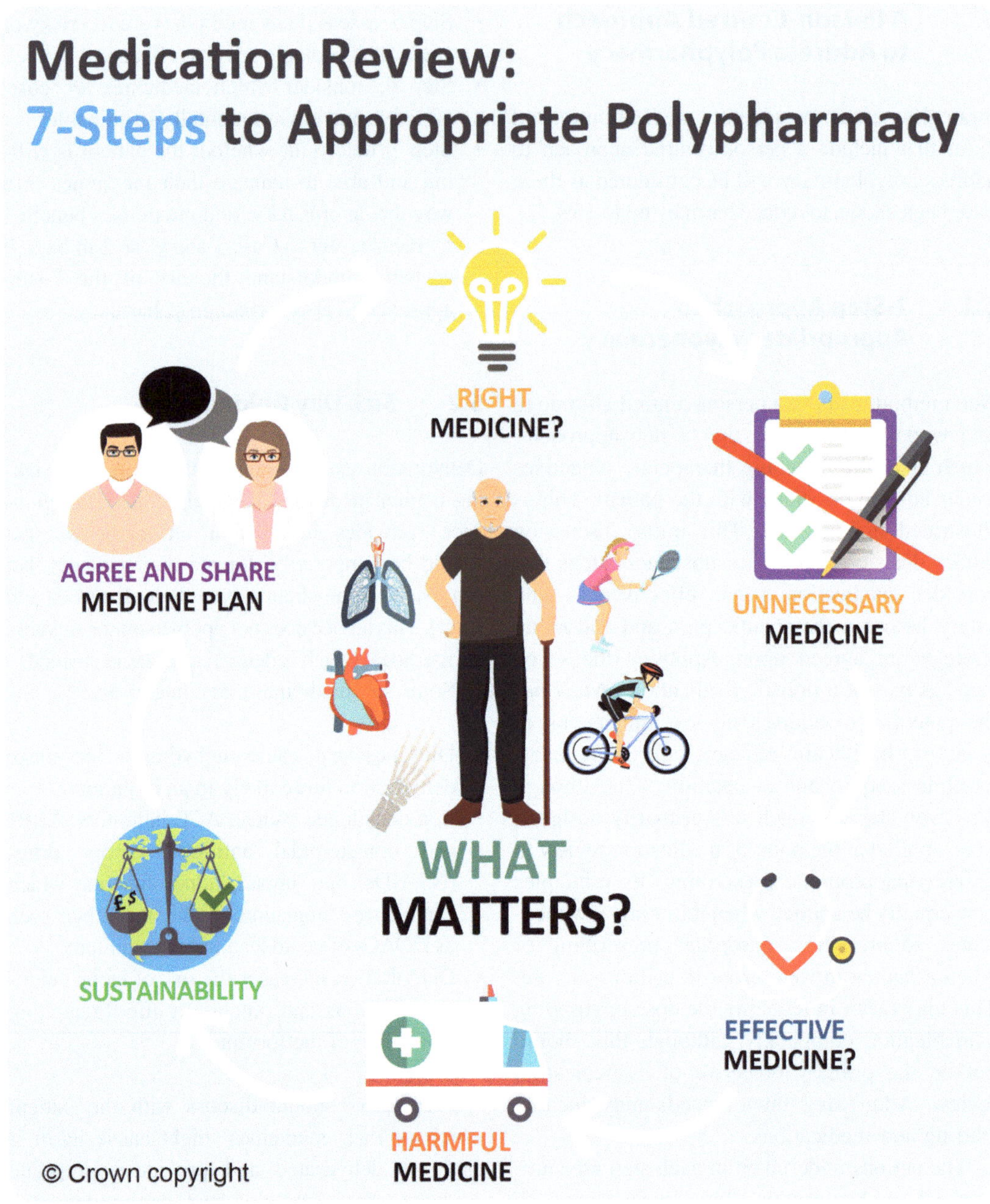
Medication Review:
7-Steps to Appropriate Polypharmacy
RIGHT
MEDICINE?
AGREE AND SHARE
MEDICINE PLAN
UNNECESSARY
MEDICINE
WHAT
MATTERS?
SUSTAINABILITY
EFFECTIVE
MEDICINE?
HARMFUL
MEDICINE
© Crown copyright

Fig. 18.2 7 steps to appropriate polypharmacy
Reproduced with permission from Scottish Government, The Scottish Polypharmacy Guidance, 2018 [7]

appropriateness of polypharmacy. The NNT is the reciprocal of the absolute risk reduction of the respective treatment versus a control (usually placebo) and is defined as the average number of patients that need to be treated for one patient to benefit. The NNT also considers the period of time required to gain benefit. A list of NNTs has been provided in the Scottish guidance [7].

Therefore, comparing the NNT for different medicines can support discussions between clinicians and patients when prioritising medicines for continuation. However, when interpreting NNTs, several questions should be considered:

- First, what is the outcome being avoided? Death is more significant than a vertebral fracture, but the importance assigned to different outcomes may vary between individuals.
- Second, over what period does the benefit accrue? Two drugs may have the same NNT, but a drug achieving the same benefit over a shorter period will be superior.
- Third, what is the likelihood and severity of harm caused by the drug? If a medicine saves the life of 1 in 25 patients but causes debilitating adverse effects for the rest, the harm it causes may outweigh the drug's benefits.
- And fourth, how applicable are the trial data to individual adults? The more similar an individual is to trial populations, the more likely it is that similar benefits will be achieved.

5.4 Shared Decision-Making

In order to take a person-centred approach, it is important to ensure that shared decision-making is in place and that resources can be shared with the patient to support this action. This is particularly important when decisions are made about the risks and benefits of medicines. Involving patients in shared decision-making around deprescribing is enabled by specific tools, such as those provided by deprescribing networks [63]. Another example is in the patient and carer tool kit which is part of the Polypharmacy Manage Medicine app [64]. The example below, in Fig. 18.3, shows how this can be set out to consider risks and benefits of benzodiazepine use. This pictorial representation can be used to illustrate the benefit an individual will get from medicines. The studies show that for every 13 people who receive a benzodiazepine, one will see an improvement in their insomnia. For every 6 people who receive a benzodiazepine, one will experience an adverse effect, e.g. memory loss, confusion, disorientation, loss of balance or falls and morning hangover effects.

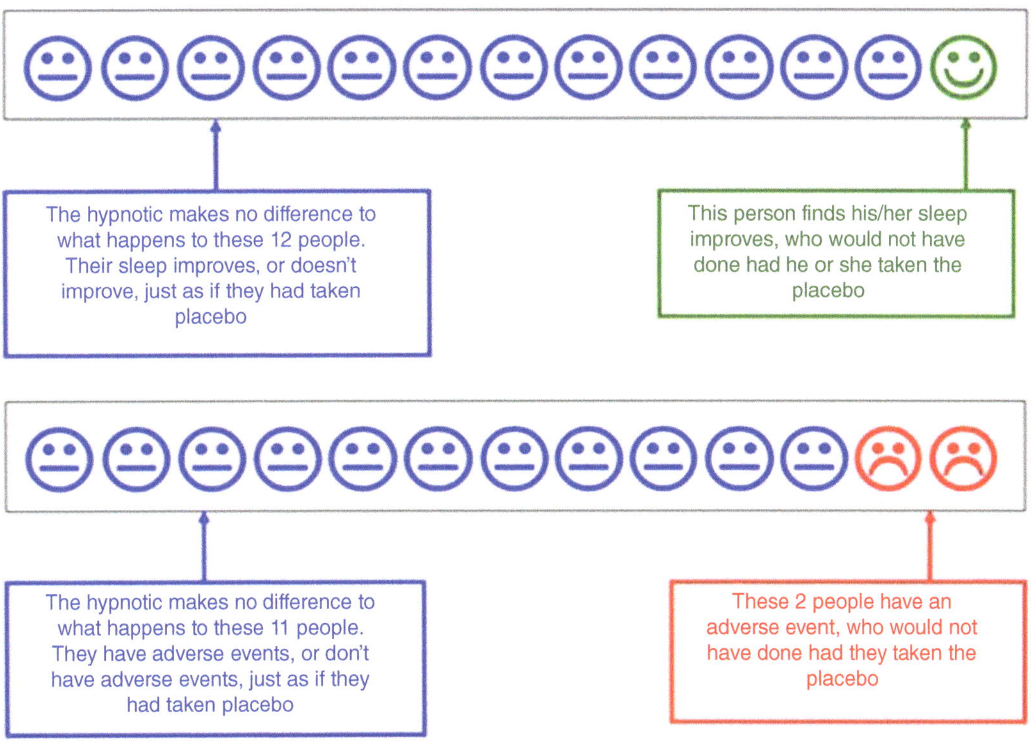

Fig. 18.3 Risks and benefits of benzodiazepine use—a shared decision-making tool. (Reproduced with permission from Effective Prescribing and Therapeutics Division – Scottish Government) [65]

5.5 Adherence

When people take multiple medications, as well as the burden of treatment, medication adherence is an important factor to consider. Non-adherence to prescribed medicines is intricately related to multimorbidity and polypharmacy. Adherence to long-term therapy for chronic illnesses in developed countries averages 50%, while in developing countries, the rates are even lower [66]. Non-adherence has been estimated to be responsible for 48% of asthma deaths, an 80% increased risk of death in diabetes and a 3.8-fold increased risk of death following a heart attack [67]. Non-adherence might be intentional or non-intentional and agreeing, and sharing the plan to manage medications will help to ensure that goals are agreed and shared, resulting in improved adherence.

5.6 Teach Back

The teach back method is a useful way to confirm that the information you provide is being understood by getting people to 'teach back' what has been discussed and what instruction has been given. This is more than saying 'do you understand?' and is more a check of how you have explained things than the patient/client understanding [68, 69]. Patients should understand that this is not a test for them. This would be useful as part of a patient sharing and agreeing with the plan and would also address where there are potential problems in understanding dosage instructions that may affect adherence.

A similar tool can be used when showing people how to carry out actions, such as where/how to apply a cream or where to give a needle. This is called 'show me'.

5.7 Deprescribing as Part of a Person-Centred Approach

As a result of reviewing medication, some medicines may be identified as no longer being appropriate and these should be stopped. This is often referred to as 'deprescribing', which is defined as the 'planned and supervised process of dose reduction or stopping of medication that might be causing harm, or no longer be of benefit' [70].

A UK-based national programme found that when taking this approach, on average 1–2 medicines were stopped per patient per review, and the rates of polypharmacy decreased [71, 72]. A Canadian multicentre study investigated a systematic intervention to deprescribe PIMs in 6000 older adults, across 11 hospitals, using MedSafer decision support [53, 73]. In this study, compared with the usual care of medication reconciliation, there was a substantial difference in the number of PIMs deprescribed in the intervention participants, from approximately 30% to over 50%, without changes to patient-reported measures such as sleep or quality of life [73].

5.8 Medication Safety Indicators

In terms of measuring for appropriate prescribing, the use of medication safety indicators is more appropriate. For example, in 2019, for the first time, the Organisation for Economic Co-operation and Development collected comparable international data on polypharmacy rates, measuring the proportion of older people chronically taking five or more medications. It was found that polypharmacy rates among older people varied more than 11-fold across 14 countries, with Turkey reporting the lowest and Luxembourg the highest rates of medication prescribing [74]. This is the first step towards benchmarking internationally which takes into account the use of safety indicators and is moving away from numbers of medications to consider appropriateness.

Twelve core quality and safety indicators were identified in a systematic review considering medication appropriateness. These included drug reactions, contraindications, drug–drug interactions and the conduct of medication reviews [75]. Countries can adopt or adapt a set of these indicators based on the context, priorities and resources available to measure inappropriate polypharmacy. Several countries have adopted indicators: one example is an indicator to identify the 'triple whammy', where the combination of an angiotensin-converting enzyme inhibitor (ACEI) or ARB plus a diuretic and a NSAID is to be avoided because of its potential to cause acute kidney injury [7].

Scottish polypharmacy guideline uses a suite of 17 quality and safety indicators to monitor appropriateness of polypharmacy nationally [7]. Figure 18.4 shows the number of people aged 65 years or older co-prescribed a NSAID, an ACE inhibitor or ARB and a diuretic, as a percentage of all people aged 65 years or older prescribed an ARB and a diuretic. Across Scotland, there are 14 different regions providing healthcare. These are known as NHS boards. This chart helps one board to benchmark against the Scottish average but also see how they are positioned against the other regional or board areas.

Canada has identified their own suite, which also include indicators related to appropriate polypharmacy, such as ensuring that people discharged from hospital after an myocardial infarction are on appropriate secondary prevention medications [76]. Similarly, Sweden has also had a suite of indicators which has been in place since 2004. The Swedish indicators include polypharmacy and covering the rational, irrational and hazardous drug use in common disorders in older people [77].

6 Barriers and Enablers to Address Inappropriate Polypharmacy

There are a number of challenges which act as barriers to actioning change from medication reviews, particularly for deprescribing which can be complex and can occur at an individual level (i.e. patient and healthcare provider), an organisational level (i.e. healthcare system and policy level) or at a cultural level, in terms of maintaining the status quo [78]. Cultural and organisational barriers identified in a recent systematic review of 40 studies across 14 countries consisted of the culture of diagnosing and prescribing; a lack of evidence-based guidelines and resources, especially for older people with multimorbidity; and a lack of shared communication with access to decision-making systems and resources [79]. The deprescribing process is considered an essential component of medication reconciliation and review [14], where inappropriate medicines which can be discontinued are identified.

The interpersonal and individual barriers included differences in professional practice; fragmented care; prescribers' and patients' reservations and fears about deprescribing; and a lack of tailored approaches to person-centred care [79]. There is often miscommunication when

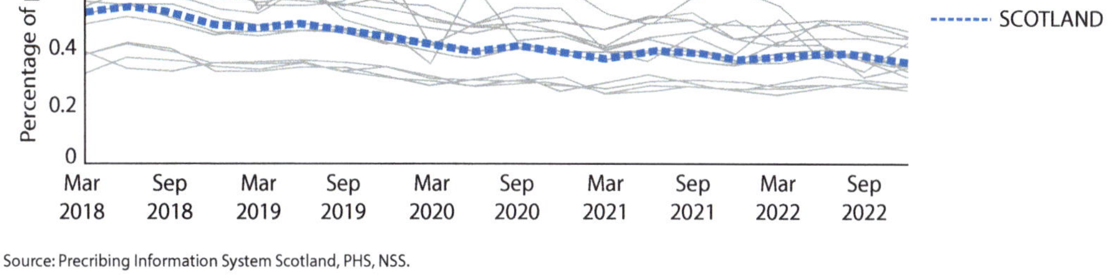

Fig. 18.4 Indicator to show the percentage of people prescribed the triple whammy combination known to cause acute kidney injury across different regions across Scotland (source accessed 29.05.2023). National therapeutic indicators data visualisation—Data to September 2022—Publications—Public Health Scotland

patients transition between providers [13]. Fear of potential for harm when stopping a medicine and a lack of knowledge of methods for optimal tapering or stopping are among other barriers given to deprescribing medicines that are no longer appropriate [80, 81].

In addition to barriers, there are a number of facilitators which need to be recognised to reviewing polypharmacy and commencing deprescribing when appropriate, as discussed throughout this chapter. These include shared decision-making, delivering person-centred care, judicious prescribing, improved communication and collaboration between patient and prescribers across different healthcare settings [78, 79]. Other facilitators include the availability of evidence-based tools and resources, formal training/teaching, an increased awareness of potential harms with continuation or benefits of stopping a medication, as well as discussions about goals of care and treatment preferences [78]. Another important facilitator of reducing or ceasing medicines includes the availability and acceptability of non-pharmacological alternatives [79]. Non-pharmacological options are not consistently considered first-line or continued once pharmacological treatments are initiated [82]. It is important that prescribers consider and recommend non-pharmacological options if appropriate. For example, heat/cold applications, massage therapy and relaxation techniques should be considered for the management of pain.

Trust between the prescriber and patient plays a complex role, as both a barrier and a facilitator [83]. Trust is necessary because of the complexity and uncertainty of decisions about changing medication regimens and is dependent on several factors such as length of time that the patient has been seeing the prescriber, repeated positive experiences of care and the perceived medical expertise of the prescriber [83]. Patients themselves can also act as either barriers and facilitators to deprescribing by unintentionally withholding information about adverse drug events and reporting their symptoms to specialists or nurses rather than their GPs, who may be mainly responsible for overall medication management [13]. Some patients are also reluctant to stop familiar medications and may not understand the need for deprescribing because of their level of education, health literacy, cognitive impairment and functional dependency [13].

The challenges of addressing inappropriate polypharmacy, especially in older people with multimorbidity and frailty, are complex and require a person-centred approach, as described. These challenges are often compounded by the involvement of several healthcare providers from different specialties, who prescribe medicines based on disease-specific guidelines which do not contain evidence on the older, frailer and multimorbid patient population [13]. It is therefore evident that an interdisciplinary approach to the treatment of these older patients needs to be implemented, ensuring that they are treated holistically. There is a growing body of evidence suggesting that deprescribing interventions led by pharmacists [84, 85] and interdisciplinary teams have successfully reduced the number of medicines, including inappropriate medicines, prescribed in older people [86]. It could be argued therefore, that for deprescribing and addressing inappropriate polypharmacy to be successfully achieved, it is essential that prescribers collaborate between themselves and with interdisciplinary team members, which include nurses, pharmacists, social workers and others [87].

Other strategies which can be used to address inappropriate polypharmacy include public involvement in changing and designing policy [88]. In addition, application of the nudge theory such as clinical decision support may help change behaviour, and there is some emerging evidence to support this [89–91]. Consideration of human factors, together with change management strategies that are scalable, is important to deliver a sustainable solution across the whole healthcare system [92].

7 Implementing Programs to Address Inappropriate Polypharmacy and Impact

The EU-funded SIMPATHY (Stimulating Innovation Management of Polypharmacy and Adherence in the Elderly) project spent 2 years studying polypharmacy management in Europe

[92]. Case studies in nine EU countries were used to determine how programs to manage polypharmacy and adherence were implemented using change-management tools such as Kotter's eight steps, PESTEL (Political, Economic, Social, Technological, Environmental and Legal), model and SWOT (Strengths, Weakness, Opportunity and Strength) analysis. In addition to a literature review, a benchmarking survey across the EU and a modified Delphi approach were used to establish an EU-wide consensus on how to address polypharmacy and a recommendation on what should be measured to demonstrate improvement [93–95]. From the modified Delphi approach, the key areas of consensus were around potential gain arising from polypharmacy management, strategic development, strategic change management, indicator measures, awareness raising and person-centred polypharmacy reviews. Notably, no consensus was achieved in relation to statements relating to the need to alter legislation in areas of healthcare delivery, remuneration and practitioner scope of practice [93].

The EU project made six key recommendations to implement programs to improve medication safety, of which polypharmacy is an essential element: (1) Use a systems approach that has multidisciplinary clinical and policy leadership; (2) nurture a culture that encourages and prioritizes the safety and quality of prescribing; (3) ensure that patients are integral to the decisions made about their medicines and are empowered and supported to do so; (4) use data to drive change and measure outcomes; (5) adopt an evidence-based approach with a bias towards action and (6) utilize, develop and share tools to support implementation.

Evidence for the outcomes of reviews and economic impact of addressing inappropriate polypharmacy is important when developing programmes to address this emerging research area. Many programmes have shown a reduction in the number of PIMs that are prescribed; however, evidence for the impact on other patient outcomes is mixed [96]. Sustainability of programmes to address inappropriate polypharmacy in the health service will be dependent on cost-effectiveness of the programs. While the economic impact of the polypharmacy reviews is mixed, some consider the savings from medicines that are stopped and others the possible indirect benefits of the review such as prevented hospital admission or ADRs avoided, against the costs of the reviews. One systematic review found evidence that an adequate system for managing, prescribing, monitoring and evaluating the use of medications is effective in reducing polypharmacy and improving adherence to medications, while decreasing drug costs, medication errors, drug-related problems, ADRs, drug–drug interactions, drug-related negative health outcomes, and hospital admissions [97]. Another systematic review looking at the economic evaluation found limited evidence for the benefit of the intervention to optimise medication outweighing implementation costs [98]. The authors recommended that there is a need to address and identify barriers when scaling up implementation.

The Scottish national polypharmacy programme implemented the learnings from programmes such as SIMPATHY [92], pharmacist-led information technology intervention for medication errors (PINCER) [99] and Data-Driven Quality Improvement in Primary Care (DQIP) [100]. The Scottish national polypharmacy programme resulted in one to two medicines reduced per patient, as well as an improvement in safety and quality indicators. The priority population were those over the age of 75 years old, chosen to prioritise the available resources which generated an average net saving of 150 euros per patient per annum, even after taking into account the cost of staff for the reviews [92]. There were additional indirect benefits in the form of cost avoidance due to fewer ADRs and hospital admissions.

Another example of a program to address inappropriate polypharmacy is the study conducted in the Basque region by Etxeberria et al. [101] This study used the multidisciplinary SIMPATHY methodology to minimise inappropriate polypharmacy in a population of 360,000 citizens. This approach, including pharmacists and physicians reviewing patients with five PIMs, resulted in statistically significant reductions in potentially inappropriate polypharmacy across primary and secondary care settings [102]. iSIMPATHY (implementing Stimulating Innovation in the

Management of Polypharmacy and Adherence Through the Years) sought to implement the SIMPATHY findings in Scotland, Northern Ireland and Ireland. The approach centred around patient partnership, "what matters to me" and shared decision-making in medicines reviews using the 7-step approach. The project demonstrated the feasibility of embedding a standardised approach to medicines review in Northern Ireland and Ireland and scaling up the Scottish work for 6,481 patients engaged in reviews in primary care, secondary care, outpatient clinics and care homes. It involved application of change management methodology and shared decision-making as part of a person-centred approach to pharmacist-led medicines use review delivery in multiple healthcare settings, with multidisciplinary team collaboration. An average of 11 interventions were made per patient, with 82% classified as clinically significant and 4% potentially preventing major organ failure or similar; 94% of interventions were accepted. The average number of medications reduced from 12 to 11 and 92% of reviews resulted in more appropriate medication use. Economic evaluation identified a positive return on investment as well as a reduction in carbon footprint of both admissions and wastage of medicines, and patient-reported outcome measures indicated improved understanding, adherence and reduced adverse effects. Together this showed a QALY gain of 7.4 per 100 patients reviewed. The iSIMPATHY [102] approach is transferable and the evidence produced supports robust policy development and recommends that barriers such as competing priorities and workforce capacity must be addressed effectively through the change management tools, and that patient awareness and empowerment to be active participants in the review is crucial. An overview of the findings is included in the Fig. 18.5 [102].

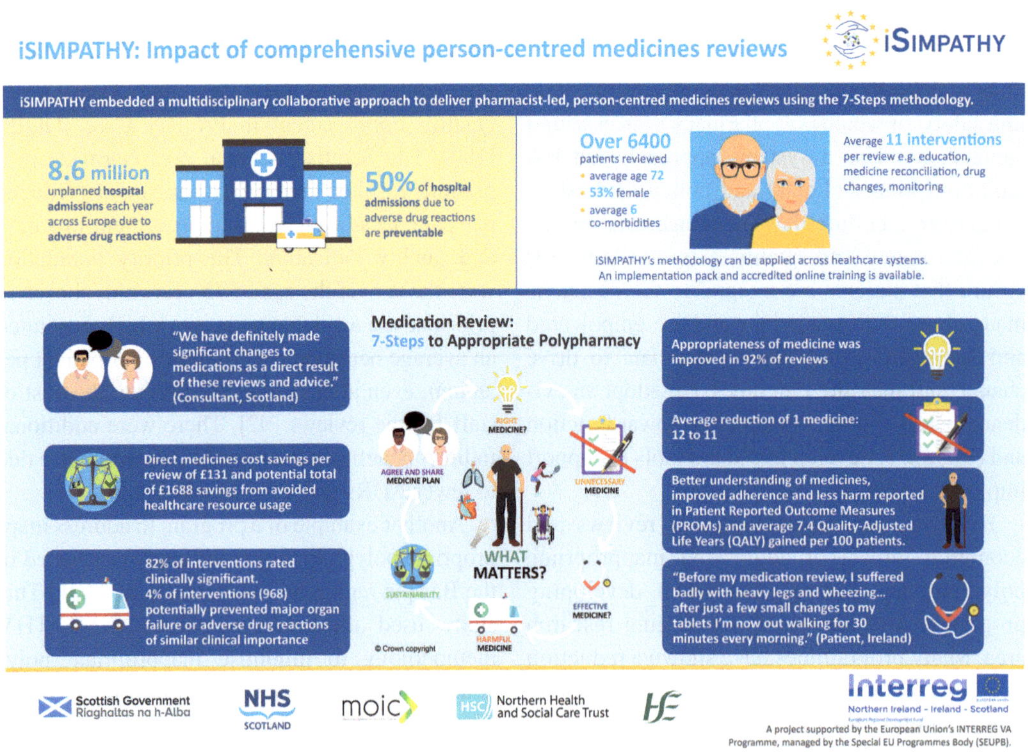

Fig. 18.5 An overview of findings from iSIMPATHY-Evaluation report

8 Summary and Conclusions

This chapter has described what constitutes inappropriate and appropriate polypharmacy and discussed strategies that are available to reduce medication-related harm focusing on a person-centred approach. The chapter also discussed which medicines have been identified to cause most harm and which patient populations are most likely to experience medication-related harm. New approaches to improving safety were discussed and include deprescribing as an outcome of medication reviews, with the most significant positive outcomes achieved with programs which include interdisciplinary teams. Some of the strategies listed are applicable to larger organisations; however, there are approaches described in the chapter and cases worked through that demonstrate how each healthcare provider at all points of the medication management pathway can reduce the risk of medication-related harm for the individual.

Research evidence are emerging in the field of polypharmacy and deprescribing on programmes that reduce inappropriate polypharmacy, but further work is needed to show impact on patient outcomes and the sustainability of national programmes across health systems. Evidence is also needed to support the review and prioritisation of medication use for people with multimorbidity. More data is also needed to show that reducing and stopping these medications that were being used to manage multimorbidity do not result in patient harm.

9 Case Studies

9.1 Case Study 1: Case Example of Polypharmacy

Consider the case of a resident in a care home with multimorbidity and polypharmacy (Ms AK), Box 18.5, keeping in mind particularly the definitions of appropriate and inappropriate polypharmacy.

Box 18.5 Case 1—Ms AK

Case summary: AK

Background (age, sex, occupation, baseline function)

- Ms AK is a 60-year-old female smoker, with heart failure following a myocardial infarction 5 years previously. Retired.

History of presentation/reason for review

- Staff at the home tell you Ms AK is a bit breathless. She is thought to have an airways condition, due to her history, and she has been started on a salbutamol inhaler. Staff also tell you she's a bit sleepier during the day since commencing zopiclone.
- Until 2 years ago, she worked in a bakery. She is a resident in a care home as she has developed early onset dementia.

Current medical history and relevant comorbidities

- Angina, hypertension, high cholesterol, type 2 diabetes mellitus, osteoarthritis.

Current medications and drug allergies obtained from Ms AK include items obtained over the counter (OTC) and herbal or complementary medicines.

- Simvastatin 40 mg daily
- Aspirin (low dose) daily
- Bisoprolol 2.5 mg daily
- Ramipril 2.5 mg daily
- Salbutamol inhaler
- Paracetamol 1000 mg, when required for pain.

She has also been recently prescribed:

- Zopiclone 3.75 mg, one to two tablets at night, for insomnia

Ms AK is living in a care home, and it would be important to assess her capacity to understand the information which is being provided to her. Due to her cognitive impairment, the clinician may need to discuss medication-related matters with the person legally responsible for making decisions about her care. Reviewing AK, the first point would be to consider 'what is important to AK?' The response is that she is breathless and that she is sleepier during the day (Box 18.6).

Taking a person-centred 7-steps approach to review Ms AK's medication, the following actions can be taken (Box 18.7).

Box 18.6 Case 1—Ms AK Continued

Lifestyle and current function, alcohol/smoking/diet/exercise

- Smoker with 20 pack year history; recently cut back to 4 pack years. She was walking but finds this hard due to breathlessness.
- 20 units per week of alcohol

'What matters to me' (patient ideas, concerns and expectations of treatment)

- What is important to Ms AK is the breathlessness and drowsiness during the day.

Results, e.g. biochemistry, other relevant investigations or monitoring

- Cholesterol, kidney function and electrolytes are within normal range.
- HbA1c is 48 mmol/Mol (6.5%)

Most recent relevant consultations

- Breathlessness raised by staff at the care home; early onset dementia

Box 18.7 Case 1—Taking the 7-Step Approach to Reviewing Ms AK's Medicines

Domain	Steps	Process	Person-specific issues to consider
Aims	1. What matters to Ms AK?	**Review diagnoses and identify therapeutic objectives with respect to:** – Identify objectives of therapy – Manage existing health problems – Prevent future health concerns	– Breathlessness and daytime drowsiness – Deterioration of dementia
Need	2. Identify essential drug therapy.	**Identify essential drugs (not to be stopped without specialist advice)** – Drugs that have essential replacement functions (e.g. thyroxine) – Drugs to prevent symptomatic decline (e.g. drugs for Parkinson's disease, heart failure)	– Essential medications are bisoprolol and ramipril, prescribed for heart failure

Domain	Steps	Process	Person-specific issues to consider
	3. Does the patient take unnecessary drug therapy?	**What is medication for?** Identify and review the (continued) need for drugs: – with temporary indications – with higher than usual maintenance doses – with limited benefit/ evidence of its use in general – with limited benefit for the patient under review (consider numbers needed to treat) [7]	– Zopiclone is unnecessary – The dose may need to be weaned gradually if Ms AK has been taking these >4 weeks. – Consider if her insomnia been caused by pain? – The indication for salbutamol is unclear and likely to be inappropriate as breathlessness is probably due to heart failure. This can be stopped. – Consider smoking history: Advise spirometry as smoking history and previous occupation may predispose Ms AK to chronic obstructive pulmonary disease (COPD) – Simvastatin is currently appropriate, however as dementia progresses and becomes severe, it would be important to review its ongoing benefits
Effectiveness	4. Are therapeutic objectives being achieved?	**Identify the need for adding/ intensifying drug therapy to achieve therapeutic objectives:** – to achieve symptom control – to achieve biochemical/ clinical targets – to prevent disease progression/exacerbation Is there more appropriate therapy that would help achieve goals?	– Review doses of ACEI (ramipril) and beta blocker (bisoprolol) and titrate to manage heart failure. – Ms AK would benefit from dose titration. – Ensure kidney function, electrolytes and BP are monitored. – Consider the different NNTs here for symptom management compared to progression.
Safety	5. Does Ms AK have adverse drug reactions (ADRs) or is at risk of ADRs?	**Identify patient safety risks by checking:** – are the targets set for the individual appropriate? – drug–disease interactions – drug–drug interactions – monitoring mechanisms for high-risk drugs – risk of accidental overdosing **Identify adverse drug effects by checking for:** – specific signs/symptoms/ laboratory markers (e.g. hypokalaemia) – cumulative adverse drug effects – drugs that may be used to treat side effects caused by other drugs	– Ensure Ms AK is not experiencing any gastrointestinal ADRs from aspirin – Zopiclone is likely to be causing drowsiness the next day – Check her weight to ensure appropriate dose of paracetamol and discuss with care home staff

Domain	Steps	Process	Person-specific issues to consider
	Does Ms AK or the care home personnel know what to do if ill with a period of acute dehydrating illness?	See Sick day guidance	– It may be appropriate to stop ACEI (ramipril) if Ms AK becomes acutely unwell. The care home staff would need training on how this is done.
Sustainability	6. Is drug therapy cost-effective and environmentally sustainable?	**Identify unnecessarily costly drug therapy:** – Consider more cost-effective alternatives. More sustainable options would be the use of dry powder inhalers rather than propellant based inhalers where these are indicated	– Balance against effectiveness, safety, convenience
Person-centred care	7. Is Ms AK willing and able to take medicines as intended?	**Does the patient understand the outcomes of the review?** – Consider 'Teach Back' **Ensure drug therapy changes are tailored to patient preferences:** – Is the medication in a form the patient can take? – Is the dose schedule convenient? – Is the patient able to take medicines as intended? Consider what assistance the patient might need and when this is available **Agree and communicate plan:** – Discuss with the patient/carer/welfare proxy objectives and priorities – Decide what medicines have an effect of sufficient magnitude to consider continuation or discontinuation – Inform relevant carers about changes in treatments	– Ensure the care staff and Ms AK understand why the medicines are being titrated up and that the inhaler is unlikely to be needed, and why zopiclone is to be weaned off

Key concepts in this case (AK)

- This patient was incorrectly diagnosed with breathing problems that were managed with salbutamol
- Although both the beta blocker (bisoprolol) and ACEI (ramipril) can be considered high-risk medicines, they are recommended to be increased to provide symptomatic relief of heart failure.
- Electrolytes and kidney function should be monitored.
- Zopiclone should be weaned and should only have been prescribed for short-term use.
- Consider non-pharmacological management, for instance, of insomnia

9.2 Case Study 2: Polypharmacy and Prescribing Cascade

Consider a case of a person living in the community with multimorbidity and polypharmacy (Mr PC), Boxes 18.8 and 18.9, particularly keeping in mind the definitions of appropriate and inappropriate polypharmacy, and for this case, the prescribing cascade.

For the second case of Mr PC, living in the community, each of the steps is set out using the 7-step process below (Box 18.10).

Box 18.8 Case 2—Mr PC

Case summary: Mr PC

Background (age, sex, occupation, baseline function)

- 76-year-old male, with type 2 diabetes mellitus. Retired. Previous football player.

History of presentation/reason for review

- Feeling light-headed and dizzy; has annoying heart burn.

Current medical history and relevant comorbidities

- Angina, hypertension, high cholesterol, type 2 diabetes mellitus, osteoarthritis.

Current medications and drug allergies, obtained from PC. Includes items obtained over the counter (OTC) and herbal or complementary medicines.

- Amlodipine 10 mg daily. The dose has been recently increased from 5 mg daily.
- Bendroflumethiazide 5 mg in the morning, recently commenced.
- Glibenclamide 15 mg daily
- Diclofenac 75 mg twice a day
- Simvastatin 40 mg at night
- Ramipril 2.5 mg in the morning

Mr PC has recently purchased Omeprazole 10 mg, which he takes daily.

Box 18.9 Case 2—Mr PC Continued

Lifestyle and current function, alcohol/smoking/diet/exercise

- Little exercise due to joint pain
- Social alcohol consumption: 4–5 units per week
- Non-smoker

'What matters to me' (patient ideas, concerns and expectations of treatment)

- Feeling light-headed and dizzy at times. Gets annoying heart burn
- Has not had a heart attack and understands his medicines may help prevent one, so he takes his medicines
- His swollen ankles are annoying

Results, e.g. biochemistry, other relevant investigations or monitoring

- BP before amlodipine dose was increased: 155/70 (sitting)
- Most recent HbA1C was 61 mmol/Mol (7.7%), and fasting blood glucose level (BGL) was 5.1 mmol/L. He does not check his own BGL via capillary (finger-prick) testing
- Kidney function is stable, although reduced (eGFR 50 mL/min/1.73 m^2) with microalbuminuria. Records have not been updated since recent additions of bendroflumethiazide and diclofenac

Most recent relevant consultations

- Community pharmacy request for relief of heartburn and discussion of symptoms. Referred for medication review.

Box 18.10 Case 2—Taking the 7-Steps Approach to Reviewing Mr PC's Medicines

Domain	Steps	Process	Person-specific issues to consider
Aims	1. What matters to PC?	**Review diagnoses and identify therapeutic objectives with respect to:** – Identify objectives of therapy – Manage existing health problems – Prevent future health concerns	– Investigate possible medication-related causes for symptoms – Avoiding future heart disease or stroke is important
Need	2. Identify essential drug therapy	**Identify essential drugs (not to be stopped without specialist advice)** – Drugs that have essential replacement functions (e.g. thyroxine) – Drugs to prevent symptomatic decline (e.g. drugs for Parkinson's disease, heart failure)	– Prescribed medicines are for long-term prevention of cardiovascular complications – Diclofenac is for managing symptoms but should be reviewed due to risk of cardiovascular complications
	3. Does PC take unnecessary therapy?	**What is medication for?** Identify and review the (continued) need for drugs: – with temporary indications – with higher than usual maintenance doses – with limited benefit/ evidence of its use in general – with limited benefit for the patient under review, consider number needed to treat (NNT) [7]	Reconsider diuretic: – commenced for ankle oedema, most likely from amlodipine and not for BP management – has potential to reduce kidney function Reason for OTC omeprazole: – possibly to manage ADRs experienced from diclofenac or amlodipine. Review diclofenac and amlodipine, considering deprescribing, with ongoing monitoring of BP.

Domain	Steps	Process	Person-specific issues to consider
Effectiveness	4. Are therapeutic objectives being achieved?	**Identify the need for adding/intensifying drug therapy to achieve therapeutic objectives:** – to achieve symptom control – to achieve biochemical/clinical targets – to prevent disease progression/ exacerbation Is there more appropriate therapy that would help achieve goals?	Investigate/exclude possible causes of heartburn – consider medication causes: amlodipine ± diclofenac – consider dose reduction of these or stopping, if appropriate – *H. pylori* eradication (if identified) – prescribe proton pump inhibitor/ eradication therapy, if appropriate, with view to 'step-down' after initial management. Add aspirin for secondary prevention of cardiovascular disease, after completing the steps above to manage heartburn – Intensify non-drug management for arthritis; use paracetamol and topical therapies; consider strict 'as required' dosing of NSAID with safer cardiovascular risk profile.
Safety	5. Does the patient have adverse drug reactions (ADRs) or is at risk of ADRs?	**Identify patient safety risks by checking:** – whether the targets set for the individual appropriate? – drug–disease interactions – drug–drug interactions (monitoring mechanisms for high-risk drugs) – risk of accidental overdosing **Identify adverse drug effects by checking for:** – specific signs/ symptoms/laboratory markers (e.g. hypokalaemia), – cumulative adverse drug effects drugs that may be used to treat side effects caused by other drugs	– Dizziness and light-headedness are non-specific symptoms: could be due to postural hypotension or low blood glucose. – if possible, check sitting and standing BP and fBGL at time of symptoms – Glibenclamide is a sulphonylurea derivative and a Potentially Inappropriate Medicine (PIM) for an older person with reduced kidney function, due to the risk of hypoglycaemia – Less stringent targets for HbA1c and fBGL are acceptable for older people with multimorbidity – Change to safer medicine, such as metformin with dose appropriate for kidney function. – Check kidney function and electrolytes (drug-drug interaction: diclofenac + bendroflumethiazide) – Drug–drug interaction: amlodipine and simvastatin. PC has maximum simvastatin dose. There are no recent cholesterol results recorded for PC. – Monitor with potential to review or reduce simvastatin dose with time.
	Does PC know what to do if ill with a period of acute dehydrating illness?	See Sick day guidance	

Domain	Steps	Process	Person-specific issues to consider
Sustainability	6. Is drug therapy cost-effective and environmentally sustainable?	**Identify unnecessarily costly drug therapy:** – Consider more cost-effective alternatives	Balance against effectiveness, safety, convenience and environmental impact
Person-centredness	7. Is the patient willing and able to take medicines as intended?	**Does the patient understand the outcomes of the review?** – Consider 'Teach Back' **Ensure drug therapy changes are tailored to patient preferences:** – Is the medication in a form the patient can take? – Is the dose schedule convenient? – Is the patient able to take medicines as intended? Consider what assistance the patient might need and when this is available **Agree and communicate plan:** – Discuss with the patient/carer/welfare proxy objectives and priorities – Decide what medicines have an effect of sufficient magnitude to consider continuation or discontinuation – Inform relevant carers about changes in treatments	– PC had no problems identified with managing the medicines as prescribed – Changes to medication regimen for PC will be undertaken systematically, to observe and monitor response, before initiating other steps in plan. – Ensure that the patient understands the importance of not taking over-the-counter NSAIDs

Key concepts in this case

- Mr PC has had medicines added that have resulted from possible ADRs from other medicines ('prescribing cascade')
- Drug–drug interactions have been identified that require more intensive monitoring
- Glibenclamide is a PIM and requires review: Symptomatic adverse effects require a change of therapy
- Avoiding a future stroke or heart attack is important for PC. Commencing an antiplatelet agent (aspirin) is appropriate, while considering and minimising the risks with including this into his current regimen.

References

1. Kongkaew C, Hann M, Mandal J, Williams SD, Metcalfe D, Noyce PR, Ashcroft DM. Risk factors for hospital admissions associated with adverse drug events. Pharmacotherapy. 2013;33(8):827–37. https://doi.org/10.1002/phar.1287.
2. Auraaen A, Slawomirski L, Klazinga N. "The economics of patient safety in primary and ambulatory care: Flying blind", OECD Health Working Papers, No. 106, OECD Publishing, Paris, 2018. https://doi.org/10.1787/baf425ad-en.
3. World Health Organization. Medication safety in polypharmacy: technical report. World Health Organization; 2019. https://www.who.int/publications/i/item/WHO-UHC-SDS-2019.11. Accessed in 2022.
4. World Health Organization. World report on ageing and health. Geneva: World Health Organization; 2015. https://www.who.int/publications/i/item/9789241565042. Accessed 2022
5. Van Lerberghe W. The world health report 2008: primary health care: now more than ever. World Health Organization; 2008. https://iris.who.int/bitstream/handle/10665/43949/9789241563734_eng.pdf?sequence=1&isAllowed=y. Accessed 2008
6. Masnoon N, Shakib S, Kalisch-Ellett L, Caughey GE. What is polypharmacy? A systematic review of definitions. BMC Geriatr. 2017;17(1):230. https://doi.org/10.1186/s12877-017-0621-2.
7. Scottish Government Polypharmacy Model of Care Group. Polypharmacy guidance, realistic prescribing. 3rd ed. Scottish Government; 2018. https://www.therapeutics.scot.nhs.uk/wp-content/uploads/2018/04/Polypharmacy-Guidance-2018.pdf. Accessed March 2022.
8. Köberlein J, Jürges H. 21 multimorbidity, incentives and the use of health services in Europe. Active ageing and solidarity between generations in Europe:243; 2013.
9. Mannucci PM, Nobili A, Pasina L, Collaborators R. Polypharmacy in older people: lessons from 10 years of experience with the REPOSI register. Intern Emerg Med. 2018;13(8):1191–200. https://doi.org/10.1007/s11739-018-1941-8.
10. Guthrie B, Payne K, Alderson P, McMurdo MET, Mercer SW. Adapting clinical guidelines to take account of multimorbidity. BMJ. 2012;345:e6341. https://doi.org/10.1136/bmj.e6341.
11. Shippee ND, Shah ND, May CR, Mair FS, Montori VM. Cumulative complexity: a functional, patient-centered model of patient complexity can improve research and practice. J Clin Epidemiol. 2012;10(65):1041–51.
12. Lu CY, Roughead E. Determinants of patient-reported medication errors: a comparison among seven countries. Int J Clin Pract. 2011;65(7):733–40. https://doi.org/10.1111/j.1742-1241.2011.02671.x.
13. Cullinan S, Raae Hansen C, Byrne S, O'Mahony D, Kearney P, Sahm L. Challenges of deprescribing in the multimorbid patient. Eur J Hosp Pharm. 2017;24(1):43–6. https://doi.org/10.1136/ejhpharm-2016-000921.
14. Frank C, Weir E. Deprescribing for older patients. CMAJ. 2014;186(18):1369–76. https://doi.org/10.1503/cmaj.131873.
15. Latimer S, Hewitt J, Teasdale T, de Wet C, Gillespie BM. The accuracy, completeness and timeliness of discharge medication information and implementing medication reconciliation: a cross-sectional survey of general practitioners. Aust J Gen Pract. 2020;49(12):854–8. https://doi.org/10.31128/AJGP-04-20-5375.
16. Rochon PA, Gurwitz JH. The prescribing cascade revisited. Lancet. 2017;389(10081):1778–80. https://doi.org/10.1016/S0140-6736(17)31188-1.
17. Cohen MR. Medication errors. 2nd ed. Washington, DC: American Pharmacist Association; 2007.
18. New South Wales Government: Clinical excellence commission high-risk medicines: A-PINCH. https://www.cec.health.nsw.gov.au/keep-patients-safe/medication-safety/high-risk-medicines/A-PINCH; 2022.
19. Agrawal M, Singh P, Joshi U. Antimicrobials associated adverse drug reaction profiling: a four years retrospective study (Pharmacovigilance study). Alexandria J Med. 2021;57(1):177–87. https://doi.org/10.1080/20905068.2021.1938425.
20. Komagamine J, Kobayashi M. Prevalence of hospitalisation caused by adverse drug reactions at an internal medicine ward of a single Centre in Japan: a cross-sectional study. BMJ Open. 2019;9(8):e030515. https://doi.org/10.1136/bmjopen-2019-030515.
21. Pirmohamed M, James S, Meakin S, Green C, Scott AK, Walley TJ, Farrar K, Park BK, Breckenridge AM. Adverse drug reactions as cause of admission to hospital: prospective analysis of 18 820 patients. BMJ. 2004;329(7456):15–9. https://doi.org/10.1136/bmj.329.7456.15.
22. Mair A, Wilson M, Dreischulte T. Addressing the challenge of polypharmacy. Annu Rev Pharmacol Toxicol. 2020;60(1):661–81. https://doi.org/10.1146/annurev-pharmtox-010919-023508.
23. Qaseem A, Wilt TJ, Kansagara D, Horwitch C, Barry MJ, Forciea MA, Clinical Guidelines Committee of the American College of P, Fitterman N, Balzer K, Boyd C, Humphrey LL, Iorio A, Lin J, Maroto M, McLean R, Mustafa R, Tufte J. Hemoglobin A1c targets for glycemic control with pharmacologic therapy for nonpregnant adults with type 2 diabetes mellitus: a guidance statement update from the American College of Physicians. Ann Intern Med. 2018;168(8):569–76. https://doi.org/10.7326/M17-0939.
24. Nazareth K, Burkhard K. Hypnotics & anxiolytics practice guide. Pract guide, All Wales Med Strateg Group, Cardiff. Vol. 20, pp. 26; 2016. http://www.wales.nhs.uk/sites3/Documents/582/Guide_Hypnotics

25. Maust DT, Kim HM, Seyfried LS, Chiang C, Kavanagh J, Schneider LS, Kales HC. Antipsychotics, other psychotropics, and the risk of death in patients with dementia: number needed to harm. JAMA Psychiatry. 2015;72(5):438–45. https://doi.org/10.1001/jamapsychiatry.2014.3018.
26. Banerjee S. The use of antipsychotic medication for people with dementia: time for action; 2009. https://psychrights.org/research/digest/nlps/banerjeereportongeriatricneurolepticuse.pdf. Accessed in 2022.
27. Risacher SL, McDonald BC, Tallman EF, West JD, Farlow MR, Unverzagt FW, Gao S, Boustani M, Crane PK, Petersen RC, Jack CR Jr, Jagust WJ, Aisen PS, Weiner MW, Saykin AJ, Alzheimer's Disease Neuroimaging I. Association between anticholinergic medication use and cognition, brain metabolism, and brain atrophy in cognitively normal older adults. JAMA Neurol. 2016;73(6):721–32. https://doi.org/10.1001/jamaneurol.2016.0580.
28. Duran CE, Azermai M, Vander Stichele RH. Systematic review of anticholinergic risk scales in older adults. Eur J Clin Pharmacol. 2013;69(7):1485–96. https://doi.org/10.1007/s00228-013-1499-3.
29. Nishtala PS, Salahudeen MS, Hilmer SN. Anticholinergics: theoretical and clinical overview. Expert Opin Drug Saf. 2016;15(6):753–68. https://doi.org/10.1517/14740338.2016.1165664.
30. Bishara D, Harwood D, Sauer J, Taylor DM. Anticholinergic effect on cognition (AEC) of drugs commonly used in older people. Int J Geriatr Psychiatry. 2017;32(6):650–6. https://doi.org/10.1002/gps.4507.
31. Chew ML, Mulsant BH, Pollock BG, Lehman ME, Greenspan A, Mahmoud RA, Kirshner MA, Sorisio DA, Bies RR, Gharabawi G. Anticholinergic activity of 107 medications commonly used by older adults. J Am Geriatr Soc. 2008;56(7):1333–41.
32. Hilmer SN, Gnjidic D. The anticholinergic burden: from research to practice. Aust Prescr. 2022;45(4):118.
33. Hilmer SN. Calculating and using the drug burden index score in research and practice. Expert Rev Clin Pharmacol. 2018;11(11):1053–5. https://doi.org/10.1080/17512433.2018.1528145.
34. Rudolph JL, Salow MJ, Angelini MC, McGlinchey RE. The anticholinergic risk scale and anticholinergic adverse effects in older persons. Arch Intern Med. 2008;168(5):508–13.
35. Lim R, Ellett LMK, Semple S, Roughead EE. The extent of medication-related hospital admissions in Australia: a review from 1988 to 2021. Drug Saf. 2022;45(3):249–57. https://doi.org/10.1007/s40264-021-01144-1.
36. Rasool MF, Rehman AU, Imran I, Abbas S, Shah S, Abbas G, Khan I, Shakeel S, Ahmad Hassali MA, Hayat K. Risk factors associated with medication errors among patients suffering from chronic disorders. Front Public Health. 2020;8:531038. https://doi.org/10.3389/fpubh.2020.531038.
37. Al Hamid A, Ghaleb M, Aljadhey H, Aslanpour Z. A systematic review of hospitalization resulting from medicine-related problems in adult patients. Br J Clin Pharmacol. 2014;78(2):202–17. https://doi.org/10.1111/bcp.12293.
38. Mullan J, Burns P, Mohanan L, Lago L, Jordan M, Potter J. Hospitalisation for medication misadventures among older adults with and without dementia: a 5-year retrospective study. Australas J Ageing. 2019;38(4):e135. https://doi.org/10.1111/ajag.12712.
39. Counter D, Millar JWT, McLay JS. Hospital readmissions, mortality and potentially inappropriate prescribing: a retrospective study of older adults discharged from hospital. Br J Clin Pharmacol. 2018;84(8):1757–63. https://doi.org/10.1111/bcp.13607.
40. Barnett S, Roderick P, Martin D, Diamond I. A multilevel analysis of the effects of rurality and social deprivation on premature limiting long term illness. J Epidemiol Community Health. 2001;55(1):44–51. https://doi.org/10.1136/jech.55.1.44.
41. Public Health Scotland. High risk drugs by age group and 2020 SIMD quintile. Public Health Scotland; 2021. https://www.isdscotland.org/. Accessed 2022.
42. Awad A, Hanna O. Potentially inappropriate medication use among geriatric patients in primary care setting: a cross-sectional study using the Beers, STOPP, FORTA and MAI criteria. PLoS One. 2019;14(6):e0218174. https://doi.org/10.1371/journal.pone.0218174.
43. Fick DM, Semla TP, Steinman M, Beizer J, Brandt N, Dombrowski R, DuBeau CE, Pezzullo L, Epplin JJ. American Geriatrics Society 2019 updated AGS Beers Criteria® for potentially inappropriate medication use in older adults. J Am Geriatr Soc. 2019;67(4):674–94.
44. O'Mahony D, O'Sullivan D, Byrne S, O'Connor MN, Ryan C, Gallagher P. STOPP/START criteria for potentially inappropriate prescribing in older people: version 2. Age Ageing. 2015;44(2):213–8. https://doi.org/10.1093/ageing/afu145.
45. Pazan F, Weiss C, Wehling M, Forta. The EURO-FORTA (Fit fOR The Aged) list: international consensus validation of a clinical tool for improved drug treatment in older people. Drugs Aging. 2018;35(1):61–71. https://doi.org/10.1007/s40266-017-0514-2.
46. Hanlon JT, Schmader KE. The medication appropriateness index: a Clinimetric measure. Psychother Psychosom. 2022;91(2):78–83. https://doi.org/10.1159/000521699.
47. Parekh N, Ali K, Davies JG, Stevenson JM, Banya W, Nyangoma S, Schiff R, Van Der Cammen T, Harchowal J, Rajkumar C. Medication-related harm in older adults following hospital discharge: development and validation of a prediction tool. BMJ Qual Saf. 2020;29(2):142–53. https://doi.org/10.1136/bmjqs-2019-009587.
48. O'Donnell LK, Reeve E, Hilmer SN. Development, validation and evaluation of the goal-directed medication review electronic decision support system (G-MEDSS)©. Res Soc Adm Pharm. 2022;18(7):3174–83.

49. O'Donnell LK, Hilmer S, Baysari M. National rollout of the Goal-directed Medication review Electronic Decision Support System (G-MEDSS)© in practice. Digital Health Week. 2022;1(1)
50. Curtin D, Gallagher P, O'Mahony D. Deprescribing in older people approaching end-of-life: development and validation of STOPPFrail version 2. Age Ageing. 2020;50(2):465–71. https://doi.org/10.1093/ageing/afaa159.
51. Nyborg G, Brekke M, Straand J, Gjelstad S, Romøren M. Potentially inappropriate medication use in nursing homes: an observational study using the NORGEP-NH criteria. BMC Geriatr. 2017;17(1):220. https://doi.org/10.1186/s12877-017-0608-z.
52. Vasilevskis EE, Shah AS, Hollingsworth EK, Shotwell MS, Mixon AS, Bell SP, Kripalani S, Schnelle JF, Simmons SF, Shed MT. A patient-centered deprescribing intervention for hospitalized older patients with polypharmacy: rationale and design of the Shed-MEDS randomized controlled trial. BMC Health Serv Res. 2019;19(1):165. https://doi.org/10.1186/s12913-019-3995-3.
53. McDonald EG, Wu PE, Rashidi B, Forster AJ, Huang A, Pilote L, Papillon-Ferland L, Bonnici A, Tamblyn R, Whitty R, Porter S, Battu K, Downar J, Lee TC. The MedSafer study: a controlled trial of an electronic decision support tool for deprescribing in acute care. J Am Geriatr Soc. 2019;67(9):1843–50. https://doi.org/10.1111/jgs.16040.
54. Choosing Wisely Canada. Choosing wisely. https://choosingwiselycanada.org/; 2022. Accessed May 2023.
55. Levinson W, Kallewaard M, Bhatia RS, Wolfson D, Shortt S, Kerr EA, Choosing Wisely International Working G. 'Choosing Wisely': a growing international campaign. BMJ Qual Saf. 2015;24(2):167–74. https://doi.org/10.1136/bmjqs-2014-003821.
56. Whitty R, Porter S, Battu K, Bhatt P, Koo E, Kalocsai C, Wu PE, Delicaet K, Bogoch II, Wu R, Downar J. A pilot study of a Medication Rationalization (MERA) intervention. CMAJ Open. 2018;6(1):E87–94. https://doi.org/10.9778/cmajo.20170134.
57. Onder G, Petrovic M, Tangiisuran B, Meinardi MC, Markito-Notenboom WP, Somers A, Rajkumar C, Bernabei R, van der Cammen TJ. Development and validation of a score to assess risk of adverse drug reactions among in-hospital patients 65 years or older: the GerontoNet ADR risk score. Arch Intern Med. 2010;170(13):1142–8. https://doi.org/10.1001/archinternmed.2010.153.
58. Parameswaran Nair N, Chalmers L, Connolly M, Bereznicki BJ, Peterson GM, Curtain C, Castelino RL, Bereznicki LR. Prediction of hospitalization due to adverse drug reactions in elderly community-dwelling patients (the PADR-EC score). PLoS One. 2016;11(10):e0165757. https://doi.org/10.1371/journal.pone.0165757.
59. Tangiisuran B, Scutt G, Stevenson J, Wright J, Onder G, Petrovic M, van der Cammen TJ, Rajkumar C, Davies G. Development and validation of a risk model for predicting adverse drug reactions in older people during hospital stay: Brighton Adverse Drug Reactions Risk (BADRI) model. PLoS One. 2014;9(10):e111254. https://doi.org/10.1371/journal.pone.0111254.
60. Yadesa TM, Kitutu FE, Tamukong R, Alele PE. Development and validation of 'Prediction of Adverse Drug Reactions in Older Inpatients (PADROI)' risk assessment tool. Clin Interv Aging. 2022;17:195–210. https://doi.org/10.2147/CIA.S350500.
61. Pharmaceutical Society of Australia. Guidelines for comprehensive medication management reviews; 2020. https://www.ppaonline.com.au/wp-content/uploads/2020/04/PSA-Guidelines-for-Comprehensive-Medication-Management-Reviews.pdf. Accessed in 2022
62. Australian Diabetes Educators Association. ADEA clinical guidelines. Australian Diabetes Educators Association;2022. https://www.adea.com.au/resources/standards-position-statements-and-other-resources/adea-clinical-guidelines/.
63. Canadian Deprescribing Network. Patient handouts on medications. https://www.deprescribingnetwork.ca/patient-handouts; 2017. Accessed June 2022.
64. Effective Prescribing and Therapeutics & Digital Health & Care Innovation Centre. Polypharmacy: manage medicines app. Patient shared decision-making app for polypharmacy reviews 2018, Scotland; 2021.
65. Effective Prescribing and Therapeutics Branch – Scottish Government. Benzodiazepine and z-hypnotic: Quality prescribing advice for adults. Accessed on 28 th March 2023. Available at https://www.therapeutics.scot.nhs.uk/wp-content/uploads/2022/03/Benoz-and-Z-d_Quality-Prescribing-Adv-FINAL-DRAFT.pdf.
66. World Health Organization. Adherence to long-term therapies. WHO; 2003. http://apps.who.int/iris/bitstream/handle/10665/42682/9241545992.pdf;jsessionid=B3EDA8A86FC93977FA35E8D7189C7F7D?sequence=1. 2022.
67. Elliott R. Non-adherence to medicines: not solved but solvable. J Health Serv Res Policy. 2009;14(1):58–61.
68. Public Health Scotland Teach back. NHS; 2022. https://www.healthliteracyplace.org.uk/toolkit/techniques/teach-back/.
69. Agency for Healthcare Research and Quality. Use the teach-back method: tool #5. AHRQ; 2020. https://www.ahrq.gov/health-literacy/improve/precautions/tool5.html. 2022.
70. CaDen. What is deprescribing? Bruyère Research Institute; 2021. https://deprescribing.org/what-is-deprescribing/. Accessed 01 May 2021.
71. Lyles LF, Hildebrandt H, Mair A. Population health management approach: integration of community-based pharmacists into integrated care systems: reflections from the U.S., achievements in Scotland

and discussions in Germany. Int J Integr Care. 2020;20(2):13. https://doi.org/10.5334/ijic.5431.
72. Mair A, Antoniadou E, Hendry A, Gabrovec B. Appropriate polypharmacy: a barometer for integrated care. J Integr Care. 2020;29:204.
73. McDonald EG, Wu PE, Rashidi B, Wilson MG, Bortolussi-Courval E, Atique A, Battu K, Bonnici A, Elsayed S, Wilson AG, Papillon-Ferland L, Pilote L, Porter S, Murphy J, Ross SB, Shiu J, Tamblyn R, Whitty R, Xu J, Fabreau G, Haddad T, Palepu A, Khan N, McAlister FA, Downar J, Huang AR, MacMillan TE, Cavalcanti RB, Lee TC. The MedSafer Study-electronic decision support for deprescribing in hospitalized older adults: a cluster randomized clinical trial. JAMA Intern Med. 2022;182(3):265–73. https://doi.org/10.1001/jamainternmed.2021.7429.
74. OECD, "Safe prescribing in older populations", in Health at a Glance 2019: OECD Indicators, 2019. OECD Publishing, Paris. https://doi.org/10.1787/c69da240-en.
75. Burt J, Elmore N, Campbell SM, Rodgers S, Avery AJ, Payne RA. Developing a measure of polypharmacy appropriateness in primary care: systematic review and expert consensus study. BMC Med. 2018;16(1):91. https://doi.org/10.1186/s12916-018-1078-7.
76. Cheng R, Yoo L, Ho C, Kadija M. Identification of medication safety indicators in acute care settings for public reporting in Ontario. Healthc Q. 2010;13 Spec No:26–34. https://doi.org/10.12927/hcq.2010.21962. PMID: 20959727.
77. Fastbom J, Johnell K. National indicators for quality of drug therapy in older persons: the Swedish experience from the first 10 years. Drugs Aging. 2015;32(3):189–99. https://doi.org/10.1007/s40266-015-0242-4.
78. Thompson W, Reeve E. Deprescribing: moving beyond barriers and facilitators. Res Social Adm Pharm. 2022;18(3):2547–9. https://doi.org/10.1016/j.sapharm.2021.04.004.
79. Doherty AJ, Boland P, Reed J, Clegg AJ, Stephani AM, Williams NH, Shaw B, Hedgecoe L, Hill R, Walker L. Barriers and facilitators to deprescribing in primary care: a systematic review. BJGP Open. 2020;4(3):bjgpopen20X1010. https://doi.org/10.3399/bjgpopen20X101096.
80. Le Bosquet K, Barnett N, Minshull J. Deprescribing: practical ways to support person-centred. Evid Based Deprescribing Pharm (Basel). 2019;7(3):129. https://doi.org/10.3390/pharmacy7030129.
81. Anderson K, Foster M, Freeman C, Luetsch K, Scott I. Negotiating "unmeasurable harm and benefit": perspectives of general practitioners and consultant pharmacists on Deprescribing in the primary care setting. Qual Health Res. 2017;27(13):1936–47. https://doi.org/10.1177/1049732316687732.
82. Rochon PA, Petrovic M, Cherubini A, Onder G, O'Mahony D, Sternberg SA, Stall NM, Gurwitz JH. Polypharmacy, inappropriate prescribing, and deprescribing in older people: through a sex and gender lens. Lancet Healthy Longevity. 2021;2(5):e290–300. https://doi.org/10.1016/s2666-7568(21)00054-4.
83. Gillespie RJ, Harrison L, Mullan J. Deprescribing medications for older adults in the primary care context: a mixed studies review. Health Sci Rep. 2018;1(7):e45. https://doi.org/10.1002/hsr2.45.
84. Farrell B, Mangin D. Deprescribing is an essential part of good prescribing. Am Fam Physician. 2019;99(1):7–9.
85. Balsom C, Pittman N, King R, Kelly D. Impact of a pharmacist-administered deprescribing intervention on nursing home residents: a randomized controlled trial. Int J Clin Pharm. 2020;42(4):1153–67. https://doi.org/10.1007/s11096-020-01073-6.
86. Seto H, Ishimaru N, Ohnishi J, Kanzawa Y, Nakajima T, Shimokawa T, Imanaka Y, Kinami S. Multidisciplinary team deprescribing intervention for polypharmacy in elderly orthopedic inpatients: a propensity score-matched analysis of a retrospective cohort study. Intern Med. 2022;61:2417. https://doi.org/10.2169/internalmedicine.8929-21.
87. Dharmarajan TS, Choi H, Hossain N, Munasinghe U, Lakhi F, Lourdusamy D, Onuoha S, Murakonda P, Skokowska-Lebelt A, Kanagala M. Deprescribing as a clinical improvement focus. J Am Med Dir Assoc. 2020;21(3):355–60.
88. Moore MH. Creating public value: strategic management in government. Harvard University Press; 1995.
89. Westbrook JI, Baysari MT. Nudging hospitals towards evidence-based decision support for medication management. Med J Aust. 2019;210(Suppl 6):S22–4. https://doi.org/10.5694/mja2.50028.
90. Nagtegaal R, Tummers L, Noordegraaf M, Bekkers V. Nudging healthcare professionals towards evidence-based medicine: a systematic scoping review. J Behav Public Admin. 2019;2(2)
91. Mollenkamp M, Zeppernick M, Schreyogg J. The effectiveness of nudges in improving the self-management of patients with chronic diseases: a systematic literature review. Health Policy. 2019;123(12):1199–209. https://doi.org/10.1016/j.healthpol.2019.09.008.
92. Mair A, Fernandez-Llimos F, Alonso A, Harrison C, Hurding S, Kempen T, Kinnear M, Michael N, McIntosh J, Wilson M. The Simpathy consortium. Polypharmacy management by 2030: A patient safety challenge. 2nd ed. SIMPATHY Consortium; 2017. https://www.simpathy.eu/sites/default/files/Managing_polypharmacy2030-web.pdf. Accessed June 2022.
93. Stewart D, Gibson-Smith K, MacLure K, Mair A, Alonso A, Codina C, Cittadini A, Fernandez-Llimos F, Fleming G, Gennimata D, Gillespie U, Harrison C, Junius-Walker U, Kardas P, Kempen T, Kinnear M, Lewek P, Malva J, McIntosh J, Scullin C, Wiese B. A modified Delphi study to determine the level of consensus across the European Union on the structures, processes and desired outcomes of the management of polypharmacy in older people. PLoS One. 2017;12(11):e0188348. https://doi.org/10.1371/journal.pone.0188348.
94. McIntosh J, Alonso A, MacLure K, Stewart D, Kempen T, Mair A, Castel-Branco M, Codina C,

Fernandez-Llimos F, Fleming G, Gennimata D, Gillespie U, Harrison C, Illario M, Junius-Walker U, Kampolis CF, Kardas P, Lewek P, Malva J, Menditto E, Scullin C, Wiese B, Consortium S. A case study of polypharmacy management in nine European countries: implications for change management and implementation. PLoS One. 2018;13(4):e0195232. https://doi.org/10.1371/journal.pone.0195232.

95. Stewart D, Mair A, Wilson M, Kardas P, Lewek P, Alonso A, McIntosh J, MacLure K, Consortium S. Guidance to manage inappropriate polypharmacy in older people: systematic review and future developments. Expert Opin Drug Saf. 2017;16(2):203–13. https://doi.org/10.1080/14740338.2017.1265503.
96. Martyn-St James M, Faria R, Wong R, Scope A. Evidence for the impact of interventions and medicines reconciliation on problematic polypharmacy in the UK: a rapid review of systematic reviews. Br J Clin Pharmacol. 2021;87(1):42–75. https://doi.org/10.1111/bcp.14368.
97. Soler O, Barreto JOM. Community-level pharmaceutical interventions to reduce the risks of polypharmacy in the elderly: overview of systematic reviews and economic evaluations. Front Pharmacol. 2019;10:302. https://doi.org/10.3389/fphar.2019.00302.
98. Laberge M, Sirois C, Lunghi C, Gaudreault M, Nakamura Y, Bolduc C, Laroche ML. Economic evaluations of interventions to optimize medication use in older adults with polypharmacy and multimorbidity: a systematic review. Clin Interv Aging. 2021;16:767–79. https://doi.org/10.2147/CIA.S304074.
99. Avery AJ, Rodgers S, Cantrill JA, Armstrong S, Cresswell K, Eden M, Elliott RA, Howard R, Kendrick D, Morris CJ, Prescott RJ, Swanwick G, Franklin M, Putman K, Boyd M, Sheikh A. A pharmacist-led information technology intervention for medication errors (PINCER): a multicentre, cluster randomised, controlled trial and cost-effectiveness analysis. Lancet. 2012;379(9823):1310–9. https://doi.org/10.1016/S0140-6736(11)61817-5.
100. Dreischulte T, Donnan P, Grant A, Hapca A, McCowan C, Guthrie B. Safer prescribing—a trial of education, informatics, and financial incentives. N Engl J Med. 2016;374(11):1053–64. https://doi.org/10.1056/NEJMsa1508955.
101. Etxeberria A, Iribar J, Vrotsou K, Rotaeche R, Barral I, Grupo de Colaboracion APAHdPyPP, Grupo de Colaboracion APAHdPPP, Barral I, Belzunegui J, Bustinduy A, Caso J, Del Bosque C, Etxeberria A, Frias O, Iribar J, Lekuona A, Lombera L, Lopez B, Nunez J, Olasagasti B, Rotaeche R, Royo I, Vrotsou K, Zapata E, Zubeldia X. Evaluation of the collaboration between primary and hospital care in order to improve inappropriate prescription. J Healthc Qual Res. 2021;36(2):91–7. https://doi.org/10.1016/j.jhqr.2020.09.005.
102. Mair A, Kirke C, Scott M, Michael N, Kanan Y, Law S, Scullin C, Fleming G, Hyder Skinner N, Kyle D. iSIMPATHY Evaluation Report, Edinburgh, iSIMPATHY Consortium; 2023. iSIMPATHY_Evaluation_report_ver8_online.pdf. iSIMPATHY Evaluation Report. Available at https://www.isimpathy.eu/uploads/iSIMPATHY_Evaluation_report_ver8_online.pdf. Accessed in March 2024.

19 Safe Prescribing and Monitoring in Pediatrics

Jeremy S. Stultz and Milap C. Nahata

Abstract

The pediatric population encompasses a wide array of vastly different patient subsets. Each subset has unique pharmacokinetic and pharmacodynamic differences that often substantially differ from other subsets and the adult population. These differences lead to the need for unique and highly patient-specific medication regimens, as well as age-specific medication safety considerations such as adverse drug event warnings and potential contraindications. Normal pediatric growth and development impacts medication-related adverse events, requiring healthcare providers to reliably assess and manage these events. The differences in the medication use process required for optimization of pediatric medication regimens may lead to an increased potential for medication errors throughout the medication use process. Implementation of medication-specific health information technologies such as the computerized provider order entry, electronic prescribing, and clinical decision support has improved the medication use process and medication safety in the pediatric population and is a vital safety measure. Practitioners should take into account the unique pediatric medication needs and implement actions to maximize efficacy and safety of medications in pediatric patients.

Keywords

Pediatrics · Children · Adverse drug events · Contraindications · Medication errors · Medication safety · Medication prescribing · Safety monitoring · Computerized provider order entry · Health information technology · Clinical decision support · Pharmacovigilance

Learning Objectives

- Delineate pharmacokinetic and pharmacodynamic differences among children of varying ages and adults
- Identify key growth and development milestones associated with occurrence of medication-related adverse events in children
- Describe important growth and development milestones impacting the assessment of related adverse drug events in children

J. S. Stultz
Department of Clinical Pharmacy and Translational Science, College of Pharmacy, University of Tennessee Health Science Center, Nashville, TN, USA

M. C. Nahata (✉)
Institute of Therapeutic Innovations and Outcomes (ITIO), Pharmacy, Pediatrics, & Internal Medicine, Pharmacy Practice and Science, Outcomes and Translational Sciences, College of Pharmacy, The Ohio State University, Columbus, OH, USA
e-mail: nahata.1@osu.edu

J. Jose et al. (eds.), *Principles and Practice of Pharmacovigilance and Drug Safety*,
https://doi.org/10.1007/978-3-031-51089-2_19

- Correlate differences in pharmacokinetics, pharmacodynamics, and growth and development with medication-related adverse events
- Indicate steps of the medication use process associated with a higher risk of medication error occurrence specifically in children
- Know potential impact of health information technology on prevention of adverse events in children
- Develop methods for prevention of adverse events when using high-risk medications in children

Key Points

- Differences in pharmacokinetics, pharmacodynamics, and pediatric growth and development result in a higher potential for adverse drug event occurrence in the pediatric versus adult population.
- Certain aspects of pharmacovigilance are more challenging in pediatric populations compared to adults.
- Studies are not always available to clearly delineate adverse drug reactions in children.
- Prescribing of medications for children is more error-prone compared to adults due to additional required steps.
- Health information technology can improve the ability to detect adverse drug events in the pediatric population.
- Health information technology can enhance the safety of prescribing medications for children by decreasing medication errors.

1 Introduction

The pediatric population is a dynamic patient cohort with distinctive pharmacovigilance needs. There are unique features of the pediatric population related to normal growth and development, drug disposition, adverse drug reaction (ADR) detection, and risk of medication errors (MEs), which must be accounted for to provide optimal drug therapy outcomes in pediatric patients. The pediatric population has been known as "therapeutic orphans" due to the lack of safety and efficacy data for many medications, despite an essential need to use the medication for a given indication. This has led to the recognition of serious ADRs after medications were used in everyday practice, in many scenarios as intended by the prescriber. Additionally, due to the error-prone, complex process surrounding medication use in a pediatric patient, catastrophic outcomes have occurred for some patients due to a ME (e.g., fatal overdoses of narrow therapeutic index medications like digoxin, potassium, and anticoagulants). This chapter will highlight the issues surrounding medication prescribing and safety monitoring in pediatric patients and specific methods for ensuring safe and effective medication utilization in this population.

There are varying pharmacovigilance terminologies used in the literature and not all definitions are suitable for the pediatric population. Throughout this chapter, select pharmacovigilance terms will be used as defined in Table 19.1. The definitions for these terms are similar to those recommended by regulatory agencies across the world (e.g., the World Health Organization and the United States Food and Drug Administration, and the Institute for Safe Medication Practices), with pediatric pharmacovigilance-specifics added [1–3]. The term adverse drug event (ADE) is intended to include both ADRs and MEs. If the term ADE is used in this chapter, then that statement is likely relevant to both an ADR and ME. If ADR or ME is used alone, it would be specific to that subcategory of ADE. Compared to the United States Food and Drug Administration (US FDA) definition for an ADR, we added the verbiage for "intended use." Other definitions use words such as "normal use," but in the pediatric population, "normal use" is difficult to define because regulatory agencies often have not approved many medications for use in the pediatric population, despite frequent use in daily practice. It is also important to note that an ADR is inherently associated with harm, but this chapter will also discuss potential ADEs or MEs which are important aspects of pharmacovigilance in the pediatric population although harm did not actually occur.

Table 19.1 Terminology[a] used in this chapter for harm[b] events associated with medication use

Terminology	Definition for this chapter	Select additional comments
Adverse drug event (ADE)[b]	Harm potentially, likely, or definitively associated with a medication when used as intended or in error	– Other definitions use this term to describe all events during the use of a medication regardless of association with the medication, but this chapter focuses on to those associated with the medication
Adverse drug reaction	Patient harm during the use of a medication as intended. The use of the medication was potentially, likely, or definitively associated with the reaction	– Other references use the term as a "normal" use of a drug, which is sometimes hard to define in pediatrics – A subcategory of an ADE
Medication error[b]	Any preventable event occurring while the medication is in the control of the healthcare professional, patient, or consumer that leads to patient harm	– May not always cause harm – It will be a subcategory of ADE, if harm occurred

[a]Terminology used is pediatric-focused, but based on definitions from: [1, 2]

[b]Pharmacovigilance also focuses on potential ADE or ME, which means that an event or scenario occurred which had a higher than normal chance for causing harm, but no harm occurred

2 Pediatric Age Terminology and Pharmacokinetic/Pharmacodynamic Differences

2.1 Age Terminology

The pediatric population encompasses numerous subcategories of dynamic patients displaying vastly different medication-related safety concerns. Typically, the pediatric population is divided into groups which tend to have similar development, physiology, and pharmacokinetic characteristics. These groups are typically based on age and/or body weight and can vary between references. Groupings usually start with the newborn or neonatal period and extend up to approximately 18 years of age for adolescents, although some advocate for increasing the upper limit to 21 years of age for patients with diseases of childhood [4, 5]. Commonly accepted groups are presented in Table 19.2, and this terminology will be used throughout this chapter.

The perinatal period is the most complicated age-group with numerous subcategories and variations in methods used for categorization. The developmental and drug disposition differences are commonly related to either gestational age (GA) at birth or birth weight in combination with postnatal age (PNA). Gestational age (GA) is defined as the number of weeks from the first day of the last menstrual cycle of the mother, with the viable age for survival of a newborn being approximately 22–23 weeks or higher of gestation at birth [6]. This is a more practical method compared to determining postconceptional age, which would be the age from the time of conception, a date often unknown. A GA of at least 37 weeks is considered full-term for a newborn. Postnatal age (PNA) refers to the age since birth. While GA may not be reliable in some patients or as applicable to those with in utero development issues, other well-accepted terminologies associated with neonatal physiology are based on the birth weight, with low birth weight neonates being considered a weight of <2500 g with additional stratifications below that weight as described in Table 19.2 [7]. It has been shown that postmenstrual (GA at birth + PNA) or postconceptional age is most correlated with appropriate dosing for medications excreted from the body primarily via the kidneys, such as vancomycin and gentamicin [8, 9]. Thus, many medication dosing recommendations are based on this descriptor, sometimes combined with the patient's birth weight.

The infant and child category can also vary. The US FDA extends the infant period up until 2 years of age, although many tertiary references and other organizations utilize an upper age range of 1 year of age [5, 7]. The terms "toddler" and "preschool age children" may also be used to

Table 19.2 Pediatric age and weight terminology

Terminology	Inclusive ages or weights	General pharmacokinetic differences compared to adults
Neonate	≤28 days PNA	– Higher Vd (inverse relationship with PMA and weight) – Slower hepatic clearance and renal elimination versus adults (direct relationship with PMA and weight) – Greater skin absorption (inverse relationship with PMA and weight) – Altered absorption for certain oral medications with pH-dependent absorption
Common terminologies describing age or weight at birth		
– Preterm	GA at birth <37 weeks	
– Term	GA at birth ≥37 weeks	
– Low birth weight	Birth weight of <2500 g	
– Very low birth weight	Birth weight of <1500 g	
– Extremely low birth weight	Birth weight of <1000 g	
Preterm infant[a]	Born <37 weeks GA, and >28 days PNA, and PMA <41 weeks[a]	
Infant (or corrected infant)	>28 days if born ≥37 weeks GA OR PMA ≥41 weeks[a] (if born preterm); one of the above and <2 years PMA[b]	– Higher Vd – Hepatic clearance may be faster depending on enzyme or conjugation mechanism – Renal elimination is usually faster than adults
Children	2 years[b]–11 years	– Hepatic clearance is usually faster for metabolic enzymes – Renal elimination is faster than adults
Adolescents	12–18 years	– Variability exists, but both renal and hepatic clearance/elimination are similar or faster than adults for most medications

GA Gestational age, *PNA* Postnatal age, *PMA* Postmenstrual age (gestational age at birth + postnatal age), *Vd* Apparent volume of distribution

[a]Some references may call preterm infants as preterm neonates. There are variations when a preterm infant is no longer considered "preterm" from a physiological perspective, with some references extending this up to 46 weeks PMA

[b]The infant categorization including ages up to 2 years is recommended by the United States Food and Drug Administration, but other references may use 1 year because drug disposition in patients 1–2 years may be similar to patients >2 years for certain medications

describe children between 1 and approximately 6 years of age (with those 7–12 years solely being considered children). Adolescents can also be further divided in certain subgroups. Importantly, these additional subgroups influence drug disposition and medication safety to a lesser extent in comparison with the neonatal subgroups, and thus, these are less utilized compared to the categories described in Table 19.2.

It is important to understand that individual patients may not fit into these categories due to developmental differences compared to population averages. For example, a patient with cerebral palsy may be 15 years old but not have the developmental or pharmacokinetic characteristics of other 15-year-old patients. Additionally, obese adolescents can present specific challenges. Typically, the maximum dosages of drugs in pediatric patients are the same as for the adult patients, but in certain scenarios this could represent undertreatment and the required pediatric dosages may exceed adult maximums for some medications [10].

2.2 Pharmacokinetic Differences Within the Pediatric Population

Pharmacokinetic differences abound within the pediatric population between the various age groups. As described in Table 19.2, neonates and preterm infants generally have higher apparent volume of distribution (Vd) due to a higher proportional amount of total body water per kilogram of body weight. Neonates and preterm infants also have lower hepatic metabolic activity for most metabolic enzymes, and slower renal elimination. This sometimes results in neonates requiring the same or higher individual dose (if the drug is concentration dependent) administered less frequently compared to older pediatric age-groups and adults. For example, for gentamicin or tobramycin, "traditional" intravenous dosing in children and adults ranges from 1 to 2.5 mg/kg/dose every 8 h. Due to larger Vd per kg in neonates compared to older patients, the dosage in neonates needed to achieve similar peak and trough concentrations as older patients is 4–5 mg/kg/dose every 24–48h depending on the PMA [11]. Neonates and young infants also have higher skin permeability and a greater skin surface area to body mass ratio [12]. This results in greater systemic concentrations after topical medication administration compared to older children and adults.

The neonatal period includes a continual process of kidney and liver development. For the first 7 days of life, serum creatinine (SCr) is typically unreliable as it is mainly reflective of SCr from the mother. Diuresis occurs over the first 1–2 weeks once renal function begins to improve. Newborns have impaired conjugation of bilirubin and potential protein binding alterations which can impact highly protein-bound medications. This can cause jaundice that in most cases is a normal physiologic process that resolves in the first 1–2 week of life without complications, but in some scenarios, this process can cause complications. Hepatic drug metabolism with certain enzymes can be compromised, although there are some enzymes functioning early into life. Generally, the most preterm neonates are expected to have the slowest renal elimination and hepatic metabolism, which increases to infant levels once they have a PMA similar to that of an infant born at full-term. This means some neonatal safety considerations are relevant to both preterm infants and neonates born at full-term. An important concept is that renal and hepatic function slowly mature with age during the neonatal and infant periods, but during childhood, renal and hepatic clearance and elimination of drugs is usually faster than that of adults. In-depth discussion on pharmacokinetics in the pediatric population has been described in the published literature [12].

2.3 Impact of Pharmacokinetic and Pharmacodynamic Differences on Drug Safety

The pharmacokinetic differences described above can create problematic medication safety considerations in the pediatric population, especially in the neonatal and infant population, resulting in unanticipated ADRs and increased MEs. Many historical experiences, sometimes labeled pediatric tragedies, occurred due to the utilization of excessive doses or formulations of medications in children due to a lack of knowledge at the time regarding pharmacokinetic differences [13, 14]. These are scenarios where drugs were available and used because they were needed, but information was not available to ensure safe use of the medications. At the time one could consider these ADRs because optimal dosing was not established, but in practice today, they would be considered an ME as more knowledge regarding appropriate dosing is now available.

While uncommonly used currently, chloramphenicol resulted in "gray-baby syndrome" (e.g., metabolic acidosis followed by cardiorespiratory collapse) when higher than required doses were used in neonates leading to toxic serum concentrations [15, 16]. This occurred because neonates and infants had slower renal elimination of the chloramphenicol sodium succinate (prodrug) leading to higher chloramphenicol concentrations, and also decreased metabolism of chloramphenicol (active drug) by the liver which was not accounted for in determining the dosage regimen. When dosed appropriately or serum concentrations monitored, toxicity could be minimized [17]. Neonates and young infants are also at risk for ADEs from inert or excipient components of medications due to pharmacokinetic differences and higher than expected exposures when normalized to body weight. Decreases in transformation of benzoic acid to hippuric acid (utilizing a hepatic conjugation) in preterm neonates and infants resulted in excessive benzoic acid and progressive metabolic acidosis, respiratory and central nervous system (CNS) depression (gasping respirations), and death with the use of benzyl alcohol as a preservative [18, 19]. This toxicity was most associated with the frequent use of 0.9% sodium chloride flushes which contained benzyl alcohol [20]. When neonates and infants received numerous daily flushes possibly in combination with other medications containing this preservative, the high mg/kg dose administered in combination with reduced clearance resulted in higher, potentially toxic concentrations and fatal "gasping syndrome" in neonates. Best practices are to avoid administration of medications containing preservatives, especially benzyl alcohol, in neonates or preterm infants when possible due to this safety concern. If it is not possible to avoid exposure, one could calculate the mg/kg/day exposure in a given patient to determine the total exposure. In adults, approximately 5 mg/kg/day has been administered without resulting toxicity. A definitive threshold has not been described in neonates, but most toxic doses described in neonates and preterm infants were 99 mg/kg/day or higher and administration of multifold smaller single doses have not resulted in toxicity [17, 20]. Older infants and children are not at risk for this toxicity with benzyl alcohol.

The inability of certain neonates to conjugate and eliminate bilirubin shortly after birth can lead to high unconjugated bilirubin concentrations. Administration of the antibiotics trimethoprim/sulfamethoxazole, dicloxacillin, and ceftriaxone can displace bilirubin attached to albumin resulting in more free bilirubin and an increased potential of kernicterus (e.g., acute and/or chronic encephalopathy due to accumulation of bilirubin in the CNS) [21]. Ceftriaxone can also chelate to calcium causing fatal deposits in the lungs and kidneys in infants when both are administered intravenously within 48 h of each other [22, 23]. These safety concerns are less relevant and limited to cases of drug–drug admixture incompatibility in patients 1 year or older. Best practices are to avoid using these medications in neonates and preterm infants (<41 weeks PMA) to prevent possible severe harm, and given other broad-spectrum cephalosporins are typically available.

The increased skin permeability and absorption/distribution differences in young pediatric patients can impact the safe use of topical or local injectable medications in neonates, infants, and young children. Use of apparent weight-based dosages or formulations of topical injections or creams/lotions can result in higher medication concentrations in the infant population (e.g., cushing syndrome and/or impact linear growth associated with corticosteroids) [24, 25]. This is especially of concern when applied to the face and diaper areas in infants where absorption is higher than other areas. Due to this pharmacokinetic difference, it is common practice to avoid the utilization of topical corticosteroids (particularly medium- and high-potency formulations) in infants and young children on the face or diaper area, and use sparingly in other parts of the body [21]. These medications are generally avoided all together topically in neonates and preterm infants and inappropriate use could now be considered an ME.

In addition to pharmacokinetic differences resulting in an ADR, some children are also more at risk for an ADR due to differences primarily focused on pharmacodynamics. For example, children and adolescents are to a greater extent predisposed to suicidal ideation upon initiation of antidepressant therapy, resulting in an FDA black box warning focused on the use of these medications in adolescents. While this is of concern, the benefits typically are believed to outweigh these risks. In order to ensure clarity with families, it is important that the practitioner, patient, and family make a shared decision about starting these medications and are made aware of the potential risks. Codeine is an example where a pharmacogenetic and pharmacodynamic difference has led to a contraindication focused on children <12 years of age and a warning in adolescents. Codeine, a prodrug, has been associated with respiratory depression and occasionally death in patients with genetic differences resulting in faster and greater conversion to the active metabolite morphine. This pharmacogenetic-derived difference also impacts adults. Some of the pharmacogenomic data is extrapolated from adults and studies are still lacking for some populations (e.g., children with decreased renal function). However, since children have higher rates of tonsillectomy and adenoidectomy procedures, they have the highest risk for a severe ADE [21]. Importantly, the use of codeine could be considered a ME in some scenarios as there are other options for pain relief posttonsillectomy and adenoidectomy.

In everyday practice, practical application of this information requires the collection and assessment of additional pediatric-specific information to appropriately prescribe or verify a dosage for a pediatric patient. It is essential to know the patient's weight (including any conversions between kg and pounds), age (including any history of preterm birth), indication, and available dosage forms that can practically be used in the pediatric population (including possible excipients). This information can then be used to identify the most appropriate dosage in medication references. These additional details must also be combined with other information commonly used when assessing medication use in adults (e.g., organ function, concomitant medications).

3 Growth and Development-Based Adverse Event Considerations

3.1 Impact of Medications on Growth and Development

Some growth and development parameters are objectively assessable (e.g., increases in height, increases in weight), while other are less so and require standardized clinical assessments (e.g., neurocognition, tooth/bone development). Importantly, growth and development are major longer-term safety outcomes commonly associated with medication use in children. This type of outcome is unique to children as adults are typically not developing substantially in regard to height or cognitive function over time, and weight gain is typically considered a negative outcome. Importantly, growth rates are individualized to the patient and based on trends over time in relation to the wide range of population norms versus being in or outside of a narrowly focused constant range.

A well-known example of medications impacting growth and development includes the use of inhaled corticosteroids, which are a cornerstone of long-term management of asthma. There are studies showing that limited systemic exposure to patients during treatments may lead to stunting of growth in children [26]. These risks are generally not considered significant (usually minimal changes seen in height at adulthood), especially in comparison to the benefits of asthma control with their use. Clinicians should be aware of this concern and prepared to have a risk versus benefit discussion with patients and families and it generally does not preclude use. Notably, as described elsewhere in this chapter, corticosteroids do have more significant risk when administered systemically in higher dosages for a prolonged period and thus should be used in that manner only when definitively needed.

Another well-described example of medication impact on growth and development is tooth discoloration as an ADR of tetracycline antibiotics. Permanent tooth discoloration has been described with prolonged and higher dose administration of tetracycline in children during the development of permanent teeth, which ends around approximately 8 years of age. While an important consideration, newer tetracyclines like doxycycline have been shown to be safe to administer in short courses (generally defined as <21 days), especially in cases of life-threatening diseases (e.g., Rocky Mountain Spotted Fever) [27].

In addition to assessing for body/skeletal growth, there is a concern that utilization of medications in young children can impact neurologic development later in life. Assessment of this outcome requires potentially subjective and multifaceted neurocognitive scales used at various time points throughout early childhood. In the neonatal period, the use of systemic dexamethasone has controversially been associated with adverse neurocognitive outcomes at 2 years. The use of this medication in neonates can help improve short-term outcomes (e.g., time to extubation) but has the possible concern for long-term neurocognitive toxicities (e.g., development delay, cerebral palsy, decreased neurocognitive scale scores) [28, 29]. Morphine use in the preterm neonatal period has also been associated with possible long-term neurocognitive ADEs that may resolve over time [30]. There is not an absolute contraindication to using these medications (and importantly they are likely a class effect), but practitioners should reserve use only for scenarios where there is a definite benefit. If the use is warranted, the lowest dose should be used for the shortest duration possible to minimize potential complications.

A challenge with long-term growth and development outcome is that it is hard to differentiate if the medication or other patient factors are impacting the development outcome that could not be controlled for. A prospective randomized controlled trail is often used to control for factors potentially impacting safety and efficacy outcomes. But this study design may take numerous years to complete in the pediatric population and prospective randomized controlled trials to evaluate adverse outcomes are ethically questionable, particularly in pediatric populations [28]. Routinely collected data, retrospective evaluative models, and healthcare registries are commonly used sources for pediatric medication safety analyses. Use of medications potentially impacting long-term neurocognitive outcomes usually involves a risk and benefit assessment to determine if the benefit to the patient would outweigh the risks of the ADR.

3.2 Impact of Growth and Development on Assessment of Safety Outcomes

Pediatric developmental milestones can also impact the ability to assess for certain ADR or harm associated with an ME [31]. Table 19.3 outlines select growth and development considerations and their impact on ADE for practical use by practitioners. For subjective assessment, a child must be able to communicate needed information regarding a possible ADR. This could be conveyed verbally or nonverbally via sign language or gestures. The age at which speech or other communication methods develop varies (generally around 2–3 years of age), but a non-communicative child cannot describe an ADR in the same way as an older child or adult. There are visual scales that allow children to pick pictures that suggest how they are feeling or the amount of pain they are in if nonverbal. Simple ADRs such as myalgias, headaches, changes in hearing, and visual field changes may not be clearly described by the patient and must be assessed during a thorough physical examination and potentially at follow-up visits relative with comparison to the baseline assessment before starting the medication.

Even after once a child is verbal, some children may not be able to describe an ADR in sufficient detail to a parent or caregiver to recognize it as such. Accurate description of subjective ADRs (e.g., headache, visual changes, pain) potentially related to the drug may not occur until 8 years of age or older. Patients who are developmentally delayed are also unable to verbalize possible ADRs for longer periods of time or at any time during their life. This makes assessment of subjective outcomes in the pediatric population difficult and potentially inaccurate. For example, long-term linezolid use has been associated with potentially severe optic and peripheral neuropathies [32]. Both of these ADRs require a patient to describe the ADR to a practitioner, making use of linezolid less desirable in children if another treatment option exists. Practitioners should be aware of medications with severe ADRs requiring subjective assessment when deciding among the available medications to use in children.

3.3 Objective Adverse Drug Reaction Assessment Considerations

In addition to subjective challenges with ADR assessment in children based on communication challenges, there are also laboratory limitations

Table 19.3 Select developmental milestones and impact on adverse drug events

Milestone	Approximate age	Impact on pediatric adverse drug events
Body movements/facial expressions	1–2 months	– Cognitive outcomes like sedation or somnolence are hard to assess when movements are minimal in the neonatal period – Assessment of pain is difficult and relies on grimacing and vital signs
Crawling	6–9 months	– Increased accuracy of assessment for joint/bone adverse events – Increased accuracy of assessment for neurologic toxicities impacting gross motor skills
Fine motor control resulting in feeding via hands	1 year of age	– Increased potential of unintentional overdoses
Walking	12–18 months	– Further increased accuracy of assessment for joint/bone issues compared to the crawling phase – Further increased accuracy of assessment for neurologic toxicity impacting gross motor skills as compared to the crawling phase
Verbal communication	– Nonspecific sounds <2 years – Nonspecific words 2–4 years	– Increased ability to communicate effectively regarding subjective adverse events (e.g., pain, vision changes)
Multiple fine, gross motor, and cognitive skills	2 years of age	– Increased ability to utilize multifaceted neurocognitive scales to assess overall development
Swallowing solid dosage forms	4–8 years (variability)	– Unable to swallow pills, increased use of liquid medications, and increased errors – Increased use of off-label compounded products – Increased reliance on intravenous and intramuscular dosage forms if liquids are not available
Cognition	8 years	– Increased ability of patient correlating adverse effects with receipt of a medication – Increased ability to describe a subjective adverse effect – Neurocognitive assessments as an outcome have increased accuracy
Completed vertical growth and reproductive organs	Fully developed in late adolescent/early adult (variable)	– Puberty allows for accurate assessment of impacts on height and reproductive organs – Prior to finishing vertical growth, growth is assessed based on trends over time as compared to others in the population without a stable baseline for comparison

that impact the determination of appropriate laboratory-based ADRs in children. Some laboratory values could require collection of 3 mL or more of blood to best conduct the required laboratory tests. Collection of numerous blood samples per day can impact the total fluid and blood volume of pediatric patients, especially neonates and preterm infants, and make providers reluctant to obtain laboratory values frequently to assess for an objective ADR. When samples are obtained, they also tend to be hemolyzed or less accurate due to limited volume issues with the sample or if they were obtained via heel sticks. Some laboratory values are also less standardized in terms of normal values for children. For example, while formulas to estimate creatinine clearance are available in children, the definition of acute kidney injury can vary substantially between recommended guideline references [33]. These practical differences make laboratory assessment of ADRs in pediatric patients more challenging than among adults.

3.4 Medications with Fewer Adverse Drug Reactions in Children

Much of pharmacovigilance in the pediatric population is focused on a higher risk of ADR in children, although it is important to highlight that some ADRs may be less common in the pediatric population due to physiologic differences. For example, *Clostridioides difficile*-associated acute colitis is less prevalent in children, especially infants <1 year of age due to possible favorable microbiota [34]. Amphotericin B conventional has been associated with less nephrotoxicity in neonates compared to adults and is considered the first-line treatment in this population [35].

3.5 Safety Data Limitations in Children and Possible Solutions

The ADR determination and assessment challenges described above impact not only daily practice but also the availability of high-quality data regarding ADRs in children. Many ADRs take years of well-designed studies and adequate sample sizes to make definite attributions. Prospective pediatric studies are commonly small in size, in part due to difficulty in recruiting sufficient patients and ethical considerations regarding undertaking clinical trials in children [36]. Because of these limitations, many prospective randomized studies are stopped early due to slow recruitment and safety analyses are based on a relatively small number of patients who received the medication. Retrospective studies after widespread utilization of a given medication are commonly performed to provide needed medication safety data.

With the enhancement of health information technology (HIT) in clinical practice around the world, there have been automated systems implemented to detect ADRs (e.g., trigger tools), electronic tracking systems developed, and large databases created in an attempt to more easily identify and quantify ADRs, including infrequent ones [23, 37, 38]. The manufacturers of new drugs without robust safety analyses done during clinical trials may be required to report additional ADR assessments longitudinally. These mechanisms have increased our knowledge regarding ADRs with the use of medications; however, a reactive approach after an occurrence of an ADR still continues due to limited knowledge of ADRs prior to widescale use of medications in the pediatric population.

4 Medication Prescribing and Safe Utilization Considerations

Pediatric medication prescribing is considered more complicated than prescribing of medications in the adult patient, with ME reported in 13% of pediatric prescriptions in the inpatient setting [39]. Major causes of prescribing errors were due to fundamental differences within pediatric age-groups and the required dosages, calculations based on age or body weight, and off-label prescribing [40]. The disparate complexity compared to adults was highlighted in a landmark study suggesting that children were at three-fold higher risk for potential ADEs compared to adults [41].

The prescription and administration phases have been reported as the two most error-prone steps in the medication use process for pediatric patients. It has been reported that 27–74% of MEs often originate at the prescription phase of the medication use process, with errors during administration comprising 13–55% [38, 41, 42]. Differences between proportional error origination are typically due to the inclusion of actual ADE vs. possible ADE (e.g., those not reaching the patient or not causing harm) and the introduction of medication safety initiatives focused on reducing errors originating at a specific phase of the medication use process (e.g., prescribing error reduction with computerized provider order entry). Importantly, MEs are often multifactorial and many errors originating at the beginning of the medication use process are propagated by other phases of the medication use process.

At institutions caring for children, it is prudent to ensure that practitioners have the needed mathematical calculation skills to safely prescribe medications for children. If an institution cares for a significant proportion of adult and pediatric patients, it is important to have a pediatric-specific medication safety officer who is well trained about pediatric-specific safety issues. Numerous studies have repeatedly illustrated reduced prescribing errors with unit-based clinical pharmacists available to assist with the prescription process at the time of prescribing [43, 44]. Thus, it is recommended that institutions caring for pediatric patients have clinical pharmacists focused on optimizing drug use in pediatric patients. The sections below and Table 19.4 outline the primary phases of the medication use process and error-prone aspects of those phases specific to the pediatric population. This information can be used to devise target educational initiatives and best utilize pharmacist and other practitioner's efforts to most effectively prevent MEs.

4.1 Prescribing Errors: Medication Selection

Prescribing of an ideal medication for a pediatric patient for a given indication can be difficult, primarily due to age-related warnings or complications, some of which were described previously in this chapter. Another example is the use of sodium phosphate rectal enema solutions which are commonly used in the adult population but can cause severe electrolyte abnormalities and acute kidney injury (even death) in infants. Thus, this medication is typically avoided in this population. Salicylate products are also not ideal for use in children when they have influenza or varicella due to the risk of Reye's syndrome. A more complete list of medications and common warnings/contraindications is provided elsewhere [21]. It is important for practitioners to know that some medications should be avoided whenever possible in certain pediatric age-groups.

In addition to many known safety concerns about medications approved by a regulatory agency for use, other complications may be relatively unknown due to the lack of data at the time of approval. Approximately 50% of FDA-approved medications in the United States with possible pediatric utilization did not have appropriate pediatric labeling, although recent initiatives have increased the number of products with pediatric labeling [45, 46]. In Europe, off-label prescribing (generally considered prescribing outside of recommendations by national or international drug regulatory agencies for drug dosing based on age and indication) can range widely from 13% to 69% in the inpatient setting and has been reported up to 100% in the outpatient setting in some countries [47]. These off-label uses can even be found in professional society-endorsed practice guidelines. For example, metronidazole remains a first-line treatment option and has been used for decades in the treatment of *Clostridioides difficile* infections in children in the United States, but it still does not have an FDA-labeled indication for use in children for this indication [48].

Medication utilization could be considered off-label due solely to the patient's age, the indication being used for, dose or regimen being used, or other reasons. Labeling requirements vary among countries. In some scenarios, medications have to be used out of clinical necessity in the pediatric population in the absence of other options. Optimal prescribing and safety considerations in the pediatric population are often unknown at the time of a new medication approval and are typically not required in most countries, although some countries have offered incentives for submitting pediatric data [45]. While many countries will have different laws regarding off-label prescribing, prescribers may need to in some scenarios inform patients that they are prescribing a medication that is not labeled by a regulatory agency for use in the specific patient for the desired indication. This may be considered compassionate use depending on the medication being prescribed. Institutions may also consider obtaining consent and assent as is commonly done when enrolling cognitively capable children in clinical trials for certain high-risk medications that have minimal data related to use in the pediatric population [49].

Table 19.4 Select medication use process stage and pediatric safety considerations

Medication process stage	Additional steps needed in the pediatric population	Resulting medication error (ME) concerns
Prescription and order verification	1. Age-/weight-related contraindications 2. Inclusion of weight and age in addition to other factors considered in adults 3. Less reliable renal function equations 4. Decreased well-designed studies in children	1. Possibly severe preventable ADE if alternatives exist 2. Increased potential of calculation errors or drug selection errors resulting in preventable ME 3. Less precise dosing in renal dysfunction 4. Increased chance of unknown event occurrence
Dispensing	1. Excipient age-/weight-specific warnings and contraindications 2. Measurement errors 3. Concentration selection errors	1. Possible selection errors resulting in harm 2. Incorrect dosage errors 3. Incorrect dosage errors
Administration	1. Lack of intravenous access 2. Possible division of IM/SQ injections 3. Inability to swallow tablets/pills 4. Patient refusal/agitation upon administration	1. Required IM/SQ administration 2. Increased injection site reactions and error potential 3. Increased risk of error due to liquid/compounded products 4. Inaccurate receipt of medication
Monitoring	1. Communication primarily with family 2. Inability to express subjective adverse events 3. Possible inability to tolerate significant volume loss needed for laboratory values	1. Missed adverse events due to nonspecific symptoms 2. Missed adverse events due to nonspecific symptoms 3. Inability to accurately assess for adverse events

ADE Adverse drug event, *IM* Intramuscular, *ME* Medication error, *SQ* Subcutaneous

4.2 Prescribing Errors: Appropriate Dosing

Once an appropriate medication is decided upon, there is also a process of prescribing a safe dose for infants and children when the appropriate dose is known. Most medications are prescribed based on a patient's weight and this calculation step can prove to be difficult. As previously described, incorrect dose determination is a large contributor to medication prescribing errors [39, 40]. This dose determination also may include converting a mg dose to an appropriate volume due to product availability and administration considerations described later in this chapter. This multiple step process can lead to significant decimal point and unit errors when prescribing a dosage (possible 10- to 100-fold over- or underdoses). Sometimes these errors can lead to disastrous outcomes for the patient [50].

In addition to manual dosing calculation errors, as in other populations, a pediatric prescriber still needs to take into account the appropriate dose based on indication, which can vary multifold between indications (e.g., pneumonia vs. meningitis) and renal function-based dose estimates [51]. Some indication-based dosing recommendations, however, may not be based on well-controlled studies in children and thus may not provide optimal outcomes.

4.3 Dispensing and Preparation Errors: Product Selection and Preparation

Many children are unable to swallow tablets or capsules, and thus, liquid formulations are commonly utilized to administer medications. Some liquid formulations may be commercially available and others may need to be compounded by pharmacists after crushing or manipulating formulations designed for use in adults [52]. Once a dose is decided upon, there can be errors during compounding and/or when calculating a measurable volume for the desired dose in a pediatric patient. If liquid formulations are commercially available, they also often come in multiple concentrations, which can increase the potential for errors. For example, liquid iron products in children can come as an elixir containing alcohol (potentially unsafe for use in neonates and young infants) or nonalcohol-based formulations (solutions and syrups). These dosage forms can have 1.25- to 10-fold different concentrations among products available within a given country [53, 54]. Additionally, the products are labeled based on the amount of ferrous sulfate versus elemental iron (a 5 times difference), but most dosage recommendations are based on the amount of elemental iron [54]. A common error is prescribing based on the wrong concentration on the bottle in addition to inadvertently selecting the wrong dosage form. Consistent and clearly labeled descriptions (in the electronic ordering system and in storage areas) of concentrations based on different quantitative measurements of a given drug are important ways to prevent these concentration errors from occurring.

Medications administrated intravenously or intramuscularly may also be associated with complications. Many intravenous products do not have available premade strengths that provide the dosage required for many younger children. Thus, medications are often manipulated from their original packaging or compounded into a new formulation before administration. For example, enoxaparin premade dosages for pediatric weight ranges are not available in the outpatient setting and require utilization of a multidose vial to get appropriate doses for younger children and even the use of concentrated dosage forms to administer to young neonates [50, 55]. These adaptations have been hallmarks of pediatric care for decades, but can increase the risk of a dosing error due to inappropriate product selection and dispensing. A common strategy to prevent this type of error is to use standardized concentrations, and some societies have suggested to use national or international standardized concentrations to avoid errors during transitions in care.

Some products containing previously described excipients (e.g., benzyl alcohol) may be administered at unsafe dosages to extremely low birth weight infants [19, 20]. Depending on the practice setting, some of the dosage form selection may be done by pharmacists, along with nurses who may administer medications from storage areas. Other settings may have specific products selected by prescribers. Appropriate labeling on the product and potentially in electronic ordering systems stating that it should not be used in neonates is an important prevention strategy.

4.4 Administration Errors: Considerations

Administration of medications also differs in the pediatric population and has been reported to cause similar or more errors than at the prescribing phase. As previously discussed, medications for oral use are often administered as liquids versus tablets due to the need to measure accurate doses based on body weight or difficulty in swallowing tablets among infants and young children. It is important for practitioners to know the volume (e.g., mL) as well as strength (e.g., mg) for appropriate administration and double check the dosage calculation. However, if a caregiver is administering the medication, the volume is likely the most relevant to focus on during patient/caregiver counseling. Administering liquids to infants and children can be challenging due to poor palatability or other unfavorable features, leading to difficulty in ensuring administration of the desired entire doses over time. Flavoring or administration with a palatable food such as apple sauce is one strategy used to help mask the taste, but the impact of flavoring or food on drug potency is often unknown.

Intramuscular and subcutaneous medications also create unique challenges in the pediatric population. Due to altered muscle/tissue size in infants and young children, gluteal and vastus lateralis muscles are often preferred for administration compared to the deltoid in adults due to increased potential of local ADRs when administered into the deltoid. Additionally, the amount of volume that can be administered via this route to an infant and young child without causing excessive pain or local tissue damage is often less and changes based on their weight. This results in the need to divide a dose into multiple injections administered at different sites, and introduces multiple additional error-prone steps during dispensing and administration.

Administration of intravenous medications can also be problematic in children. While use of infusion pumps can increase safety of administering intravenous medications, errors may occur with infusion pump programming. Ideally the infusion pumps should be integrated with an electronic medical record and institutional standards should be set for common concentrations utilized [56]. The infusion pumps used may also have variability in flow rates which can delay administration of desired dose volumes at low rates and attainment of desired peak concentration of medications with short half-lives, leading to unintentional outcomes [57]. The strategy to avoid infusion pump issues is to dilute the medication from the initial concentration. While this prevents pump administration issues, it also could lead to mathematical errors or errors related to utilizing the incorrect product or programming the intravenous pump incorrectly. Some organizations (e.g., the Institute for Safe Medical Practices) have recommended flow rates to try and systemically combat this issue, but institutions may still have rate limits for use at their specific institutions. These issues illustrate examples of medication administration being more complex among infants and children compared to adults. Focused training for practitioners related to common mathematical calculations with respect to drug administration is necessary to avoid calculation errors during administration.

4.5 Health Information Technology and Pediatric Medication Use

Health information technology (HIT) adoption has greatly improved the safe use of medications in the pediatric population, although errors still persist and new types of errors occur possibly related to the HIT [58, 59]. The major innovations with prescribing have been with electronic medication administration records, computerized provider order entry (CPOE or electronic prescribing in the outpatient setting), and clinical decision support (CDS) functionalities [60–62]. While these were at times implemented together, they can be considered separate medication safety-related HIT advancements.

The transition to CPOE or electronic prescribing has been shown to make an impact primarily on preventing errors of manual transcription during prescribing (e.g., omitting information needed or handwriting misinterpretations) [61]. While implementation success has varied, CPOE is considered to have improved patient care and reduced ADEs [58, 63]. Importantly, implementation and modifications of CPOE systems require a large, multidisciplinary team-based approach to ensure all involved in the medication use process have input on the design and implementation. Inclusion of specific pediatric needs within the system is important. Some important aspects include common pediatric drug concentrations, pediatric-specific prescription order sentences, and other pediatric-centric HIT functionalities. This is especially important when the institution cares for adult and pediatric patients. It is highly recommended that pediatric practitioners are involved directly in building and customization of a system to ensure the system fits specific institutional needs and practices. After implementation, updates and continual practitioner educational efforts related to the appropriate use of the HIT are vital to ensure safe and effective use and prevent MEs using HIT.

CDS functionalities are meant to target errors in decision-making such as dosing calculation errors, drug interaction errors, unsafe drug selection errors, or prescribing of suboptimal treatments. A CDS functionality can include dosage calculators, order sets, interruptive and noninterruptive alerts to practitioners, drug-interaction alerts, and duplicate therapy alerts, to name a few [62]. In many systems, some of the CDS functionalities are capable of only alerting certain practitioners (e.g., prescribers, pharmacists, nurses). Many successful CDS implementations

Table 19.5 Medication use process and health information technology functionalities

Medication process stage	Pediatric health information technology functionality focused on error prevention
Prescription and verification	– Order sets and order sentences – Mandatory and pre-populated order entry fields (e.g., frequency, route, dose) – Automated dosage calculators – Dose and frequency range alerts – Automated renal function calculators – Renal function alerts – Highlighted antibiotic susceptibility reports and abnormal laboratory values
Dispensing	– Medication barcoding – Automated dispensing cabinets and medication carousels (it is important to note that some medications, like opioids, may not be legally allowed to be stored in these dispensing systems) – Prepopulated medication product selection fields – IV admixture compounders (e.g., PN compounder, robotic IV preparations) – Gravimetric scale technology for intravenous medication preparation – Standardizing concentrations of medications within an institution or within nearby institutions
Administration	– Automated infusion rate calculators – IV administration pumps (with or without preset limits on dosages and rates) – Electronic medication administration record with administration reminders – Patient and medication barcoding – Prepopulated administration considerations (e.g., warnings regarding administration of ciprofloxacin via gastric tube labeled on the medication administration record) – Prepopulated dosage forms or calculators for code situations (may also be considered to be related to prescribing)
Monitoring	– Formatting for lab value reporting with normal ranges – Prepopulated laboratory value orders within order sets for medications – Lab monitoring alerts within the electronic health record

PN Parenteral nutrition, *IV* Intravenous

have been described, although there is variability between functionalities and institutional customization is usually needed to apply CDS to local patient care settings [64, 65]. Dosing calculators and dosing alerts are the most pediatric-focused CDS functionalities and have led to decreases in dosing errors independent of CPOE. Use of calculator assistance is highly recommended at institutions caring for pediatric patients, although calculation training should still be utilized to ensure understanding of the system and prevent inappropriate use.

Table 19.5 provides some examples of HIT strategies to prevent errors at various phases of the medication use process. Alert-based CDS has the risk of causing alert fatigue due to too many unnecessary alerts, especially if not optimally designed or implemented [51, 66]. Customization of CDS systems to meet the unique patient needs at specific institutions has improved medication safety. Although improvements have been made, it's important for practitioners to know that after extensive adoption of HIT and CDS, 50% of errors are still likely not preventable by available HIT functionalities (e.g., due to HIT rule logic limitations and difficulties integrating HIT within clinical workflow) [38].

5 Summary and Conclusions

Medication safety is an essential component of medication utilization in the pediatric population. Care providers must be cognizant that the process of medication for ADR assessment and the type of ADRs that occur in the pediatric population are different when compared to other populations. These differences are largely due to developmental impacts on patient assessment, drug distribution, and possible drug toxicities. Providers should also be aware that the medication use process from prescription to administration usually involves more steps and thus is more error-prone in the pediatric population. Advancements in HIT have improved the safety of medication use in the pediatric population, although clinicians should still be aware that no system can fully prevent medication safety incidents.

6 Case Studies

6.1 Case Study 1

A care team is considering use of a betamethasone dipropionate 0.05% ointment (a topical high-potency corticosteroid) in a 9-month-old child with moderate severity eczema across 20% of the body, including some in the diaper area. The current prescription has two daily administrations to the affected area for 2 months.

1. *What are the most relevant pharmacokinetic differences compared to adults that impact the use of the medication in this patient?*
   (a) Infants <1 year of age have higher absorption of medications through their skin comparatively to adults leading to higher systemic exposure for topically administered corticosteroids.
2. *If the patient's team feels the patient requires this medication to treat their condition, what are the methods to minimize the possibility of an ADE in this patient?*
   (a) Potentially administer only as needed versus scheduled two times per day.
   (b) Do NOT apply this steroid to the diaper or face area. Consider a lower dose topical corticosteroid for eczema in those areas.
   (c) Avoid wrapping the area, which would increase absorption.
   (d) Ensure it is not the augmented form of betamethasone dipropionate.
   (e) Recommend consideration of other forms.
3. *What are the possible issues with assessing this patient for an ADE related to this medication?*
   (a) Since the patient is 9 months old, assessing for adverse events (e.g., growthstunting) could take months/years to assess for and are dependent on accurate weight and height measurements.
   (b) Subjective issues like headache due to intracranial hypertension, insomnia, or neurologic toxicities from corticosteroid use would be difficult to obtain.
4. *What are the possible methods to overcome the ADE assessment issues?*
   (a) Ensure weight and height measurements are done accurately and often to obtain a trend over time. Importantly, ensure the patient is weighed in a dry diaper each time for consistent assessment.
   (b) Consider frequent monitoring for hypothalamus pituitary adrenal function via cortisol stimulation tests.

6.2 Case Study 2

A team utilized morphine in a 2-month-old (8 weeks postnatal) former 27-week GA at birth during a procedural sedation for pain control/sedation. The prescriber verified with the team that patient didn't have significant prior opioid exposure and that the patient's weight was 5.4. The dosing guide the prescriber had on hand said morphine was typically dosed up to 0.6–0.8 mg/kg for infants <6 months, so the prescriber verbally ordered 3.3 mg IV to get faster onset and since the patient was NPO. Ten minutes later, the nurse entered the order in the computer system and got an alert that the dosage was too high but overrode the alert with an override reason that the patient is being monitored.

Thirty minutes after the dose, just as the procedure was being completed, the patient had decreased respiratory rate and oxygen saturations and required naloxone for reversal of opioid toxicity. When the team discussed what happened, the team realized the dosing weight used was in pounds versus kilograms. When double-checking the prescriber's reference and verifying with a pharmacist, it was realized that the dosing range used for calculations was for oral and not intravenous morphine, and the ranges were also for a total daily dose versus a single dose.

1. *What pediatric pharmacokinetic/pharmacodynamic considerations were important in this scenario?*
   (a) The patient was an infant based on age, but because the patient was born preterm the pharmacokinetics likely would resemble that of a neonate due to a PMA of only 35 weeks.
   (b) Neonates and preterm infants have decreased metabolism of morphine which can increase the chance of toxicities due to morphine.
   (c) Neonates/preterm infants are also more susceptible to respiratory depression with opioids compared to infants and children.
2. *Describe the pediatric factors associated with the error and resulting adverse event?*
   There were multiple calculation errors in this case leading to a ~13-fold overdose in this patient, which typically would receive up to 0.1 mg/kg/dose or 0.25 mg of IV morphine. Some of these are not as relevant when prescribing the same medication in adults.
   - The patient's weight in pounds was used instead of converting to kg, which is a 2.2-fold dosing error.
   - The oral dosage range was used instead of the intravenous range, which is at least a twofold higher dose.
   - The total daily dose range was used instead of the single dose range, which resulted in a four- to six-fold higher dose.
3. *During what stage(s) of the medication use process did this error start at?*
   This was a two-fold error, although the origin is most likely associated with the prescription phase. The incorrect interpretation of dosing recommendations and resulting calculation errors were clearly associated with decision-making during prescription. But there also was an error during the documentation and communication phase which led to the use of the incorrect dosing weight.
4. *What other stages of the medication use process were involved in the propagation of this error?*
   (a) Inappropriate communication/documentation was also involved in the error related to identifying the appropriate weight.
   (b) The error was continued/propagated by not being caught in the verification phase and administration phase (e.g., by nurses and others in the room).
5. *What is a prevention strategy for each stage of this process?*
   (a) Prescribing
   - Consider utilizing prepopulated dosing cards based on an accurate weight for common medications used during procedures.
   - Consider requiring entry of prescriptions in the computer system before administration unless it is an absolute emergency situation.

   (b) Verifying
   - Require double-checks or read backs for high-alert medications.
   - Consider requiring entry of prescriptions in the computer system with verification before administration unless it is an absolute emergency situation.
   - It appears alerts were available but not utilized at the appropriate time in this scenario. Education regarding alert overrides and the possibility for alert fatigue, especially for high-alert medications, should be done.

   (c) Dispensing
   - While not discussed in this case in detail, the correct morphine product without benzyl alcohol should be included in the automated dispensing cabinet for procedures involving preterm infants or neonates.
   - Consider nursing double-check when medications are being pulled from surgical boxes or medication storage machines outside of the pharmacy.

   (d) Administration
   - Ensure barcoding of correct product which may have caught that an incor-

rect vial size or number of vials was utilized.

(e) Documentation
- Ensure consistency between kg and pounds documentation in charts and also consider weight-based normal ranges with alerts as entry of a 5.5 kg 35-week PMA child would be on the higher end of normal or above the 95% for weight.

(f) Monitoring
- While an error was not made here as monitoring did occur, patients on high-risk medications should undergo appropriate monitoring (e.g., oxygen saturation and vitals in this scenario). This could be a required field or policy as part of an order set for some medications.

References

1. Nebeker RJ, Barach P, Samore MH. Clarifying adverse drug events: a clinician's guide to terminology, documentation, and reporting. Ann Intern Med. 2004;140(10):795–801. https://doi.org/10.7326/0003-4819-140-10-200405180-00009.
2. World Health Organization. Safety of medicines: a guide to detecting and reporting adverse drug reactions; 2002. https://www.who.int/publications/i/item/WHO-EDM-QSM-2002-2. Accessed 2 May 2023.
3. US Department of Health and Human Services, Food and Drug Administration, Center for Drug Evaluation and Research, Center for Biologics Evaluation and Research. Guidance for industry and investigators safety reporting requirements for INDs and BA/BE studies; 2012. https://www.fda.gov/media/79394/download. Accessed 2 May 2023.
4. Hardin AP, Hackell JM, Committee on Practice & Ambulatory Medicine. Age limit of pediatrics. Pediatrics. 2017;140(3) https://doi.org/10.1542/peds.2017-2151.
5. US Department of Health and Human Services, Food and Drug Administration, Center for Devices and Radiological Health. Guidance for industry and FDA staff: pediatric expertise for advisory panels; 2003. https://www.fda.gov/media/72451/download. Accessed 11 May 2022.
6. Engle WA, American Academy of Pediatrics Committee on the Fetus & Newborn. Age terminology during the perinatal period. Pediatrics. 2004;114(5):1362–4. https://doi.org/10.1542/peds.2004-1915.
7. World Health Organization. International statistical classification of diseases and related health problems (11th ed); 2023. https://icd.who.int/. Accessed 2 May 2023.
8. Landers S, Berry PL, Kearns GL, Kaplan SL, Rudolph AJ. Gentamicin disposition and effect on development of renal function in the very low birth weight infant. Dev Pharmacol Ther. 1984;7(5):285–302. https://doi.org/10.1159/000457178.
9. Lisby-Sutch SM, Nahata MC. Dosage guidelines for the use of vancomycin based on its pharmacokinetics in infants. Eur J Clin Pharmacol. 1988;35(6):637–42. https://doi.org/10.1007/BF00637600.
10. Ross EL, Heizer J, Mixon MA, Jorgensen J, Valdez CA, Czaja AS, Reiter PD. Development of recommendations for dosing of commonly prescribed medications in critically ill obese children. Am J Health Syst Pharm. 2015;72(7):542–56. https://doi.org/10.2146/ajhp140280.
11. Avent ML, Kinney JS, Istre GR, Whitfield MB. Gentamicin and tobramycin in neonates: comparison of a new extended dosing interval regimen with a traditional multiple daily dosing regimen. Am J Perinatol. 2002;19(8):413–20. https://doi.org/10.1055/s-2002-36836.
12. Kearns GL, Abdel-Rahman SM, Alander SW, Blowey DL, Leeder JS, Kauffman RE. Developmental pharmacology--drug disposition, action, and therapy in infants and children. N Engl J Med. 2003;349(12):1157–67. https://doi.org/10.1056/NEJMra035092.
13. Shirkey H. Therapeutic orphans. Pediatrics. 1999;104(3 Pt 2):583–4.
14. Shirkey, H. C. (2006). Therapeutic orphans—everybody's business. Ann Pharmacother, 40(6), 1174. doi:https://doi.org/10.1345/aph.140023.
15. Lietman PS. Chloramphenicol and the neonate—1979 view. Clin Perinatol. 1979;6(1):151–62.
16. Weiss CF, Glazko AJ, Weston JK. Chloramphenicol in the newborn infant. A physiologic explanation of its toxicity when given in excessive doses. N Engl J Med. 1960;262:787–94. https://doi.org/10.1056/NEJM196004212621601.
17. Nahata MC. Serum concentrations and adverse effects of chloramphenicol in pediatric patients. Chemotherapy. 1987;33(5):322–7. https://doi.org/10.1159/000238516.
18. LeBel M, Ferron L, Masson M, Pichette J, Carrier C. Benzyl alcohol metabolism and elimination in neonates. Dev Pharmacol Ther. 1988;11(6):347–56. https://doi.org/10.1159/000457714.
19. Nahata MC. Safety of "inert" additives or excipients in paediatric medicines. Arch Dis Child Fetal Neonatal Ed. 2009;94(6):F392–3. https://doi.org/10.1136/adc.2009.160192.
20. Gershanik J, Boecler B, Ensley H, McCloskey S, George W. The gasping syndrome and benzyl alcohol poisoning. N Engl J Med. 1982;307(22):1384–8. https://doi.org/10.1056/NEJM198211253072206.

21. Meyers RS, Thackray J, Matson KL, McPherson C, Lubsch L, Hellinga RC, Hoff DS. Key potentially inappropriate drugs in pediatrics: the KIDs list. J Pediatr Pharmacol Ther. 2020;25(3):175–91. https://doi.org/10.5863/1551-6776-25.3.175.
22. Bradley JS, Wassel RT, Lee L, Nambiar S. Intravenous ceftriaxone and calcium in the neonate: assessing the risk for cardiopulmonary adverse events. Pediatrics. 2009;123(4):e609–13. https://doi.org/10.1542/peds.2008-3080.
23. Christensen ML, Zareie P, Kadiyala B, Bursac Z, Reed MD, Mattison DR, Davis RL. Concomitant ceftriaxone and intravenous calcium therapy in infants. J Pediatr Pharmacol Ther. 2021;26(7):702–7. https://doi.org/10.5863/1551-6776-26.7.702.
24. Deboer MD, Boston BA. Failure-to-thrive in an infant following injection of capillary hemangioma with triamcinolone acetonide. Clin Pediatr (Phila). 2008;47(3):296–9. https://doi.org/10.1177/0009922807308744.
25. Tempark T, Phatarakijnirund V, Chatproedprai S, Watcharasindhu S, Supornsilchai V, Wananukul S. Exogenous Cushing's syndrome due to topical corticosteroid application: case report and review literature. Endocrine. 2010;38(3):328–34. https://doi.org/10.1007/s12020-010-9393-6.
26. Zhang L, Prietsch SO, Ducharme FM. Inhaled corticosteroids in children with persistent asthma: effects on growth. Cochrane Database Syst Rev. 2014;7:CD009471. https://doi.org/10.1002/14651858.CD009471.pub2.
27. Stultz JS, Eiland LS. Doxycycline and tooth discoloration in children: changing of recommendations based on evidence of safety. Ann Pharmacother. 2019;53(11):1162–6. https://doi.org/10.1177/1060028019863796.
28. Demauro SB, Dysart K, Kirpalani H. Stopping the swinging pendulum of postnatal corticosteroid use. J Pediatr. 2014;164(1):9–11. https://doi.org/10.1016/j.jpeds.2013.10.020.
29. Doyle, L. W., Cheong, J. L., Hay, S., Manley, B. J., & Halliday, H. L. (2021). Early (<7 days) systemic postnatal corticosteroids for prevention of bronchopulmonary dysplasia in preterm infants. Cochrane Database Syst Rev, 10, CD001146. doi:https://doi.org/10.1002/14651858.CD001146.pub6.
30. Steinhorn R, McPherson C, Anderson PJ, Neil J, Doyle LW, Inder T. Neonatal morphine exposure in very preterm infants-cerebral development and outcomes. J Pediatr. 2015;166(5):1200–1207 e1204. https://doi.org/10.1016/j.jpeds.2015.02.012.
31. Zubler JM, Wiggins LD, Macias MM, Whitaker TM, Shaw JS, Squires JK, et al. Evidence-informed milestones for developmental surveillance tools. Pediatrics. 2022;149(3) https://doi.org/10.1542/peds.2021-052138.
32. Nambiar S, Rellosa N, Wassel RT, Borders-Hemphill V, Bradley JS. Linezolid-associated peripheral and optic neuropathy in children. Pediatrics. 2011;127(6):e1528–32. https://doi.org/10.1542/peds.2010-2125.
33. Sutherland SM, Byrnes JJ, Kothari M, Longhurst CA, Dutta S, Garcia P, Goldstein SL. AKI in hospitalized children: comparing the pRIFLE, AKIN, and KDIGO definitions. Clin J Am Soc Nephrol. 2015;10(4):554–61. https://doi.org/10.2215/CJN.01900214.
34. Tang P, Roscoe M, Richardson SE. Limited clinical utility of Clostridium difficile toxin testing in infants in a pediatric hospital. Diagn Microbiol Infect Dis. 2005;52(2):91–4. https://doi.org/10.1016/j.diagmicrobio.2005.01.003.
35. Pappas PG, Kauffman CA, Andes DR, Clancy CJ, Marr KA, Ostrosky-Zeichner L, et al. Clinical Practice guideline for the Management of Candidiasis: 2016 update by the Infectious Diseases Society of America. Clin Infect Dis. 2016;62(4):e1–50. https://doi.org/10.1093/cid/civ933.
36. Benjamin DK Jr, Kaufman DA, Hope WW, Smith PB, Arrieta A, Manzoni P, et al. A phase 3 study of micafungin versus amphotericin B deoxycholate in infants with invasive candidiasis. Pediatr Infect Dis J. 2018;37(10):992–8. https://doi.org/10.1097/INF.0000000000001996.
37. Stockwell DC, Bisarya H, Classen DC, Kirkendall ES, Landrigan CP, Lemon V, et al. A trigger tool to detect harm in pediatric inpatient settings. Pediatrics. 2015;135(6):1036–42. https://doi.org/10.1542/peds.2014-2152.
38. Stultz JS, Nahata MC. Preventability of voluntarily reported or trigger tool-identified medication errors in a pediatric institution by information technology: a retrospective cohort study. Drug Saf. 2015;38(7):661–70. https://doi.org/10.1007/s40264-015-0303-y.
39. Ghaleb MA, Barber N, Franklin BD, Wong IC. The incidence and nature of prescribing and medication administration errors in paediatric inpatients. Arch Dis Child. 2010;95(2):113–8. https://doi.org/10.1136/adc.2009.158485.
40. Conn RL, Kearney O, Tully MP, Shields MD, Dornan T. What causes prescribing errors in children? Scoping review. BMJ Open. 2019;9(8):e028680. https://doi.org/10.1136/bmjopen-2018-028680.
41. Kaushal R, Bates DW, Landrigan C, McKenna KJ, Clapp MD, Federico F, Goldmann DA. Medication errors and adverse drug events in pediatric inpatients. JAMA. 2001;285(16):2114–20. https://doi.org/10.1001/jama.285.16.2114.
42. McClead RE Jr, Catt C, Davis JT, Morvay S, Merandi J, Lewe D, et al. An internal quality improvement collaborative significantly reduces hospital-wide medication error related adverse drug events. J Pediatr. 2014;165(6):1222–1229 e1221. https://doi.org/10.1016/j.jpeds.2014.08.063.
43. Kaushal R, Bates DW, Abramson EL, Soukup JR, Goldman DA. Unit-based clinical pharmacists' prevention of serious medication errors in pediatric inpatients. Am J Health Syst Pharm. 2008;65(13):1254–60. https://doi.org/10.2146/ajhp070522.

44. Wang JK, Herzog NS, Kaushal R, Park C, Mochizuki C, Weingarten SR. Prevention of pediatric medication errors by hospital pharmacists and the potential benefit of computerized physician order entry. Pediatrics. 2007;119(1):e77–85. https://doi.org/10.1542/peds.2006-0034.
45. Burckart GJ, Kim C. The revolution in pediatric drug development and drug use: therapeutic orphans no more. J Pediatr Pharmacol Ther. 2020;25(7):565–73. https://doi.org/10.5863/1551-6776-25.7.565.
46. Sachs AN, Avant D, Lee CS, Rodriguez W, Murphy MD. Pediatric information in drug product labeling. JAMA. 2012;307(18):1914–5. https://doi.org/10.1001/jama.2012.3435.
47. Schrier L, Hadjipanayis A, Stiris T, Ross-Russell RI, Valiulis A, Turner MA, et al. Off-label use of medicines in neonates, infants, children, and adolescents: a joint policy statement by the European Academy of Paediatrics and the European society for Developmental Perinatal and Pediatric Pharmacology. Eur J Pediatr. 2020;179(5):839–47. https://doi.org/10.1007/s00431-019-03556-9.
48. McDonald LC, Gerding DN, Johnson S, Bakken JS, Carroll KC, Coffin SE, et al. Clinical Practice guidelines for Clostridium difficile infection in adults and children: 2017 update by the Infectious Diseases Society of America (IDSA) and Society for Healthcare Epidemiology of America (SHEA). Clin Infect Dis. 2018;66(7):e1–e48. https://doi.org/10.1093/cid/cix1085.
49. Lagler FB, Hirschfeld S, Kindblom JM. Challenges in clinical trials for children and young people. Arch Dis Child. 2021;106(4):321–5. https://doi.org/10.1136/archdischild-2019-318676.
50. Ghaleb MA, Barber N, Franklin BD, Yeung VW, Khaki ZF, Wong IC. Systematic review of medication errors in pediatric patients. Ann Pharmacother. 2006;40(10):1766–76. https://doi.org/10.1345/aph.1G717.
51. Stultz JS, Porter K, Nahata MC. Sensitivity and specificity of dosing alerts for dosing errors among hospitalized pediatric patients. J Am Med Inform Assoc. 2014;21(e2):e219–25. https://doi.org/10.1136/amiajnl-2013-002161.
52. Nahata MC, Morosco RS, Brady MT. Extemporaneous sildenafil citrate oral suspensions for the treatment of pulmonary hypertension in children. Am J Health Syst Pharm. 2006;63(3):254–7. https://doi.org/10.2146/ajhp050208.
53. Mattiello V, Schmugge M, Hengartner H, von der Weid N, Renella R, et al. Diagnosis and management of iron deficiency in children with or without anemia: consensus recommendations of the SPOG Pediatric Hematology Working Group. Eur J Pediatr. 2020;179(4):527–45. https://doi.org/10.1007/s00431-020-03597-5.
54. Wang M. Iron deficiency and other types of anemia in infants and children. Am Fam Physician. 2016;93(4):270–8.
55. Bauman ME, Black KL, Bauman ML, Belletrutti M, Bajzar L, Massicotte MP. Novel uses of insulin syringes to reduce dosing errors: a retrospective chart review of enoxaparin whole milligram dosing. Thromb Res. 2009;123(6):845–7. https://doi.org/10.1016/j.thromres.2008.09.001.
56. Ni Y, Lingren T, Huth H, Timmons K, Melton K, Kirkendall E. Integrating and evaluating the data quality and utility of smart pump information in detecting medication administration errors: evaluation study. JMIR Med Inform. 2020;8(9):e19774. https://doi.org/10.2196/19774.
57. Snijder RA, Egberts TC, Lucas P, Lemmers PM, van Bel F, Timmerman AM. Dosing errors in preterm neonates due to flow rate variability in multi-infusion syringe pump setups: an in vitro spectrophotometry study. Eur J Pharm Sci. 2016;93:56–63. https://doi.org/10.1016/j.ejps.2016.07.019.
58. van Rosse F, Maat B, Rademaker CM, van Vught AJ, Egberts AC, Bollen CW. The effect of computerized physician order entry on medication prescription errors and clinical outcome in pediatric and intensive care: a systematic review. Pediatrics. 2009;123(4):1184–90. https://doi.org/10.1542/peds.2008-1494.
59. Walsh KE, Adams WG, Bauchner H, Vinci RJ, Chessare JB, Cooper MR, et al. Medication errors related to computerized order entry for children. Pediatrics. 2006;118(5):1872–9. https://doi.org/10.1542/peds.2006-0810.
60. Jani YH, Ghaleb MA, Marks SD, Cope J, Barber N, Wong IC. Electronic prescribing reduced prescribing errors in a pediatric renal outpatient clinic. J Pediatr. 2008;152(2):214–8. https://doi.org/10.1016/j.jpeds.2007.09.046.
61. Potts AL, Barr FE, Gregory DF, Wright L, Patel NR. Computerized physician order entry and medication errors in a pediatric critical care unit. Pediatrics. 2004;113(1 Pt 1):59–63.
62. Stultz JS, Nahata MC. Computerized clinical decision support for medication prescribing and utilization in pediatrics. J Am Med Inform Assoc. 2012;19(6):942–53. https://doi.org/10.1136/amiajnl-2011-000798.
63. Han YY, Carcillo JA, Venkataraman ST, Clark RS, Watson RS, Nguyen TC, et al. Unexpected increased mortality after implementation of a commercially sold computerized physician order entry system. Pediatrics. 2005;116(6):1506–12. https://doi.org/10.1542/peds.2005-1287.
64. Kazemi A, Ellenius J, Pourasghar F, Tofighi S, Salehi A, Amanati A, Fors UG. The effect of computerized physician order entry and decision support system on medication errors in the neonatal ward: experiences from an Iranian teaching hospital. J Med

Syst. 2011;35(1):25–37. https://doi.org/10.1007/s10916-009-9338-x.
65. Stultz JS, Nahata MC. Appropriateness of commercially available and partially customized medication dosing alerts among pediatric patients. J Am Med Inform Assoc. 2014;21(e1):e35–42. https://doi.org/10.1136/amiajnl-2013-001725.
66. Cash JJ. Alert fatigue. Am J Health Syst Pharm. 2009;66(23):2098–101. https://doi.org/10.2146/ajhp090181.

Further Reading

Pain Scales for Non-verbal Children

Trottier ED, Ali S, Doré-Bergeron MJ, Chauvin-Kimoff L. Best practices in pain assessment and management for children. *Paediatr Chiler*. Health. 2022;179(4):27(7):429-448. https://doi.org/10.1093/pch/pxac048.

Ethical Considerations for Children in Research

Cayouette F, O'Hearn K, Gertsman S, Menon K. Operationalization of assent for research participation in pre-adolescent children: a scoping review. BMC Med Ethics. 2022;23(1):106. https://doi.org/10.1186/s12910-022-00844-2.

Example Recommendations for Standardized Drug Concentrations for Use in the Pediatric Population

American Society for Health Systems Pharmacists Standardize 4 Safety. Pediatric Continuous Infusion Standards; updated March 2024. Accessed 4/10/2024. Available at: https://www.ashp.org/-/media/assets/pharmacy-practice/s4s/docs/Pediatric-Infusion-Standards.pdf. Accessed 10 April 2024

Safe Prescribing and Monitoring in the Older Person

20

Alpana Rajesh Mair, Amil Rajesh Mair, Sarah N. Hilmer, and Lisa Kouladjian O'Donnell

Abstract

This chapter will consider the main factors that increase the risk of adverse drug reactions and events in older people. This will include changes in physiology that affect the older person. It will also outline how older people should be prioritized for medication review and the monitoring that is needed to minimize harm, while optimizing patient outcomes from the use of medications. The chapter will also discuss the essential factors to be considered while prescribing and the monitoring that is needed to improve medication use and safety in this group. Various tools and methods that could be employed when prescribing and selecting medications that are considered appropriate for this population, including tools to review appropriate prescribing, monitoring of medication use, at the various levels of delivery of patient care and at a systems level, will be discussed. Medications which require special consideration among this group of patients will also be discussed, including review of existing medication and, in particular, the importance of patient prioritization due to high-risk medication use. Case studies will be used to illustrate how a person-centered approach can be taken in the reviews, including shared decision-making.

A. R. Mair (✉)
Prescribing and Therapeutics Division, Scottish Government, Edinburgh, UK

Edinburgh Napier University, Edinburgh, UK
e-mail: alpana.mair@gov.scot

A. R. Mair
Emergency Medicine, NHS North East England, BMJ Best Practice Clinical Champion, Newcastle-Upon-Tyne, UK

S. N. Hilmer
Kolling Institute, The University of Sydney and Northern Sydney Local Health District and Departments of Clinical Pharmacology and Aged Care, Royal North Shore Hospital, St Leonards, Australia

L. Kouladjian O'Donnell
School of Pharmacy, Faculty of Medicine and Health, The University of Sydney, Sydney, Australia

Laboratory of Ageing and Pharmacology, Kolling Institute, The University of Sydney and Northern Sydney Local Health District, St Leonards, Australia

Keywords

Older person · Person-centered · Medication-related harm · Pharmacokinetics and pharmacodynamics · Prescribing safety · Monitoring · Medication safety culture · Geriatric syndrome · Polypharmacy · Deprescribing

Learning Objectives

- Understand the factors that predispose the older person to medication-related harm
- Understand how medicines can impact healthy aging and geriatric syndromes

J. Jose et al. (eds.), *Principles and Practice of Pharmacovigilance and Drug Safety*,
https://doi.org/10.1007/978-3-031-51089-2_20

- Apply the principles of structured medication review and monitoring to improve medication safety
- Adopt strategies and tools to implement person-centered medication review
- Understand the importance of multidisciplinary team decision-making and safe prescribing culture

Key Points

- Multimorbidity increases with age and affects pharmacokinetics and pharmacodynamics. Consequently, older people have a high prevalence of medication use and medication-related harm.
- Adverse effects of medications frequently present as non-specific geriatric syndromes, such as falls, delirium, incontinence, or frailty.
- In clinical practice involving older persons, pharmacovigilance is critical to prevent, detect, and manage medication-related harm.
- Reporting of unexpected or severe adverse drug events seen clinically in older patients is important since post-marketing surveillance is a major source of information on medication effects in this population.
- Tools to inform pharmacovigilance include prescribing tools to guide clinical medication reviews and quality indicators at a health service level.
- Medication safety in older people requires constant review, good communication, and shared decision-making between all members of the clinical team in collaboration with the patient.

1 Introduction

Prescribing and safe use of medications in the older person poses a unique challenge. With an aging population and the presence of comorbidities with aging, the number of older people taking multiple medications is increasing. This, together with the associated age-related changes in physiology, puts the older person at an increased risk of medication-related harm. Regular review of medications is important at initiation of treatment, but also when patients transition across different levels of care.

Therefore, to prevent harm due to medications, clinical management of older people will require:

- Review of existing medications to consider whether the presenting problem is the result of medication-related harm, and before new medications are added
- Assess if doses may need to be adjusted to accommodate changes in aging physiology
- Identify the medications most likely to cause harm in this group
- Use of tools to guide prescribing and deprescribing
- A person-centered approach
- Involve the older person and their family in their care to support shared decision-making and adherence

This chapter introduces readers to how medication use is different in older people, the steps to be taken at various stages of medication use to ensure that harm is minimized, and the need for a multidisciplinary approach in managing this special group of patients.

2 Global Aging and Consequences

The proportion of the global population over 60 years old will increase from 12% in 2015 to 22% in 2050 [1]. During this period, their number in developing countries is projected to increase 250%, compared to 71% in developed countries [1], so that in 2050, 80% of older people will be living in low- and middle-income countries. In Europe, advances in healthcare, education, and socioeconomic circumstance mean that in most countries people can now expect to live beyond the age of 80 [2]. However, evidence shows that the average healthy life years (HLY) for EU citizens is only 61 years, meaning that many people are living for around 20 years in suboptimal health. One aspect that can affect HLY is medication, which can have an impact on both physical and cognitive capacity of the older person.

3 Increasing Multimorbidity with Age

Multimorbidity is defined by the World Health Organization (WHO) as the co-occurrence of two or more chronic health conditions in one person [3]. Patients with multimorbidity may require medicines to treat each condition, which can lead to polypharmacy. Currently around 50 million EU citizens are estimated to have multimorbidity. Most of them are 65 years of age and over, and this number is expected to continue to increase [4]. Epidemiological data indicates that multimorbidity increases markedly with age. In a Scottish study, multimorbidity was prevalent in 81.5% of individuals aged 85 years and over, with a mean number of 3.62 morbidities [5]. The most common morbidities are noncommunicable diseases, which occur 10–15 years earlier in deprived areas than in more affluent. Ornstein et al. found that the most prevalent chronic conditions in primary care were hypertension (33.5%), hyperlipidemia (33.0%), and depression (18.7%) [6]. The presence of multiple morbidities is associated with multiple symptoms, impairments, and disabilities.

Multimorbidity may result in a combined negative effect on physical and mental health, and can have a major impact on a person's quality of life, limiting daily activities and reducing mobility [7, 8]. The need to take multiple medications can be just as problematic, resulting in frequent healthcare contacts and an increase in the likelihood of medication-related harm [9]. The population aged over 60 consumes nearly three times more medicines as the general population, but with an adherence to long-term medication ranging only between 25% and 70% [10]. Age and the number of medications taken are the two major predictors of the risk of experiencing a medication-related harm [11].

Furthermore, multimorbidity imposes a large economic burden to the health service due to patients' complexity of healthcare needs and frequent interaction with health services, which may be fragmented, ineffective, and incomplete [12]. People with multimorbidity utilize twice as many primary care services and are three times as likely to be hospitalized than their non-multi-morbid counterparts [13]. Other factors to consider are those with underlying illness such as the management of blood-borne viruses (e.g., hepatitis, HIV), cancer, and vascular disease, as these individuals are living longer due to the improved treatment and subsequent survival. As a consequence, these older people will be taking medications for multiple chronic diseases. A fourfold increase in drug interactions is observed in older people living with HIV [14].

Case study 1 discusses the case of an elderly lady with multiple morbidities and potential medication-related harm to understand the related issues.

4 Impact of Aging on Pharmacokinetics and Pharmacodynamics

The physiological changes of aging affect how the body handles drugs (pharmacokinetics) and how drugs affect the body (pharmacodynamics). Pharmacokinetic changes in aging are better characterized than pharmacodynamic changes and are summarized in Fig. 20.1. The most significant pharmacokinetic changes in old age are reduced drug metabolism and excretion. Consequently, maintenance dose may need to be reduced to obtain similar serum concentrations of drugs to those seen in younger people. Toxicity can be seen in older people who use usual adult therapeutic doses of chronic medications.

Age is only one of many variables that impact on clinical pharmacokinetics. Other factors persist with increasing age, e.g., sex, weight, smoking, alcohol use, and there may be increased exposure over a long life. Multimorbidity and polypharmacy increase in old age and are responsible for drug–disease and drug–drug interactions. Many clinical conditions influence

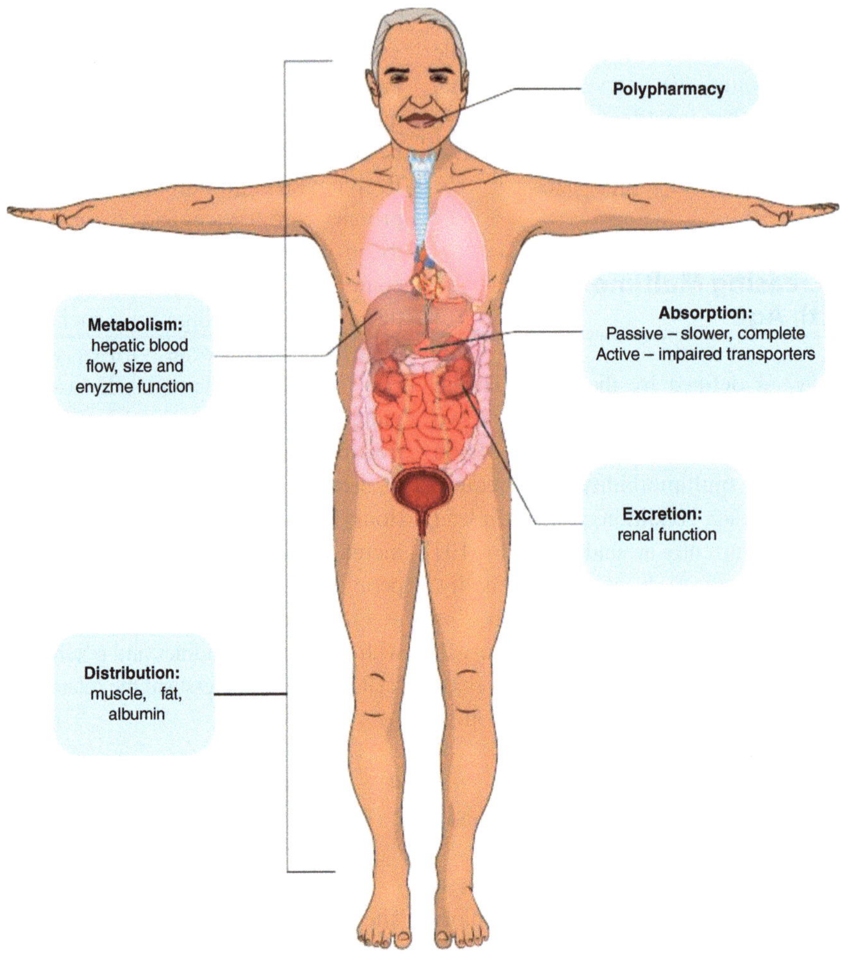

Fig. 20.1 Common pharmacokinetic changes in drug use, absorption, distribution, metabolism, and excretion in old age

pharmacokinetics and pharmacodynamics [15, 16]. There is limited research characterizing the effects of frailty as a source of variability in pharmacokinetics and pharmacodynamics among older people [17].

Digoxin provides an example of the complexity of pharmacokinetics and pharmacodynamics in old age. Clearance of digoxin, which is predominantly excreted unchanged by the kidneys, is reduced by age-related decline in glomerular filtration and tubular secretion, compounded by the effects of common chronic diseases in old age such as diabetes, hypertension, and cardiovascular disease, and exacerbated by acute renal failure during acute illness or injury. Drug interactions may occur by blockage of renal transporters involved in active secretion of digoxin by commonly used drugs in older people, such as erythromycin or verapamil, resulting in digoxin toxicity. Pharmacodynamically, the most serious adverse effects of digoxin are cardiac arrhythmias. Susceptibility to these is likely to be increased with the increased prevalence of underlying cardiovascular disease in old age and the increased prevalence of hypokalemia and hypomagnesemia, which are very common with concurrent use of diuretics or proton pump inhibitors. Even the less serious adverse effects of digoxin, such as nausea, can precipitate serious malnutrition in an older person. Safe use of a narrow therapeutic index drug like digoxin requires constant vigilance with frequent clinical and therapeutic drug monitoring and proactive dose adjustment.

5 Aging, Medication-Related Harm, and Pharmacovigilance

One of the consequences of polypharmacy in older adults is medication-related harm, which can include harm from adverse drug reactions (ADRs), nonadherence, and medication errors. Factors such as age-related changes in pharmacokinetics and pharmacodynamics, reduced physiological reserve, and a higher prevalence of cognitive impairment can predispose older adults to medication-related harm.

Between 1988 and 2021, 250,000 hospital admissions in Australia were medication-related, with an associated cost of AUD$1.4 (€920) billion annually [18]. Importantly, two-thirds of the medication-related hospitalizations were potentially preventable. In the UK, it was estimated that there are 237 million medication errors in England over a year period [19], and preventable ADRs were estimated to cost the National Health Service (NHS) £98.5 (€115) million per annum, consume 181,626 bed days, and cause/contribute to 1708 deaths during initial hospitalization. Additionally, certain environments may increase patients' risks of developing medication-related problems. These include transitions of care, such as transition from hospital to the home or residential care, due to changes in medications, poor communication between transition, and problems with medication adherence. A systematic review found that 17–51% of community dwelling patients discharged from hospital within 30 days experienced medication-related harm [20]. The effects of medication-related harm include disability, hospitalization, and death [20]. It is estimated that in the USA, adverse drug events will be responsible for at least 4.6-million hospitalizations of older people and as many as 150,000 premature deaths over the next decade, with economic cost of medical care to treat adverse drug events about $62 billion [21]. The Organisation for Economic Cooperation and Development (OECD) found older people in long-term care settings were at an increased risk of medication-related harm [4]. Interestingly, a Norwegian study reported that more medication-related problems were found for patients who were frail, receiving nursing home care in their own homes, rather than those residents in nursing homes [22].

Specific to the older person, there are many challenges prescribers face that can impede appropriate prescribing, especially with multiple prescribers and multiple patient comorbidities. Avoiding the "prescribing cascade" is one such challenge—when a new medicine is prescribed to "treat" a side effect of another medicine, in the mistaken belief that a new medical condition requiring treatment has developed [23]. In younger individuals, side effects may be easier to differentiate; however, given the complexities of older adults, multimorbidity and polypharmacy, a side effect can be misdiagnosed as a new condition. For example, dihydropyridine calcium channel blockers, such as amlodipine, are commonly prescribed for hypertension and can often result in peripheral edema in the individual. Treatment of peripheral edema with loop diuretics, such as furosemide, can increase the risk of adverse events such as falls and hospitalization, and can potentially decrease quality of life [24]. A simpler solution for addressing the peripheral edema would be to reduce the dose of amlodipine, while monitoring for side effects and blood pressure goals, considering if an alternative medication should be prescribed in place.

Identifying medications that may predispose an older person to medication-related harm can be challenging for healthcare practitioners. Several tools have been developed to identify high-risk or potentially inappropriate medications, and these include explicit and implicit criteria, such as The Beers Criteria [25] and the Screening Tool of Older Person's Prescriptions/ Screening Tool to Alert Doctors to the Right Treatment (STOPP/START) [26]. These criteria have been studied extensively in older people to evaluate their effects on medication-related harm and ADRs [27, 28]. Other tools such as The Drug Burden Index (DBI); a measure of the cumulative exposure to anticholinergic and sedative medications in an older person can be used to estimate the impact of high-risk medications on clinical measures such as physical function [29]. In practice, these measures are all potentially useful clinical risk assessment and screening tools. However, clinical decisions require assessment of the risk of harm in the individual (which is variable) and the potential benefit of treatment.

Case study 2 discusses about an older person with high anticholinergic and sedative burden to understand the contribution of multimorbidity and polypharmacy on medication-related harm and the role of pharmacovigilance in reducing it.

6 Undertaking Person-Centered Medication Review

When undertaking medication reviews, it is important to involve the older person and their carer in the decision-making about the medications they are taking, considering "what matters to you." One example is the seven-step approach taken to review medication [30] (Fig. 20.2: *Seven steps to appropriate polypharmacy)*. The seven-step approach starts by matching therapeutic objectives to current life priorities with the patient. This initial discussion guides decision-making in subsequent steps that consider medication need, effectiveness, and safety before a therapeutic plan and follow-up strategy are agreed upon. Determining the therapeutic objectives with the patient's current life priorities (step 1) allows decision about whether the right medication has been chosen, followed by assessing whether the medicines are essential (step 2) or unnecessary (step 3), whether therapeutic objectives that matter to the patient are achieved (step 4), which medicines are too risky or cause unacceptable adverse effects (step 5), which medicines are not cost-effective or more harmful to the environment (step 6), and whether the patient is willing and able to manage their medicines in a way that avoids harm and maximizes benefit (step 7).

Medication reviews can be conducted in multiple settings, such as within the home, residential aged care facility, or hospital, and by multiple practitioners, including pharmacists, general practitioners, and specialist physicians. There are various models of medication review service provision internationally. In the USA, the Medication Therapy Management (MTM) service aims to ensure the best therapeutic outcomes for patients and includes five elements: medication therapy review, a personal medication record, a medication-related action plan, intervention or referral, and documentation and follow-up [31]. In a study that evaluated the collaboration between physicians and pharmacists providing the MTM service for 150 patients, physicians accepted 47–50% of recommendations made by pharmacists to stop or change medications for patients with polypharmacy and demonstrated that patients benefited from collaboration between physicians and pharmacists [32]. The Home Medicines Review (HMR) and Residential Medication Management Review (RMMR) are two established, government-funded pharmacist-led medication review services available in Australia [33]. A study that aimed to evaluate RMMRs on medication use appropriateness in 223 aged care residents demonstrated a reduction in inappropriate prescribing among aged care residents [34]. Across the UK health services, there are GP practice pharmacists who are working as part of the multidisciplinary teams, and part of their roles will be to undertake medication reviews. In Scotland, in 2012, policy was introduced for pharmacists to work as part of the multidisciplinary teams to undertake polypharmacy reviews using the seven-step process, and was also introduced as part of the GP contract for those patients who needed anticipatory care plans [35]. Many pharmacists across the UK are independent prescribers, which allows for the prescribed medications to be altered and amended by the reviewing pharmacist. Across England, medicines optimization services have been developed for pharmacists to deliver structured medication reviews as part of contracted enhanced services [36].

While undertaking medication reviews, it is important to consider the older person's goals and preferences, together with their current medical conditions and medications. Shared decision-making during medication review can open the conversation with older people, allowing them to express their preferences and improve patient

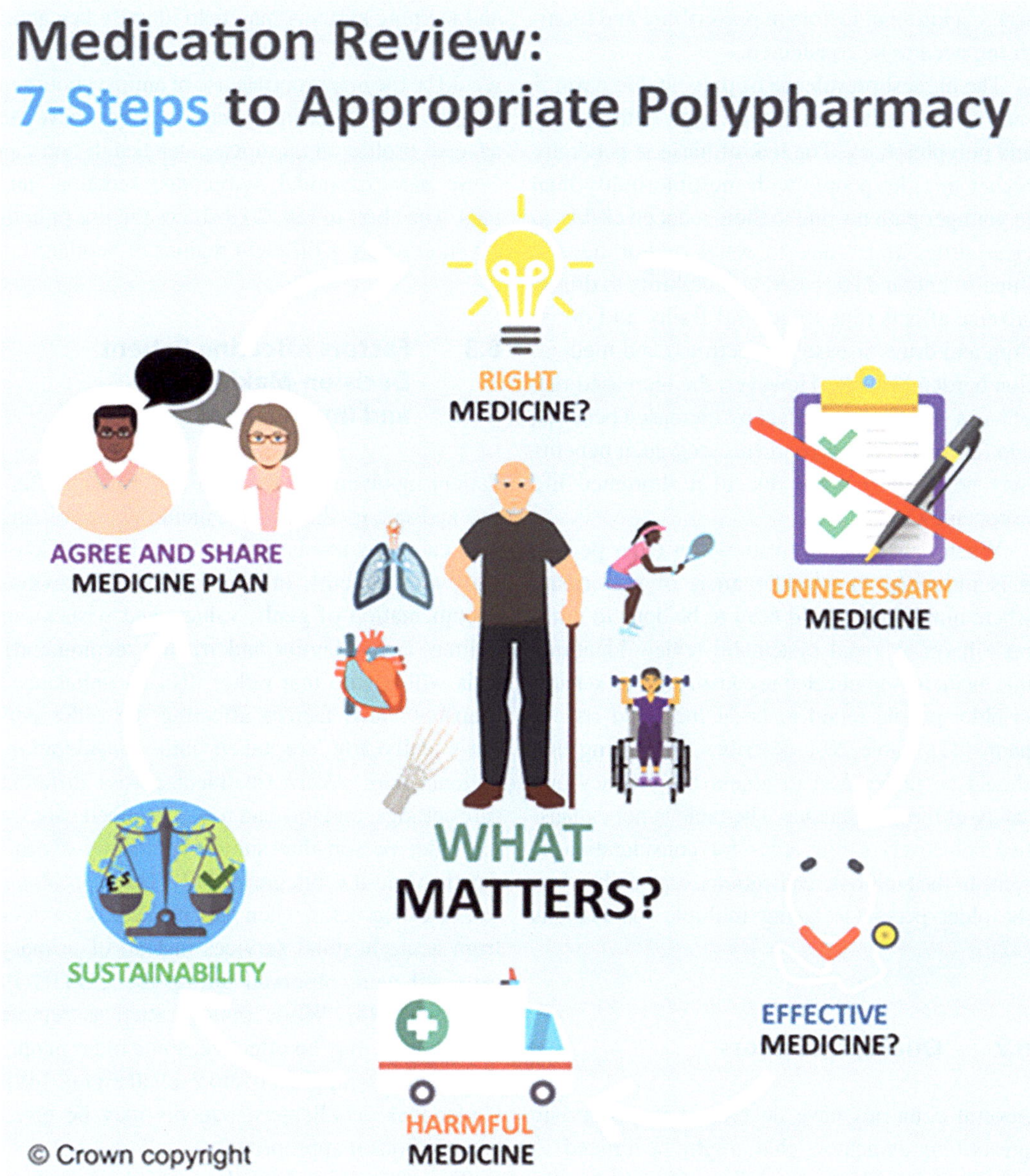
Medication Review:
7-Steps to Appropriate Polypharmacy
RIGHT
MEDICINE?
AGREE AND SHARE
MEDICINE PLAN
UNNECESSARY
MEDICINE
WHAT
MATTERS?
SUSTAINABILITY
EFFECTIVE
MEDICINE?
HARMFUL
MEDICINE
© Crown copyright

Fig. 20.2 Seven-step process to person-centered approach for appropriate prescribing (reproduced with permission from Scottish Government, Effective Prescribing and Therapeutics Division [30])

autonomy, which is important for all decisions including deprescribing [37]. A recently developed tool called the PREparing Patients for Active Involvement in medication Review (PREPAIR) can support active involvement of patients during medication review within general practice [38].

Case studies 1 and 2 discuss the importance of undertaking person-centered medication review.

6.1 Monitoring and Review of High-Risk Medicines in Older People

In the earlier sections of this chapter, we have considered the changes in physiology that predispose the older person to increased medication-related harm. Incidence of frailty further complicates this issue, and particular attention needs to be given to the groups of medication where additional factors in prescribing and monitoring need to be considered.

The highest prevalence of preventable harm is seen in the older person, with high comorbidity and polypharmacy. The risk of harm is generally higher in older people with multimorbidity than in younger patients due to their reduced ability to clear drugs (e.g., due to renal and/or hepatic impairment) and increased vulnerability to drugs' adverse effects (due to general frailty and drug–drug and drug–disease interactions) and medication burden [39, 40]. However, the increased risk of harm is not always offset by increased benefits, and for many preventive medicines, such benefits may never be realized due to a shortened life expectancy.

When reviewing medications for older people, it is important to consider areas of prescribing where monitoring would need to be done to minimize harm. A rapid systematic review identified that medicines implicated in causing the most harm in older people found to be at increased risk of harm [41]. Table 20.1 describes monitoring that should be undertaken to assess the efficacy and safety of these medicines. The table is not exhaustive but covers a few areas for consideration of some of the high-risk medications, especially when the older person is taking multiple medications [42].

6.2 Quality Indicators

Several countries have developed inappropriate prescribing indicators that might be related to either the number of medications used, specific medications, or specific medication combinations used for older persons [30, 43–45]. Some jurisdictions also have indicators for identification of medication-related harm and process indicators for medication review [45, 46]. The use of quality indicators is helpful to establish benchmarks but then to also drive improvement and sustain change.

These indicators should be chosen to address country-specific prescribing challenges that need addressing for the older person. National prescribing data or national pharmacovigilance reporting and learning systems may help identify key areas to address. One example of a quality indicator would be the inappropriate use of antipsychotics in people with dementia. Antipsychotics have an adverse profile on cardiovascular health and can cause extrapyramidal symptoms, sedation, and falls. The chart in Fig. 20.3 shows the use of antipsychotics across different regions of Scotland.

6.3 Factors Affecting Patient Decision-Making and Involvement

Patient involvement is crucial for making effective and safe medical plans, including optimizing medication regimens. This may be direct (discussion with patient), informed (through previous documentation of goals, values, and wishes), or indirect (what family and friends recommend). This will ensure that rather than an unbalanced snapshot view, factors affecting the older person's daily life are taken into consideration. Patients may access treatment across different care settings, and this can result in siloed care for the older person that should be ideally coordinated so that it is integrated [47]. These problems can be exacerbated when patients access services from acute hospital services instead of primary care and were observed during the COVID-19 pandemic [48]. While options such as remote consultation may be effective, some older people may find this approach more challenging [49]. Under these challenges, patients may be given prescriptions inappropriately.

There are several mechanisms that can help instigate involvement of older patients in the acute setting to ensure optimal, safe patient decisions [50]:

- Ensure involvement of the multidisciplinary team to assess frailty and function prior to acute illness and aim to restore patient to this level of function if possible.
- Involve pharmacists to help assess appropriateness of medication by obtaining the best possible medication history and medication review, to avoid inappropriate polypharmacy

Table 20.1 Common medication classes that have the potential to cause harm in the older person and a summary of monitoring that should be undertaken to optimize safety and effectiveness of treatment

Medication class with potential to cause harm	Monitoring to be done to assess efficacy	Monitoring that should be done to avoid and detect harm (with comments)
Simple analgesics (e.g., acetaminophen/ paracetamol)	Onset of pain relief is approximately 30 min after oral administration and 5–10 min after IV infusion Chronic pain can take up to 3 months to control	• Elevated aminotransferases • Factors that may predispose to hepatotoxicity: prolonged fasting or malnutrition, hepatic enzyme inducers, severe renal/liver impairment, chronic alcohol intake • Adherence/medication error contributes to toxicity in old age, with cumulative exposure from different formulations available over the counter
Commonly used antibiotics For example: piperacillin/ tazobactam, amoxicillin/ clavulanic acid, gentamicin, ciprofloxacin	Systemic (e.g., fever, white cell count, and inflammatory markers) and local evidence (e.g., wound) of bacterial infection	• Liver and renal function—inform dose and may be signs of toxicity • Other toxic effects—ototoxicity, gastrointestinal side effects (e.g., *Clostridium difficile*) • Antibiotic allergy: immediate (e.g., urticaria, angioedema, anaphylaxis) or delayed (e.g., Stevens–Johnson syndrome) • Use as per local antimicrobial formulary with reference to local resistance patterns and take in depth drug allergy history
Antithrombotics including aspirin, clopidogrel, and other antiplatelet drugs, Factor Xa inhibitors, low molecular weight heparin, warfarin	Relevant coagulation measure (e.g., INR for warfarin), clinical conditions (vessel imaging may be required), patient status	• Renal function, liver function • Consider pharmacokinetic and pharmacodynamic drug interactions • Note an increased risk of hemorrhage with multiple antithrombotics, e.g., combination of aspirin and clopidogrel
Anti-inflammatory (NSAIDs)	Check the impact on pain relief/ symptoms after initiating the treatment	• Risk of gastrointestinal bleeding is exacerbated by a history of peptic ulcer disease and the pharmacodynamic interactions of several medicines, including other NSAIDs, antiplatelets, anticoagulants, corticosteroids, and selective serotonin reuptake inhibitors • Decisions to use NSAIDs in older patients, alone or in combination, should be restricted to scenarios where there are no alternatives. When unavoidable, consider gastroprotection: • May increase cardiovascular risk • Consider topical preparation
Antidepressants	Begin with a low dose, increasing gradually over 2–4 weeks as tolerated Full effect may take 6–8 weeks, but improvement is often seen within 1–3 weeks. "Start low and go slow" with frequent consultations to monitor for efficacy	• Older people may have slow response to treatment with a higher risk of recurrence • Hypernatremia, falls, and anticholinergic effects are common adverse effects of antidepressants in old age • Older adults are at increased risk of long QT syndrome • Mirtazapine and sertraline seem ineffective for depression in people with dementia • Optimize nonpharmacological interventions

(continued)

Table 20.1 (continued)

Medication class with potential to cause harm	Monitoring to be done to assess efficacy	Monitoring that should be done to avoid and detect harm (with comments)
Antiepileptics	"Start low and go slow" with frequent consultations to monitor for clinical efficacy Tailor the dose of all antiepileptic drugs to clinical response. With some agents (e.g., phenytoin, carbamazepine), monitoring plasma concentrations may be useful	• For seizure-free older patients, altering the dose to bring apparently subtherapeutic plasma concentrations into the therapeutic range can induce toxicity • Falls and fracture risk may be increased by CNS adverse effects • Hyponatremia is common with carbamazepine and oxcarbazepine and hypernatremia is common with phenytoin • Can be used for neuropathic pain and should not be used for generalized pain—evaluate appropriateness
Antipsychotics	Antipsychotic response may occur in 1–2 weeks; however, allow 2–3 months for full trial "Start low and go slow" because of greater risk for adverse effects (e.g., hypotension, confusion, anticholinergic effects, and acute Extra Pyramidal Side [EPS] effects)	• Associated with increased risk of stroke and death (increased risk with higher doses and first-generation antipsychotics) • Treat for the shortest possible time to minimize the risk of tardive dyskinesia and death • Avoid if possible, in people with dementia • Falls and anticholinergic effects are common adverse effects of antipsychotics in old age • Older adults are at increased risk of long QT syndrome
Cardiovascular: antiarrhythmics (e.g., atenolol, bisoprolol)	Review response to medication after initiation in terms of cardiovascular symptoms, Heart Rate, BP, and ECG/ 24-h ECG monitoring as appropriate for indication	• Be aware of drug–drug interactions that may precipitate heart block (e.g., other antiarrhythmics, cholinesterase inhibitors) • Consider cardiovascular disease or drug side effects with falls, syncope, and breathlessness
Corticosteroids	Review of clinical condition and whether there is ongoing indication for prolonged therapy of oral (e.g., >7.5 mg daily of prednisolone or equivalent for >3 months) and inhaled forms	Prolonged corticosteroid therapy can lead to osteoporosis, glaucoma, and cataracts; increased infections; and changes in blood chemistry/ physiology, blood sugar, and blood pressure (Cushing's-like syndrome) Acute corticosteroid therapy can precipitate delirium in older people
Hypnotics	Monitor effects on sleep Tolerance develops to the hypnotic effects of benzodiazepines in weeks	• The pharmacological action of benzodiazepines, through positive allosteric modulation of the GABA-A receptors increasing GABAergic transmission, impair memory, increase sedation, cause inattentiveness, ataxia, and motor impairment, providing a pathway for their association with dementia, delirium, and falls • Multidisciplinary review of falls prevention interventions to minimize impact of drug-induced falls

(continued)

Table 20.1 (continued)

Medication class with potential to cause harm	Monitoring to be done to assess efficacy	Monitoring that should be done to avoid and detect harm (with comments)
Centrally acting analgesics: e.g., opioids, gabapentinoids	Review indication regularly: avoid long-term use of opioids for chronic noncancer pain Monitor pain and be aware of tolerance Check that simple analgesics are used optimally Set realistic goals regarding pain management and ensure use of multidisciplinary interventions	• Monitor for potential dependency and withdrawal reaction (while dose is being reduced) • Monitor people taking opioids for constipation and prevent with aperients (bulk-forming laxatives) • Review multidisciplinary falls prevention interventions to minimize impact of drug-induced falls
Diuretics	Onset of action following oral administration is 4–6 h Monitor fluid balance (e.g., weight) and symptoms/signs (e.g., peripheral or pulmonary edema)	• Older adults are more susceptible to electrolyte imbalance, orthostatic hypotension, and urinary incontinence with diuretics. Urinary incontinence may reduce adherence • If deprescribed, then wean slowly to prevent rebound fluid retention and heart failure
Respiratory: prednisolone and inhaled corticosteroids; inhaled beta-agonists; inhaled anticholinergics	Review of clinical condition with examination and use of investigation such as peak flow and spirometry	• Review inhaler technique to avoid oral thrush and ensure effectiveness • Review side effects of steroids (as above) and encourage patient education for adherence and appropriate weaning regimens • Consider beta agonist effect in patients with tachycardia or palpitations • Side effects of long-acting muscarinic receptor antagonists (LAMA), e.g., glaucoma

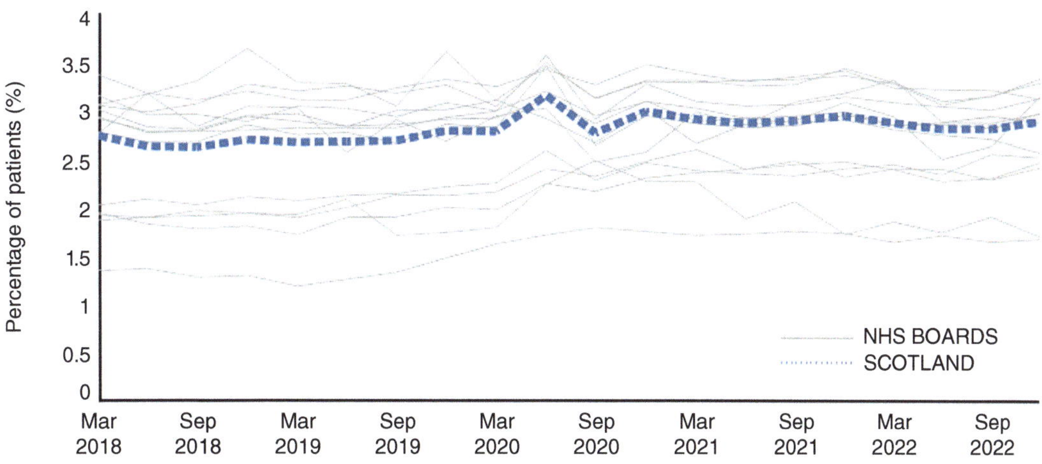

Source: Prescribing Information System Scotland, PHS, NSS.

Fig. 20.3 Proportion of people aged 75 years and over prescribed an antipsychotic medication as a percentage of all people aged 75 years and over (from Mar 2018 to Sept 2022)

as well as ensure crucial medications are not being missed [30, 51, 52].

- One way to avoid harm is to have prearranged emergency healthcare plans (anticipatory care plans) in place, which are documents detailing patient goals and wishes and past medical history [51]. It is also important to consider any legal documents that may have been put in place to support the older person and avoid unnecessary hospital prescriptions and potential admissions. This would have a dual effect in optimizing patient care and reducing the burden on hospital services.
- Appropriately direct patients to the most relevant care service to help ensure best practice treatment and most effective continuity of care, e.g., clinical pharmacists supporting review of prescribing.
- Empower patients to become their own healthcare champion to help alleviate the strain built up due to service provision. For example, having an accurate medication list held by the patient or a "health passport" can enhance the medication history that should be integrated as part of every consultation.
- Conduct a thorough medication review that includes reconciliation when the patient crosses care transitions to enable safer medication prescribing.
- Enhanced, streamlined documentation, online prescribing, shared access to notes between primary and secondary care, as well as patient involvement documented clearly allow primary and secondary care to efficiently communicate and ensure safe medication-related decisions are made while considering patient views.

6.4 Impact of Medicines on Healthy Aging

Successful aging focuses on expanding healthy, functional years of life [53]. This includes avoiding disease and disability, having high cognitive and physical function, high social engagement, a positive mood, and feeling in control. Currently available therapeutic drugs play important roles in prevention and management of disease. Pharmacovigilance studies suggest that medications can affect healthy aging in either direction. Some medicines (e.g., those with anticholinergic and sedative effects) have negative impacts on cognitive, mental, and physical function [29]. Medicines may also affect social engagement, for example, people may avoid outings because of incontinence precipitated by diuretics, or be better able to interact socially because their breathlessness is well controlled by medicines treating chronic cardiac or respiratory disease, allowing them to talk more easily.

Internationally, development or repurposing of medicines that target aging biology itself to improve health span is underway, with the emergence of geroscience research [54]. Geroscience investigates the effects of interventions, including licensed therapeutic medications, on modifying the hallmarks of aging, such as DNA instability, telomere attrition, epigenetic alterations, loss of proteostasis, deregulated nutrient-sensing, mitochondrial dysfunction, cellular senescence, stem cell exhaustion, and altered intercellular communication [55]. For example, in preclinical studies, metformin and rapamycin have shown some effects on some of these hallmarks and have reduced the incidence of age-related disease and increased some measures of healthspan. In the absence of rigorous clinical data and of a regulatory framework, no medications are currently recommended to target healthy aging. Some older people already take medications and/or supplements in the hope that they may improve healthspan. It is important to ask patients about these since they may interact with the patient's medications and medical conditions. The future use of effective therapies that target healthy aging will need to consider all issues in safe prescribing for older adults discussed in this chapter and ultimately may impact on the prevalence of multimorbidity and polypharmacy in old age.

Pharmacovigilance is a key tool for identification of associations between drug use and markers of successful aging [56]. It is important to test the effects of real-world drug use in complex older people on not only lifespan but also health span. This can be done with cross-sectional and longitudinal pharmacoepidemiology studies, analyzing data on drug use and on components of successful aging, including incident diagnoses of chronic disease, objective functional measures, measures of social activity and mood. For example, among people with diabetes, metformin, which acts on key pathways in the biology of aging, is associated with slower cognitive decline and reduced risk of dementia [57].

6.4.1 Geriatric Syndromes

Geriatric syndromes are nonspecific, multifactorial conditions and are common presentations among older people (e.g., cognitive impairment, frailty, falls, incontinence). Geriatric syndromes have a bidirectional relationship with medication-related problems. The most reversible causes of geriatric syndromes are ADRs. Therefore, it is important to consider this possibility when older people present with conditions such as cognitive impairment, falls, incontinence, and frailty. A medication is more likely to cause an acute presentation when there has been a change in prescribing (new drug or dose, affecting person directly or indirectly through drug interaction) or an acute increase in concentration (e.g., acute renal or hepatic failure, reducing clearance).

Geriatric syndromes also increase the risk of non-adherence, medication errors, and adverse drug effects. For example, people with cognitive impairment may have difficulty remembering and following medication regimens, and medication management may involve formal and/or informal carers. Frail older people with multimorbidity are more likely to have multiple prescribers, which can result in a lack of care co-ordination, unrecognized drug–drug and drug–disease interactions, and complex management regimens. Various tools are available to assess frailty, for example the Rockwood Frailty Index [58] including electronic versions available at the point of care [59], which measure accumulation of age-associated deficits across multiple domains. These are helpful to inform anticipatory or emergency care planning and have conversations about patients' objectives and priorities for treatment, as well as raising awareness of additional care required to treat these complex, vulnerable people, who are at increased risk of severe adverse drug effects.

Much of the evidence on the association between medication use and geriatric syndromes comes from pharmacovigilance [56]. This includes spontaneous case reporting and pharmacoepidemiologic studies of associations between medication use and these outcomes. There are also observational studies demonstrating differences between people with and without geriatric syndromes in adherence with single disease treatment guidelines [60] and prevalence of drug interactions [61].

The signals from these pharmacovigilance studies are supported by mechanistic pharmacological data and interventional studies. Mechanistically, medications with anticholinergic and sedative actions have well-studied pharmacological mechanisms that explain the observed associations of the use of these medication classes with geriatric syndromes. Short-term interventional studies of treatment with single drugs demonstrate direct drug effects relevant to geriatric syndromes. For example, single-dose studies of tricyclic antidepressants, which have anticholinergic properties, result in deficits in attention and reaction time, although these effects may vary with dose, with development of tolerance during long-term treatment [62]. These effects may be cumulative when multiple anticholinergic drugs are administered together [63].

For some medication classes, interventional studies have demonstrated a reduction in these syndromes when medications are withdrawn and ceased (deprescribed) [46]. For example, a randomized trial demonstrated that withdrawal of psychotropic drugs reduced the risk of falling in older people [64].

The combined data from pharmacovigilance, mechanistic, and interventional studies are used to inform clinical assessment. If a patient presents with a geriatric syndrome, it is important to look for a potentially reversible drug-related cause.

7 Avoiding Harm and the Role of the Healthcare Professional

7.1 Prescribing Culture

Organizational culture is complex, affects all the building blocks within the healthcare system, and can help or hinder the implementation of safe patient management and new innovation. It includes the values, assumptions, and beliefs held by those within the organization; more simply put, the way in which things are accepted to be done in practice [65, 66]. Results from the European Union (EU)-funded Stimulating Innovation Management of Polypharmacy and Adherence in the Elderly (SIMPATHY) Delphi study supported this understanding of organizational culture [67]. In fact, the failure to account for organizational culture is one of the main reasons cited when evaluating why planned change initiatives are unsuccessful. For example, an open patient safety culture is essential for discussions among health professionals reviewing and challenging prescribing appropriateness. Case study 3 illustrates challenges that are present for junior prescribers, which can include pharmacists and nurses as well as doctors, and particularly the pressure to prescribe medicines either out with their competence or what would be appropriate for the older person.

7.2 Factors to Consider to Address the Culture and Avoid Medication-Related Harm

When considering prescribing within a team, there are several integral and interrelated elements that should be considered by all involved to ensure safe and effective patient care, as set out in Fig. 20.4.

Using appropriate tools with reference to policies allows safety issues to be addressed in an understanding and accountable culture, empowering players to become role models for change among the team they work; this leads to improvement of services while setting the standard for future care.

Tools for avoiding harm include guidance documents for reviewing treatment in older people taking multiple medications and addressing medication safety [30, 68] and also professional guidance on safe management of patients [69]. To ensure general robustness to avoid harm, there are common areas to be vigilant about when prescribing. These are presented in Fig. 20.5, particularly considering management of pain for the older person particularly in the acute setting. It is worth noting that these areas are common areas of uncertainty in clinical practice and require attention to detail to ensure decisions are made in a patient's best interest [70].

8 Education, Training, and Tools to Guide Prescribing

Medication-related harm is a major cause of hospital admissions and costs worldwide [50]. It is therefore essential that healthcare providers at different levels and specialities are empowered from the start of their training to become best practice prescribers. As detailed earlier, healthcare systems across the board are under immense pressures to cope with the ever-increasing clinical demand; more appropriate and safer prescribing would reduce adverse effects and therefore the burden on already stretched services. Figure 20.6 illustrates how vigilant prescribing can enhance patient safety and experience.

One aspect of minimizing medication-related harm in the older person can be through focused teaching and training of prescribers to prescribe and review appropriately with necessary input. This helps to create a culture that values the multifaceted aspects required for vigilant prescribing (Fig. 20.6). Although the focus of prescribing education tends to be on medical practitioners, other healthcare practitioners such as nurse practitioners and pharmacists also play a fundamental role and need to be exposed to equivalent training [71]. A "competent prescriber" is defined as a prescriber who embodies the four stages of the

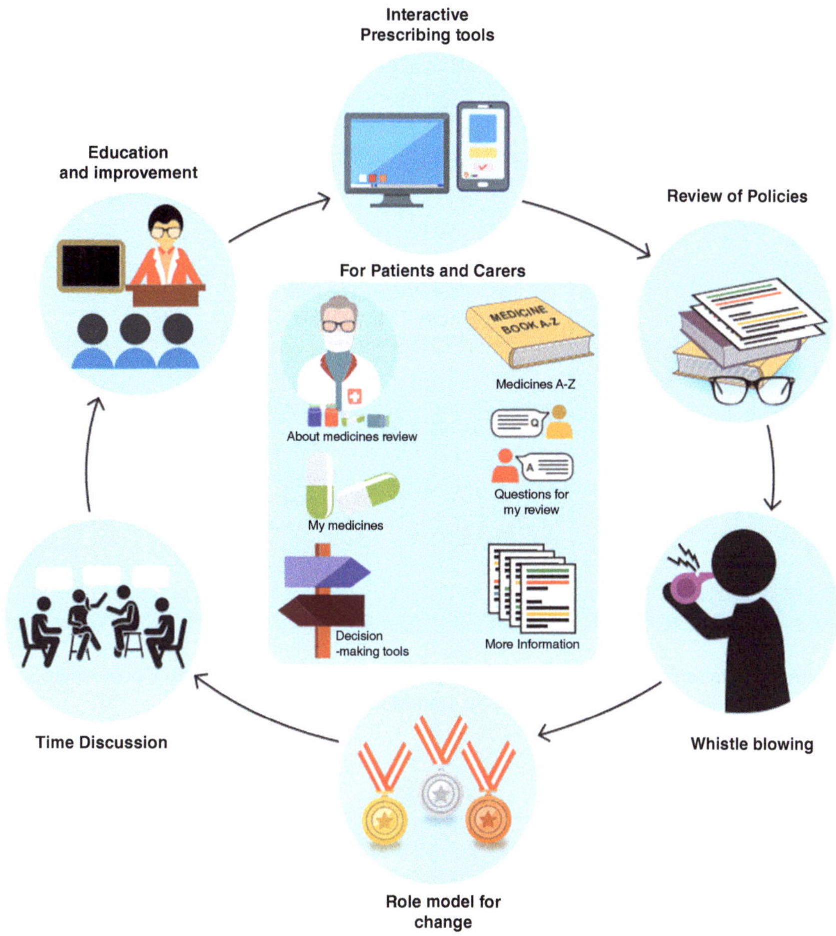

Fig. 20.4 Avoiding harm when prescribing: components required to avoid harm when prescribing in clinical practice for the multidisciplinary team (designed by Amil Mair)

prescribing process—information gathering, clinical decision-making, communication, and monitoring and review [72].

The International Union of Basic and Clinical Pharmacology's international curriculum on geriatric clinical pharmacology for medical schools highlights key domains for knowledge, skills, and attitudes: (1) biology, physiology, and pathophysiology; (2) pharmacokinetics/pharmacodynamics; (3) communication; (4) quality use of medicines; (5) individualization of therapy; (6) polypharmacy and deprescribing; (7) adverse drug events and drug interactions; and (8) drug development, evaluation, and regulation [73].

In the UK, there is a competency framework for all prescribers on prescribing that is led by the Royal Pharmaceutical Society of Great Britain [74], and national guidance on medicines optimization and review of medication [30, 75].

8.1 Prescribing and the Multidisciplinary Team

Continued integration of pharmaceutical care training in various job roles, with tools and updates to implement current clinical guidance, enables consistent application of vigilant prescribing.

No clinician works or should ever try to work in isolation. There has rightly been a shift from

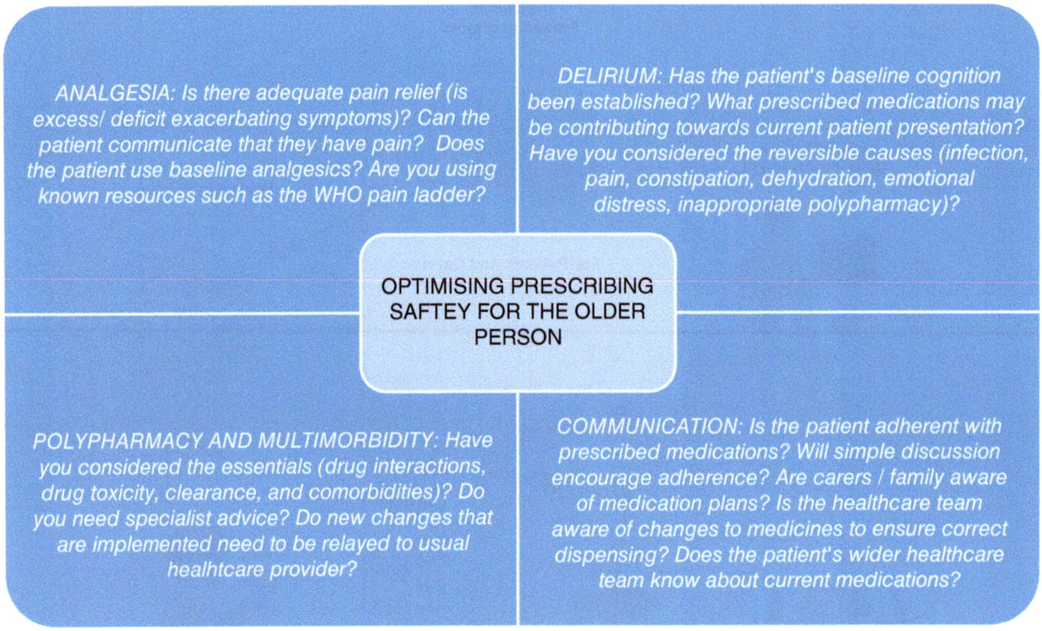

Fig. 20.5 Optimizing prescribing safety for the older person: figure demonstrates how prescribing safety could be optimized for the older person with pain (designed by Amil Mair)

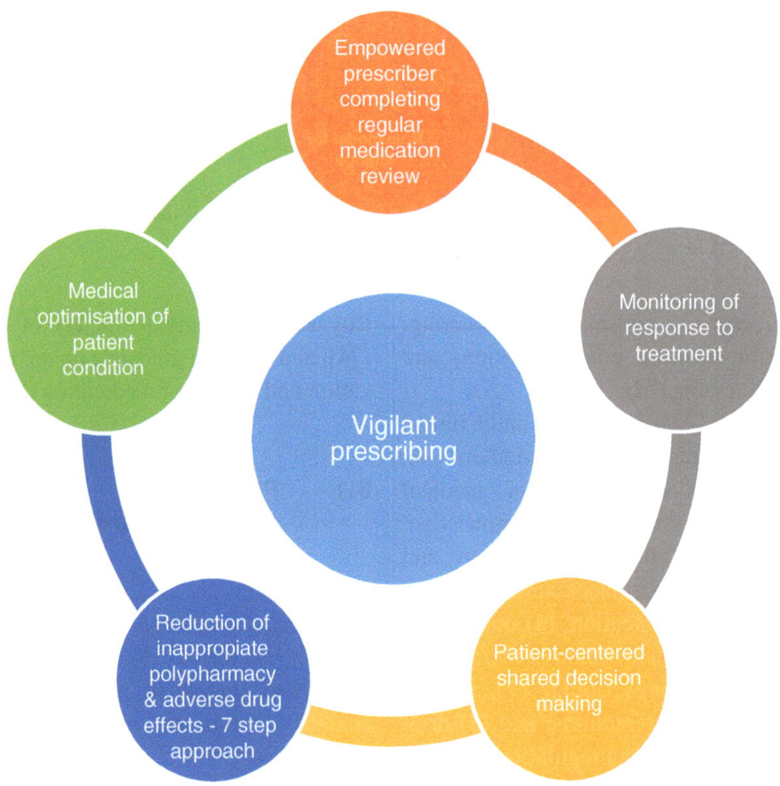

Fig. 20.6 Steps in vigilant prescribing: illustrates how prescribers can optimize medication safety (designed by Amil Mair) (to be used alongside Fig. 20.2: The seven-step process for appropriate polypharmacy)

doctor-led hierarchy to one which recognizes and appreciates the skills and attributes of other highly skilled healthcare professionals. This shift has led to increased pharmacy team presence in primary and secondary care, as well as increased roles of allied healthcare professionals such as specialist diabetic nurses and specialist frailty nursing teams. This approach allows supplemental training and expertise to be brought to areas where prescribing is often overlooked or poorly understood. Discussing these in a multidisciplinary setting allows a 360°, holistic management of patient care and prescribing [69]. However, multiple prescribers bring additional risks around communication, responsibility, and care co-ordination, which need to be addressed proactively. Section 6 described multidisciplinary approaches that have been effective in addressing inappropriate prescribing for the older person.

8.2 Person-Centered Decision-Making Tools

Provision and integration of person-centered decision-making tools into prescribing and clinical planning system that can be used by the healthcare team are essential. There already exists a variety of different tools such as the Scottish polypharmacy guidance [30], local healthcare trust guidance, national guidance [75] for medication prescribing, as well as internationally accredited clinical decision-making tools which incorporate patient comorbidities (such as the British Medical Journal Best Practice) [76]. Integrating these into the ever-evolving clinical documentation and prescribing systems with appropriate warnings for high-risk medications in computerized clinical decision support tools can reduce risks of unsafe prescriptions as well as guide to safest and most holistic management [69].

9 Summary and Conclusions

The key points for consideration when prescribing for older people are set out in Table 20.2.

Table 20.2 Key points for clinical practice to ensure medication safety and monitoring in the older person

- Aging increases multimorbidity and affects many aspects of clinical pharmacology. Consequently, older people have a high prevalence of medication use and of medication-related harm
- Some medications are known to affect both cognitive and physical capacity in the older person and are considered modifiable risk factors that can be addressed by undertaking a person-centered medication review, e.g., seven-step medication review
- When considering prescribing for the older person, consider pharmacokinetics and pharmacodynamics as these can be altered with aging
- In addition, when considering initiation of medication, consider the benefit to the older person using Number Needed to Treat and harm using Number Needed to Harm, and considering if they are applicable ensures treatment which will benefit the individual while minimizing harm.
- The level of frailty using available scales should be used to help informed decision-making on appropriates of prescribing
- Adverse effects of medications frequently present as nonspecific geriatric syndromes, such as falls, delirium, incontinence, or frailty
- In order to support the review of medication and prevent any medication-related harm, healthcare professionals should work with each other to address medication safety culture in the work place
- In clinical practice, pharmacovigilance is critical to prevent, detect, and manage medication-related harm
- Reporting of unexpected or severe adverse drug events seen clinically in older patients is important since postmarketing surveillance is a major source of information on medication effects in this population
- Tools to inform pharmacovigilance include prescribing tools to guide clinical medication reviews and quality indicators at a health service level. Safety indicators can be used to drive improvement
- Medication safety in older people requires constant review, good communication, and shared decision-making between all members of the clinical team in collaboration with the patient

This chapter has set out the contributing factors that predispose the older person to a higher risk of medication-related harm. These are multifactorial and include increasing multimorbidity with age and changes in physiology that affect pharmacodynamics and pharmacokinetics. Therefore, the importance of monitoring for effectiveness in clinical practice is discussed, highlighting some medicines commonly causing harm in the older person, including those that can contribute to falls, cognitive impairment, and/or frailty.

The importance of reviewing the dose of medicines and the effectiveness of medications for the older person needs to be considered. Person-centered approaches that allow for shared decision-making on prescribing and deprescribing with older patients are important. Multidisciplinary strategies for medication management are outlined, together with the education and training that is needed for healthcare professionals who prescribe and review treatment of the older person, including medication safety culture. The three case studies in the chapter provide practical and clinical application of key themes raised in this chapter.

A better evidence base is needed to guide safe and effective use of medicines in the older person, particularly for the older person with multimorbidity and frailty. Pharmacovigilance research is key to understanding real-world outcomes in this population. A key advance on the horizon is representative inclusion of patients in clinical drug development trials, so that efficacy and safety of drugs is rigorously evaluated in the frail older people who will use them so that the numbers needed to treat (NNT) can help assess whether the benefits outweigh the risks. This evidence will inform robust clinical prescribing decisions with older people and improve quality use of medicines. Further research is also needed to understand the role of an individual's goals and values of care in the context of being prescribed multiple medications.

10 Case Studies

10.1 Case Study 1: Multimorbidity, Pain Management and Falls

A 78-year-old lady with multiple morbidities and medication-related harm

Mrs. M, a 78-year-old woman with type 2 diabetes and cardiovascular disease, presents with pain to her general practitioner (GP). Her blood pressure is well controlled and is 142/78 mmHg and cholesterol is 4.8 mmol/L. Recent urea and electrolytes are within normal range, as are liver function tests. Latest glycated hemoglobin concentration (HbA1c) is 67 mmol/mol (8.3%). This HbA1c level is within the target range agreed with Mrs. M.

Mrs. M presents at her most recent consultation with pain that the GP tells her is likely to be due to her diabetes and "nerve" pain. Mrs. M has previously tried codeine 30 mg (up to four times a day) which helped a bit with pain but made her feel dizzy and constipated.

Medical history	Current medications
Type 2 diabetes	Simvastatin 40 mg daily
Cardiovascular disease	Ramipril 10 mg daily
Hypertension	Aspirin 75 mg daily
Hyperlipidemia	Metformin 500 mg three times a day
Pain	Bisoprolol 5 mg daily
Insomnia	Amlodipine 5 mg each morning
	Paracetamol when needed for pain

Her GP prescribes pregabalin, 75 mg twice daily. Mrs. M is not keen to take these tablets, but reluctantly agrees. Mrs. M tells her family that the new medications make her feel dizzy. The family notifies the GP, who says that she needs to take them for neuropathic pain and persevere.

Mrs. M has a fall. Her GP tells her that this is probably not due to the pregabalin. Mrs. M continues the pregabalin and has another fall. The GP stops the pregabalin.

Mrs. M doesn't have any more falls. However, she loses confidence, stops going outside, and becomes low in her mood.

Her GP discusses the option of adding an antidepressant. Mrs. M asks if they will make her dizzy and when her GP explains that they might, Mrs. M decides she wants to "see how she goes."

Mrs. M continues to complain of pain and also presents with weakness in her legs.

On reviewing Mrs. M, medication-related events have more than likely to have been caused by the pregabalin and it's important to review all her medications. The possible causes of harm and suggested actions are set out as follows:

1. *What are the possible causes of harm in Mrs. M? Mention the suggested action/s to minimize the harm in Mrs. M.*

If we consider Mrs. M, the things that are important to her are that she "doesn't want to fall and her mood is low." The fall happened after she started the pregabalin.

- While Mrs. M agreed to the trial of pregabalin, when on monitoring it became clear that it was causing unacceptable side effects; it was appropriate to stop the medication.
- Review of appropriateness of the treatment of her medicines for secondary prevention of cardiovascular disease (which had been prescribed for almost 15 years) found no evidence of hypotension or postural hypotension, indicating that these medicines were unlikely to be contributing to her falls. These are therefore appropriate to continue for secondary prevention of cardiovascular disease.
- After minimizing medication-related precipitants of her falls, consider referral to a physiotherapist for strength and balance training to reduce her risk of falling further and so reduce her fear of falling.

10.2 Case Study 2: Addressing Anticholinergic and Sedative Burden

An 81-year-old man with high anticholinergic and sedative burden

Mr. JL, 81 year old, lives with his wife at home. Recently diagnosed with Parkinson's disease, his wife notices that he has been more forgetful and unsteady on his feet. He even tripped in the lounge room on the way to his chair. He has also been complaining of constipation.

Medical history	Current medications
Parkinson's disease	Levodopa/carbidopa 100 mg/25 mg three times daily
Hypertension	Telmisartan 80 mg in the morning
Hyperlipidemia	Rosuvastatin 10 mg at night
Chronic back pain	Tapentadol 50 mg twice daily
Insomnia	Temazepam 10 mg at night
Diabetes	Glibenclamide 5 mg daily

His medications are packed into a dosing administration aid by the local pharmacy to improve adherence. Recent pathology tests reveal a high HbA1 of 9% (75 mmol/mol). During the home visit, the consultant pharmacist discovers several missed doses of the lunchtime levodopa/carbidopa. Mr. JL does not mention that he is in pain.

A review of Mr. JL's medication would identify medication-related problems. These are set out as follows:

1. *What are the medication-related problems identified in Mr. JL through a person-centered medication review? Suggest suitable recommendations in resolving the identified medication-related problems in Mr. JL.*

   If we consider Mr. JL, "what's important" to him and his wife is to address his issues: he is more forgetful, unsteady on his feet, and has bouts of constipation. Key medication-related problems may include:

   - High anticholinergic and sedative burden (tapentadol, temazepam in addition to recently initiated levodopa/carbidopa) may contribute to his forgetfulness and high falls risk.
   - Tapentadol possibly contributing to constipation, and over prolonged period of time lead to addiction, dependence, and tolerance.
   - Uncontrolled hyperglycemia and prescribed glibenclamide, which should be avoided when possible in older people due to greater risk of hypoglycemia which can lead to falls.

Recommendations:

- Aim to cease tapentadol. Taper down the dose to avoid any withdrawal effects. Introduce regular paracetamol and nonpharmacological treatments (e.g., massage, heat packs) to manage chronic back and osteoarthritic pain. Refer to a physiotherapist.

- Aim to cease temazepam. Taper down the dose slowly to avoid any withdrawal effects. Educate on good sleep hygiene practices (e.g., avoiding caffeine, optimal sleep environment). If pharmacotherapy is needed, melatonin may be considered.
- Switch from glibenclamide to metformin for better glucose control. Sulfonylureas are not recommended in those over the age of 75 due to increased risk of hypoglycemia. Monitor for renal function before and after initiating metformin and adjust the dose accordingly. Ensure that the dose of metformin is increased gradually to minimize any gastrointestinal side effects. Repeat HbA1c in 3–6 months to assess impact on overall glucose control.

10.3 Case Study 3: An Ethical Dilemma

Ward round has just ended for the junior doctor on the surgical ward. Robert is a 79-year-old gentleman who has been admitted following a hip fracture. He has no cognitive past medical history and nursing staff are concerned that he is confused and "making too much noise," disturbing the other patients. The senior nurse requests that a hypnotic is prescribed, albeit off license, so that nursing staff can work peacefully and other patients can rest. On informed reflection, the junior doctor is concerned that a prescription of such a medication would not be appropriate and may cause medication-related harm if used. He appreciates the disruption that complex and challenging patients can have. Patient review reveals a gentleman who does not appear to be a risk to himself or others, and he suggests initially to attempt verbal de-escalation. The junior doctor discusses the case with an experienced hospital pharmacist and the medical registrar who agree with his assessment. There is concern that the patient is mildly delirious (acute) due to increased pain from the fracture and possible constipation due to previous opioids. It is identified that a more effective, appropriate analgesic review could be useful. Tactful discussion and reference to guidance by the junior doctor with the member of staff who asked for the prescription do not end with a mutual agreement, albeit the decision to prescribe lies with the medical team. Later that day, he reflects on this experience: he felt he made the right informed team decision, but will this staff member resent him or portray him in a negative light?

1. *What are the factors to be considered during such a challenging situation to ensure that you are functioning as a responsible and pharmacovigilant prescriber?*

The use of prescribing tools, continued training and education, and working well within the multidisciplinary team are all integral aspects toward a healthcare professional's practice. It is crucial that the prescribing healthcare professional is aware that ultimately they are responsible for their own practice and they need to ensure that it is robust.

A pharmacovigilant prescriber is one who does not work in isolation, taking into account the opinions and idea of others, and makes evidence-based decisions to ensure safe and effective patient care. They are not afraid to make difficult decisions and prioritize patient safety, making use of necessary support systems to make these challenging choices. There are several interlinked concepts for safe prescribing that need to function well, with each individual committed to being involved at every stage. Maintaining a smooth cycle (shown in Fig. 20.4) reduces the risk of harm and means the healthcare professional is a proactive champion to bring positive change when required. This involves taking appropriate written and verbal advice as well as proactively raising areas of concern and improving systems through education and review [70].

References

1. World Health Organization. 10 facts on ageing and health; 2022. https://www.who.int/news-room/fact-sheets/detail/10-facts-on-ageing-and-health
2. Rechel B, Grundy E, Robine JM, Cylus J, Mackenbach JP, Knai C, McKee M. Ageing in the European union. Lancet. 2013;381(9874):1312–22. https://doi.org/10.1016/S0140-6736(12)62087-X.
3. World Health Organization. The world health report 2008 : primary health care now more than ever. Geneva: World Health Organization; 2008.
4. OECD. OECD health working paper no. 121, the economics of patient safety part III: long-term care; 2020. http://www.oecd.org/officialdocuments/publicdisplaydocumentpdf/?cote=DELSA/HEA/WD/HWP(2020)6&docLanguage=En
5. Barnett K, Mercer SW, Norbury M, Watt G, Wyke S, Guthrie B. Epidemiology of multimorbidity and implications for health care, research, and medical education: a cross-sectional study. Lancet. 2012;380(9836):37–43. https://doi.org/10.1016/S0140-6736(12)60240-2.
6. Ornstein SM, Nietert PJ, Jenkins RG, Litvin CB. The prevalence of chronic diseases and multimorbidity in primary care practice: a PPRNet report. J Am Board Fam Med. 2013;26(5):518–24. https://doi.org/10.3122/jabfm.2013.05.130012.
7. Boyd CM, Fortin M. Future of multimorbidity research: how should understanding of multimorbidity inform health system design? Public Health Rev. 2010;32(2):451–74. https://doi.org/10.1007/BF03391611.
8. Wister A, Kendig H, Mitchell B, Fyffe I, Loh V. Multimorbidity, health and aging in Canada and Australia: a tale of two countries. BMC Geriatr. 2016;16(1):163. https://doi.org/10.1186/s12877-016-0341-z.
9. Doos L, Roberts EO, Corp N, Kadam UT. Multi-drug therapy in chronic condition multimorbidity: a systematic review. Fam Pract. 2014;31(6):654–63. https://doi.org/10.1093/fampra/cmu056.
10. World Health Organization. Failure to take prescribed medicine for chronic diseases is a massive, worldwide problem. News; 2003.
11. Nguyen TL, Leguelinel-Blache G, Kinowski JM, Roux-Marson C, Rougier M, Spence J, et al. Improving medication safety: development and impact of a multivariate model-based strategy to target high-risk patients. PLoS One. 2017;12(2):e0171995. https://doi.org/10.1371/journal.pone.0171995.
12. Picco L, Achilla E, Abdin E, Chong SA, Vaingankar JA, McCrone P, et al. Economic burden of multimorbidity among older adults: impact on healthcare and societal costs. BMC Health Serv Res. 2016;16:173. https://doi.org/10.1186/s12913-016-1421-7.
13. de Gruyter, W. (2012). Active ageing and solidarity between generations in Europe: first results from SHARE after the economic crisis.
14. Ruellan AL, Bourneau-Martin D, Joyau C, Secher S, Fialaire P, Hitoto H, et al. Assessment of drug-drug interaction in an elderly human immunodeficiency virus population: comparison of 3 expert databases. Br J Clin Pharmacol. 2021;87(3):1194–202. https://doi.org/10.1111/bcp.14491.
15. Dumbreck S, Flynn A, Nairn M, Wilson M, Treweek S, Mercer SW, et al. Drug-disease and drug-drug interactions: systematic examination of recommendations in 12 UK national clinical guidelines. BMJ. 2015;350:h949. https://doi.org/10.1136/bmj.h949.
16. Rawlins MD, Thompson JW. Pathogenesis of adverse drug reactions. In textbook of adverse drug reactions. Oxford: Oxford University Press; 1977.
17. Hilmer SN, Kirkpatrick CMJ. New horizons in the impact of frailty on pharmacokinetics: latest developments. Age Ageing. 2021;50(4):1054–63. https://doi.org/10.1093/ageing/afab003.
18. Lim R, Ellett LMK, Semple S, Roughead EE. The extent of medication-related hospital admissions in Australia: a review from 1988 to 2021. Drug Saf. 2022;45(3):249–57. https://doi.org/10.1007/s40264-021-01144-1.
19. Elliott RA, Camacho E, Jankovic D, Sculpher MJ, Faria R. Economic analysis of the prevalence and clinical and economic burden of medication error in England. BMJ Qual Saf. 2021;30(2):96–105. https://doi.org/10.1136/bmjqs-2019-010206.
20. Parekh N, Ali K, Page A, Roper T, Rajkumar C. Incidence of medication-related harm in older adults after hospital discharge: a systematic review. J Am Geriatr Soc. 2018;66(9):1812–22. https://doi.org/10.1111/jgs.15419.
21. Lown I. Medication overload: America's other drug problem: how the drive to prescribe is harming older adults; 2019. https://lowninstitute.org/wp-content/uploads/2019/08/medication-overload-lown-web.pdf
22. Devik SA, Olsen RM, Fiskvik IL, Halbostad T, Lassen T, Kuzina N, Enmarker I. Variations in drug-related problems detected by multidisciplinary teams in Norwegian nursing homes and home nursing care. Scand J Prim Health Care. 2018;36(3):291–9. https://doi.org/10.1080/02813432.2018.1499581.
23. Kalisch LM, Caughey GE, Roughead EE, Gilbert AL. The prescribing cascade. Aust Prescr. 2011;34:162–6.
24. Morris EJ, Brown JD, Manini TM, Vouri SM. Differences in health-related quality of life among adults with a potential dihydropyridine calcium channel blocker-loop diuretic prescribing cascade. Drugs Aging. 2021;38(7):625–32. https://doi.org/10.1007/s40266-021-00868-0.
25. By the American Geriatrics Society Beers Criteria Update Expert, P. American Geriatrics Society 2019 updated AGS beers criteria(R) for potentially inappropriate medication use in older adults. J Am Geriatr Soc. 2019;67(4):674–94. https://doi.org/10.1111/jgs.15767.
26. O'Mahony D. STOPP/START criteria for potentially inappropriate medications/potential prescribing omis-

sions in older people: origin and progress. Expert Rev Clin Pharmacol. 2020;13(1):15–22. https://doi.org/10.1080/17512433.2020.1697676.
27. Lavan AH, O'Mahony D, Gallagher P, Fordham R, Flanagan E, Dahly D, et al. The effect of SENATOR (Software ENgine for the Assessment and optimisation of drug and non-drug Therapy in Older peRsons) on incident adverse drug reactions (ADRs) in an older hospital cohort - trial protocol. BMC Geriatr. 2019;19(1):40. https://doi.org/10.1186/s12877-019-1047-9.
28. Parekh N, Ali K, Davies JG, Rajkumar C. Do the 2015 beers criteria predict medication-related harm in older adults? Analysis from a multicentre prospective study in the United Kingdom. Pharmacoepidemiol Drug Saf. 2019;28(11):1464–9. https://doi.org/10.1002/pds.4849.
29. Hilmer SN, Mager DE, Simonsick EM, Cao Y, Ling SM, Windham BG, et al. A drug burden index to define the functional burden of medications in older people. Arch Intern Med. 2007;167(8):781–7. https://doi.org/10.1001/archinte.167.8.781.
30. Scottish Government, editor. Polypharmacy guidance, realistic prescribing. 3rd ed. Scottish Government Polypharmacy Model of Care Group; 2018.
31. CDC. Community pharmacists and medication therapy management; 2021. https://www.cdc.gov/dhdsp/pubs/guides/best-practices/pharmacist-mtm.htm
32. Doucette WR, McDonough RP, Klepser D, McCarthy R. Comprehensive medication therapy management: identifying and resolving drug-related issues in a community pharmacy. Clin Ther. 2005;27(7):1104–11. https://doi.org/10.1016/s0149-2918(05)00146-3.
33. Chen TF. Pharmacist-led home medicines review and residential medication management review: the Australian model. Drugs Aging. 2016;33(3):199–204. https://doi.org/10.1007/s40266-016-0357-2.
34. Koria LG, Zaidi TS, Peterson G, Nishtala P, Hannah PJ, Castelino R. Impact of medication reviews on inappropriate prescribing in aged care. Curr Med Res Opin. 2018;34(5):833–8. https://doi.org/10.1080/03007995.2018.1424624.
35. Lyles LF, Hildebrandt H, Mair A. Population health management approach: integration of community-based pharmacists into integrated care systems: reflections from the U.S., achievements in Scotland and discussions in Germany. Int J Integr Care. 2020;20(2):13. https://doi.org/10.5334/ijic.5431.
36. NHS. Structured medication reviews and the primary care network multidisciplinary approach; 2022. https://www.england.nhs.uk/gp/case-studies/structured-medication-reviews-and-the-primary-care-network-multidisciplinary-approach/
37. Jansen J, Naganathan V, Carter SM, McLachlan AJ, Nickel B, Irwig L, et al. Too much medicine in older people? Deprescribing through shared decision making. BMJ. 2016;353:i2893. https://doi.org/10.1136/bmj.i2893.
38. Sandbaek A, Moller MCR, Bro F, Hoj K, Due Christensen L, Mygind A. Involving patients in medicines optimisation in general practice: a development study of the "PREparing patients for active involvement in medication review" (PREPAIR) tool. BMC Prim Care. 2022;23(1):122. https://doi.org/10.1186/s12875-022-01733-8.
39. Guthrie B, Payne K, Alderson P, McMurdo ME, Mercer SW. Adapting clinical guidelines to take account of multimorbidity. BMJ. 2012;345:e6341. https://doi.org/10.1136/bmj.e6341.
40. Shippee ND, Shah ND, May CR, Mair FS, Montori VM. Cumulative complexity: a functional, patient-centered model of patient complexity can improve research and practice. J Clin Epidemiol. 2012;65(10):1041–51. https://doi.org/10.1016/j.jclinepi.2012.05.005.
41. Hodkinson A, Tyler N, Ashcroft DM, Keers RN, Khan K, Phipps D, et al. Preventable medication harm across health care settings: a systematic review and meta-analysis. BMC Med. 2020;18(1):313. https://doi.org/10.1186/s12916-020-01774-9.
42. Mair A, Wilson M, Dreischulte T. Addressing the challenge of polypharmacy. Annu Rev Pharmacol Toxicol. 2020;60:661–81. https://doi.org/10.1146/annurev-pharmtox-010919-023508.
43. Fastbom J, Johnell K. National indicators for quality of drug therapy in older persons: the Swedish experience from the first 10 years. Drugs Aging. 2015;32(3):189–99. https://doi.org/10.1007/s40266-015-0242-4.
44. Health Quality & Safety Commission New Zealand. Polypharmacy in people aged 65 and over; 2021. https://www.hqsc.govt.nz/assets/Our-data/Publications-resources/Methodology_polypharmacy_2021.pdf
45. NSW Therapeutic Advisory, G. Resource kit for measuring strategies to reduce harm from polypharmacy in Australian Hospitals: QUM indicators, patient reported experience measures and risk stratification tools; 2020. https://www.nswtag.org.au/wp-content/uploads/2020/11/Resource-Kit-for-Measuring-Strategies-to-Reduce-Harm-from-Polypharmacy_Nov2020.pdf
46. Wu H, Kouladjian O'Donnell L, Fujita K, Masnoon N, Hilmer SN. Deprescribing in the older patient: a narrative review of challenges and solutions. Int J Gen Med. 2021;14:3793–807. https://doi.org/10.2147/IJGM.S253177.
47. World Health Organization. Integrated care for older people: guidelines on community-level interventions to manage declines in intrinsic capacity; 2017. https://www.who.int/publications/i/item/9789241550109
48. Anandaciva S. What does the NHS England review of waiting times mean for accident and emergency departments?; 2019. https://www.kingsfund.org.uk/publications/nhs-england-review-waiting-times-accident-emergency
49. General Medical, C. Good practice in prescribing and managing medicines and devices; 2022. https://www.gmc-uk.org/-/media/documents/prescribing-guidance-updated-english-20210405_pdf-85260533.pdf

50. World Health Organization. Global patient safety action plan 2021–2030: towards eliminating avoidable harm in health care. Retrieved from Geneva World Health Organization; 2021.
51. Northern Cancer, A. Emergency Health Care Plan: Guide for Professionals; 2021. https://www.northerncanceralliance.nhs.uk/wp-content/uploads/2021/05/Professional-Guidance-EHCP-FINAL-April-2021.pdf
52. RCEM. The Royal College of Emergency Medicine Best Practice Guideline: emergency department out of hours discharge medications; 2019. https://rcem.ac.uk/wp-content/uploads/2021/10/RCEM_Emergency_Department_Out_of_Hours_Discharge_Medications_Final.pdf
53. Urtamo A, Jyvakorpi SK, Strandberg TE. Definitions of successful ageing: a brief review of a multidimensional concept. Acta Biomed. 2019;90(2):359–63. https://doi.org/10.23750/abm.v90i2.8376.
54. Kennedy BK, Berger SL, Brunet A, Campisi J, Cuervo AM, Epel ES, et al. Geroscience: linking aging to chronic disease. Cell. 2014;159(4):709–13. https://doi.org/10.1016/j.cell.2014.10.039.
55. López-Otín C, Blasco MA, Partridge L, Serrano M, Kroemer G. The hallmarks of aging. Cell. 2013;153:1194–217. https://doi.org/10.1016/j.cell.2013.05.039.
56. Hilmer SN, Gnjidic D, Abernethy DR. Pharmacoepidemiology in the postmarketing assessment of the safety and efficacy of drugs in older adults. J Gerontol A Biol Sci Med Sci. 2012;67(2):181–8. https://doi.org/10.1093/gerona/glr066.
57. Campbell JM, Stephenson MD, de Courten B, Chapman I, Bellman SM, Aromataris E. Metformin use associated with reduced risk of dementia in patients with diabetes: a systematic review and meta-analysis. J Alzheimers Dis. 2018;65(4):1225–36. https://doi.org/10.3233/JAD-180263.
58. Rockwood K, Song X, MacKnight C, Bergman H, Hogan DB, McDowell I, Mitnitski A. A global clinical measure of fitness and frailty in elderly people. CMAJ. 2005;173(5):489–95. https://doi.org/10.1503/cmaj.050051.
59. Clegg A, Bates C, Young J, Ryan R, Nichols L, Teale EA, et al. Development and validation of an electronic frailty index using routine primary care electronic health record data. Age Ageing. 2018;47(2):319. https://doi.org/10.1093/ageing/afx001.
60. Gnjidic D, Bennett A, Le Couteur DG, Blyth FM, Cumming RG, Waite L, et al. Ischemic heart disease, prescription of optimal medical therapy and geriatric syndromes in community-dwelling older men: A population-based study. Int J Cardiol. 2015;192:49–55. https://doi.org/10.1016/j.ijcard.2015.05.045. PMID: 25988541.
61. Bennett A, Gnjidic D, Gillett M, Carroll P, Matthews S, Johnell K, et al. Prevalence and impact of fall-risk increasing drugs, polypharmacy, and drug-drug interactions in robust versus frail hospitalised falls patients: a prospective cohort study. Drugs Aging. 2014;31(3):225–32. https://doi.org/10.1007/s40266-013-0151-3. PMID: 24452921.
62. Tannenbaum C, Paquette A, Hilmer S, Holroyd-Leduc J, Carnahan R. A systematic review of amnestic and non-amnestic mild cognitive impairment induced by anticholinergic, antihistamine, GABAergic and opioid drugs. Drugs Aging. 2012;29(8):639–58. https://doi.org/10.2165/11633250-000000000-00000; doi: 10.1007/BF03262280.
63. Taylor-Rowan M, Edwards S, Noel-Storr AH, McCleery J, Myint PK, Soiza R, et al. Anticholinergic burden (prognostic factor) for prediction of dementia or cognitive decline in older adults with no known cognitive syndrome. Cochrane Database Syst Rev. 2021;5:CD013540. https://doi.org/10.1002/14651858.CD013540.pub2.
64. Campbell AJ, Robertson MC, Gardner MM, Norton RN, Buchner DM. Psychotropic medication withdrawal and a home-based exercise program to prevent falls: a randomized, controlled trial. J Am Geriatr Soc. 1999;47(7):850–3. https://doi.org/10.1111/j.1532-5415.1999.tb03843.x.
65. Cameron KS, Quinn RE. Diagnosing and changing organizational culture. 3rd ed. John Wiley & Sons; 2011.
66. Deal TE, Kennedy AA. Corporate cultures: the rites and rituals of corporate life. New York: Cambridge Perseus; 2000.
67. Mair A, Fernandez-Llimos F, Alonso A, Harrison C, Hurding S, Kempen T, et al.. Polypharmacy management by 2030: a patient safety challenge; 2017. http://www.simpathy.eu/sites/default/files/Managing_polypharmacy2030-web.pdf.
68. Mair, A. Optimising patient care with Dr Amil Mair, North East England; 2021a. https://bestpractice.bmj.com/info/customerstory/optimising-patient-care-with-dr-amil-mair/
69. Mair A. World Health Organisation: Medication Safety in Polypharmacy Technical Report. Retrieved from Geneva, Switzerland; 2019. https://apps.who.int/iris/rest/bitstreams/1235792/retrieve
70. Mair A. Safe best practice management of patients; 2021b. https://bestpractice.bmj.com/info/safe-best-practice-management-of-patients
71. Kouladjian O'Donnell L, Sawan MJ. Deprescribing needs to be considered in the pharmacists' prescribing role. Med J Aust. 2020;212(3):141–141 e141. https://doi.org/10.5694/mja2.50461.
72. Lum E, Mitchell C, Coombes I. The competent prescriber: 12 core competencies for safe prescribing. Aust Prescr. 2013;36:13–6.
73. Kashyap M, Thuermann P, Le Couteur DG, Abernethy DR, Hilmer SN. IUPHAR international geriatric clinical pharmacology curriculum for medical students. Pharmacol Res. 2019;141:611–5. https://doi.org/10.1016/j.phrs.2019.01.032.
74. Royal Pharmaceutical, S. A competency framework for all prescribers; 2021. https://www.rpharms.com/Portals/0/RPS%20document%20library/Open%20access/Prescribing%20Competency%20

Framework/RPS%20English%20Competency%20 Framework%203.pdf?ver=mctnrKo4YaJDh2nA8N5 G3A%3d%3d
75. National Institute for Health and Care Excellence, N. Medicines optimisation: the safe and effective use of medicines to enable the best possible outcomes; 2015. https://www.nice.org.uk/guidance/ng5
76. BMJ. BMJ Best Practice; 2022. https://bestpractice.bmj.com/info/

Further Reading

Hilmer SN, Agency for Clinical Innovation NSW Optimising Medication Management for Frailty Reference Group. Medication review for people living with frailty | Agency for Clinical Innovation (nsw.gov.au); https://aci.health.nsw.gov.au/networks/frailty-taskforce/resources/medication-review

Mair A, Wilson M, Dreischulte T. Addressing the challenge of polypharmacy. Annu Rev Pharmacol Toxicol. 2020;60:661–81. https://doi.org/10.1146/annurev-pharmtox-010919-023508 .

Mair A, Alonso A, International Organisation of Integrated Care. Polypharmacy and integrated care. In: Handbook of integrated care. 2nd ed. Springer; 2020. 978-3-030-69261-2. https://doi.org/10.1007/978-3-030-69262-9_27.

Patient Shared Decision Making App for Polypharmacy Reviews 2018. Effective prescribing and therapeutics & digital health & care innovation centre (DHI). Polypharmacy: manage medicines (version 3.0.3) [Mobile app]; 2020.

21 Safe Prescribing and Drug Use in Pregnancy and Breastfeeding

Hedvig Nordeng, Eva Jirsová, and Olav Spigset

Abstract

This chapter focuses on the special challenges related to pharmacovigilance and drug safety for pregnant and breastfeeding women. It takes the reader through the principles of drug safety and pharmacotherapy among pregnant and breastfeeding women and presents examples relevant for clinical practice. It also addresses how evidence on drug safety specific to pregnant and breastfeeding women is generated and how drug safety in these populations is surveyed (i.e., perinatal pharmacovigilance).

H. Nordeng (✉)
PharmacoEpidemiology and Drug Safety Research Group, Department of Pharmacy, Faculty of Mathematics and Natural Sciences, University of Oslo, Oslo, Norway
e-mail: h.m.e.nordeng@farmasi.uio.no

E. Jirsová
Pharmacovigilance Department, State Institute for Drug Control, Prague, Czech Republic

O. Spigset
Department of Clinical and Molecular Medicine, Faculty of Medicine and Health Sciences, Norwegian University of Science and Technology, Trondheim, Norway

Department of Clinical Pharmacology, St. Olav University Hospital, Trondheim, Norway

Keywords

Pregnancy · Breastfeeding · Teratology Malformation · Breast milk · Perinatal pharmacovigilance

Learning Objectives

- Describe principles of
  - Pharmacological treatment in pregnancy and breastfeeding
  - Drug teratogenicity
  - Drug transfer into breast milk
- Give examples of
  - Teratogenic drugs and drugs increasing the risk of pregnancy complications
  - Drugs that should be avoided when breastfeeding and the reason why
- Reflect on
  - How benefits are weighted against risks of drug use among pregnant and breastfeeding women, and how a balanced benefit–risk assessment should be presented to the woman
  - Why the product label can differ from clinical guidelines
- Describe
  - How evidence specific to pregnant and breastfeeding women is generated

J. Jose et al. (eds.), *Principles and Practice of Pharmacovigilance and Drug Safety*,
https://doi.org/10.1007/978-3-031-51089-2_21

– How surveillance of drug safety in these populations is undertaken (i.e., perinatal pharmacovigilance)
- Know
  – Which questions are important for causality assessments of new signals of drug teratogenicity

Key Points
- Few drugs are proven teratogens and strictly contraindicated in pregnancy.
- Prescribing during pregnancy is often challenging due to missing and/or inconsistent information.
- Teratogenicity of a drug depends on several factors other than its mechanism of action, such as dose, administration form, duration of exposure, timing in pregnancy, and genetic susceptibility. Teratogenic effects include birth defects, embryo-fetal death, growth retardation, functional defects (e.g., reduced cognition), or impaired health in offspring later in life (e.g., cancer).
- Therapeutic drug monitoring (TDM) is recommended for certain drugs that commonly require dose adjustments in pregnancy. This is because physiological changes in pregnancy affect pharmacokinetics and pharmacodynamics.
- Most women who use a drug may breastfeed, because the benefits of breastfeeding outweigh or exceed the disadvantage of drug exposure to the infant. In most cases, the drug amount transferred to the breast milk is too small to exert any clinically important effects on the infant. Often, the combination of available information and clinical experience is sufficient to provide specific advice.
- Adverse drug reactions in infants via breast milk exposure are rare and depend on several factors related to the pharmacodynamic (e.g., inherent toxicity) and pharmacokinetic properties of the drug, the dose and treatment duration as well as maternal-infant characteristics (e.g., genetic polymorphisms, infant age, prematurity, health status of the infant), and extent of breastfeeding.
- Surveillance of drug safety in pregnancy and breastfeeding starts prior to marketing authorization and continues throughout the entire drug lifecycle. Perinatal pharmacoepidemiologic studies are essential in the postmarketing setting.

1 Introduction

Avoiding all drugs in pregnancy and during breastfeeding is unrealistic and may even be dangerous. Untreated diabetes, epilepsy, severe mental illnesses, and infections in pregnancy are examples where the underlying disease in itself may be more harmful to the woman and the fetus/infant than the drug and thus require treatment. Consequently, we need to know which drugs are safe and how drugs are used by pregnant and breastfeeding women. Moreover, health care professionals need to know how to find and interpret available scientific data.

The prevalence of drug use in pregnancy ranges from approximately 25–99% with analgesics, anti-infectives, antacids, antiemetics, and respiratory drugs being most frequently used [1]. By far, paracetamol (acetaminophen) is the most commonly used over-the-counter (OTC) drug during pregnancy, used by almost half of all pregnant women. Similarly, drug use is common among breastfeeding women, with analgesics, anti-infectives, and oral contraceptives as the most frequently used.

Pregnant and breastfeeding women generally tolerate drugs as well as nonpregnant individuals. Drugs should only be prescribed in the lowest effective dose, when clinically needed and according to prescribing guidelines. The information needs in pregnant women, however, are different, often with questions related to pregnancy and their disease, ranging from their ability to become pregnant, how symptoms of the underlying disease might change during pregnancy, how the disease and the use of medicines may affect their unborn or breastfed child, and their ability to breastfeed and care for their baby. Studies show that both pregnant women and health care professionals tend to overestimate risks of drugs when used in pregnancy [2, 3]. In many countries, Teratology Information Services (TIS) provide the public and health professionals with tailor-made information on drug risks in pregnancy or breastfeeding. An overview of TIS centers members of the European Network of Teratology Information Services (ENTIS) can be found at www.entis-org.eu.

2 Drugs in Pregnancy

2.1 Principles of Pharmacological Management of Pregnant Women

Pregnancy may affect the woman's disease and vice versa; the disease may impact a woman's pregnancy by, for example, increasing the risk of pregnancy complications or adverse pregnancy outcomes [4]. Disorders like migraine and some rheumatic diseases tend to improve in some patients during pregnancy, potentially due to high estrogen and progesterone levels. Other diseases including cardiovascular and mental health disorders, and diseases with episodic manifestations (e.g., systemic lupus erythematosus, multiple sclerosis), may worsen, relapse, or flare when the woman becomes pregnant. Some disorders increase the risk of pregnancy complications in themselves. A well-known example is diabetes. Poor glucose control during pregnancy increases the risk of birth defects, macrosomia (birth weight >4500 g), miscarriage, and stillbirths, among others. Acute conditions (e.g., infections) and pregnancy-related ailments (e.g., nausea) may also require pharmacological treatment. In sum, pharmacological treatment in pregnancy may help prevent birth defects and other adverse maternal-fetal health outcomes, as well as help to avoid impaired maternal-fetal health [4].

Decisions about pharmacological treatment with drugs during pregnancy require an individual benefit–risk assessment. Such an assessment should be based upon factors including the woman's prior treatment response, severity of disorder, risk of relapse, and the availability of data on drug effects in pregnancy. Drugs' adverse drug reaction (ADR) profiles should also be considered as these may be particularly unfavorable for the pregnant woman (Box 21.1). Women with chronic disease and pregnancy-related complications should be followed-up by multidisciplinary teams of health care professionals in pregnancy.

Box 21.1 Unfavorable Adverse Drug Reaction Profiles for Drugs When Used in Pregnant Women

- Nausea → worsening of nausea and vomiting in pregnancy (many antidepressants)
- Metabolic impairment (e.g., reduced glucose tolerance) → gestational diabetes, gestational hypertension, preeclampsia (some antipsychotics, especially olanzapine, clozapine, and quetiapine)
- Weight gain → excessive weight gain in pregnancy* → gestational diabetes (some antipsychotics including olanzapine, clozapine, and quetiapine)
- Sedation → excessive tiredness (first-generation antihistamines, hypnotics)
- Hemorrhage → increased blood loss at delivery (nonsteroidal anti-inflammatory drugs; NSAIDs)

**Most pregnant women gain approximately 10–12 kg in pregnancy, putting on most of the weight after week 20*

Generally, the most restrictive prescribing is recommended during the first trimester, when the bases for the organs are formed. In the fetal period (second and third trimesters), some drugs may negatively impact fetal growth and functional maturation and should therefore also be avoided after the first trimester [e.g., tetracyclines, angiotensin-converting enzyme (ACE) inhibitors]. In addition, some drugs may cause pharmacological effects in the newborn when given shortly before labor (e.g., sedatives, anesthetics), and some drugs might also cause withdrawal symptoms in the newborn (e.g., opioids, benzodiazepines).

2.1.1 Therapeutic Drug Monitoring

Physiological changes in pregnancy may lead to altered pharmacokinetics resulting in difficulty in predicting the appropriate drug dosage. Pharmacokinetic changes are mainly due to altered metabolic activity in the liver with increased (most common) or decreased drug metabolism and enhanced renal excretion due to increased renal perfusion. Other physiological changes include increased fluid volume and decreased plasma albumin concentration, which may also to some extent impact the plasma concentrations of drugs. These changes may appear already during the first trimester but are often most pronounced in the second and third trimesters.

For drugs with a broad therapeutic range, these changes have no or little clinical significance (e.g., for commonly used antibiotics). For other drugs, an increased dosage could be necessary to ensure adequate treatment effect (see list of examples below). When available, therapeutic drug monitoring (TDM) is commonly recommended for such drugs to optimize drug dosing regimens in pregnancy.

Examples of drugs where monitoring in pregnancy is generally recommended:

- Anticonvulsants, e.g., lamotrigine
- Antiretroviral drugs, e.g., HIV drugs
- Opioids, e.g., methadone

Because of individual differences, it is advisable to monitor the plasma concentration of the drug at baseline (prior to pregnancy) as well as several times in pregnancy, depending on the woman's clinical symptoms and the previously measured plasma levels.

Within the first week or so after birth, the woman's drug elimination returns to baseline state, and consequently, doses that have been increased during pregnancy must be reduced again to avoid risk of overdose and adverse drug reactions.

Box 21.2 summarizes the prescribing principles in pregnancy.

Box 21.2 Principles of Drug Prescribing in Pregnancy

- Offer counseling to all women with chronic disorders before pregnancy
- Ensure that women with chronic disorders are followed-up by the appropriate specialists during pregnancy. The pattern and the severity of the underlying disease may change
- Perform a benefit–risk assessment on an individual patient basis and prescribe a drug in pregnancy only if the expected benefits outweigh the potential risks to the mother and child
- Avoid known human teratogens
- Be aware that some teratogenic drugs should be stopped long before conception. The length of this period varies depending on the specific drug
- Communicate clearly and ensure that the woman is informed of known benefits and risks of both taking and *not* taking the drug
- Use the lowest effective dose for the shortest required duration—bear in mind that *effective* is more important than *lowest*
- Prefer nonpharmacological treatments, if available and effective (e.g., for the treatment of nausea and vomiting in pregnancy)
- Prefer topical administration over systemic administration when possible (e.g., for asthma, allergy, and dermatological disorders)
- Monitor effect and adverse drug reactions closely and consider the need for therapeutic drug monitoring, as changes in drug metabolism and excretion during pregnancy may require dose adjustments
- Ensure that patients treated with drugs with unfavorable adverse drug reactions related to pregnancy (e.g., nausea, weight gain, metabolic effects) are specifically monitored for pregnancy-related complications
- Remember that absence of information for a drug does not imply that the drug is safe

2.2 Birth Defects and Other Adverse Pregnancy Outcomes

2.2.1 Birth Defects

Every pregnancy starts out with a 2–4% risk of resulting in a major birth defect (a congenital malformation) [5]. This is called the background risk. Birth defects can occur during any stage of pregnancy, but the vast majority originate in the first trimester (Fig. 21.1). Some birth defects (e.g., cleft lip) are clearly visible at birth, whereas others (e.g., heart defects, vision and hearing impairments) are detected through examinations or tests, such as echocardiography or visual and auditory tests.

Birth Defect

Abnormality that arises because of an abnormal developmental process during intrauterine life. Birth defects are also known as congenital abnormalities or congenital malformations. They can be defined as structural anomalies (e.g., limb reduction) or functional anomalies (e.g., hearing impairments). Broadly, congenital refers to the existence at or before birth.

About 80% of birth defects have unknown etiology. Among the remaining 20% with known etiology, almost all are due to genetic or chromosomal abnormalities. Notably, less than 1% of all birth defects are due to teratogenic agents, making teratogenicity of drugs rare in clinical practice [6]. Of note, medications that are suspected teratogens based on animal studies are generally contraindicated in humans, making them rarely used. In such situations, it is difficult (both ethically and practically) to study them and determine their safety in humans.

Other common adverse pregnancy outcomes include miscarriage, premature delivery, and low birth weight (Fig. 21.1). In Europe, the estimated background risk of miscarriages in clinically recognized pregnancies is 10–20% [7], while approximately 6–8% of infants are born prematurely (<37 completed gestational weeks) and 4–8% are born with a low birth weight (<2500 g) [8].

2.2.2 Passage of Drugs Through the Placenta

There is a close connection between the woman's blood and fetal blood through the placenta. Even though a "placenta barrier" with drug transporters and metabolic enzymes exists, most drugs have the ability to cross the placenta to the fetus via passive diffusion if administered in sufficiently high doses for a sufficiently long duration. The exceptions are drugs with very high molecular weights [above a few thousand Dalton (Da)], such as insulin and heparin, which do not cross the placenta this way. In principle, any drug that reaches the fetal circulation has the biological potential to affect fetal development.

Some substances can be transferred to the fetus via active transport mechanisms across the placenta. An example is antibodies of immunoglobulin G (IgG) type that passes from the mother to the fetus via pinocytosis toward the end of pregnancy. Such active transfer of maternal IgG antibodies gives the infant passive immunity and protects it against various infectious diseases in the first 6 months of life. For example, if the mother has been vaccinated or has had COVID-19 and has SARS-CoV-2 antibodies, she will transfer these to the fetus. Maternal pertussis vaccination in pregnancy uses this principle to protect the newborn against pertussis. Of note, other immunoglobulins, mainly of IgM type, do not pass the placental barrier.

The fetus itself metabolizes drugs to a very small degree, but excretes drugs mainly via the placenta.

2.2.3 Teratogenicity

A teratogen is generally defined as a substance that causes birth defects or can disturb the development of an embryo or fetus. Examples of teratogenic effects are birth defects, fetal death (i.e., miscarriage or stillbirth), growth retardation, and functional defects later in life [9]. As of today, only 30–40 drugs have been proved to be major teratogens in humans (Table 21.1).

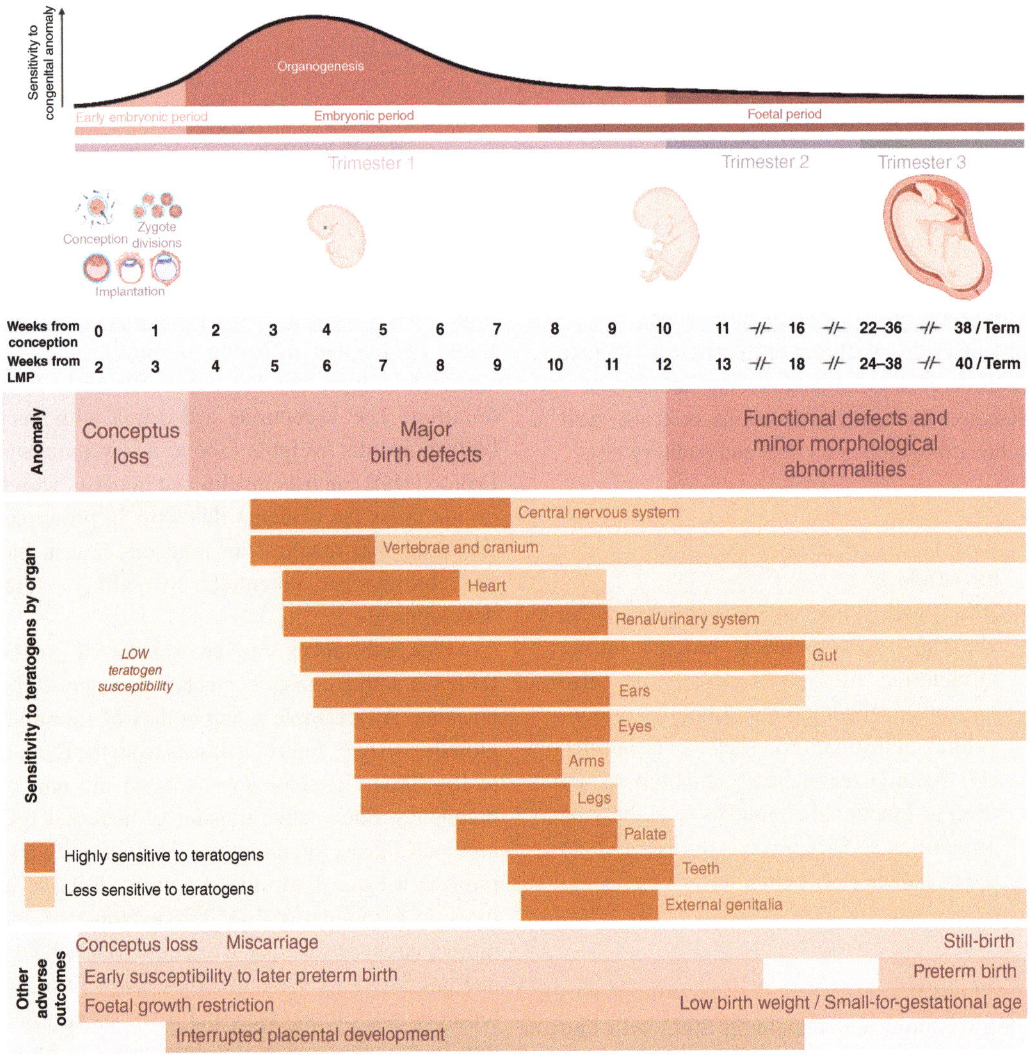

Fig. 21.1 Risk of birth defects and other adverse outcomes vary by timing in pregnancy
LMP last menstrual period. In teratology, weeks are numbered from the time of conception, whereas in obstetrics, weeks are numbered from the first day of the last menstrual period. (Figure created with BioRender.com. Adapted from Moore KL: The Developing Human: Clinically Oriented Embryology, fourth ed. Saunders, 1988. Elsevier)

Teratogen
An agent that causes birth defects or can disturb the structural or functional development of an embryo or fetus.

The timing and duration of drug use are of great importance in relation to the risk for fetal harm (Fig. 21.1). For example, neural tube defects do not occur after week 6, i.e., after closure of the neural tube. Use of tetracyclines will not affect dental and skeletal development before the fourth month of pregnancy, only by later use, as these organs form later in fetal life.

Drugs have been linked to six main distinct teratogenic mechanisms [10]:

- Folate antagonism (carbamazepine, methotrexate, phenytoin, trimethoprim, valproic acid)
- Neural crest cell disruption (retinoic acid, tretinoin, isotretinoin)

Table 21.1 Examples of known human teratogens that increase the risk of structural malformations [5, 9]

Drug	Main identified malformation(s)	Risk[a]
Diethylstilbestrol (DES)	Vaginal and cervical cancer, genital defects	~40% risk of genital defects
Isotretinoin	CVD, ear anomalies, skeletal defects, cognitive dysfunction	~40% overall risk of malformations
Lithium	CVD (Ebstein's anomaly)	5% risk of CVD (~10 times increased risk of Ebstein's anomaly)
Methotrexate	Skeletal defects	5% overall risk of malformations
Misoprostol[b]	Facial defect: Moebius syndrome (paralysis of sixth and seventh cranial nerves), limb defects	~30 times increased risk of Moebius syndrome
Mycophenolate	Facial defects, CVD, cleft lip	~10–20% overall risk of malformations. 40–50% risk of miscarriage
Phenytoin	Facial defects, cognitive dysfunction, "fetal hydantoin syndrome"	5–10% risk for "fetal hydantoin syndrome" ~7 times increased risk for cognitive dysfunction
Thalidomide	Limb anomalies (phocomelia), CVD	20–30% malformation risk after exposure on days 34–50 of gestation
Valproic acid	NTD, neurodevelopmental impairments	1–2% risk of NTD. Risk of neurodevelopmental delays, including reduced IQ. Dose-dependent with highest risks with doses >700 mg/day
Warfarin	Multiple malformations, "fetal warfarin syndrome"	Up to 25% risk of "fetal warfarin syndrome"

CVD cardiovascular defects, *IQ* intelligence quotient, *NTD* neural tube defects
[a]Baseline risk of malformations: any malformation: 2–4%, NTD: 0.1%, CVD: 1% (Ebstein's anomaly 1 in 20,000), Moebius syndrome 1 in 50,000–100,000
[b]Misoprostol in combination with mifepristone is used to induce miscarriage and is 95% effective when used in the first 9 weeks of pregnancy

- Endocrine disruption [cytotoxic agents, sex hormones, diethylstilbestrol (DES)]
- Oxidative stress (thalidomide, phenytoin, valproic acid, antiarrhythmic agents, chemotherapeutic agents)
- Vascular disruption (misoprostol, ergotamine, thalidomide)
- Specific receptor- or enzyme-mediated teratogenesis, e.g.,
  - Inhibitors of enzymes or receptors of the renin–angiotensin system (ACE inhibitors and angiotensin II receptor antagonists)
  - Inhibitors of cyclooxygenase [nonsteroidal anti-inflammatory drugs (NSAIDs)]

Many drugs classified as teratogens are associated with several of these mechanisms.

2.2.4 Harmful Effects Beyond the First Trimester

Some medications can disrupt normal fetal development if used in the second or third trimester of pregnancy. Some well-known examples are ACE inhibitors, angiotensin II receptor antagonists, and NSAIDs.

ACE inhibitors and angiotensin II receptor antagonists may impair the blood flow to the placenta and can cause low levels of amniotic fluid surrounding the fetus. This can induce poor lung development, poor growth, poor development of the skull bones, problems with the development of the kidneys, and, in the most severe cases, death of the developing fetus.

NSAIDs are from gestational week 20 associated with fetal renal dysfunction leading to oligohydramnios (low level of amniotic fluid). When used in the third trimester of pregnancy, NSAIDs may induce premature closure of the ductus arteriosus (a blood vessel essential for fetal blood circulation), which may result in persistent pulmonary hypertension in the newborn.

Some medicines should not be used close to delivery because they may affect the delivery or the newborn (e.g., NSAIDs). Moreover, newborns may develop respiratory, suckling, or other motor problems or show signs of withdrawal reactions if the woman has used benzodiazepines or opioids close to delivery.

The central nervous system is vulnerable to neurotoxic drugs throughout pregnancy (Fig. 21.1). **Behavioral teratology** focuses on neurotoxicity induced during development of the brain and has received increasing attention in the last decade. Adverse neurodevelopmental outcomes include, for example, behavioral disorders (e.g., ADHD), cognitive impairment, and delayed language and motor development. These are outcomes that are essential for children's daily lives, and as such, important outcomes in pregnancy safety studies.

2.2.5 Medication and Impaired Fertility

Medicines can impair fertility through a variety of mechanisms. For example:

Altering hormone levels: Some drugs, such as hormonal contraceptives, can alter the levels of sex hormones, which can disrupt the normal menstrual cycle and make it more difficult to conceive. Drugs that raise prolactin levels (e.g., metoclopramide, most antipsychotics, and some antidepressants) can affect ovulation, thereby reducing fertility.

Damaging reproductive tissues: Cytotoxic drugs, for example, cisplatin, can damage the function of the ovaries or testes, thereby impairing fertility.

Disrupting sperm production: Certain drugs, such as anabolic steroids, can reduce sperm production or impair sperm motility.

Affecting implantation: Some drugs, such as NSAIDs, can impair implantation of the fertilized egg in the uterus, making it more difficult to achieve pregnancy.

3 Drug Safety During Breastfeeding

Human milk represents the ideal primary source of nutrients for infants and offers also other health advantages to both mother and child. Given the range of benefits of breastfeeding, the World Health Organization (WHO) recommends that children should be exclusively breastfed for the first 6 months of life. As the infant should not unnecessarily be denied the benefits of breastfeeding, health care professionals should tailor pharmacological treatment and support women who wish to breastfeed whenever possible.

In clinical practice, prescribers need to weigh the potential risk to the infant of drug exposure through the milk against the disadvantage of not being breastfed. Other options, such as not initiating or stopping pharmacotherapy might be even more harmful, taking into account the risk for the mother and thereby indirectly also for the infant if the mother is not receiving adequate treatment.

The lack of knowledge on drug safety during breastfeeding among health care professionals may result in unnecessary cessation of breastfeeding in women who need to take drugs. Despite the lack of clinical studies, the sum of available information in combination with clinical experience will in most cases be sufficient to provide specific advice about the use of drugs during breastfeeding [11–13].

Specific questions to clarify the benefit–risk ratio of using drugs when breastfeeding are given in Table 21.2.

Answers to these questions require knowledge about principles for transfer of drugs to breast milk and the situations in which this transfer may entail a risk of adverse effects in breastfed infants. They also often depend on the individual maternal-child characteristics.

Any drug used by the mother must pass several steps to exert an effect in a breastfed infant (Fig. 21.2). In reality, most drugs are transferred to breast milk in amounts well below a level expected to exert any pharmacological effect on the breastfed infant [11, 12]. Nevertheless, during long-term maternal treatment, particularly when the infant is premature or newborn, also low doses ingested via breast milk may exert a pharmacological effect to the infant due to immature elimination pathways causing accumulation of the drug.

Table 21.2 Questions that should be asked to clarify the benefit–risk ratio of using a drug when breastfeeding

Drug factors:

- Is the drug formally contraindicated during breastfeeding?
- Have any adverse effects been previously reported in breastfed infants?
- What can the safety profile of the drug tell us about the potential to cause ADRs relevant for infants?
- How much drug will the infant ingest via breast milk (i.e., are there data on the relative infant dose [RID], the levels in breast milk, and/or plasma levels in the infant available)?
- If levels in breast milk are known, how does the drug dose ingested via breast milk compare to a therapeutic dose for infants?
- If data are missing, what breast milk exposure could be expected based on pharmacokinetic characteristics (e.g., molecular weight, bioavailability, elimination half-life)?
- Are there any alternative drugs that would be safer for the infant?

Maternal factors:

- What are the mother's breastfeeding intentions?
- How necessary is the drug for the mother?
- What is the mother's drug dose, the frequency of administration, the duration of treatment, and the route of administration?

Infant factors:

- How old is the infant?
- Was the infant born prematurely?
- Is the infant fully breastfed?
- Is the infant healthy?

The steps that the drug has to pass in order to exert an effect in the infant are the following (Fig. 21.2):

Step 1: The drug must be absorbed systemically in the woman to achieve a certain plasma concentration. Drugs taken orally or injected are those that are most often found in the milk. Many locally acting drugs (dermatological preparations, inhalational drugs, eye drops, nasal sprays, vaginal suppositories, etc.) will in general not be detectable in the woman's plasma in significant concentrations, and thereby neither in the milk.

Step 2: Most drugs transfer between maternal plasma and breast milk based on the principles of passive diffusion through lipid membranes and will therefore follow a gradient from a high to a low concentration of free (unbound) drug (Fig. 21.3). Passive diffusion from plasma to milk (and vice versa) depends on the pharmacokinetic (PK) properties of the substance: The drugs that most easily diffuse into breast milk have high concentrations in maternal plasma, are fat-soluble, have relatively low molecular weights (<500 Dalton), and relatively low plasma protein binding.

It is a common misconception that the drug remains in the milk and that the women therefore should pump out and discard milk after having taken a drug that may affect her infant. The breast is not a reservoir where substances may accumulate, like the urinary bladder, but rather a compartment in dynamic equilibrium with maternal plasma. As the drug is gradually eliminated by the woman and the maternal plasma concentration of the drug declines, it will diffuse from breast milk back to the maternal plasma. Pumping and discarding milk is therefore necessary only in exceptional cases, for example, when the mother uses a contraindicated drug over a short period and needs to pump herself to maintain lactation and avoid breast engorgement.

For drugs with short elimination half-lives, the time interval between drug intake and breastfeeding is a key determinant for the drug concentration in the milk. When the concentration reaches its peak level in the plasma, it will, with a short delay, also reach its highest level in the milk.

As an example, the hypnotic drug zolpidem (elimination half-life 0.8–4 h) is rapidly eliminated from maternal plasma/milk. Consequently, the risk of adverse effects in the infant can be reduced by breastfeeding at times when the concentration in breast milk is at its lowest level. This can generally be achieved, e.g., by taking the daily dose in the evening and avoiding breastfeeding during the night.

Step 3: At a given drug concentration in milk, the amount of milk that the infant ingests at that time will be decisive for the drug dose to the infant. Standard milk volumes used in calculations of drug intake via milk amount to 30 mL/kg body weight in a meal and 150 mL/kg body weight in a day.

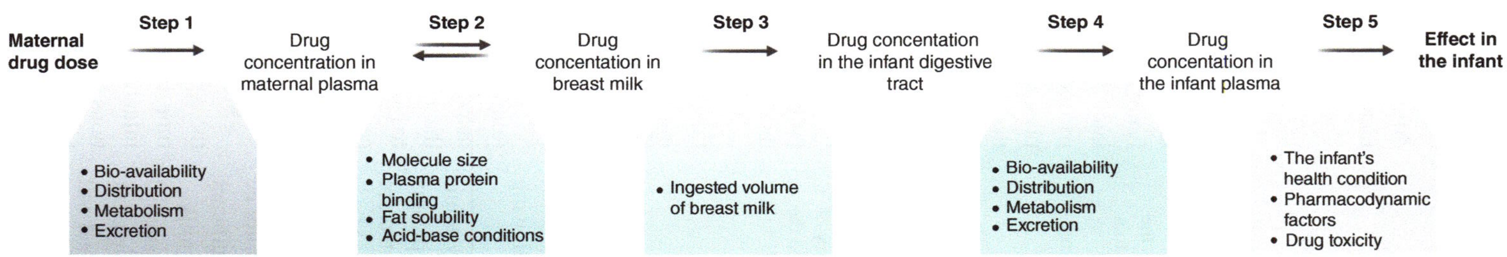

Fig. 21.2 Pharmacological pathway for infant drug exposure via breast milk. (Figure created with BioRender.com)

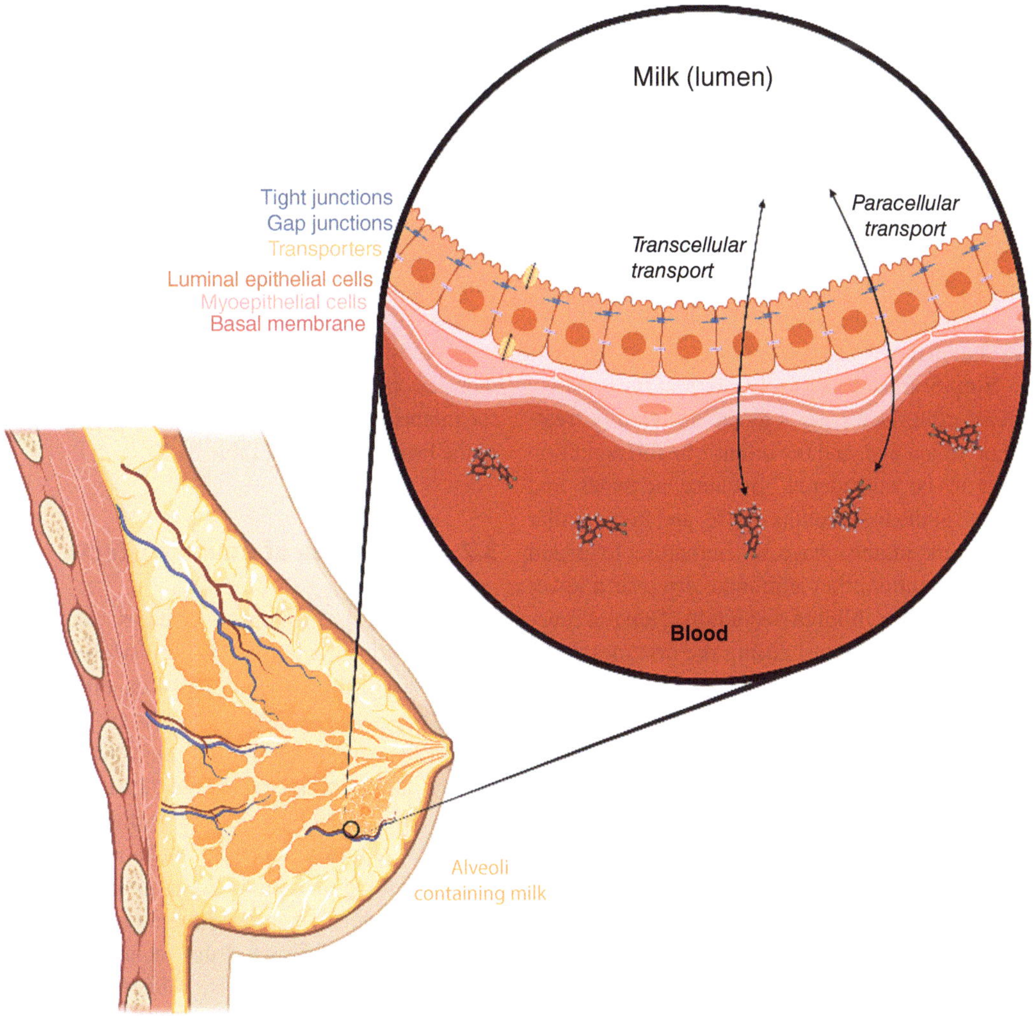

Fig. 21.3 Transport of drug to breast milk
The mammary epithelium consists of lobes, containing alveoli and milk ducts. The luminal epithelial cells secrete milk into the lumen of the alveolus. The surrounding myoepithelial cells contract under the stimulation of oxytocin and cause excretion of the milk into the ducts. Transport of drug to breast milk is possible via passive or active transport mechanisms. Transcellular transport implies crossing of cell membranes, whereas paracellular transport occurs via the confined spaces between cells. (Figure created with BioRender.com)

Step 4: The drug must subsequently be absorbed from the infant's digestive tract before it can enter the bloodstream. A high molecule weight restricts this absorption, and drugs which are proteins, such as insulin, will be degraded in the gastrointestinal tract. Drugs that are not at all or very poorly absorbed from infant's gastrointestinal tract would not cause any systemic effects in the infant. However, they could have local effects in the gut leading, e.g., to gastrointestinal discomfort or diarrhea.

Step 5: In addition to the amount ingested via breast milk, factors such as the duration of treatment, infant age, and the infant's health condition need to be considered. Because neonates and infants in the first months of life, and in particular premature infants, have an immature liver and kidney function, they eliminate drugs at a lower rate than older children and adults. Hepatic function gradually matures during the first months of life, and after about 3–4 months of age, the metabolic capacity reaches adult levels. In contrast, renal function is not fully developed until the infant is 6–9 months old. Therefore, drugs with a high degree of renal elimination, such as lithium, are of particular concern related to accumulation in young infants.

In addition to the pharmacokinetic aspects, premature or seriously ill infants will often be more sensitive than healthy infants and have a lower tolerance to the pharmacological action of drugs, including possible unfavorable effects.

3.1 Infant Dose

In scientific literature and clinical guidelines, it is common to express infant exposure as the infant's weight-adjusted relative dose (relative infant dose, RID), which is the calculated dose the infant ingests per kilogram bodyweight in relation to the maternal dose per kilogram bodyweight (see Case Example 2 Lamotrigine during breastfeeding). Infant exposure is regarded as minimal when the relative dose is below 2%, small when the relative dose is 2–5%, moderate when the relative dose is 5–10%, and high when the relative dose is above 10% [11, 12]. With relative doses above 10%, it is generally considered that a risk of pharmacological effects in the infant does exist, if the infant is fully breastfed [11, 12]. Comparing the drug dose ingested via breast milk to the therapeutic dose for infants will help evaluating the risk of effects in the breastfed infant (Table 21.2).

3.2 Evidence of Adverse Effects

Adverse effects in breastfed infants caused by maternal drug treatment are rare. Moreover, in about 80% of the cases with adverse effects, the infant was younger than 2 months of age [14]. This is in accordance with the expected gradual maturation of hepatic and renal function during the first months of life and clearly illustrates that infant age is a critical factor to take into account when assessing the individual infant risk.

Breastfeeding is contraindicated only for a few drugs. Examples of such drugs include cytotoxic agents, radiopharmaceuticals, iodine-based X-ray contrast fluids, and gold compounds. Some drugs are contraindicated because they may interfere with milk production or the process of lactation. Examples are dopamine agonists (cabergoline, bromocriptine) as they inhibit prolactin secretion; in fact, such drugs are used therapeutically to inhibit lactation when breastfeeding is contraindicated (e.g., due to maternal HIV infection) or after stillbirth.

It is far more common to advise caution with the use of a drug during breastfeeding (on the basis of the pharmacological effects or the drugs' ability to pass into the breast milk) and a careful follow-up of the infant. Examples include long-term use of antipsychotics, opioids, benzodiazepines, and several antiepileptics. This approach is generally considered more appropriate than refraining from initiating breastfeeding or weaning for precautionary reasons (see Box 21.3 Principles of drug prescribing during breastfeeding). Most commonly, ADRs in a breastfed infant will develop gradually. Therefore, it is important to inform the mother about which symptoms to observe for. If symptoms possibly indicating ADRs occur in the infant, a change in drug, a decrease in dose, or interrupted breastfeeding is warranted.

The most frequently reported ADRs in breastfed infants are sedation, sleepiness, poor feeding, failure to thrive, irritation, crying, gastrointestinal effects, and rash. In a few specific cases, hematotoxicity (e.g., thrombocytopenia and leukopenia) or hepatotoxicity has been reported [11, 12]. For some drugs, a potential effect on growth and maturation (e.g., for corticosteroids) or neurodevelopmental disorders (e.g., for some antiepileptics) has been proposed, but not demonstrated in humans. Breastfed newborns with suspected ADRs will also often have been exposed in utero, making it possible that symptoms are related to pregnancy exposures rather than drug exposure in breast milk.

Mixed nutrition (i.e., partial breastfeeding) may be suggested in some situations to reduce the infant's drug dose per day. These situations could occur when the woman uses a drug that could potentially affect the infant over a longer period while breastfeeding an infant younger than 3 months of age.

Box 21.3 provides an overview of the principles that are important to take into account before prescribing drugs to breastfeeding patients.

Box 21.3 Principles of Drug Prescribing During Breastfeeding

The principles of drug prescribing during pregnancy apply also during breastfeeding (e.g., benefit–risk assessment, use of lowest effective dose, preferred nonpharmacological options, or local administration forms). There are, however, some additional prescribing principles during breastfeeding that are important to know:

- If the medication has been prescribed to a woman during pregnancy, it can most likely also be used during breastfeeding
- Before prescribing, ensure that you know the woman's breastfeeding intentions
- Acknowledge the benefits of breastfeeding for the mother and child. Recommending weaning without clear evidence, just to be "on the safe side," is poor practice
- Prefer drugs with a low relative infant dose (RID) and avoid drugs with a high RID (>10%)
- Be most restrictive with prescribing psychotropic medications to breastfeeding women with infants less than 3 months, as they account for most reported ADRs in breastfed infants
- Ensure that breastfeeding women using medications where infant follow-up is recommended know which symptoms to monitor for (e.g., drowsiness, poor feeding, rash, bruising, and diarrhea)
- Avoid prescribing drugs with high toxicity to breastfeeding women. If prescribing requires breastfeeding interruption, ensure the woman knows when she can reinitiate breastfeeding after the last drug intake

4 Regulatory Perinatal Pharmacovigilance

Information about drug safety is often limited or missing at the time of marketing authorization, especially in the areas of pregnancy and breastfeeding. This lack of data has also had an impact on the information in the drug labels. A review of the labels of 213 drugs approved by the U.S. Food and Drug Administration (FDA) between 2003 and 2012 found that 98% of the drugs had missing information about safety in pregnancy [15]. There were no data on breastfeeding in 48% of the labels, animal milk data were available in 43% of the labels, whereas breast milk data from humans were available in less than 5% of the labels [15]. On average, it took 27 years to obtain data on safety in pregnancy [16].

Note: All drug labels [called Summary of product characteristics (SmPC) in European countries] have a specific section where data on pregnancy and breastfeeding, as well as animal reproductive toxicity data, are summarized. The SmPC is updated by the marketing authorization holders when significant new information becomes available as per the guidelines of the regulatory agencies. See an example in Box 21.4.

Box 21.4 Example of a Summary of Product Characteristics (SmPC) Document for the SARS-CoV-2 (COVID-19) Virus Vaccine Comirnaty (last revised March 2023, www.medicines.org.uk)

Pregnancy

A large amount of observational data from pregnant women vaccinated with Comirnaty during the second and third trimester have not shown an increase in adverse pregnancy outcomes. While data on pregnancy outcomes following vaccination during the first trimester are presently limited, no increased risk for miscarriage has been seen. Animal studies do not indicate direct or indirect harmful effects with respect to pregnancy, embryo/fetal development, parturition, or postnatal development. Comirnaty can be used during pregnancy.

Breastfeeding

No effects on the breastfed newborn/infant are anticipated since the systemic exposure of breastfeeding women to Comirnaty is negligible. Observational data from women who were breastfeeding after vaccination have not shown a risk for adverse effects in breastfed newborns/infants. Comirnaty can be used during breastfeeding.

Fertility

Animal studies do not indicate direct or indirect harmful effects with respect to reproductive toxicity.

In the European Union (EU), pharmaceutical companies have since 2012 been required to have an RMP to ensure that more information is collected in the postmarketing setting (see Chap. 6). If data on safety in pregnancy or breastfeeding are missing, suspected, or identified, the RMP will reflect measures considered necessary to identify, characterize, and/or minimize the drugs' important risks for pregnant and breastfeeding woman, women of childbearing age, and fathers to be (when paternal exposures should be avoided). When major risks with use in pregnancy have been identified, a set of risk minimization measures (RMMs) are required to avoid exposure in utero, including, if relevant, a pregnancy prevention program (PPP). A PPP includes a range of RMMs to minimize the risk of pregnancy during drug exposure. The most commonly used additional RMMs are educational materials to health care professionals and patients, contraceptive requirements, and pregnancy testing. However, PPPs vary between the different teratogenic products. See some examples in Table 21.3.

Table 21.3 Examples of drugs with proven teratogenicity according to additional RMMs (as of July 2022, www.medicines.org.uk)

	Contraindication in the SmPC	PPP	Contraception, women	Contraception, men	Pregnancy testing[a]	Supply restrictions[a]	Educational material and forms (for HCPs and patients)
Thalidomide	Yes	Yes	Yes	Yes	Monthly	Yes	Yes
Valproic acid	For bipolar disorder: yes For epilepsy: exception possible[b]	Yes	Yes	–	Regularly	Yes	Yes
Isotretinoin	Yes	Yes	Yes	–	Monthly	Yes	Yes
Mycophenolate	Yes. Exception possible[b]	Yes	Yes	Yes	Initially	–	Yes
Fingolimod	Yes	–	–	–	Regularly	–	Yes
Brentuximab	No	–	Yes	Yes	–	–	Yes

RMMs risk minimization measures, *SmPC* summary of product characteristics, *PPP* pregnancy prevention program, *HCP* health care professional
[a]Controlled access at prescribing level to ensure that a pregnancy test is carried out and negative results are verified by the health care professional before drug prescription
[b]If no suitable alternative treatment exists

In the USA, the FDA can request a risk evaluation and mitigation strategy (REMS, see definition) from the pharmaceutical company if there is a concern related to teratogenicity of a prescription medication. One example is The iPLEDGE® REMS, which is a safety program to manage the risk of isotretinoin's teratogenicity and to minimize fetal exposure (https://ipledgeprogram.com/). A recent study based on data from the FDA's REMS database with information up to 09/2021 found that 11 out of 61 REMS programs (18%) had been requested to minimize teratogenic risks for ten drugs (ambrisentan, bosentan, isotretinoin, lenalidomide, macitentan, mycophenolate, phentermine–topiramate, pomalidomide, riociguat, thalidomide) [17]. This study showed, however, significant variation in requirements related to the use of contraceptives and pregnancy testing [17].

These measures aim to ensure that health care professionals and patients have information available to make informed decisions about drug use in pregnancy and during breastfeeding.

PPP: Pregnancy Prevention Program: a set of risk minimization measures put in place by the European Medicines Agency to reduce risk of exposure to medical products during pregnancy that are teratogenic or have an adverse neurological effect on the child in utero.

REMS: Risk Evaluation and Mitigation Strategy: a drug safety program that the U.S. Food and Drug Administration (FDA) requires for certain medications with serious safety concerns to help ensure the benefits of the medication outweigh its risks. Teratogenicity is a common reason for the FDA to request a REMS.

5 Generating Evidence on Drug Safety

A wide variety of studies are used to generate evidence relevant for pregnant and breastfeeding women. Considering all available evidence from different fields (triangulation) can strengthen causal inference and support clinical recommendations.

Animal studies: Before a drug is approved and introduced into clinical practice it has to be tested for teratogenicity on at least two different mammalian species, of which typically one is a rodent [18]. This is based on the expectation that animal exposure would predict human experience. While this has worked in some important cases (e.g., isotretinoin), it has failed in others (e.g., thalidomide, as it was only tested in one species, rats). On the other hand, all established human teratogens have been teratogenic in at least one animal species. For example, whereas thalidomide was found not to be teratogenic in rodents, it was later proven teratogenic in rabbits and nonhuman primates. Notably, the dosage used in animals is usually much higher than used in humans, which may lead to false-positive findings. On the other hand, some species may eliminate drugs at a considerably higher rate than in humans, causing false-negative findings if the dose is not sufficiently high. One illustrating example is the discussion related to corticosteroid treatment regarding local vs. systemic administration, dose–effect relationships when used systemically, and the possible risk of cleft lip and palate [19]. In conclusion, interspecies differences may lead to both false-negative and false-positive conclusions. Moreover, animal studies are often not suited to reveal (long-term) effects related to, e.g., behavioral teratogenicity or certain maternal effects such as preeclampsia.

Studies on drug passage into animal breast milk are also performed during drug development. These, however, cannot be used to inform safety or transfer to breast milk in humans, as no clear correlation between drug dose in animal and human milk is known.

Case reports and case studies: Several human teratogens have been identified through small case studies. If a certain drug has a high rate of specific, otherwise rare, birth defect(s), case reports can be extremely useful. Teratogenicities of thalidomide, warfarin, isotretinoin, and mycophenolate were all discovered this way (see Sect. 2.2.3). Analyses of suspected adverse reactions based on spontaneous reports are routinely done, in the EU through the EudraVigilance system [20], and globally by the Uppsala Monitoring Centre (UMC) for the WHO [21]. UMC stores all reports of suspected adverse reactions to medicinal products in the database, VigiBase [21].

Randomized controlled trials (RCTs). RCTs often exclude pregnant women due to ethical and/or legal concerns of harmful fetal exposure. The COVID-19 pandemic, however, represented a shift with that respect, demonstrating how RCTs including pregnant and breastfeeding women using COVID-19 vaccines could be performed in a robust and ethical way. The example below is one of the first RCTs specifically focusing on pregnant women.

Example: *Study to Evaluate the Safety, Tolerability, and Immunogenicity of SARS CoV-2 RNA Vaccine Candidate (BNT162b2) Against COVID-19 in Healthy Pregnant Women 18 Years of Age and Older*. This study is a Phase 2/3, randomized, placebo-controlled, observer-blind study evaluating the safety, tolerability, and immunogenicity of 30 μg of BNT162b2 or placebo administered in 2 doses, 21 days apart, in approximately 350 healthy pregnant women 18 years of age or older vaccinated at 24–34 weeks' gestation [22].

Epidemiological studies: Epidemiological studies are central in the evaluation of drug safety in pregnancy. Typically, drug safety studies aim to investigate associations between in utero exposures to specific drugs and pregnancy outcomes, such as malformations, stillbirths, birth weight, or even sometimes long-term development in children. In practice, rigorously designed and well-conducted pharmacoepidemiological studies provide the best feasible way of evaluating whether drug use during pregnancy has adverse effects on the developing fetus in the postmarketing setting.

Epidemiological studies, however, are subject to inherent limitations, given their nonrandomized design. Often confounding by the maternal underlying indication for drug use, concomitant drug treatment, socio-economic and lifestyle risk factors cannot be ruled out. Moreover, misclassification of drug exposure, confounders, and/or pregnancy outcomes may occur and bias the effect estimates. Issues that are particularly relevant to drug safety studies in pregnancy are sample size (i.e., rare exposures and outcomes), errors in measurement of drug use in relation to timing in pregnancy, and lack of information about the validity of the pregnancy outcome studied. History has shown us that several drugs such as the antiemetic Bendectin (pyridoxine/doxylamine) [23] have falsely been labeled as teratogens due to signals in epidemiological studies [24]. Moreover, conflicting results, such as for antidepressants and child neurodevelopment, make evidence-based benefit–risk assessments particularly challenging.

In recent years, increasing attention has been given to analyzing large databases like prescription databases, claims databases, or medical records databases compiled for administrative purposes by health authorities or medical reimbursement organizations. These registries are based upon prescriptions dispensed from pharmacies or from submitted drug refund claims. Their main strengths are their size and the fact that they do not depend on recall of drug use. Furthermore, after initial establishment, drug registries are relatively inexpensive. Prescription (or more strictly, pharmacy filling) registries are found in North America and in a large number of European countries and are used in recent large initiatives to increase the knowledge about drug safety in pregnancy and breastfeeding (e.g., the IMI ConcePTION project, www.imi-conception.eu). The prescription registry must be linked to a birth registry or other data sources where pregnancies can be identified. Prescription registries, however, often fail to include over-the-counter and herbal drugs, and in some countries, also nonrefundable prescription drugs. Moreover, issuance of a prescription or a filling at a pharmacy does not guarantee actual use due to an often unknown degree of nonadherence.

Although birth defects are the adverse pregnancy outcome most focused on when studying drug safety, there are several other adverse pregnancy outcomes that can take place. Some examples are summarized here:

- During pregnancy
  - Spontaneous abortions (e.g., mycophenolate, misoprostol)
  - Intrauterine growth restriction or small-for-gestational age (e.g., beta-blockers, immunosuppressants)
  - Prematurity (e.g., statins, immunosuppressants)
  - Stillbirths (e.g., warfarin)
  - Gestational diabetes (e.g., antipsychotics including olanzapine, clozapine, and quetiapine)
  - Hypertension/preeclampsia (serotonin and noradrenalin reuptake inhibitors)
- At or after delivery
  - Postpartum hemorrhage (e.g., NSAIDs)
  - Neonatal side effects (e.g., CNS depression and poor suckling due to sedatives)
  - Withdrawal reactions in the neonate (e.g., opioids and benzodiazepines)
- Long term
  - Impaired neurodevelopment (e.g., valproic acid)

5.1 Causality Assessment of Safety Signals in Pregnancy

Perinatal pharmacovigilance includes detection and assessment of risks of drugs in pregnancy and breastfeeding. Safety signals or concerns can arise from nonclinical or clinical data/studies throughout the lifecycle of the drug. Interpreting these data, including performing causality assessments and deciding on risk-proportionate measures, is an important regulatory activity performed by the competent medicines agencies. In the EU, the Pharmacovigilance Risk Assessment Committee (PRAC) at the European Medicines Agency (EMA) is responsible for assessing and monitoring the safety of human medicines. In 2022, a topiramate referral was initiated at the request of the French medicines agency, under Article 31 of Directive 2001/83/EC [25] (see Box 21.5).

Box 21.5 Topiramate (Safety) Referral

The European Medicines Agency's (EMA's) Safety Committee (PRAC) started a review of topiramate and the risk of neurodevelopmental disorders in children whose mothers were taking this drug during pregnancy. The review was triggered by an epidemiological study which suggested a possible increase in the risk of neurodevelopmental disorders, in particular autism spectrum disorders and intellectual disability, in children whose mothers were taking topiramate during pregnancy. The study was based on data from several nordic registries (Denmark, Finland, Iceland, Norway, and Sweden) and included information from more than 24,000 children exposed in utero to at least one antiepileptic drug. Of these children, 471 were exposed to topiramate alone, including 246 children born to mothers who had epilepsy [26]. The PRAC started reviewing the study results as part of a Safety Signal Assessment in July 2022.

Box 21.6 provides an overview of questions that may aid causality assessments of signals of drug teratogenicity. Jointly, these questions may help to answer the question: Does the total weight of the evidence support a causal association? If the answer to the question is "yes," then a decision about the appropriate risk-proportionate measures needs to be taken.

Box 21.6 Questions That May Aid Causality Assessments When Drug Teratogenicity Is Suspected

1. **Strength:** How strong is the effect? The stronger the association [i.e., the higher effect estimate, e.g., relative risk (RR), odds ratio (OR), or hazard ratio (HR)], the more likely it is to be causal. Statistical significance should not be mistaken for evidence of a substantial association, and precision should not be mistaken for validity.

2. **Biological plausibility:** Does the association make biological sense? A biological mechanism to support the association makes it more likely that it is causal.

3. **Specificity/pattern of birth defects:** Is there a specific syndrome or pattern of malformation? Teratogens induce specific malformations rather than a general increase in all types of birth defects.

4. **Analogy:** If the drug has the same mechanism of action or is in the same class as a known teratogen, it is more likely that a similar finding is causal.

5. **Consistency:** Is there consistency across human studies? Associations should be consistent across time and in different populations, using different methods.

6. **Temporal relationship:** Did the exposure occur when the birth defect could originate? (e.g., sensitive time periods for fetal development). The cause must come before the effect.

7. **Biological gradient:** Is there a dose–response relationship? Teratogenic effects are usually dose-dependent. A confirmed dose–response relationship increases the chance that the association is causal.

8. **Animal studies:** Is there any supportive evidence from animal studies? Teratogenicity in animals is important, but not essential.

9. **Alternative explanations:** Can there be alternative explanations for the finding? Other plausible explanations should be ruled out. This includes genetic/chromosomal disorders. For epidemiological studies, bias and confounding by, e.g., the underlying maternal condition, lifestyle, and health-related factors should be considered.

Epidemiological studies (i.e., drug utilization studies) have also an important role in evaluating the impact of regulatory actions on prescribing practices to pregnant and breastfeeding women. Such studies have also been able to provide important information on whether regulatory risk mitigation measures [e.g., Pregnancy Prevention Programs (*Guideline on good pharmacovigilance practices (GVP): Module XVI Addendum III—Pregnancy prevention programme and other pregnancy-specific risk minimisation measures*, [27, 28]) or clinical guidelines] are being followed.

Example: A study that examined trends in valproic acid use among women of childbearing potential in Ireland following two regulatory warnings in 2014 and 2018 found no evidence of change after the 2014 intervention [29]. A numerically small, but statistically significant decline in the use of valproic acid was observed after the 2018 intervention ($p = 0.03$), which the authors attributed to the introduction of new contraindication measures in 2018.

5.2 Breastfeeding Studies

Historically, surveillance of spontaneous reports and published cases has been the main pharmacovigilance activity to assess drug safety during breastfeeding.

Published case reports of possible ADRs in breastfed infants, however, often suffer from severe methodological limitations that impair causal inference. It is often not possible to separate potential drug effects from the infant's normal state or from concurrent disease. Moreover, reports are often confounded by in utero exposure, i.e., the breastfed infant was also exposed to the drug during pregnancy. That said, case series can also be valuable if performed and reported properly. Use of tools like the Naranjo scale can help standardize the causality assessment (see Chap. 8). When an adverse reaction is suspected in a breastfed infant, having a plasma concentration measurement of the drug from the infant will greatly improve causality assessment.

So far, postauthorization studies in breastfed infants are rare. A recently updated EMA guideline recommends that for drugs that are widely used among breastfeeding women and have an unknown potential for serious adverse reactions in breastfed children, postauthorization studies among breastfeeding women and their infants should be considered. This may include a clinical lactation study and/or a prospective study following infants exposed to a specific drug through breast milk. Use of pregnancy registries to follow-up of breastfed infants is also possible.

Box 21.7 Updating SmPCs When New Data Occurs: The Oxcarbazepine Case

For the antiseizure medication oxcarbazepine, the original product information recommended the drug should not be used during breastfeeding, as the effects on breastfed infants were not known. When a new study became available [30], the recommendation on use during breastfeeding was re-evaluated.

The study described 6 nursing mothers treated with oxcarbazepine. Blood samples for the analysis of oxcarbazepine were obtained at about the same time from the mothers and the infants. None of the infants had blood levels above the lower limit of quantification of the analytical method. By estimation, median infant blood levels were 0.3% of the maternal levels. Although the number of infants assessed in this study is relatively small, the sample size is larger than had been available previously. Moreover, the study was well performed. Therefore, the information on breastfeeding in product information was changed from "*oxcarbazepine should not be used during breastfeeding*" to "*a decision must be made whether to discontinue breastfeeding taking into account the benefit of breastfeeding for the child and the benefit of the therapy for the woman.*"

It should also be noted that the information on oxcarbazepine available in an expert domain [Oxcarbazepine—Drugs and Lactation Database (LactMed) [11]—NCBI Bookshelf (nih.gov)] is even more reassuring: *Oxcarbazepine is not expected to cause any adverse effects in breastfed infants, a safety scoring system finds it possible to use cautiously during breastfeeding*. When health care professionals are making decisions about treatment of a breastfeeding woman, they should complete the basic information from product information with data from the expert domain and also take into account the individual maternal and infant characteristics of the specific case (Table 21.2).

6 Evidence-Based Information Sources

Clinicians should use a variety of reliable and evidence-based information sources to support prescribing and clinical decision-making when treating pregnant and breastfeeding patients. Table 21.4 includes some examples of recommended information sources. It is important to critically evaluate the information obtained from these sources and consider the relevance and applicability of the information to the specific patient and clinical context.

Table 21.4 Examples of evidenced-based information sources about medication use in pregnancy and lactation

Type	Example
Clinical practice guidelines	**The American College of Obstetricians and Gynecologists (ACOG)**: ACOG provides guidelines on medication use during pregnancy and breastfeeding. Available at www.acog.org
	The Royal College of Obstetricians and Gynecologists (RCOG) publish "Green-top Guidelines". Available at www.rcog.org.uk/guidance/browse-all-guidance/green-top-guidelines
	The National Institute for Health and Care Excellence (NICE): NICE provides guidance on the management of health conditions during pregnancy and breastfeeding, including the use of medications. Example: Hypertension in pregnancy: Diagnosis and management (NICE guideline NG133). Available at www.nice.org.uk/guidance/ng133
Professional organizations, general information	**The United Kingdom Teratology Information Service (UKTIS)**. Evidence-based safety information about medications, vaccines, chemical and radiological exposures in pregnancy. Available at www.uktis.org
	The Organization of Teratology Information Specialists (OTIS): OTIS provides evidence-based information on medication use during pregnancy and breastfeeding through their MotherToBaby program. Fact sheets are available at https://mothertobaby.org
	Association for promotion of and cultural and scientific research into breastfeeding (APILAM): APILAM maintains an online evidence-based database on whether the medication is compatible with breastfeeding. Available at https://e-lactancia.org
Professional organizations, specific disorders	**International League Against Epilepsy (ILAE):** The ILAE has published guidelines on the management of epilepsy in pregnancy. Available at Guidelines // International League Against Epilepsy (ilae.org)
	The American College of Rheumatology (ACR) has published guidelines on the management of rheumatic disease during pregnancy and lactation. Available at Reproductive Health in Rheumatic & Musculoskeletal Diseases Guideline (rheumatology.org)
Textbooks, including e-text books	Hale TW. Krutsch K. **Drugs and mothers' milk**. 20th ed. Amarillo, TX New York, NY: Pharmasoft Medical Pub. Springer Publishing Company. 2023. ISBN: 9780826160638
	Schaefer C, Peters PWJ, Miller RK. **Drugs during pregnancy and lactation: Treatment options and risk assessment**. Third ed. Amsterdam, Boston: Elsevier Academic Press; 2015. ISBN: 9780124080782.
	Briggs, GG. Freeman, RK; Tower, CV Forinash AB. **Brigg's Drugs in Pregnancy and Lactation**: A Reference Guide to Fetal and Neonatal Risk. 12th ed. Lippincott Williams&Wilkins, 2021. ISBN/ISSN:9781975162375.
Health authorities	The U.S. **Centers for Disease Control and Prevention (CDC)**: The CDC provides guidance on medication use during pregnancy and breastfeeding through their treating for two initiative. Example: Influenza antiviral medications: Summary for clinicians. Available at https://www.cdc.gov/flu/professionals/antivirals/summary-clinicians.htm
Online medical libraries	National library of Medicines. Drugs and Lactation Database (**LactMed®**): Evidence-based safety information about medications and breastfeeding, available at www.ncbi.nlm.nih.gov/books/NBK501922

As illustrated in Box 21.7, it is important to be aware of the fact that clinical guidelines and textbooks will often differ from drug labels in their recommendations. Another example is presented in Box 21.8. These differences are caused by the strict regulatory requirements for information presented in the drug label. Also, guidelines and textbooks can take into account the risk of untreated maternal illness and the availability of safer treatment options when providing pregnancy and breastfeeding recommendations [18]. Health care professionals should explain this to patients when prescribing a drug that may be recommended in a clinical guideline, but warned against in the product label and package information leaflet. As recommendations in different information sources may differ, it is advisable to check several sources before making decisions about drug prescription during pregnancy and breastfeeding.

Box 21.8 Difference in Regulatory vs. Expert Breastfeeding Recommendation: The Rituximab Case

Rituximab is a monoclonal antibody commonly used for rheumatoid arthritis. As this is a condition affecting women of childbearing potential, it is clinically important to have recommendations about rituximab use and breastfeeding.

SmPC of rituximab products reads, about breastfeeding:

"Limited data on rituximab excretion into breast milk suggest very low rituximab concentrations in milk (relative infant dose less than 0.4%). Few cases of follow-up of breastfed infants describe normal growth and development up to 2 years. However, as these data are limited and the long-term outcomes of breastfed infants remain unknown, breastfeeding is not recommended while being treated with rituximab and optimally for 6 months following rituximab treatment."

The wording is restrictive due to limited data and warns against breastfeeding 6 months following the treatment due to rituximab's long elimination half-life.

In contrast to the SmPC wording, recent clinical guidelines consider rituximab to be acceptable for use during breastfeeding [31–33].

In general, monoclonal antibodies are large molecules and as such they are not expected to be excreted in breast milk in significant amounts; moreover, if present in breast milk, the absorption from the infant's gastrointestinal tract is probably minimal. Thus, considering pharmacokinetic properties, rituximab should be safe to use while breastfeeding.

When making decisions about medications for breastfeeding individuals, it is important to consider different data sources (see Table 21.4) and tailoring the information to the individual patient.

7 Communicating Information About Drugs to Pregnant and Breastfeeding Women

Concerns about the risks of drug use to the fetus and breastfed infant are widespread among pregnant and breastfeeding women [8, 28]. This may result in anxiety, poor drug adherence, discontinuation of drug, early cessation of breastfeeding, relapse, or worsening of the underlying condition and may put both the mother and child at risk. Understanding a woman's beliefs, information needs and health literacy level are important for health care professionals to appropriately counsel women in these important periods of life.

Health care professionals need to be able to provide information that in plain language summarizes what is known about the risks to the fetus or breastfed infant if the drug is taken. It is equally important to clearly communicate the risks of *not* taking the drug. When communicating with the pregnant woman, it is important to explain that if treatment is crucial for her wellbeing, it generally also benefits her unborn child (see also Chaps. 11 and 17).

Relative risks (RRs), odds ratios (ORs), and hazard ratios (HRs) are easily misinterpreted and are generally not appropriate for conveying risk estimates to patients. A large increase in the RR for a rare defect may not imply a large increase in absolute risk. If it is desirable to quote the relative risk, always include baseline rates of the particular pregnancy outcome.

For example, in a cohort study including 1.8 million pregnancies, first trimester ondansetron use was associated with an increased risk of oral clefts with an adjusted relative risk of 1.24 (95% CI 1.03–1.48) [19]. With a baseline risk of oral clefts of 11 per 10,000, this represented 3 additional cases per 10,000 ondansetron-treated women. The benefits for the mother and child of adequately treating *hyperemesis gravidarum* may by far outweigh this risk, and ondansetron is generally recommended as a second-line treatment for this most severe form of nausea and vomiting in pregnancy [34].

In 2015, the FDA removed the former pregnancy risk letter categories in drug labels (category A–D and X) as clinicians and patients were often confused by the meaning of these categories. The new labeling system, called "Pregnancy and Lactation Labeling Rule" (PLLR), instead includes more comprehensive and drug-specific information discussing the potential risks and benefits to the mother and the fetus, as well as information about the background risk, to contextualize the risk. A background risk statement could be "*In the general population, the estimated background risk of major birth defects and miscarriage in clinically recognized pregnancies is 2–4% and 15–20%, respectively*." Moreover, the PLLR requires information about a pregnancy exposure registry if it exists. More details about the old and current labeling requirements can be found at the FDA website: https://www.fda.gov/drugs/labeling-information-drug-products/pregnancy-and-lactation-labeling-drugs-final-rule.

In conclusion, it is essential for health care professionals to provide information in a way that supports informed decision-making and promotes patient involvement in decisions about drug use during pregnancy and while breastfeeding. Decision support tools, including visual aids such as pictograms or graphs, may enhance the understanding of risks.

8 Summary and Conclusions

Few drugs are proven teratogenic or harmful to breastfed infants. Prescribing drugs during pregnancy and breastfeeding, however, is often challenging due to missing and/or inconsistent information about safety to the fetus or breastfed infant. Postmarketing pharmacoepidemiologic studies are important to generate information about safety among pregnant and breastfeeding women as clinical studies tend to exclude these individuals. Teratogenicity of a drug depends on its mechanism of action, dose, administration form, duration of exposure, timing in pregnancy, and genetic susceptibility. Teratogenic effects include birth defects, embryo-fetal death, growth retardation, and functional defects later in life. Most medications are transferred into breast milk in too small amounts to exert any clinically important effects on the infant. Drug labels and clinical guidelines/textbooks may differ in their recommendations to pregnant and breastfeeding women due to strict regulatory requirements for data in the drug labels. Explaining risks to the mother in a clear way is essential to promote optimal drug use during pregnancy and while breastfeeding.

9 Case Studies

9.1 Case Study 1: Lamotrigine in Pregnancy

Miriam is a 31-year-old woman who has been diagnosed with epilepsy since childhood. In the last 8 years, she has been treated with lamotrigine 400 mg/day. The plasma concentration of lamotrigine has been fairly stable with this dose, varying between 8 and 12 mg/L [therapeutic range 3–15 mg/L (10–60 µmol/L)]. She and her husband now plan to have a child, but are concerned about how a pregnancy would affect her epilepsy, and how her medication could affect the baby. Miriam now has an appointment with the neurologist and wants to discuss her drug treatment and how to handle it during the pregnancy. She also wants to know if there are any vitamins or supplements that could be helpful.

1. *What do you think is the important general information the neurologist should give her?*

   The neurologist explains to Miriam that lamotrigine has been used in more than 13,000 pregnancies and that there is no indication that its use increases the risk of birth defects compared to women with epilepsy not using any antiseizure medications. Moreover, he tells her that studies show that lamotrigine use in pregnancy does not increase the risk of miscarriage, stillbirth, preterm birth, or low birth weight. He also explains Miriam the importance of high adherence to the treatment regime; if she skips lamotrigine anytime during pregnancy and experiences an epileptic seizure, the risk for the fetus would be higher than any theoretically possible risk of continuing lamotrigine.

2. *What would be your answer to Miriam's question regarding vitamins or supplements?*

   The neurologist is aware that lamotrigine, like many other antiseizure drugs, is a folate antagonist and that folate is important for normal early development of the central nervous system. Thus, folic acid supplementation in women using such drugs reduces the risk of neural tube defects, including spina bifida. As these malformations originate early in pregnancy, even before the woman would be aware of her pregnancy, it is important to start with folic acid already when the woman is trying to conceive. The dose needed is high, 5 mg/day, so the woman usually needs a prescription of 5 mg tablets. In contrast, the doses of tablets available over the counter are usually just about one tenth of this, 0.4–0.6 mg, which are too low to protect properly against neural tube defects when using folate antagonists. Such low-dose tablets are therefore not an option for Miriam. (In many countries, low-dose tablets with folic acid are recommended for all women from at least 1 month prior to conception and during the first trimester of pregnancy. In some countries, flour is fortified with folic acid to reduce the rate of neural tube defects.)

   The neurologist explains to Miriam that although lamotrigine is considered safe during pregnancy, it is a weak folate antagonist, and as an extra precaution, he recommends that she uses folic acid 5 mg/day while trying to become pregnant and during the first trimester of pregnancy.

3. *Do you think there is a need to arrange any extra monitoring during pregnancy?*

   During pregnancy, Miriam is followed with monthly clinical controls for her epilepsy, which also includes measuring plasma concentrations of lamotrigine. As the concentrations are steadily decreasing—just as expected due to the pregnancy-induced increase in its metabolism and excretion—the lamotrigine dose is gradually increased to 700 mg/day. She is also followed with regular prenatal care visits and the progress of the pregnancy was completely normal.

   In gestational week 35, she gives birth to a premature but otherwise healthy boy with no signs of any malformation, weighing 2650 g.

9.2 Case Study 2: Lamotrigine During Breastfeeding

Shortly after delivery, Miriam has some trouble with establishing breastfeeding, so the first 2 weeks postpartum the boy is given additional milk from other sources. However, her milk production gradually improves, and the infant, who is now 4 weeks old, has been fully breastfed for 2 weeks.

The last few days, Miriam has observed that the boy has become drowsy and that he also has some trouble with suckling. She contacts the maternity unit at the hospital. There, they wonder whether the symptoms could be caused by lamotrigine transferred to the infant via breast milk—although her lamotrigine dose has been gradually decreased again after birth and is now 550 mg/day.

1. *What would be your first step to do in this situation?*

   They decide to measure drug concentrations in maternal and infant plasma as well as in breast milk.

   The lamotrigine plasma concentration in the infant is 5.6 mg/L, whereas the maternal plasma concentration is 18 mg/L (therapeutic range 3–15 mg/L). The breast milk concentration is 6.2 mg/L.

2. *What would be the relative infant dose (RID) in this case? Is this a high or a low RID? The maternal body weight is 77 kg and the standard estimated infant milk intake is 0.150 L/kg/day.*

   The infant daily dose per kg body weight would be 6.2 mg/L × 0.150 L/kg/day = 0.93 mg/kg/day. The maternal daily dose per kg body weight was 550 mg/day divided by 77 kg = 7.14 mg/kg/day. Thus, the

RID would be 0.93 divided by 7.14 = 0.13 = 13%. As the RID is above 10%, it indicates a high infant exposure, just as expected based on data from the literature.

3. *How likely do you think that lamotrigine is causing the symptoms in the breastfed infant? How do you handle the situation now?*

   The physician at the maternity unit considers that it is likely that the infant symptoms are caused by the transfer of lamotrigine to the infant via breast milk. Due to the high maternal plasma concentration the maternal dose is reduced to the prepregnant level of 400 mg/day. As the mother still has a strong desire to breastfeed her infant, the physician and the mother agree that she should try partial breastfeeding and partial formula feeding for a week. During this period, the infant's symptoms would expect to wane and finally disappear. Thereafter she could gradually increase breastfeeding again.

4. *What would be your expectations related to the drug concentrations in maternal and infant plasma when the dose is reduced from 550 to 400 mg/day?*

   A dose reduction from 550 to 400 mg/day is a reduction of 28%. It would then be expected that the maternal plasma concentration is reduced by 28% as well, i.e., down to 13 mg/L. This concentration is within the therapeutic range.

   Such a maternal dose reduction (and provided that the infant is again fully breastfed), the infant plasma concentration could also be expected to decrease by 28%, i.e., down to 3.0 mg/L, which is just at the lower limit of the therapeutic interval. Hopefully, the dose of 400 mg/day would therefore be too low to cause any infant symptoms.

5. *If the infant symptoms do not disappear after dose reduction to 400 mg/day, what could be the next step to consider?*

   If a concentration of 3.0 mg/L (when exclusively breastfed) would not be sufficiently low to remove the symptoms, a further dose reduction (e.g., down to 350–300 mg/day) could be a possibility, particularly as the maternal plasma concentration is still well within the therapeutic range. However, before physician at the maternity unit makes any decision of reducing the dose below 400 mg/day, he would discuss this option with the neurologist. If the infant symptoms do not disappear despite further dose reductions, it seems that formula feeding will be the best alternative.

   It turns out that after a dose reduction to 400 mg/day, the symptoms did not reappear when full breastfeeding was reintroduced. Further dose reductions were therefore not needed, and the mother was very satisfied with the situation.

   As a final note, since pregnancy-induced increases in drug clearance and volume of distribution normalize within a week or so after labor, dose reduction of lamotrigine had been unnecessarily slow in this case. A faster lamotrigine tapering after birth could possibly have prevented the infant symptoms.

References

1. Nordeng H, van Gelder M. Chapter 3.3.1. Drug utilization studies in pregnant women. In: Drug utilization research—methods and applications. Wiley; 2024.
2. Ceulemans M, Lupattelli A, Nordeng H, Odalovic M, Twigg M, Foulon V. Women's beliefs about medicines and adherence to pharmacotherapy in pregnancy: opportunities for community pharmacists. Curr Pharm Des. 2019;25(5):469–82. https://doi.org/10.2174/1381612825666190321110420.
3. Petersen I, McCrea RL, Lupattelli A, Nordeng H. Women's perception of risks of adverse fetal pregnancy outcomes: a large-scale multinational survey. BMJ Open. 2015;5(6):e007390. https://doi.org/10.1136/bmjopen-2014-007390.
4. Mahmood T, Savona-Ventura C, Messinis I, Mukhopadhyay S. The EBCOG postgraduate textbook of obstetrics and gynaecology. Cambridge: Cambridge University Press; 2021.
5. Schaefer C, Peters PWJ, Miller RK. Drugs during pregnancy and lactation: treatment options and risk assessment. 3nd ed. Amsterdam: Elsevier Academic Press; 2014.
6. Feldkamp ML, Carey JC, Byrne JLB, Krikov S, Botto LD. Etiology and clinical presentation of birth defects: population based study. BMJ. 2017;357:j2249. https://doi.org/10.1136/bmj.j2249.
7. Magnus MC, Wilcox AJ, Morken NH, Weinberg CR, Haberg SE. Role of maternal age and pregnancy history in risk of miscarriage: prospective register based

study. BMJ. 2019;364:l869. https://doi.org/10.1136/bmj.l869.
8. Euro-Peristat. European Perinatal Health Report. Core indicators of the health and care of pregnant women and babies in Europe in 2015. www.europeristat.com. https://www.europeristat.com/images/EPHR2015_web_hyperlinked_Euro-Peristat.pdf.
9. Shepard TH. Catalog of teratogenic agents. 13th ed. Baltimore: Johns Hopkins University Press; 2010.
10. van Gelder MM, van Rooij IA, Miller RK, Zielhuis GA, de Jong-van den Berg LT, Roeleveld N. Teratogenic mechanisms of medical drugs. Hum Reprod Update. 2010;16(4):378–94. https://doi.org/10.1093/humupd/dmp052.
11. Drugs and Lactation Database (LactMed) 2023. National Library of Medicine www.toxnet.nlm.nih.gov/cgi-bin/sis/htmlgen?LACT.
12. Hale TW, Krutsch K. Hale's medications and mothers' milk. 20th ed. New York: Springer Publishing Company; 2023.
13. Ito S. Drug therapy for breast-feeding women. N Engl J Med. 2000;343(2):118–26.
14. Anderson PO, Pochop SL, Manoguerra AS. Adverse drug reactions in breastfed infants: less than imagined. Clin Pediatr (Phila). 2003;42(4):325–40. https://doi.org/10.1177/000992280304200405.
15. Mazer-Amirshahi M, Samiee-Zafarghandy S, Gray G, van den Anker JN. Trends in pregnancy labeling and data quality for US-approved pharmaceuticals. Am J Obstet Gynecol. 2014;211(6):690–11. https://doi.org/10.1016/j.ajog.2014.06.013.
16. Adam MP, Polifka JE, Friedman JM. Evolving knowledge of the teratogenicity of medications in human pregnancy. Am J Med Genet C Semin Med Genet. 2011;157C(3):175–82. https://doi.org/10.1002/ajmg.c.30313.
17. Brown BL, Kesselheim AS, Sarpatwari A. Analysis of risk evaluation and mitigation strategies for teratogenic drugs: variation in primary and secondary prevention measures. PLoS Med. 2023;20(3):e1004190. https://doi.org/10.1371/journal.pmed.1004190.
18. CHMP guideline on risk assessment of medicinal products on human reproduction and lactation: from data to labelling, EMEA/CHMP/203927/2005, 2005. https://www.ema.europa.eu/en/documents/scientific-guideline/guideline-risk-assessmentmedicinal-products-human-reproduction-and-lactation-data-labelling_en.pdf.
19. Huybrechts KF, Hernandez-Diaz S, Straub L, Gray KJ, Zhu Y, Patorno E, Bateman BT. Association of maternal first-trimester ondansetron use with cardiac malformations and oral clefts in offspring. JAMA. 2018;320(23):2429–37. https://doi.org/10.1001/jama.2018.18307.
20. Postigo R, Brosch S, Slattery J, van Haren A, Dogne JM, Kurz X, Arlett P. EudraVigilance medicines safety database: publicly accessible data for research and public health protection. Drug Saf. 2018;41(7):665–75. https://doi.org/10.1007/s40264-018-0647-1.
21. Star K, Sandberg L, Bergvall T, Choonara I, Caduff-Janosa P, Edwards IR. Paediatric safety signals identified in VigiBase: methods and results from Uppsala Monitoring Centre. Pharmacoepidemiol Drug Saf. 2019;28(5):680–9. https://doi.org/10.1002/pds.4734.
22. Nana M, Hodson K, Lucas N, Camporota L, Knight M, Nelson-Piercy C. Diagnosis and management of Covid-19 in pregnancy. BMJ. 2022;377:e069739. https://doi.org/10.1136/bmj-2021-069739.
23. Koren G. Medication safety in pregnancy and breastfeeding: the evidence-based A-to-Z clinician's pocket guide. New York: McGraw-Hill Medical; 2007.
24. Schwarz EB, Moretti ME, Nayak S, Koren G. Risk of hypospadias in offspring of women using loratadine during pregnancy: a systematic review and meta-analysis. Drug Saf. 2008;31(9):775–88.
25. PRAC-CMDh. Topiramate (safety) referral_Art31. 2022. https://www.ema.europa.eu/en/medicines/human/referrals/topiramate.
26. Bjork MH, Zoega H, Leinonen MK, Cohen JM, Dreier JW, Furu K, Christensen J. Association of prenatal exposure to antiseizure medication with risk of autism and intellectual disability. JAMA Neurol. 2022;79(7):672–81. https://doi.org/10.1001/jamaneurol.2022.1269.
27. European Medicines Agency (EMA). Guideline on good pharmacovigilance practices (GVP): Module XVI Addendum III—pregnancy prevention programme and other pregnancy-specific risk minimisation measures. 2023. https://www.ema.europa.eu/en/documents/regulatory-procedural-guideline/draft-guideline-good-pharmacovigilance-practices-gvp-module-xvi-addendum-iii-pregnancy-prevention_en.pdf.
28. Raguideau F, Mezzarobba M, Zureik M, Weill A, Ricordeau P, Alla F. Compliance with pregnancy prevention plan recommendations in 8672 French women of childbearing potential exposed to acitretin. Pharmacoepidemiol Drug Saf. 2015;24(5):526–33. https://doi.org/10.1002/pds.3763.
29. Murphy S, Bennett K, Doherty CP. Prescribing trends for sodium valproate in Ireland. Seizure. 2016;36:44–8. https://doi.org/10.1016/j.seizure.2016.01.019.
30. Birnbaum AK, Meador KJ, Karanam A, Brown C, May RC, Gerard EE, MONEAD Investigator Group. Antiepileptic drug exposure in infants of breastfeeding mothers with epilepsy. JAMA Neurol. 2020;77(4):441–50. https://doi.org/10.1001/jamaneurol.2019.4443.
31. Dobson R, Rog D, Ovadia C, Murray K, Hughes S, Ford HL, Brex P. Anti-CD20 therapies in pregnancy and breast feeding: a review and ABN guide-

lines. Pract Neurol. 2023;23(1):6–14. https://doi.org/10.1136/pn-2022-003426.
32. Russell MD, Dey M, Flint J, Davie P, Allen A, Crossley A, Guidelines Working, Group. British Society for Rheumatology guideline on prescribing drugs in pregnancy and breastfeeding: immunomodulatory anti-rheumatic drugs and corticosteroids. Rheumatology (Oxford). 2023;62(4):e48–88. https://doi.org/10.1093/rheumatology/keac551.
33. Sammaritano LR, Bermas BL, Chakravarty EE, Chambers C, Clowse MEB, Lockshin MD, D'Anci KE. 2020 American College of Rheumatology guideline for the management of reproductive health in rheumatic and musculoskeletal diseases. Arthritis Rheumatol. 2020;72(4):529–56. https://doi.org/10.1002/art.41191.
34. Royal College of Obstetricians and Gynaecologists. Management of nausea and vomiting of pregnancy and hyperemesis gravidarum (Green-top Guidelines No. 69). 2016. www.rcog.org.uk.

Further Reading

The European Network of Centres for Pharmacoepidemiology and Pharmacovigilance (ENCePP). Guide on Methodological Standards in Pharmacoepidemiology. 2023. https://encepp.europa.eu/document/download/51d343d5-cd71-4e9b-a455-235d8a03ccba_en?filename=methodologicalGuideAnnex2.pdf - Chapter on 'Methods for evaluation of Medicines in pregnancy and lactation'.

European Medicines Agency (EMA). Guideline on good pharmacovigilance practices (GVP): product- or population-specific considerations III: pregnant and breastfeeding women. 2020. https://www.ema.europa.eu/en/documents/scientific-guideline/draft-guideline-good-pharmacovigilance-practicesproduct-population-specific-considerations-iii_en.pdf.

22 Safe Prescribing in Patients with Kidney and Hepatic Diseases

Wubshet Tesfaye, Ronald L. Castelino, Monica Zolezzi, and Fatima Small

Abstract

Safe prescribing in kidney disease, particularly chronic kidney disease (CKD), requires careful monitoring of the use of nephrotoxic medications and dosage adjustments for those that are predominantly cleared by the kidneys. Generally, to minimize the risk of adverse effects and toxicity, medication selection in people with CKD should consider a host of factors, such as medications' route of clearance, nephrotoxicity potential, therapeutic window, and their adverse effect profile. For medications that are predominantly cleared by the kidneys, dosage adjustment decisions are made based on residual kidney function, which is typically determined using equations that provide an estimated glomerular filtration rate.

The hepatic system also plays a crucial role in the metabolism of many medications by converting them into active and inactive metabolites as well as elimination of exogenous substances. Rates of hepatic elimination and therapeutic window of medications are important aspects to consider in people with reduced hepatic function. The Child–Pugh score and the Model for End-stage Liver Disease are some of the tools used to assess and score levels of hepatic impairment, with implication for medication choice and dosing.

In summary, prescribing decisions in people with kidney or hepatic diseases should be made based on several clinical and patient factors, as well as considering functional and biochemical markers.

Keywords

Kidney disease · Chronic kidney disease
Nephrotoxicity · Hepatic impairment
Hepatotoxicity · Hepatic diseases
Dosage adjustment · Dose adjustment
Drug-induced liver injury

Learning Objectives

Part I

- Describe how reduced kidney function affects absorption, distribution, metabolism, and elimination of medicines.

W. Tesfaye (✉)
School of Pharmacy, The University of Queensland, Brisbane, Australia

School of Pharmacy, Faculty of Medicine and Health, The University of Sydney, Sydney, NSW, Australia
e-mail: Wubshet.Tesfaye@sydney.edu.au; w.tesfaye@uq.edu.au

R. L. Castelino
School of Pharmacy, Faculty of Medicine and Health, The University of Sydney, Sydney, NSW, Australia

Pharmacy Department, Blacktown Hospital, WSLHD, Blacktown, NSW, Australia

M. Zolezzi
College of Pharmacy, QU Health, Qatar University, Doha, Qatar

F. Small
Pharmacy Department, Blacktown Hospital, WSLHD, Blacktown, NSW, Australia

J. Jose et al. (eds.), *Principles and Practice of Pharmacovigilance and Drug Safety*,
https://doi.org/10.1007/978-3-031-51089-2_22

- Recognize medicines that require monitoring in people with reduced kidney function.
- Outline the effects of medicines in the context of kidney disease, including nephrotoxicity.
- Identify high-risk medicines that can cause acute kidney injury and understand the need for medication dosage adjustments.
- Explain the effect of dialysis on medicines and support clinicians with medicines optimization.

Part II

- Describe how hepatic impairment affects absorption, distribution, metabolism, and elimination of medicines.
- Discuss pharmacokinetic and pharmacodynamic changes in people with hepatic impairment.
- Identify medications that require monitoring in people with hepatic impairment.
- Outline the effects of medicines on the hepatic system, including drug-induced hepatic impairment and its management.
- Discuss the prescribing and dosing considerations in people with hepatic impairment.

Key Points

- Several medications require dosage adjustment in people with kidney or hepatic diseases.
- Kidney function is often determined using equations that estimate glomerular filtration rate, which is used to adjust the dosage of various medications.
- Unlike kidney disease, there is no single parameter for adjusting dosages in hepatic impairment.
- The Child–Pugh score and the Model for End-stage Liver Disease are common methods used to assess and score levels of hepatic impairment, with implications for medication dosing and selection.
- Optimal prescribing for people with reduced kidney or hepatic function should consider residual organ function, medication pharmacokinetics and pharmacodynamics, potential for organ toxicity, therapeutic window, comorbidities, safety profile, and patient comorbidity status, among other factors.

1 Introduction

Drug therapy is critical to the medical management of people with kidney and liver diseases. Not only are drugs used to prevent and treat a range of kidney and liver diseases and their complications, but they are also required to manage several complex comorbidities commonly seen in patients affected with these conditions.

Drug management and prescribing in people with kidney and liver diseases can be challenging because of the important role of kidneys and liver in the metabolism and excretion of endogenous and exogenous compounds. Impaired kidney and liver function can result in significantly altered drug pharmacokinetics and pharmacodynamics, putting people with kidney and liver diseases at a significantly higher risk of experiencing adverse drug effects. When prescribing drugs for these patients, it is important that clinicians take these changes into consideration to avoid predictable serious adverse effects and maximize therapeutic benefits.

To identify a safe and effective drug dose regimen in people with kidney and liver disease, healthcare professionals ideally require data and information derived from these patient populations. However, as these people are often excluded from clinical studies leading to limited literature, clinical judgment is often required.

This chapter has been developed specifically to provide healthcare professionals with concise practical information to assist decision-making process for the safe use of drugs in people with kidney and hepatic disease.

2 Part One: Safe Prescribing in Patients with Kidney Disease

2.1 Background

Kidney disease presents in many different forms with varied prevalence, presentation, outcomes, and personal and societal impact. It is typically diagnosed using blood and urine tests, in combination with relevant history and physical examinations. Estimation of glomerular filtration rate (GFR), assessment of serum creatinine (SCr), newer markers such as serum cystatin C, and urine tests for albuminuria are some of the basic diagnostic evaluations employed in clinical settings. Several additional immunological tests, imaging, and biopsy may be necessary to provide a specific diagnosis, reflect the level of disease severity, and guide a more tailored treatment of the disease.

Chronic kidney disease (CKD) is defined as a sustained kidney damage (presence of protein in urine) and/or reduced kidney function [estimated glomerular filtration rate (eGFR) of <60 mL/min/1.73 m^2] lasting for at least 3 months [1]. It affects around 10% of the adult population worldwide, and its prevalence has increased by 30% over the past three decades, with high-income countries affected more than developing nations [2]. As shown in Fig. 22.1, CKD is traditionally classified into five stages based on eGFR and albuminuria (classification based on Kidney Disease Improving Global Clinical Outcome [KDIGO] organization) [3]. Acute kidney injury (AKI), on the other hand, is characterized by a sudden deterioration of kidney function over a period of hours to days [4]. It is clinically defined through an increase in SCr or decrease in urine output with accumulation of metabolic wastes and/or the development of complications such as acidosis and hyperkalemia. Table 22.1 presents the diagnosis and staging criteria for AKI.

Assessment of kidney function is essential for safe prescribing as the ability of the kidneys to handle medications is significantly altered during kidney disease. Kidney disease can affect the absorption, distribution, metabolism, and elimination (ADME) of a medicine and can also result in pharmacodynamic changes. Many medications and some active metabolites are eliminated by the kidneys, either through glomerular filtration or tubular secretion. Furthermore, people with kidney disease often take multiple medications, increasing the potential for adverse effects due to interactions and

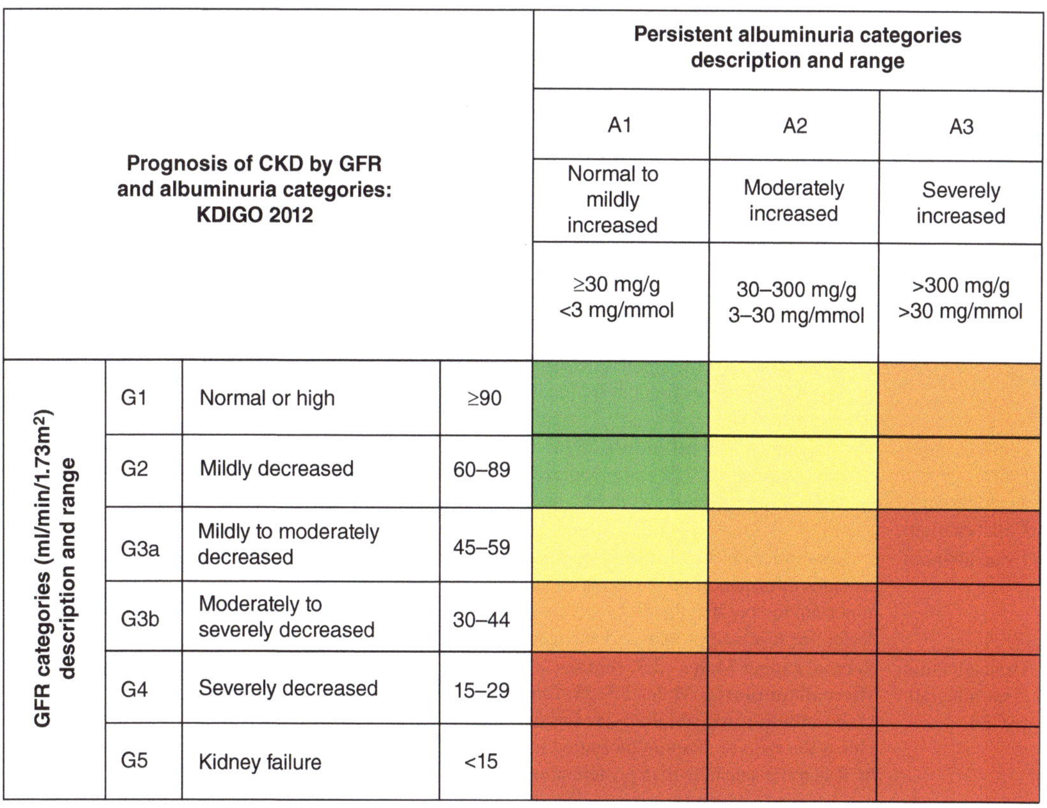

Fig. 22.1 Staging of chronic kidney disease based on eGFR and albuminuria [3]

Table 22.1 Key laboratory tests used for routine diagnosis or monitoring of kidney disease [5–9]

Test	Comments	
Serum creatinine (SCr)	**Normal range: 60–110 μmol/L** Creatinine is a product of muscle metabolism. It is a waste product freely filtered by the kidneys with no tubular reabsorption but undergoes tubular section. As creatinine is produced at a constant rate, serum creatinine (SCr) levels have been used to estimate glomerular filtration rate (GFR). Creatinine concentrations are higher in men compared to women and people with a large muscle bulk. Drugs including trimethoprim that inhibit creatinine secretion will raise creatinine levels and so results should be interpreted with care.	
Potassium	**Normal range: 3.5–5.3 mmol/L** Hyperkalemia is a common problem in both Acute Kidney Injury (AKI) and Chronic Kidney Disease (CKD) and is frequently monitored owing to the risk of arrhythmias. Many drugs also affect the potassium levels and should be used cautiously in people with kidney disease (e.g., spironolactone, angiotensin-converting enzyme inhibitors, angiotensin receptor blockers).	
Urinalysis	A urine dipstick test for hematuria, proteinuria, leucocytes, and glucose is recommended to detect glomerulonephritis, acute pyelonephritis, and interstitial nephritis. However, dipstick tests should be interpreted with caution in people with catheters because of the possibility of false-positive results (e.g., dipstick hematuria because of simple trauma). Strongly positive results, for example, 2+ blood, 2+ protein usually indicates glomerular pathology. Increased white cells are nonspecific but may suggest infection (most common) or interstitial nephritis.	
Additional tests	Several immunology tests such as antinuclear antibody (ANA), double-stranded DNA, serum immunoelectrophoresis, complement tests (e.g., C3 and C4) are often ordered in patients presenting with kidney disease where renal pathology is suspected (e.g., lupus nephritis, myeloma).	
Diagnosis and staging of AKI		
Diagnosis	• Increase in SCr by ≥0.3 mg/dL (≥26.5 μmol/L) within 48 h; or • Increase in SCr to ≥1.5 times baseline, which is known or presumed to have occurred within the prior 7 days; or • Urine volume <0.5 mL/kg/h for 6 h	
Staging	Serum creatinine	Urine output
1	1.5–1.9 times baseline OR ≥0.3 mg/dL (≥26.5 μmol/L) increase	<0.5 mL/kg/h for 6–12 h
2	2.0–2.9 times baseline	<0.5 mL/kg/h for ≥12 h
3	3.0 times baseline OR increase in SCr ≥4.0 mg/dL (≥35.36 μmol/L) OR initiation of kidney replacement therapy	<0.3 mL/kg/h for ≥24 h OR anuria for ≥12 h
Additional key tests for diagnosis, monitoring, and staging of CKD		
Urea	**Normal range: 2.5–7.8 mmol/L** Urea is a waste product produced by the liver. It is filtered by the kidneys, undergoes tubular reabsorption with some amount excreted in the urine. On its own, it is a relatively insensitive marker for kidney function but frequently measured with SCr. Urea levels are increased when dehydrated.	
eGFR (using CKD Epidemiology Collaboration)	**Normal range: >90 mL/min/1.73 m²** Used for staging of CKD and is reported with every SCr request in most laboratories. eGFR with cystatin C or combination with SCr and cystatin C are also employed in some countries.	
Urine albumin	Urinary protein is often used as an initial screening test for the presence of kidney disease and provides information on the cause of kidney disease (e.g., glomerulonephritis). However, it is important to note that dipsticks are usually used to screen overt proteinuria and do not usually detect low levels of protein and are semiquantitative.	
Urine albumin creatinine ratio (ACR)	**Normal range: Male: <2.5; female: <3.5** **Microalbuminuria: Male: 2.5–25; female: 3.5–35** **Macroalbuminuria: Male: >25; female: >35** This is the ratio of albumin measured in mg in the urine to SCr in mmol. ACR is more sensitive than protein creatinine ratio (PCR) and is used in CKD staging.	

(continued)

Table 22.1 (continued)

Test	Comments
Protein creatinine ratio (PCR)	This is the ratio of protein in the urine in mg to SCr measured in mmol PCR is used to quantify and monitor higher levels of proteinuria, e.g., when ACR is >70 mg/mol
Hemoglobin	**Normal range: 130–180 g/L (male); 125–160 g/L (female)** Hemoglobin should be monitored in people with eGFR <45 mL/min/1.73 m^2 to identify renal anemia. In patients receiving erythropoietin-stimulating agents (ESAs), the target hemoglobin is 100–120 g/L
Iron studies	Along with Hb, iron studies are frequently monitored in people with CKD. It is recommended to maintain a ferritin level of 200–500 mcg/L and transferrin saturation of 20–30% in people on ESAs
Serum calcium	**Normal range: 2.15–2.55 mmol/L** Serum calcium should be monitored in all people with stage 4 and 5 CKD to identify and monitor for bone and mineral disease of CKD
Serum phosphate	**Normal range: 0.8–1.4 mmol/L** Serum phosphate concentrations are measured in people with stage 4 and 5 CKD due to the accumulation in kidney disease and its impact on the development of renal bone disease
Parathyroid hormone (PTH)	Serum PTH concentrations are monitored in people with stage 4 and 5 CKD. PTH, controls calcium levels, is often increased in kidney disease, and may be checked to help determine if enough calcium and vitamin D are being taken to prevent bone damage and for hyperparathyroidism. However, optimum levels of PTH in CKD are yet to be determined
Bicarbonate	**Normal range: 22–29 mmol/L** Serum bicarbonate levels are measured to assess metabolic acidosis. Acidosis can be a problem in people with advanced stages of CKD (predialysis) and in AKI. However, oral bicarbonate supplementation is usually not necessary in patients on kidney replacement therapy (dialysis).

accumulation in reduced kidney function. The main factor that determines the need for and the extent of any dose reduction is the GFR and its impact on drug clearance. In practice, GFR is usually estimated from SCr and it may be unreliable in patients with rapidly changing kidney function, e.g., in those with AKI. The first part of this chapter focuses on medication use considerations in kidney disease, some of the key tests involved in assessing kidney function, handling of medications in people with kidney disease, when and how alteration of medication dosage is necessary including discussion on some of the medications that could cause a reduction in kidney function.

2.2 Medicine Use Considerations in Patients with Kidney Disease

Kidney disease affects the way medicines are handled and hence affects both the choice of medicine and the method of administration. The pharmacokinetics and pharmacodynamics of many medications are altered by kidney disease. An understanding of why and how these processes are impacted by kidney disease is essential to optimize medicines safely.

2.2.1 Absorption and Bioavailability

Absorption of orally administered medicines may be reduced in people with impaired kidney function because of vomiting and diarrhea associated with uremia [10, 11]. Uremia can also result in an increase in gut pH from increased gastric ammonia production, which reduces the bioavailability of medicines requiring an acidic environment for absorption. Additionally, coadministration of medicines that increase gastric pH (histamine-2-receptor antagonists) or the use of chelating agents such as those for binding phosphate in kidney disease can also affect the absorption of medicines [11, 12]. There is relatively little quantitative information regarding the influence of kidney disease on medication absorption and bioavailability, as these are not routinely altered to factor these changes but must be considered as a holistic picture.

2.2.2 Distribution

The distribution of many medications is affected in people with kidney disease because of changes in the fluid status, protein, and tissue binding. Changes in the fluid status are common in people with AKI or later stages of CKD or critically ill patients receiving intravenous fluids. These factors can result in edema, pleural effusion, and fluid overload and subsequently lead to an increase in volume of distribution (*Vd*) and a decrease in serum concentrations [13]. It is also important to know hydration status of patients when performing therapeutic drug monitoring and interpreting the results. Some examples of medications that may be impacted include hydrophilic medications such as gentamicin [14].

Likewise, distribution of medicines may be affected by alteration in the protein binding which may be due to low albumin. This may be the case in nephrotic syndrome or due to uremia, accumulation of metabolites and endogenous substances which compete for binding to albumin. Protein binding may also be affected due to altered structural arrangement of albumin possibly reducing the affinity or number of binding sites for medicines [15]. Alterations in protein binding is clinically important for highly protein-bound medicines (>80%) such as phenytoin, which can result in a higher proportion of unbound and active medicine in the plasma [11, 12].

2.2.3 Metabolism

Phase I and phase II metabolisms are slower in kidney disease [11, 16]. The effect of this is increase in serum concentrations of the parent medicine. This may lead to a higher risk of adverse effects and toxicity where medicines are usually metabolized to inactive metabolites. The kidney itself acts as the site of metabolism for some medicines. An example of metabolism being affected in kidney disease includes that of insulin, whereby diabetic patients' insulin requirements may be less [11, 16].

2.2.4 Elimination

The kidneys are involved in the elimination of medicines and metabolites. This occurs through the filtration of unbound drug from plasma at the glomerulus and for some drugs, secretion and reabsorption in renal tubules [11]. In people with kidney disease, all these functions are reduced, resulting in a slower rate of elimination for medicines which are cleared by the kidneys. The reduction in glomerular filtration and tubular secretion results in higher plasma levels of medicine and the reduction in reabsorption results in higher concentrations of medicine in the urine. The extent to which medicines are affected depends on the fraction of the dose excreted unchanged [16]. Hence, to optimize medications in people with kidney disease, an assessment of kidney function is required [11].

2.2.5 Pharmacodynamic Changes

It is also known that kidney disease due to its effects on multiple organ systems can alter a pharmacodynamic response or physiological process that in turn may affect a clinical response. Examples include (1) the inability of the kidney to activate vitamin D precursors renders vitamin D2 and vitamin D3 therapy less effective in people with CKD, (2) people with kidney disease also have coagulopathy because of uremic effect on platelet function and may be prone to the bleeding complications from anticoagulant and antiplatelet therapy, and (3) an increased risk of hyperkalemia with medicines such as potassium-sparing diuretics [17].

2.3 Diagnosis of Kidney Disease

A range of blood and urine tests are used to determine how well the kidneys are functioning. These tests may be requested in people at risk of kidney disease or in people with signs and symptoms of kidney disease and to monitor progression. Assessing the kidney function usually involves an estimation of GFR [5]. GFR cannot be measured directly, so it is estimated from the clearance of an exogenous or endogenous solute present in stable concentration in the plasma and freely filtered by the kidney. The solute ideally used should not be secreted or reabsorbed by the renal tubule. Endogenous solutes used for determining kidney functioning include urea, creatinine, and cystatin C [5–7]. Urea is an insensitive marker for kidney function, while SCr is a widely used marker despite overestimating GFR by 10–20 mL/min/1.73 m^2 due to tubular secretion and being influenced by factors like age, sex, race, and weight [5, 7, 18]. Cystatin C appears to be a more accurate marker than creatinine, less affected by external factors, and is combined with creatinine in an estimating equation (eGFRcr-cys) for better accuracy. However, disease states like hypo/hyperthyroidism and drugs such as corticosteroids can affect cystatin C values [7, 18].

Although SCr and serum cystatin C are commonly used to estimate kidney function and guide the dosages of medications cleared by the kidneys, other tests can also be used to diagnose and detect kidney disease or monitor the progression of kidney disease over time. A summary of these tests and their implication can be found in Table 22.1. Healthcare professionals can use these tests to support the selection of appropriate treatments for patients with kidney disease.

2.3.1 Kidney Function Assessment Methods

There are two methods for determining GFR: measured GFR (mGFR) and estimated GFR (eGFR). mGFR is determined from the urinary or plasma clearance of an exogenous filtration marker such as inulin, but it is not used in routine clinical practice due to its limited precision and cumbersome procedure [7]. However, it may be used as a confirmatory test in special circumstances and research studies [7]. On the other hand, eGFR is determined from estimating equations that incorporate the steady-state serum concentration of one or more endogenous filtration markers such as SCr or cystatin C. GFR estimating equations also include demographic and clinical variables as surrogates of non-GFR determinants affecting the serum concentrations of these markers [6, 7]. In situations such as assessing a potential living kidney donor or infrequent medication dosing for critical drugs like chemotherapy, mGFR may be considered. Alternatively, plasma clearance of iohexol and urinary and plasma clearance of Cr-EDTA are alternative clearance methods and filtration markers that have shown strong to moderate evidence of accuracy.

2.3.2 Serum Creatinine-Based Kidney Function Estimation

There are several methods available for estimating GFR including the CKD epidemiology collaboration (CKD-EPI) formula, the Modification of Diet in Renal Disease (MDRD), and the Cockcroft–Gault equation (eCrCl) [7, 10, 13] (Table 22.2). Each method has its own strengths and limitations.

The Cockcroft–Gault formula was developed in 1976 using data from 249 men to estimate creatinine clearance from approximately 30–130 mL/min. It is not adjusted for body surface area and standardized SCr and is not accurate for very young or old populations, AKI, pregnancy, and other special circumstances [7]. It should not be used for patients with kidney failure or receiving kidney replacement therapy (KRT) and does not account for variation among different races. The MDRD Study equation was developed in 1999

Table 22.2 Formulae used for estimating GFR or estimating CrCl [7, 18]

CKD-EPI equation (2009):

eGFR (mL/min/1.73 m^2) = 141 × min (SCr/K, 1)$^{\alpha}$× max (SCr/K, 1)$^{-1.209}$ × 0.993^{age}

[× 1.018 if female] [× 1.159 if African American]

where:

- SCr = serum creatinine in mg/dL
- K = 0.7 for females and 0.9 for males
- α = −0.329 for females and − 0.411 for males
- min (SCr/K, 1) indicates the minimum of SCr/K or 1
- max (SCr/K, 1) indicates the maximum of SCr/K or 1

MDRD equation:

eGFR (mL/min/1.73 m^2) = 170 × (serum creatinine) − 0.999 × (age) − 0.176 × (0.762 if female) × (1.180 if African American) × [serum urea nitrogen] − 0.170 × [Alb] + 0.318

Cockcroft–Gault equation:

Creatinine clearance (mL/min) = {((140−age) × weight (kg)) ÷ (72 x SCr)} × 0.814 (× 0.85 if female)

De-indexed eGFR (mL/min) = eGFR (mL/min/1.73 m^2) × patient's body surface area ÷ 1.73

Body surface area (m^2) (this is for use in having de-indexed values of eGFR reported by laboratories, for example, in drug dosing decision in people with moderate-to-severe obesity) = 0.007184 × weight in kg$^{0.425}$ × height in cm$^{0.725}$

Ideal body weight (kg) (this can be in Cockroft-Gault instead of actual body weight; as a rule of thumb, use whichever of the two is lower for clinical decision-making) = (height − 152.4) × 0.9 + 45.5 (+ 4.5 if male)

based on data on 1628 CKD patients aged 18–70 years. It is more accurate than the Cockcroft–Gault formula but underestimates mGFR at higher values of eGFR and is less accurate than CKD-EPI when eGFR exceeds 60 mL/min/1.73 m^2. The CKD-EPI equation was developed in 2009 to overcome limitations of the MDRD equation in a cohort of 8254 people and was validated in a cohort of 3771 people from 16 studies. The CKD-EPI equation, adjusted for BSA and utilizing SCr, age, sex, and race as variables, allows reporting of numeric values across the entire GFR range and is as accurate as the MDRD Study equation in the subgroup with estimated GFR <60 mL/min/1.73 m^2. In 2021, a new equation was redeveloped from the same development dataset as the 2009 equation, but without inclusion of race, and was validated in 4050 participants in 12 studies. Therefore, GFR can now be estimated using serum creatinine, age, and sex alone [7].

Historically, the Cockcroft and Gault equation has been used to estimate creatinine clearance and guide drug dosing. However, the CKD-EPI formula is now the preferred method for estimating GFR and calculating medication doses in most patients with kidney disease [7]. It should be noted, however, that this eGFR method may not be appropriate in certain situations, such as for drugs with a narrow therapeutic index, older adults, and those with extreme muscle mass, where calculation of creatinine clearance (CrCl) or de-indexed eGFR with correction for body surface area is recommended [18].

Limitations of Creatinine-Based Estimates

eGFR based on SCr including the eGFR-CKD EPI are limited by the fact that SCr is influenced by other factors, including differences in muscle mass and diet, as well as differences in the rate of tubular secretion. Both eCrCl and eGFR are inaccurate in individuals at the extremes of body weight or muscle mass. These estimates also require kidney function to be stable and must be interpreted with great care in an unwell patient with rapidly changing kidney function, e.g., in an AKI context [19].

2.3.3 Serum Cystatin C-Based Kidney Function Estimation

Cystatin C is another endogenous solute that can be used to estimate GFR [7]. However, the test is not yet universally offered by all pathology laboratories in different countries. Cystatin C is less influenced by muscle mass and some studies show that serum levels of cystatin C are more highly correlated with GFR than SCr alone, so it may be advantageous in certain group of patients, such as those at the extremes of body weight. An alternative CKD-EPI formula has been developed to incorporate cystatin C. The combination of cystatin C and creatinine combined in an estimating equation (eGFRcr-cys) is more accurate than either eGFRcr or eGFRcys [7].

2.4 Prescribing Principles in People with Kidney Disease Including Kidney Replacement Therapies

It is always important for healthcare professionals to accurately collect a detailed history of all medications including reviewing regimens for any potential interactions or nephrotoxins. Physical and laboratory parameter details indicating volume status, height, weight, and the presence of other disease states such as liver disease should also be collected.

2.4.1 Estimating Kidney Function for Drug Dosing

Accurately estimating kidney function is crucial in determining the appropriate drug dosage for patients with kidney disease. The degree of kidney impairment determines the extent of dosage modification needed. Generally, medication dosage does not need adjustment until GFR is <60 mL/min/1.73 m^2 for most drugs used in clinical practice [20]. However, different literature sources use varying classification systems for renal impairment, such as CrCl values or qualitative measurements like "mild," "moderate," or "severe," and it is important to follow these systems to avoid errors in dosage adjustments [21]. Another limitation of many kidney function estimates is their inaccuracy in rapidly changing kidney function, which can lead to over- or underestimation of kidney function and subsequently result in underdosing or overdosing of medications. For example, in severe AKI, GFR can decline so rapidly that dosing should be based on a GFR of less than 10 mL/min. Conversely, in patients with rapidly improving kidney function after AKI, dosage adjustments may need to be decreased or even stopped entirely. Hence, clinical decision-making is essential to each individual case as dosage adjustment is not precise science [14].

To minimize the potential problems with adverse effects and toxicity, it is important to carefully choose medications for patients with kidney disease. Ideally, medications should (1) not be nephrotoxic, (2) not require kidney metabolism to be converted to an active form, (3) not depend on kidney excretion of active medicine or active metabolites, (4) not be affected by fluid balance changes, (5) have a wide therapeutic index, (6) have low adverse effect profile, and (7) be able to reach the site of action in high enough concentrations even in the presence of kidney disease.

Avoid nephrotoxins. Nephrotoxicity can occur with many different drugs or combination of drugs (Table 22.3). Sometimes, the nephrotoxicity can be idiosyncratic (e.g., interstitial nephritis [22, 26]; Case 1) which is unpredictable and independent of dose. Use of nephrotoxic drugs, however, may be acceptable in people who are on hemodialysis (HD) who do not have potential for further loss of kidney function.

Effect of kidney disease on pharmacodynamic changes. Kidney disease can alter the pharmaco-

Table 22.3 Examples of drug-induced kidney damage and potential mechanisms [20, 22–25]

Kidney damage	Drugs involved	Potential mechanism
Pseudo-AKI	Cimetidine, dexamethasone, dronedarone, trimethoprim	Inhibit tubular secretion of creatinine
Acute tubular necrosis	Aminoglycosides, radiographic contrast media, cisplatin, and amphotericin B	Proximal tubular damage, cationic charge of the drugs leads to binding to tubular epithelial cells, uptake, and toxicity Renal ischemia, renal vasoconstriction, direct tubular toxicity by reactive oxygen species Complex; direct tubular toxicity Arterial vasoconstriction, direct proximal and distal tubular toxicity
Functional (hemodynamically mediated) AKI	ACEIs/ARBs/NSAIDs/ cyclosporine and tacrolimus	Decreased intraglomerular pressure through vasoconstriction of afferent arteriole and vasodilation of efferent arterioles
Tubulointerstitial disease (can be acute or chronic)		
Acute allergic interstitial nephritis	Penicillins	Interstitial inflammation, tubulitis, edema, and in certain cases interstitial fibrosis
	NSAIDs	Inhibit prostaglandins production (especially during states of volume depletion, older age, hypercalcemia, and effective arterial volume depletion such as cirrhosis, heart failure, nephrotic syndrome)
Chronic interstitial nephritis	Lithium	Toxicity results from a duration-related decrease in response to antidiuretic hormone after long-term use
Postrenal (obstructive) nephropathy		
Renal tubular obstruction	Statin	Rhabdomyolysis leading to intratubular precipitation of myoglobin
	Acyclovir	Drug precipitation
Extrarenal urinary tract obstruction	Cyclophosphamide	Bladder outlet or ureteral obstruction from fibrosis after hemorrhagic cystitis
Glomerular disease	NSAIDs, gold	Proteinuria is the hallmark of glomerular disease and may occur with or without a decrease in GFR

dynamic response or physiological processes which can in turn alter the clinical response. For example, vitamin D_2 and D_3 activation is impaired in people with later stages of CKD [20].

Kidney excretion of active drug (and active or toxic metabolite). The greater the fraction of the active drug or metabolite excreted unchanged by the kidneys (fe), the greater the need for dose modification. Dose modification is usually necessary only if the fe of the active drug is >25–50%. Active or toxic metabolites should be assessed separately for their dependence on kidney excretion in the same way as the parent drug [20].

Fluid balance changes. Many patients with kidney disease are intolerant of sodium loading, which can promote fluid overload and hypertension. Medicines with high infusion volume and sodium content and those that promote sodium and water retention should be used cautiously [20].

Therapeutic index. For many antibiotics (e.g., penicillins), dose modification is often not necessary, due to their wide therapeutic window despite elimination by the kidney. However, for drugs with narrow therapeutic window such as digoxin, dose modification is critical to avoid toxicity [20].

Drugs that can aggravate the metabolic effects of kidney disease. Many drugs do not have direct nephrotoxic effects but when used in kidney disease they can aggravate the metabolic consequences of kidney failure. For example, hyperkalemia can be worsened by angiotensin-converting enzyme inhibitors (ACEIs)/angiotensin II receptor blockers (ARBs) [20].

Drug concentration at the site of action. Reduced kidney function can significantly alter drug concentrations at the site of action. For example, diuretics, some antibiotics, and sodium glucose cotransport inhibitors (SGLT2i) may be less effective in patients with advanced stages of CKD, as they do not achieve adequate concentration of drugs at the site of action, the renal tubules [8, 20].

Although these are some of the ideal characteristics of a medication in people with kidney disease, it is rarely possible to find a medicine that fits all these criteria. Hence, sound clinical judgment and clinical condition of the patient should override theoretical concerns with close monitoring of response to therapy to guide dose titration.

2.4.2 Methods to Optimize Medications in Kidney Disease

If nonkidney clearance accounts for >50% elimination, then no adjustment needs to be made to the dose or frequency of administration for most drugs. Toxic medications which are mainly excreted in active form by the kidney (unchanged or active metabolites) may need to be modified to avoid accumulation [18, 27].

Loading Dose

In general, for most drugs, steady-state concentrations are usually reached after about 5 drug half-lives. Loading doses are sometimes necessary to reduce the time required to reach the steady state. Presence of kidney disease prolongs the half-life of a drug, thereby prolonging the time to achieve steady state if drug dose is reduced. Hence, the loading dose need not be changed provided the desired concentration and *Vd* are not changed. For example, in the case of antibiotics, a loading dose will enable therapeutic levels to be attained quickly [10, 13, 18, 27].

Loading dose can be calculated from the product of desired plasma concentration (mg/mL) and *Vd* (mL/kg) and is independent of clearance.

Maintenance Dose

If a medicine is normally excreted via the kidney, its maintenance dose will need to be adjusted in patients with reduced kidney function to produce a plasma level that will normally be achieved in the absence of kidney disease.

There are two ways of adjusting the maintenance dose:

- Increase the dosing interval, while the dose remains unchanged: The total delivered dose is reduced by administration of the same dose at reduced frequency. This is important for drugs where size of the dose and peak concentration are important for efficacy (e.g., aminoglycosides).

- Decrease the dose, while the dosing interval remains unchanged: Alternatively, a smaller dose may be administered at the usual dosing interval. This method is usually employed where the size of a dose and peak concentrations are less critical [10, 13, 18, 27].

In some cases, a combination of both methods may be employed especially for drugs with narrow therapeutic index like digoxin, where a tight control of concentration is required. Several medications require dosage adjustment or caution in people with kidney disease. Few important examples are provided in Table 22.4.

Table 22.4 Examples of medications which require dosage adjustments and precautions in decreased kidney function [8, 27, 28]

Drug class	Classes/agents requiring dosage adjustment
Antibiotics	Almost all antibiotics require dosage adjustment (exceptions: ceftriaxone, clindamycin, linezolid, metronidazole, macrolides)
Anticoagulants	Enoxaparin, fondaparinux, apixaban, rivaroxaban, dabigatran
Cardiac medications	Atenolol, ACEIs, ARBs, digoxin, moxonidine, sotalol; caution with potassium-sparing diuretics
Lipid-lowering therapy	Fenofibrate, statins (particularly rosuvastatin)
Narcotics	Codeine, tramadol, avoid pethidine and morphine; other agents may also accumulate
Antipsychotic and antiepileptic agents	Gabapentin, levetiracetam, lithium, pregabalin, primidone, topiramate, trazodone, vigabatrin, duloxetine, desvenlafaxine, venlafaxine
Antidiabetic agents	SGLT2is, gliptins (except linagliptin), GLP-1 agonists, sulfonyl urea, insulin, metformin
Antivirals	Lamivudine, adefovir, emtricitabine, stavudine, tenofovir, zidovudine, acyclovir, valaciclovir, valganciclovir, famciclovir, nirmatrelvir/ritonavir
Others	Allopurinol, colchicine, denosumab, bisphosphonates, NSAIDs, H_2 receptor antagonists

2.4.3 Prescribing in People with Kidney Replacement Therapy

Dialysis drug clearance may significantly reduce drug efficacy if not accounted for [29, 30]. Some medicines will be removed from the blood via different dialysis modalities, while some will not be removed at all. Some general principles that will impact on whether the drug will be removed by dialysis include (1) renal clearance—medicines or metabolites that are not cleared by the kidney normally are unlikely to be removed by dialysis, (2) molecular size—small molecules are likely to be removed by dialysis while larger molecules (e.g., proteins, monoclonal antibodies) are unlikely to diffuse across the dialysis membrane, (3) volume of distribution—drugs with large *Vd* will distribute into the lipid tissues resulting in a smaller portion of the drugs being distributed in the blood and available for clearance. Conversely, drugs with a smaller *Vd* will be primarily distributed in the blood and therefore be cleared, and (4) protein binding—drugs that are protein bound are too large to be removed by dialysis. Medicines with low protein binding affinity are free in the blood to be removed [29–33].

Medicine Dosing in Dialysis

If a medication is removed from the body through dialysis, the dose and timing of the medication may need to be adjusted. In general, medications that are not cleared by the kidneys do not need to be adjusted in dialysis patients since they are metabolized and eliminated by other mechanisms, such as hepatic metabolism. Adjusting medication dosage is typically only necessary if clearance via the kidney accounts for over 30% of the total body clearance of that particular medication. Medications that are eliminated during dialysis do not require a higher dose than normal, since dialysis treatment is not more efficient than normally functioning kidneys.

HD drug clearance occurs mainly by passive diffusion along a concentration gradient but also by convectional movement of soluble drug with ultrafiltrate plasma water [33]. Medicines that are removed by HD should be administered after a dialysis session (also referred to as post-HD). This is especially important for once daily medicines rather than more frequent medicines (e.g., three to four times daily). Many drug properties that affect removal by HD also apply to peritoneal dialysis (PD), but PD is usually less efficient. For most drugs, there is little evidence of significant removal during chronic PD. For significant removal by PD, the drug must in general have a very low *V*d and low protein binding [32].

Drug clearance by Continuous Kidney Replacement Therapy (CKRT) differs from intermittent HD. CRRT can result in clearance of larger molecules; however, large *V*d and protein binding will still prevent removal of drugs from CRRT [31]. There are limited studies on drug clearance in CRRT in comparison to other modalities and clinicians must rely on judgment, physicochemical properties of the drugs, and more importantly the clinical response of the patient. For medicine-specific advice, there are several resources which provide guidance on medicine dosing in patients on HD and PD [31].

2.5 Summary and Conclusions

Medicine dosing in people with kidney disease is a complex area. It is important to understand how medicine use may be altered in kidney disease and KRT, and on the limitations of the calculations often used to estimate kidney function to help make informed decisions on medicine doses. Where possible, clinicians and health professionals should consult textbooks on medicine dosing in renal impairment and make use of specialist pharmacists, who have clinical experience with these patients. In all cases, once a medicine regimen has been prescribed, it is important to monitor the patient for efficacy, adverse effects, and signs of toxicity.

2.6 Case Studies

2.6.1 Case Study 1: Identifying and Managing Drug-Related Kidney Disease

Presenting complaint: A 76-year-old lady presents with a month-long history of nausea, lethargy, excessive thirst, and weight loss of 5 kg over the past month. Patient reported a normal appetite with fluid intake of about 2 L daily with no other symptoms. Her past medical history included a transient ischemic attack 5 years ago, osteopenia, and osteoarthritis. Patient was treated with cephalexin for *E. coli* sensitive urinary tract infection 2 weeks prior to presentation with no difference in symptoms. Patient's blood pressure on presentation was 140/60 mmHg, heart rate of 60 beats per minute, and no elevation of jugular venous pressure. Patient had no other significant finding on physical examination and reported being a non-smoker and with social alcohol consumption. Her regular medications included aspirin 100 mg once daily, rosuvastatin 10 mg once daily, vitamin D 25 μg one daily, polyethylene glycol sachets once daily, meloxicam 15 mg one daily when needed (4–5 per week). Further information revealed meloxicam was started a month ago, prior to which she used to take ibuprofen 200 mg one daily intermittently for 6 years.

Relevant investigations:

Urea: 9.6 mmol/L; SCr: 167 μmol/L, eGFR: 25 mL/min/1.73 m^2.

Baseline: SCr: 70 μmol/L, eGFR: 73 mL/min/1.73 m^2 (10 months ago).

Urine: UACR; 17.6 mg/mmol; no hematuria; presence of pyuria.

Hemoglobin: 113 g/L.

Renal biopsy report: The light microscopy revealed features of active tubular interstitial nephritis. Given the presence of a few scattered eosinophils, it raises the possibility of drug-induced interstitial nephritis. Correlation with the clinical findings is suggested.

Final diagnosis: Acute interstitial nephritis due to meloxicam. Patient was treated with prednisolone for 12 weeks and 3 months post treatment SCr was 80 μmol/L, eGFR: 62 mL/min/1.73 m^2.

1. *How do you determine whether this is induced by meloxicam?*

   Patient's kidney function recovered substantially after the patient was started on prednisolone. Although cephalexin can also potentially cause acute interstitial nephritis, the renal team ruled it out as a cause as her symptoms started following the commencement of meloxicam approximately a month ago. More importantly, the improved kidney function after stopping meloxicam (dechallenge) confirms the cause of the kidney injury.

2. *What are the most common analgesics that could cause an AKI?*

   NSAIDs are among the most commonly identified medications implicated in drug-induced AKI. While the patient in this case used ibuprofen, this was only on intermittent basis and was ruled out by the renal team as a possible cause of the interstitial nephritis in this case.

3. *What are the major risk factors for an AKI, particularly that caused by medications like NSAIDs?*

   Pre-existing chronic kidney disease, volume depletion, concomitant use of other medications like renin–angiotensin system inhibitors (ACEIs/ARBs), older age, and electrolyte abnormalities like hypercalcemia may increase risk of AKI, especially one caused by NSAIDs.

4. *What are some of the management strategies for an AKI?*

   The management of AKI involves identifying the etiology of AKI, treating reversible causes such as hypotension, volume depletion or urinary tract obstruction, removing any active insults (e.g., ongoing use of nephrotoxic drugs like NSAIDs), and identifying and managing serious complications including those that require KRT if AKI is not resolved.

3 Part Two: Safe Prescribing in Patients with Hepatic Disease

3.1 Background

The liver plays a pivotal role in drug metabolism. This is crucial as most drugs must traverse the liver for the conversion of prodrugs into their active metabolites or the transformation of active drugs into inactive forms. These processes occur before the drugs enter the systemic circulation for elimination. This chemical alteration of drugs, often referred to as biotransformation, is a key step in drug processing. The majority of orally administered drugs are absorbed in the small intestine. They are then transported to the liver via the portal vein, which accounts for approximately 75% of the total liver blood flow, through the mesenteric vessels [34]. This process is known as first-pass metabolism or first-pass effect [35].

Drug metabolism in the liver involves several mechanisms that can be generally categorized into three phases [36]. **Phase I** metabolism involves chemical modification through functionalization reactions, such as hydrolysis, hydroxylation, oxidation, reduction, demethylation, which are mediated by cytochrome P450 (CYP450) enzymes. These enzymes derive their name from the fact that they contain a heme pigment that absorbs light at a wavelength of 450 nm when exposed to carbon monoxide and are bound to membranes within the cell [35, 37]. Although there are more than 30 distinct cytochrome P450 enzymes that are grouped according to biochemical relatedness, the most important ones in drug metabolism are CYP1A2, CYP2C, CYP2D6, and CYP3A4 [37]. **Phase II** metabolism involves the binding of hydrophilic molecules to either the original molecule or the metabolite derived from the Phase I reactions. The final product is typically inert and water-soluble, making it easy to clear or excrete from the body. Phase II reactions include glucuronidation, sulfation, acetylation, methylation, and conjugation with glutathione and amino acids, such as glycine, taurine, and glutamic acid [38]. **Phase III** metabolism refers to the uptake of compounds into hepatocytes through drug transporters and their efflux into bile [36]. It involves additional modification, transporter-mediated detoxification, and excretion of the drug and/or conjugated metabolites after Phase II.

Due to the crucial role of the hepatic system in the metabolism of several drugs, liver dysfunction, including mild-to-moderate hepatic impairment, can affect drug metabolism. Liver disease or hepatic impairment not only reduces the clearance of a drug metabolized through hepatic enzymes but can also affect plasma protein binding due to reduced synthesis of albumin and other drug-binding proteins. On the other hand, drugs can also have a direct effect on the liver or alter hepatic blood flow, potentially leading to hepatic impairment including organ failure [35]. It is, therefore, important to recognize the signs and symptoms of hepatic failure in patients and identify possible causes including the presence of detrimental drug interactions. Furthermore, once a patient is diagnosed with liver disease or failure, it is a clinical imperative to select the right medicines, carefully monitor, and individualize treatments to reduce ADRs.

Patients with hepatic impairment often require drug therapy. Since the liver is primarily responsible for detoxification and elimination, patients with reduced hepatic function must be carefully assessed for the need and appropriateness of individual treatments. If a drug is needed for a patient with hepatic disease, the choice of drug, its dose, and duration of therapy must be carefully considered in order to avoid adverse effects. Ideally, it is better to choose a drug that has higher therapeutic index, has lesser pharmacokinetic and pharmacodynamic interactions, is devoid of hepatotoxic effects, and is predominantly eliminated via the kidney. However, the ideal drug with these properties is often not available, and in such cases, the dose and drug should be individualized to the patient, who should then be carefully monitored, and the drug used for the shortest period possible. In this chapter, we will look in detail drugs that need to be either avoided or dose modified in patients with hepatic disease, with the view to improve the safe prescribing of drugs in people with hepatic diseases.

3.2 Hepatic Diseases: Their Effect on Drug Metabolism

Table 22.5 outlines types of hepatic diseases, which have various etiologies (including infections, inherited/autoimmune conditions, and alcohol/drug-induced) and can result in a wide range of pathophysiological changes in hepatic function (both catabolic and anabolic) [39, 40]. Regardless of the specific cause, injury to hepatic tissues can trigger an inflammatory reaction known as hepatitis. Liver diseases can be acute, occurring over relatively short periods like acute hepatitis, or chronic, developing over months to years and eventually leading to cirrhosis and end-stage liver disease [39]. Patients with chronic liver diseases (CLDs) may experience an acute decompensation of hepatic function and/or develop acute hepatic failure due to the effect of various precipitants, a condition that is known as acute-on-CLD [40]. CLD is estimated to affect approximately 1.5 billion people worldwide, with about 2 million deaths attributed to the condition annually [41, 42]. Furthermore, the 2019 disability-adjusted life years caused by CLD have increased by 33.0% over the past three decades, accounting for 1.8% of the global burden [43].

Table 22.5 General classification of liver diseases

Etiology	Examples of hepatic disease
Infections (bacterial and viral)	Hepatitis A, B, C
Inherited	Wilson's disease
Impaired bile flow	Cholestatic liver disease
Drug-induced	Antitubercular/methotrexate-induced liver disease
Neoplasms	Hepatocellular carcinoma
Metabolic	Nonalcoholic fatty liver disease

Upon progression of hepatic disease, scar tissue develops, leading to a complication known as hepatic fibrosis. While early fibrosis is often asymptomatic, advanced and progressive hepatic fibrosis or "cirrhosis" is associated with increasing loss of hepatocyte density and function and intrahepatic resistance to blood flow [44]. This leads to an increase in portal vein pressure followed by portal hypertension. In the absence of complications, cirrhosis is known as being "compensated." However, silent progression of portal hypertension and hepatocellular dysfunction can lead to the development of a rapidly progressive "decompensated" phase, which is characterized by debilitating complications including ascites (fluid accumulation in the abdomen caused by alterations of splanchnic circulation driven by portal hypertension), hepatic encephalopathy (driven by impaired detoxification and accumulation of neurotoxins), jaundice, and increased risk of bleeding (from esophageal or gastric varices, resulting from portal hypertension, and impaired synthesis of coagulation factors) [44].

As explained earlier, the liver is the major site of action of the CYP450 hemoproteins, a group of enzymes responsible for the metabolism of most drugs in humans. As such, hepatic disease may affect how the body manages and eliminates drugs by reducing drug-metabolizing capacity, reducing the synthesis of plasma proteins, and altering hepatic blood flow [39]. As presented by Blaschke [39] in Table 22.6, the pathophysiological changes associated with hepatic disease can impair drug metabolism and disposition in a variety of ways, which is highly correlated with the type and severity of hepatic diseases [39, 45]. For example, in patients with chronic hepatitis without cirrhosis, or those with hepatocellular carcinoma, hepatic drug metabolism is generally comparable to that of subjects with normal hepatic function [46]. For the most part, CLD is more predictably associated with impaired metabolism of drugs than acute hepatic dysfunction, with the exemption of acute hepatic failure [47]. Similarly, hepatic injury due to viral hepatitis appears to have minimal impact on hepatocellular metabolic function [39]. However, in patients with liver cirrhosis, hepatic drug clearance is in most cases significantly reduced. Therefore, most literature addresses the concerns in relation to the impairment of drug disposition in people with liver cirrhosis [45].

Alcohol-associated hepatic disease is one of the major causes of CLD [48, 49]. In alcoholic hepatic disease, drug metabolism is more complex as it could be inhibited or induced. For example, with acute ingestion of alcohol, a drug's metabolism may be inhibited by competing for the same set of metabolizing enzymes [47]. With chronic excessive alcohol ingestion, there may be occurrence of hepatic enzyme induction of the CYP2E1 variant, resulting in increased clearance of certain drugs (such as benzodiazepines). These enzymes often remain inhibited/induced for several weeks even after cessation of drinking [47]. Furthermore, certain enzymes induced by chronic alcohol consumption transform some drugs into toxic compounds that can damage the liver; for example, the induction of CYP2E1 increases the generation of *N*-acetyl-*p*-benzoquinone imine, a toxic metabolite of paracetamol [47, 50].

Hepatic steatosis, or fat in the liver, is another common feature of different hepatic diseases that can affect hepatic drug metabolism and occurs largely because of metabolic processes such as insulin resistance, diabetes, and hyperlipidemia [51]. The same processes can also result in nonalcoholic fatty liver disease (NAFLD) and nonalcoholic steatohepatitis (NASH). It has been suggested that changes in liver drug transporters may have a hepatoprotective effect in CLDs through the facilitation of efflux transporters and repression of uptake transporters. These changes may also result in increased plasma drug concentration in NASH patients [51].

Table 22.6 Pathophysiological changes associated with liver disease

	Pathophysiological changes			
Liver disease	Total hepatic blood flow	Hepatocellular function	Albumin concentration	Bilirubin
Cirrhosis (moderate to severe)	Decreased	Decreased	Decreased	Increased
Viral hepatitis	Unchanged or increased	Decreased	Unchanged	Unchanged or increased
Alcoholic liver disease	Unchanged or decreased	Decreased	Unchanged or decreased	Significantly increased

Modified from: Blaschke TF [39]

3.3 Assessment of Hepatic Impairment

As illustrated by Talal and colleagues [51] (see Fig. 22.2), hepatic injury of various etiologies can cause deposition of collagen, leading first to liver fibrosis and ultimately cirrhosis, which in turn results in hepatocyte loss which, as discussed earlier, affects the liver's ability to metabolize and transport medications. As such, assessment of hepatic function is important to understand the stage and severity of hepatic disease to help clinicians guide drug prescribing and overall management of the condition.

As explained above, for medications cleared by the kidneys, the serum creatinine concentration and the glomerular filtration rate are used to guide dosage adjustments; however, there is not a single reliable laboratory parameter to guide dosage regimens for patients with hepatic dysfunction [47, 52]. Both noninvasive methods (which assess structural changes within the liver) and functional measurements via a combination of indices (such as Child–Pugh, Model of End-Stage Liver Disease, National Cancer Institute Index) are used to assess hepatic dysfunction (as illustrated in Fig. 22.2) [51].

Although not necessarily serve as direct measures of hepatic dysfunction, elevated hepatic enzymes (commonly referred to as liver function tests or LFTs) may indicate abnormality of hepatic dysfunction that needs to be confirmed with further investigations [47]. For example, a predominant rise in aspartate aminotransferase (AST) and alanine aminotransferase (ALT) signals hepatocellular injury. This can be caused by drug reactions or toxicity (e.g., paracetamol), viral hepatitis, autoimmune hepatitis, alcoholic hepatitis, ischemic hepatitis secondary to profound hypotension, and rare causes such as Wilson's disease [35]. An obstructive pattern has a rise predominantly of alkaline phosphatase (ALP) and gamma-glutamyl transferase (GGT); these are canalicular enzymes and suggest cholestasis. This is caused by obstruction, either calculi or tumor (primary biliary, pancreatic or metastases), and hepatic diseases such as primary biliary cirrhosis [35].

The Child–Pugh score (CPS) is the most used method to assess hepatic impairment, particularly in patients with cirrhosis [47, 51, 52]. The current parameters used to calculate the score include serum concentrations of bilirubin and albumin, prothrombin time, severity of hepatic encephalopathy, and ascites [53]. As presented in Table 22.7, the CPS characterizes hepatic disease severity as class A (mild, score 5–6 points), B (moderate, score 7–9

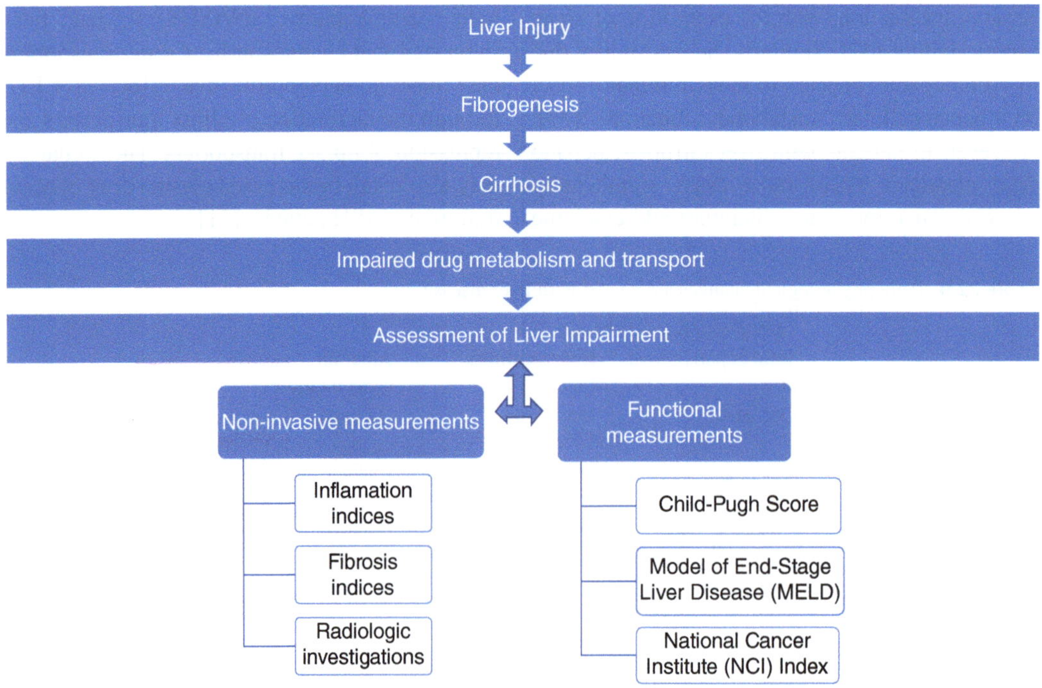

Fig. 22.2 Assessment of hepatic dysfunction (Modified from: Talal AH, Venuto CS, Younis I [51])

Table 22.7 The Child–Pugh Scoring System for classification of hepatic impairment

	Assigned score based on parameters' findings		
Parameter	1	2	3
Serum bilirubin	<2 mg/dL (<34 μmol/L)	2–3 mg/dL (34–51 μmol/L)	>3 mg/dL (>51 μmol/L)
Serum albumin	>3.5 g/dL (>35 g/L)	2.8–3.5 g/dL (28–35 g/L)	<2.8 g/dL (<28 g/L)
Prothrombin time (seconds prolonged) or international normalized ratio (INR)	<4 s INR <1.7	4–6 s INR = 1.7–2.3	>6 s INR >2.3
Ascites	Absent	Mild	Moderate to severe
Encephalopathy grade[a]	0	1 or 2	3 or 4

Modified from: Gardner KN, Bostwick JR [52]

[a]Grade 0: Normal consciousness, personality, neurological examination, electroencephalogram; Grade 1: restless, sleep disturbed, irritable/agitated, tremor, impaired handwriting, 5 CPS waves; Grade 2: lethargic, time-disoriented, inappropriate, asterixis, ataxia, slow triphasic waves; Grade 3: somnolent, stuporous, place-disoriented, hyperactive reflexes, rigidity, slower waves; Grade 4: unrousable coma, no personality/behavior, decerebrate, slow 2–3 CPS delta activity

points), or C (severe or 10–15 points). CPS class A is considered compensated cirrhosis, whereas class B and C reflect decompensated cirrhosis [52, 53]. Drug information resources may include possible dose recommendations relative to the CPS; however, this serves only as an estimate since the score does not provide information on the ability of the liver to metabolize specific drugs [52].

The Model for End-stage Liver Disease (MELD) is another scoring system, which is commonly employed to rank candidates for liver transplantation [51]. The MELD was initially created to predict survival among patients undergoing transjugular intrahepatic portosystemic shunt (TIPS) placement [54]. It contains three objective variables: international normalized ratio (INR), creatinine, and total bilirubin. Studies comparing the CPS to MELD suggest that both scoring systems have similar prognostic significance, although each score may have different predictive capacity in different situations [55].

The National Cancer Institute (NCI) index is mostly used to grade hepatic dysfunction in patients undergoing trials of cancer chemotherapy [51]. The NCI index uses two laboratory-based parameters to grade hepatic dysfunction: total bilirubin and AST. Based on the NCI criteria, normal to mild hepatic dysfunction often corresponds to a CPS class A, while moderate-severe hepatic dysfunction corresponds to a CPS class B or C [51]. Therefore, patients in the latter NCI-based group may require chemotherapy dose modification, while those in the first group are unlikely to need one. The use of readily available laboratory values by the NCI makes it likely to be implemented in routine clinical practice for dosing decisions of approved oncology compounds, even though the dosing recommendations in a product label is more likely to be based on CPS classification [56].

3.4 Pharmacokinetic and Pharmacodynamic Changes in Hepatic Disease

The impact of hepatic impairment on drug disposition is related to the type and severity of hepatic diseases, as well as the physiochemical and pharmacokinetic characteristics of individual drugs [51]. Knowledge of the pharmacokinetic and pharmacodynamic profile of a drug is essential to guide clinical decision-making in patients with a range of hepatic diseases [52]. Therefore, below we discuss the different pharmacokinetic and pharmacodynamic changes associated with hepatic diseases, including those with implication for dosage adjustment considerations.

3.4.1 Pharmacokinetic Changes

To have a better understanding of the effect of hepatic impairment on different stages of drug pharmacokinetics, we have summarized below the major changes on drug absorption, distribution, metabolism, and excretion induced by decreased hepatic function.

Absorption: In general, drug absorption remains unchanged in patients with cirrhosis, although the absorption rate may be reduced [51]. However, in hepatic failure, absorption is typically affected by delayed gastric emptying, diarrhea, and increased gastric transit time [35]. Patients with cholestatic disease usually experience impaired bile flow from the liver to the duodenum [52], which can lead to reduced efficacy of lipophilic drugs that rely on bile salts [57].

Distribution: Hepatic dysfunction can cause fluid retention leading to edema and ascites, often seen in patients with liver cirrhosis, increasing the *Vd*, particularly for hydrophilic drugs, resulting in reduced plasma concentration and slower elimination [35, 50, 52]. If a loading dose is needed in these patients, larger doses may be required [52]. Furthermore, as hepatic disease progresses, protein synthesis may be reduced. As these proteins are important as binding sites for drugs, this may alter the amount of free drug available, the *Vd*, the half-life, and the duration of action of highly protein-bound (>90%) drugs [35, 52]. Hyperbilirubinemia may also cause displacement of protein-bound drugs [35, 52].

Metabolism: In general, and as previously discussed, drug metabolism is least affected in people with CLD without cirrhosis, moderately affected in compensated cirrhosis, and most affected in those with decompensated cirrhosis and acute hepatic failure, particularly fulminant hepatitis [52, 58]. The bioavailability of medications can be substantially altered in hepatic disease depending on (1) the route of metabolism, (2) whether a medication is a prodrug that needs to be metabolized to become active, and (3) the hepatic extraction ratio of the medication [52]. In hepatic failure, as the degree of metabolism is reduced, drugs that undergo the "first-pass effect" by the liver will have reduced extraction ratio, and thus, more drug will reach the systemic circulation, increasing their systemic bioavailability [35].

The hepatic extraction ratio of a drug (i.e., the measure of efficiency of the liver to remove a drug from the systemic circulation) and the degree of hepatic intrinsic clearance of the drug (i.e., the enzyme-mediated biotransformation of the drug) are important determinants in how hepatic dysfunction affects drug metabolism [51]. Drugs can be categorized based on their extraction ratios, which can be high (>0.7) or low (<0.3). Most drugs have low extraction ratios (<0.3), indicating poor permeability and limited clearance due to reduced metabolism rather than blood flow [35]. On the other hand, medications with high extraction ratios should be used with caution since they may result in higher and unpredictable steady-state levels compared to drugs with lower extraction ratios [52].

Variable and nonuniform reductions in drug-metabolizing activities are commonly observed in CLD. Glucuronidation is often considered to be affected to a lesser extent than CYP450-mediated reactions in mild-to-moderate cirrhosis but can also be substantially impaired in patients with advanced cirrhosis [52, 59]. It has been reported that in noncholestatic hepatic disease the activity of CYP1A2, CYP2C19, and CYP3A4 may be reduced relative to the activity of CYP2D6, CYP2C9, and CYP2E1 [60]. In contrast, primary biliary cirrhosis is associated with less effect on CYP3A4 activity compared to noncholestatic liver disease [52]. Interestingly, patients with nonalcoholic steatohepatitis and other inflammatory diseases may exhibit an upregulation of CYP2E1; however, the impact of this on medication prescribing is not likely clinically significant since the fraction of drug (e.g., acetaminophen) metabolized is often unchanged as long as the phase I metabolic pathways are preserved and unsaturated [52, 60].

The efficacy of a prodrug depends on successful conversion to the active moiety, oftentimes by hepatic enzymes. Depending on the metabolic requirement for a successful conversion (e.g., de-acetylation, hydrolysis, etc.), hepatic disease may lead to impaired ability or failure to form an active metabolite [52]. Thus, in patients with reduced hepatic function, prodrugs may have diminished therapeutic efficacy [46]. As such, prodrugs should be used cautiously since higher, yet unpredictable, steady-state levels are more likely to occur than in case of non-prodrugs; however, this too depends on the nature of the prodrug and site of metabolism/activation [46, 52].

Elimination: Assessing drug elimination impairment in individuals with hepatic disease can be challenging [58, 59]. There is a lack of simple endogenous marker to predict hepatic function regarding the elimination capacity of particular drugs [59]. However, it is crucial to consider whether a particular drug has significant hepatic elimination, i.e., accounting for over 20% of total elimination. In such cases, the therapeutic range of the compound should be carefully reviewed [47].

The impact of hepatic disease on alternative routes of elimination including biliary excretion, enterohepatic circulation, and kidney-based elimination should also be considered. For example, cirrhotic patients often present with kidney disease (e.g., hepatorenal syndrome) [58]. Studies have shown that serum creatinine concentrations tend to be low and that calculated or measured creatinine clearances often overestimate GFR, possibly because of impaired hepatic synthesis of creatinine, reduced muscular mass, and increased tubular secretion of creatinine in cirrhosis [50]. Thus, drugs eliminated primarily by the kidney with a narrow therapeutic range should be used with caution in patients with hepatic cirrhosis and ascites, even when creatinine clearance is normal. Also, agents eliminated through biliary excretion or recycled through enterohepatic circulation should be avoided in patients who present with cholestatic disease [35, 52].

3.4.2 Pharmacodynamic Changes

Hepatic disease can cause pharmacodynamic changes that affect the way certain drugs interact with the body, particularly in the central nervous system and kidney [39]. Tissue responsiveness to the pharmacological action of some drugs may be modified in people with CLD, as evidenced by the increased susceptibility of the central nervous system to many psychoactive agents, especially in patients with cirrhosis [50, 61]. This increased sensitivity can result in a heightened risk of adverse effects from medications like morphine and benzodiazepines, as well as NSAIDs, which can negatively affect kidney function, whereas the sensitivity to the natriuretic effect of loop diuretics was found to be reduced [47, 57]. Additionally, individuals with hepatic disease are more vulnerable to the potential nephrotoxic effects of aminoglycosides, so these medications should be avoided in this population [61].

The use of any benzodiazepines has been associated with the development of encephalopathy, a condition that can be reversed with the use of a benzodiazepine antagonist. It is important to exercise caution when prescribing benzodiazepines, particularly those with long half-lives that are metabolized through phase I reactions, such as diazepam, especially as hepatic disease progresses. Patients with TIPS are at an increased risk of developing encephalopathy due to the diversion of blood flow away from the liver [52]. Therefore, extra vigilance is necessary when considering the use of benzodiazepines in this patient population.

Drugs may also interfere with adaptive physiological processes induced by hepatic disease, as is the case of the ACEIs and NSAIDs. These drugs counteract the enhanced activity of the renin–angiotensin system in advanced hepatic disease, thereby generating a high risk of excessive hypotension and AKI, respectively [50, 52, 61]. Although no clinical data have been published for selective cyclo-oxygenase (COX)-2 inhibitors, it is prudent to avoid this class of drugs in cirrhotic patients with ascites, since COX-2 inhibitors have been shown to impair renal perfusion in salt-depleted, healthy individuals [50, 61].

Finally, there may be pharmacological effects that overlap with some pathophysiological modifications related to the process of hepatic disease, such as an increased portal pressure produced by some calcium antagonists, or hypoprothrombinemia related to the inhibition of synthesis of vitamin K-dependent clotting factors by some beta-lactam antibacterial agents. Accordingly, the use of these drugs should be carefully considered in advanced hepatic disease. It is important to note that reduced drug metabolism in patients with hepatic impairment does not seem to have a significant impact on the frequency of drug-induced hepatotoxicity. Special caution should be exercised; however, in patients with alcoholic hepatic disease, excessive alcohol intake may potentiate the hepatotoxic effect of paracetamol [61].

3.5 Medication Management in People with Hepatic Impairment

The effects of hepatic impairment on the pharmacokinetics of drugs are complex, inconsistent, unpredictable, and drug specific [61]. Problems in predicting drug kinetic behavior could be further, depending on individual patient's circumstances, complicated by concurrent impairment of kidney function (frequently encountered in patients with advanced hepatic disease), and the unpredictability of GFR using customary methods in patients with cirrhosis [61]. Further, much of the focus on dosage optimization in patients with hepatic diseases has been on alterations in the pharmacokinetics of drugs eliminated largely by hepatic metabolism. Less consideration has been given to changes in the plasma concentration—response relationships (pharmacodynamics) associated with the diseases [39].

Overall, there are two important considerations to keep in mind when discussing drugs and the hepatic system. First consideration is related to drugs that can inherently cause hepatotoxicity, while the other consideration is related to drugs that may need to be avoided or their doses adjusted in people with hepatic impairment. This section discusses these two prescribing considerations citing important drug and drug classes that are applicable in both scenarios.

3.5.1 Drug-Induced Hepatotoxicity: Cause, Type, and Epidemiology

Drug-induced liver injury (DILI), which is characterized either as acute or chronic, can be caused by various drugs (including nonprescription drugs), toxins, natural products, or dietary supplements. While jaundice commonly presents as one of the major symptoms, DILI presentations can be asymptomatic and be detected opportunistically [62]. Clinically, DILI can be functionally categorized as hepatocellular, cholestatic, or mixed, with different liver test abnormalities, histological findings and etiological factors used to further classify DILI [63]. For example, alkaline phosphatase is elevated in cholestatic injury, while AST and ALT are elevated in hepatocellular pattern; all enzymes will be elevated in mixed injury [64]. Most patients affected with DILI recover and will have normal liver function tests; however, there are also incidents of developing chronic DILI like cirrhosis and fulminant hepatic failure [65, 66].

Some of the drugs implicated in inducing different hepatic abnormalities and the respective histologic patterns are shown in Table 22.8. A more comprehensive source to understand drugs that may cause liver damage are comprehensively documented in the database named LiverTox [67], which lists the drugs that could lead to DILI along with their underlining mechanism.

The true extent of DILI is challenging to determine due to the lack of consensus on the criteria that define this condition. However, estimates suggest that nearly 1 in 20 people may be affected, with a crude annual incidence rate of 19.1% (95% CI 1.54–23.3%) [63]. Antibiotics like amoxicillin with clavulanate, isoniazid, and NSAIDs are among major contributors to DILI incidents [63].

Although several drugs have been identified as having hepatotoxic potential, much less is known as to whether the use of such drugs exacerbate existing liver damage [68]. In fact, other complications such as drug-induced kidney injury, gastrointestinal bleeding, and hepatic encephalopathy are more likely to occur in people with hepatic disease rather than the DILI itself [69]. This underscores the importance of considering multiple factors to fully understand the causes and consequences of hepatic impairment.

Table 22.8 Drugs implicated in different abnormalities and associated histologic patterns [67]

Liver test abnormalities	Drugs implicated
Hepatocellular	Acetaminophen, aspirin, allopurinol, amiodarone, baclofen, bupropion, ciprofloxacin, HAART, imatinib, isoniazid, ketoconazole, lisinopril, losartan, methotrexate, NSAIDs, rifampin, statins, tetracyclines, valproic acid
Cholestasis	Amoxicillin/clavulanate, anabolic steroids, chlorpromazine, clopidogrel, erythromycin, estrogen, irbesartan, oral contraceptive
Mixed	Amoxicillin/clavulanate, anabolic steroids, azathioprine, carbamazepine, clindamycin, enalapril, erythromycin, nitrofurantoin, phenytoin, sulfonamides, trazodone, TMP-SMX, verapamil
Histologic patterns	
Drug-induced autoimmune hepatitis	Atorvastatin, halothane, hydralazine, ipilimumab, methyldopa, minocycline, nitrofurantoin, TNF-alpha antagonists, vemurafenib
Steatohepatitis	Amiodarone, tamoxifen, valproic acid
Steatosis	Methotrexate, NRTIs, tetracycline, valproic acid
Granulomatous	Allopurinol, amiodarone, carbamazepine, diltiazem, hydralazine, penicillamine, procainamide, phenytoin, sulfonamides
Fibrosis	Methotrexate
Nodular regenerative hyperplasia	Azathioprine, bleomycin, cyclophosphamide, chlorambucil, doxorubicin, interleukin 2 receptor antagonists, trastuzumab

HAART highly active antiretroviral therapy, *NRTI* nucleoside reverse transcriptase inhibitor, *NSAID* nonsteroidal anti-inflammatory drug, *TMP-SMX* trimethoprim-sulfamethoxazole, *TNF* tumor necrosis factor

Management of DILI

Effective management of DILI necessitates routine monitoring of hepatic function markers, both before and during treatment. In particular, it is critical to assess for pre-existing hepatic diseases or viral infections before initiating therapies with drugs that have the potential to cause liver damage.

DILI is a significant contributor to hepatic impairment in several clinical settings and may result from the use of several medications. Effective management of DILI involves identifying the offending agent and the mechanism of injury and may involve specific or general approaches. For instance, specific hepatotoxicity caused by agents like acetaminophen can be managed by rapidly acting before it affects the liver or treating with the antidote *N*-acetylcysteine to minimize hepatic injury once it has occurred [64, 65]. While *N*-acetylcysteine is primarily used for acetaminophen toxicity, it may also have some benefit in other forms of idiosyncratic DILI, although the evidence and recommendations for this purpose remain largely inconclusive [65, 67]. Notably, the use of *N*-acetylcysteine has been associated with improvements in transplant-free survival in individuals with early-stage nonacetaminophen acute hepatic failure [70].

To manage DILI, it is important to consider the different complications of the injury that are manifested during patient presentations. Management strategies can range from the use of topical agents and antihistamines to manage intense pruritus to the use of corticosteroids in the event of severe DILI [59, 70, 71]. Further, there are general treatment approaches for non-specific DILI, which may include detoxification using extracorporeal devices, the use of liver regeneration techniques with agents like growth factors, or liver transplantation depending on the stage and disease prognosis [65].

3.5.2 Drug Dosage Adjustment in Hepatic Impairment

As explained in Sect. 4, hepatic diseases can indirectly impact drug metabolism by affecting various metabolic enzymes or drug transporters, leading to altered drug concentrations and clinical response [72]. The liver contains a high concentration of enzymes that are responsible for the metabolism of many drugs [59, 73], including the CYP450 enzymes, which are primarily responsible for the phase I metabolism of several drugs. These enzymes are primarily located in the liver and their function may be affected in the presence of hepatic diseases. Similarly, other hepatic enzymes like the glucuronyl transferases, *N*-acetyl transferases, and glutathione-*S*-transferases are responsible for phase II metabolism by the liver, although the phase II enzymes are less affected by hepatic conditions than the CYP450 enzymes.

Liver damage can lead to suboptimal or excessive clinical response depending on the severity of the hepatic condition that affects the plasma concentration of drugs. In prodrugs, for instance, impaired hepatic function may lead to reduced conversion of drugs to active metabolites, potentially leading to suboptimal pharmacodynamic response. In contrast, if the metabolism of active drugs is affected, this may lead to increased probability for toxicity. Prescribing in hepatic impairment therefore needs to consider various drug alternatives with the view to avoid drugs that may exacerbate liver damage. People with various hepatic diseases particularly require careful monitoring of doses and associated outcomes, with the frequency and nature of the monitoring depending on the drug or drug class involved [69].

Some clinical and drug factors should be considered to determine if drugs require dosage reduction or be avoided in people with hepatic impairment. This includes whether the drug is considerably metabolized by the liver, its therapeutic index, hepatic extraction ratio of the drug, and its potential for causing hepatotoxicity. According to the Food and Drug Administration (FDA) [74], there are generally three major pharmacokinetic considerations to consider in people with reduced hepatic function. This includes when the drug under consideration has ≥20% hepatic elimination; has an unknown elimination profile; and when the drug has a narrow therapeutic window [74]. While pharmacokinetic studies of drugs should consider the CPS or other mechanisms to assess and classify hepatic impairment before making dosage adjustments, the hepatotoxicity tendency of the drugs should also be considered to avoid further toxicity in those with pre-existing hepatic conditions.

Table 22.9 Some of the drugs that should be closely monitored in people with certain hepatic diseases [72, 75–77]

Drugs/drug classes	Rationale
Phenytoin, theophylline, antipsychotics	Hepatic clearance decreased because of high extraction ratio
Warfarin, phenindione	Inhibit clotting factor synthesis
Corticosteroids, NSAIDs	Lead to excess sodium and water retention
Corticosteroids, diuretics	Lead to potassium loss
Hypnotics/sedatives, lithium, loop diuretics, opioids, NSAIDs	May precipitate hepatic encephalopathy
Proton pump inhibitors, H2-receptor antagonists	Increased risk of spontaneous bacterial peritonitis
ACEIs (hypotension), aminoglycosides (nephrotoxicity), cimetidine (confusion), NSAIDs (kidney injury and GI bleeding), oral antidiabetics (hypoglycemia), quinolones (CNS toxicity)	Enhanced risk of adverse drug reactions
Antitubercular agents (isoniazid, rifampin, pyrazinamide, dapsone)	Largely unknown (idiosyncratic reactions)
Anticancer drugs (tretinoin, imatinib, flutamide)	Reduced clinical response or enhanced adverse reactions
Antifungal agents (itraconazole, ketoconazole, terbinafine, voriconazole, griseofulvin)	Largely unknown
Antiretroviral therapies (ritonavir, indinavir, lamivudine, lopinavir–ritonavir, nevirapine, efavirenz)	Mitochondrial toxicity (NRTIs), direct cholestatic injury, and hypersensitivity reaction (NNRTIs)

ACEIs angiotensin-converting enzyme inhibitors, *NSAIDs* nonsteroidal anti-inflammatory drugs, *NRTIs* nucleoside reverse transcriptase inhibitors, *NNRTIs* nonnucleoside reverse transcriptase inhibitors

Some of the drugs and drug classes that need monitoring in the event of hepatic impairment are highlighted in Table 22.9, while a more comprehensive list of drugs and the need for hepatic monitoring can be accessed from an article published by Tice et al. [75].

3.6 Prescribing Considerations in People with Hepatic Impairment

In contrast to kidney disease, there is no single parameter for determining dosage adjustment in people with hepatic impairment, despite the availability of various liver function tests. Abnormal liver function tests may be absent in certain hepatic diseases or may have an extrahepatic origin [78]. The CPS, which considers ascites, encephalopathy, total bilirubin, albumin, and prothrombin time [79], is not only used for assessing the severity of hepatic diseases during drug development, but it can also be employed for dosage adjustment considerations, according to recommendations from the FDA and European Medicines Agency [74, 80]. Although it may not provide full information on the liver's drug-metabolizing ability, the CPS has been used by pharmacists in hospital settings to suggest drug and dosage adjustments in people with hepatic impairment [81].

The MELD and its pediatric version, the Pediatric End-stage Liver Disease (PELD), are alternative tools for assessing hepatic impairment, especially in cases of severe impairment [82]. These scores consider serum bilirubin, serum creatinine, and the INR to determine hepatic impairment severity. While these scores are primarily used clinically to predict the probability of death from liver disease and determine the need for transplantation [83], it has been shown to be a feasible screening tool for determining hepatic impairment in hospital settings and recommending drug dosage adjustments [72].

Hepatic impairment may have tremendous impact on clinical responses to certain drugs. An important consideration is people with hepatic conditions, particularly those with severe hepatic diseases, may have multiple coexisting conditions that require multiple medication use. Therefore, the selection of drugs should consider the potential adverse event(s) associated with individual drugs before starting or continuing medications used for treating other medical conditions. Clinical decision-making should generally involve consideration of indication, pharmacokinetics, presence and safety of alternative medications, comorbidities (particularly kidney disease), potential for drug–drug interactions, and severity of the hepatic disease, among other things.

Anticancer drugs are a good example because there are several of them that are hepatically metabolized and/or have narrow therapeutic window ranges [72]. While prodrugs that need to be transformed into active metabolites like cyclophosphamide may have reduced clinical response in the event of hepatic impairment, drugs like everolimus may lead to overexposure unless doses are adjusted [72]. Similarly, in patients with cirrhosis, agents like antipsychotics, benzodiazepines, diuretics, and NSAIDs are among medications that require careful consideration either because they undergo extensive hepatic metabolism or due to their narrow therapeutic window [72]. Some drugs like lithium, loop diuretics, opioids, and NSAIDs may precipitate hepatic encephalopathy [76], and hence the need for their careful considerations in high-risk individuals. It is also important to consider that hepatic impairment may enhance risk of adverse drug reactions associated with some drugs, including hypotension because of ACEIs, nephrotoxicity due to aminoglycosides, hypoglycemia due to antidiabetics, or central nervous system toxicity due to quinolone antibiotics [76].

The use of antitubercular drugs is another example that presents a clinical challenge when managing CLD due to the inherent hepatotoxicity associated with some first-line treatments for tuberculosis. Although guidelines for antituberculosis agent use in CLD lack clarity, a CPS of ≤ 7 (for CLD or cirrhosis with stable liver function), 8–10 (for advanced hepatic impairment), and ≥ 11 (for very advanced hepatic impairment) are used as cutoff values to determine the use of two, one, or no antitubercular drugs in people with hepatic diseases [84]. Additionally, it is crucial to provide adequate education and information to patients on the correct administration of drugs, particularly for those taking high-risk drugs like methotrexate (i.e., once a week instead of once daily), to prevent potential overdose and hepatotoxicity.

Finally, an important factor to consider when prescribing drugs that undergo hepatic metabolism is the influence of genetic polymorphisms. For example, when using drugs such as isoniazid as part of an antitubercular treatment, individual variations in the *N*-acetyl transferase (NAT2) enzyme, responsible for metabolizing this drug, can lead to variations in drug concentrations and clinical response. Although the literature presents mixed findings, a meta-analysis has provided evidence that individuals with reduced NAT2 expression, known as slow acetylators, are at a higher risk of experiencing isoniazid-induced hepatotoxicity [85]. This highlights the importance of further study to understand the role of precision medicine in determining whether personalized isoniazid dosage can improve safety outcomes.

3.7 Summary and Conclusions

Dosing adjustment for people with hepatic impairment is not straightforward and traditionally relied on expert opinion. However, reducing drug dosage and closely monitoring biochemical and functional markers of hepatic function can help minimize adverse consequences of certain drugs. Prescribing for hepatic impairment should consider the extent of drug elimination via the liver. For drugs that are heavily metabolized and eliminated by the hepatic system, therapy should be individualized based on the remaining hepatic function. Drugs that are minimally metabolized or have a wide therapeutic window may not require dosage adjustment.

While CPS is an important indicator often used in drug development, other factors such as a drug's hepatic extraction ratio and plasma protein binding affinity should also be considered when deciding the right treatment strategy. In the case of hepatic diseases, the liver's intrinsic ability and hepatic blood flow are crucial variables. Moreover, free drug concentration in the plasma should be considered to minimize adverse reactions.

It is also essential to consider comorbidities that are closely related to or affected by hepatic disease. For instance, in patients with complex conditions like hepatorenal syndrome, typical kidney function markers such as creatinine may be overestimated, making it necessary to carefully consider dosage adjustment requirements, particularly for drugs that are excreted by the kidneys in their unchanged form. Prescribing for hepatic impairment should, therefore, be guided by multiple factors, including indications for drug use, drug pharmacokinetics, coexisting conditions such as kidney disease, severity of hepatic impairment, and concurrent drug use.

3.8 Case Studies

3.8.1 Case Study 1: Identifying and Managing Drug-Related Problems in Hepatic Disease

Presenting complaint: A 76-year-old Caucasian male patient presents to the emergency department following a fall incident. He says his hip and shoulder are very sore and that he is unsteady on his feet. He also reports suffering increasing shortness of breath and swelling of his ankles over the past week.

Past medical history: He is long-term patient of the hospital, having had numerous admissions over recent years for problems related to alcoholic liver disease: ascites, withdrawal seizures, and recurrent falls.

Medications on hospital admission:

Phenytoin 400 mg each morning

Propranolol 80 mg twice daily

Furosemide 40 mg daily

Spironolactone 50 mg twice daily

Lactulose 20 mL three times daily

Mylanta® 20 mL when required; an antacid preparation

Patient was noted to be slightly jaundiced and had spider nevi on his face and abdomen. Pitting edema was present in both ankles and his abdomen was grossly distended. His weight is 79 kg, and his height is 165 cm.

Laboratory tests:

Biochemistry

Sodium: 133 mmol/L (135–145 mmol/L)

Potassium: 5.5 mmol/L (3.5–5.0 mmol/L)

Urea: 3.0 mmol/L (3.8–9.6 mmol/L)

Creatinine: 119 μmol/L (60–120 μmol/L)

Liver function tests
Bilirubin (total): 68 μmol/L (3–20 μmol/L)
Alk Phos: 460 U/L (35–120 U/L)
ALT: 163 U/L (8–60 U/L)
GGT: 337 U/L (5–55 U/L)
Other biochemistry
Glucose: 5.1 mmol/L (<5.5 mmol/L)
Albumin: 25 g/L (35–45 g/L)
Total protein: 57 g/L (63–80 g/L)
Toxicology
Phenytoin: 8.5 mg/L (10–20 mg/L)
Coagulation profile
INR: 1.6 (0.8–1.2)
Diagnosis:
Fall: Severely bruised right hip and shoulder,
Decompensated alcoholic liver disease

1. *After reviewing the patient's pathology results, can you explain potential reason for the liver function abnormalities?*

   The liver function abnormalities like ALP, ALT, GGT, and bilirubin indicate that this patient has hepatic disease, likely due to multiple lifestyle and medical factors.
2. *Can you identify the list of drug-related problems, especially considering his hepatic impairment?*

   Even though phenytoin levels look low, it is important to consider that phenytoin is highly protein bound. In the event of hepatic impairment, albumin is reduced; hence, the free phenytoin levels are increased. Therefore, a small change in dosage may result in a disproportionately large change in phenytoin concentration because of saturation of its hepatic metabolism. Consider measuring free phenytoin (not bound to albumin) in patients with low albumin concentration or CKD. If this measurement is not readily available, an estimate can be calculated; contact your local laboratory service for advice.
3. *What special considerations apply when using analgesics and diuretics in people with alcoholic liver disease?*

   Analgesics and diuretics have to be used with caution as they can precipitate hepatic encephalopathy. Diuretics can also precipitate hepatorenal syndrome. Generally, start with low doses of analgesics and consider increasing dosing interval, especially in those with decompensated alcoholic liver failure. For example, the maximum daily recommended paracetamol dose in hepatic disease is 2 g, as opposed to the 4 g for those without hepatic dysfunction.

References

1. Kidney Health Australia 2019. National Strategic Action Plan for Kidney Disease. https://kidney.org.au/get-involved/advocacy/national-strategic-action-plan-for-kidney-disease.
2. Hill NR, Fatoba ST, Oke JL, Hirst JA, O'Callaghan CA, Lasserson DS, et al. Global prevalence of chronic kidney disease—a systematic review and meta-analysis. PLoS One. 2016;11(7):e0158765.
3. Inker LA, Astor BC, Fox CH, Isakova T, Lash JP, Peralta CA, et al. KDOQI US commentary on the 2012 KDIGO clinical practice guideline for the evaluation and management of CKD. Am J Kidney Dis. 2014;63(5):713–35.
4. Khwaja A. KDIGO clinical practice guidelines for acute kidney injury. Nephron Clin Pract. 2012;120:c179–84. https://doi.org/10.1159/000339789.
5. Stevens LA, Levey AS. Measurement of kidney function. Med Clin N Am. 2005;89(3):457–73.
6. Mole DR, Mason PD. Assessment of renal function. Medicine. 2003;31:5–10.
7. National Kidney Foundation. Frequently asked questions about GFR estimates. 2022. https://www.kidney.org/sites/default/files/441-8491_2202_faqs_about-gfr_v5.pdf. Accessed 18th Oct 2022.
8. Chronic Kidney Disease (CKD). Management in primary care. 4th ed. Melbourne: Kidney Health Australia; 2020. https://kidney.org.au/uploads/resources/CKD-Management-in-Primary-Care_handbook_2020.1.pdf
9. Palevsky PM, Liu KD, Brophy PD, Chawla LS, Parikh CR, Thakar CV, et al. KDOQI US commentary on the 2012 KDIGO clinical practice guideline for acute kidney injury. Am J Kidney Dis. 2013;61(5):649–72.
10. Lea-Henry TN, Carland JE, Stocker SL, Sevastos J, Roberts DM. Clinical pharmacokinetics in kidney disease: fundamental principles. Clin J Am Soc Nephrol CJASN. 2018;13(7):1085–95.
11. Gabardi S, Abramson S. Drug dosing in chronic kidney disease. Med Clin N Am. 2005;89(3):649–87.
12. Aweeka FT. Dosing of drugs in renal failure. In: Koda-Kimble MA, Young LY, editors. Applied therapeutics: the clinical use of drugs. 7th ed. Philadelphia: Lippincott Williams & Wilkins; 2001. p. 32.1–32.21.
13. Roberts DM, Sevastos J, Carland JE, Stocker SL, Lea-Henry TN. Clinical pharmacokinetics in kidney dis-

ease: application to rational design of dosing regimens. Clin J Am Soc Nephrol CJASN. 2018;13(8):1254–63.
14. Whittlesea C, Hodson K, editors. Clinical pharmacy and therapeutics. 6th ed. London: Churchill Livingstone; 2018.
15. Nolin TD. A synopsis of clinical pharmacokinetic alterations in advanced CKD. Semin Dial. 2015;28(4):325–9.
16. Matzke GR, Frye RF. Drug administration in patients with renal insufficiency. Minimising renal and extrarenal toxicity. Drug Saf. 1997;16(3):205–31.
17. Aronson JK. Drugs and renal insufficiency. Medicine. 2003;31:103–9.
18. Stefani M, Singer R, Roberts D. How to adjust doses in chronic kidney disease. Australian Prescriber. 2019;42:5.
19. Faull R, Lee L. Prescribing in renal disease. Australian Prescriber. 2007;30:17–20.
20. Reidenberg MM. Kidney function and drug action. N Engl J Med. 1985;313(13):816–8.
21. Khanal A, Castelino RL, Peterson GM, Jose MD. Dose adjustment guidelines for medications in patients with renal impairment: how consistent are drug information sources? Intern Med J. 2014;44(1):77–85.
22. Awdishu L. Drug-induced kidney disease in the ICU: mechanisms, susceptibility, diagnosis and management strategies. Curr Opin Crit Care. 2017;23(6):484–90.
23. Awdishu L, Mehta RL. The 6R's of drug induced nephrotoxicity. BMC Nephrol. 2017;18(1):124.
24. Perazella MA. Pharmacology behind common drug nephrotoxicities. Clin J Am Soc Nephrol CJASN. 2018;13(12):1897–908.
25. Perazella MA, Rosner MH. Drug-induced acute kidney injury. Clin J Am Soc Nephrol. 2022;17(8):1220–33.
26. Moledina DG, Perazella MA. Drug-induced acute interstitial nephritis. Clin J Am Soc Nephrol CJASN. 2017;12(12):2046–9.
27. Manski-Nankervis J, McMorrow R, Nelson C, Jesudason S, Sluggett J. Prescribing and deprescribing in chronic kidney disease. AJGP. 2021;50:4.
28. Bell JS, Blacker N, Leblanc VT, Alderman CP, Phillips A, Rowett D, et al. Prescribing for older people with chronic renal impairment. Austral Fam Physician. 2013;42(1–2):24–8.
29. Johnson CA. Dialysis of drugs. Verona: CKD Insights; 2009.
30. Matzke GR, Comstock TJ. Influence of renal function and dialysis on drug disposition. In: Burton ME, Shaw LM, Schentag JJ, et al., editors. Principles of therapeutic drug monitoring. 4th ed. Philadelphia: Lippincott Williams & Wilkins; 2006.
31. Bohler J, Donauer J, Keller F. Pharmacokinetic principles during continuous renal replacement therapy: drugs and dosage. Kidney Int Suppl. 1999;72:S24–8.
32. Paton TW, Cornish WR, Manuel MA, Hardy BG. Drug therapy in patients undergoing peritoneal dialysis. Clinical pharmacokinetic considerations. Clin Pharmacokinet. 1985;10(5):404–25.
33. Lee CS, Marbury TC. Drug therapy in patients undergoing haemodialysis. Clinical pharmacokinetic considerations. Clin Pharmacokinet. 1984;9(1):42–66.
34. Talevi A, Quiroga A. ADME processes in pharmaceutical sciences. Cham: Springer; 2018.
35. Vaja R, Rana M. Drugs and the liver. Anaesth Intensive Care Med. 2020;21(10):517–23.
36. Almazroo OA, Miah MK, Venkataramanan R. Drug metabolism in the liver. Clin Liver Dis. 2017;21(1):1–20.
37. Gregg CR. Cytochrome P450. In: Johnson LR, editor. Encyclopedia of gastroenterology. Elsevier; 2004. p. 542–3.
38. Gibson GG, Skett P. Pathways of drug metabolism. Introduction to drug metabolism. Boston: Springer; 1996. p. 1–34.
39. Blaschke TF. Effect of liver disease on dose optimization. International Congress Series. Elsevier; 2001.
40. Zhang Y-Y, Meng Z-J. Definition and classification of acute-on-chronic liver diseases. World J Clin Cases. 2022;10(15):4717.
41. Man L, Wang ZQ, Zhang L, Zheng H, Liu DW, Zhou MG. Burden of cirrhosis and other chronic liver diseases caused by specific etiologies in China, 1990–2016: findings from the Global Burden of Disease Study 2016. Biomed Environ Sci. 2020;33(1): 1–10.
42. Moon AM, Singal AG, Tapper EB. Contemporary epidemiology of chronic liver disease and cirrhosis. Clin Gastroenterol Hepatol. 2020;18(12):2650–66.
43. Asrani SK, Devarbhavi H, Eaton J, Kamath PS. Burden of liver diseases in the world. J Hepatol. 2019;70(1):151–71.
44. Tsochatzis EA, Bosch J, Burroughs AK. Liver cirrhosis. Lancet. 2014;383(9930):1749–61.
45. Palatini P, De Martin S. Pharmacokinetic drug interactions in liver disease: an update. World J Gastroenterol. 2016;22(3):1260.
46. Morgan DJ, McLean AJ. Clinical pharmacokinetic and pharmacodynamic considerations in patients with liver disease. Clin Pharmacokinet. 1995;29(5):370–91.
47. Sloss A, Kubler P. Prescribing in liver disease. Aust Prescr. 2009;32(2):32–5.
48. Johnson AL, Hayward KL. Managing medicines in alcohol-associated liver disease: a practical review. Aust Prescr. 2021;44(3):96.
49. Singal AK, Mathurin P. Diagnosis and treatment of alcohol-associated liver disease: a review. Jama. 2021;326(2):165–76.
50. Delco F, Tchambaz L, Schlienger R, Drewe J, Krähenbühl S. Dose adjustment in patients with liver disease. Drug Saf. 2005;28(6):529–45.
51. Talal AH, Venuto CS, Younis I. Assessment of hepatic impairment and implications for pharmacokinetics of substance use treatment. Clin Pharmacol Drug Dev. 2017;6(2):206–12.
52. Gardner KN, Bostwick JR. Medication prescribing in liver dysfunction. Ment Health Clin. 2014;4(3): 131–7.

53. Pugh R, Murray-Lyon I, Dawson J, Pietroni M, Williams R. Transection of the oesophagus for bleeding oesophageal varices. Br J Surg. 1973;60(8):646–9.
54. Malinchoc M, Kamath PS, Gordon FD, Peine CJ, Rank J, Ter Borg PC. A model to predict poor survival in patients undergoing transjugular intrahepatic portosystemic shunts. Hepatology. 2000;31(4):864–71.
55. Peng Y, Qi X, Guo X. Child–Pugh versus MELD score for the assessment of prognosis in liver cirrhosis: a systematic review and meta-analysis of observational studies. Medicine. 2016;95(8):e2877.
56. Giri N, Masters JC, Plotka A, Liang Y, Boutros T, Pardo P, et al. Investigation of the impact of hepatic impairment on the pharmacokinetics of dacomitinib. Investig New Drugs. 2015;33(4):931–41.
57. Keiding S. Drug administration to liver patients: aspects of liver pathophysiology. In: Seminars in liver disease. Thieme Medical Publishers Inc.; 1995.
58. Nguyen H, Cutie A, Pham D. How to manage medications in the setting of liver disease with the application of six questions. Int J Clin Pract. 2010;64(7):858–67.
59. Verbeeck RK. Pharmacokinetics and dosage adjustment in patients with hepatic dysfunction. Eur J Clin Pharmacol. 2008;64(12):1147–61.
60. Frye RF, Zgheib NK, Matzke GR, Chaves-Gnecco D, Rabinovitz M, Shaikh OS, et al. Liver disease selectively modulates cytochrome P450—mediated metabolism. Clin Pharmacol Ther. 2006;80(3):235–45.
61. Westphal J-F, Brogard J-M. Drug administration in chronic liver disease. Drug Saf. 1997;17(1):47–73.
62. Wang YP, Shi B, Chen YX, Xu J, Jiang CF, Xie WF. Drug-induced liver disease: an 8-year study of patients from one gastroenterological department. J Digest Dis. 2009;10(3):195–200.
63. Leise MD, Poterucha JJ, Talwalkar JA. Drug-induced liver injury. Mayo Clin Proc. 2014;89(1):95–106.
64. Giordano C, Rivas J, Zervos X. An update on treatment of drug-induced liver injury. J Clin Transl Hepatol. 2014;2(2):74.
65. Andrade RJ, Aithal GP, Björnsson ES, Kaplowitz N, Kullak-Ublick GA, Larrey D, et al. EASL clinical practice guidelines: drug-induced liver injury. J Hepatol. 2019;70(6):1222–61.
66. Smith IDM, Simpson KJ, Garden OJ, Wigmore SJ. Non-paracetamol drug-induced fulminant hepatic failure among adults in Scotland. Eur J Gastroenterol Hepatol. 2005;17(2):161–7.
67. Hoofnagle JH. LiverTox: a website on drug-induced liver injury. In: Drug-induced liver disease. Elsevier; 2013. p. 725–32.
68. Benson GD, Koff RS, Tolman KG. The therapeutic use of acetaminophen in patients with liver disease. Am J Ther. 2005;12(2):133–41.
69. Lewis J, Stine J. Prescribing medications in patients with cirrhosis—a practical guide. Aliment Pharmacol Ther. 2013;37(12):1132–56.
70. Lee WM, Hynan LS, Rossaro L, Fontana RJ, Stravitz RT, Larson AM, et al. Intravenous *N*-acetylcysteine improves transplant-free survival in early stage non-acetaminophen acute liver failure. Gastroenterology. 2009;137(3):856–64.
71. Czaja AJ. Drug-induced autoimmune-like hepatitis. Digest Dis Sci. 2011;56(4):958–76.
72. Krens SD, Lassche G, Jansman FG, Desar IM, Lankheet NA, Burger DM, et al. Dose recommendations for anticancer drugs in patients with renal or hepatic impairment. Lancet Oncol. 2019;20(4):e200–e7.
73. Pá D. The cytochrome P450 superfamily: biochemistry, evolution and drug metabolism in humans. Curr Drug Metab. 2002;3(6):561–97.
74. Food and Drug Administration. Pharmacokinetics in patients with impaired hepatic function: study design, data analysis and impact on dosing and labeling. 2013.
75. Tice SA, Parry D. Medications that require hepatic monitoring. Hosp Pharm. 2004;39(6):595–608.
76. Pirmohamed M. Prescribing in liver disease. Medicine. 2015;43(10):577–80.
77. Qin F, Jiang J, Qin C, Huang Y, Liang B, Xu Y, et al. Liver damage in patients living with HIV on antiretroviral treatment with normal baseline liver function and without HBV/HCV infection: an 11-year retrospective cohort study in Guangxi, China. BMJ Open. 2019;9(4):e023140.
78. Friedman LS, Chopra S, Travis A. Approach to the patient with abnormal liver biochemical and function tests. Up to Date. 2014:4.
79. Heidelbaugh JJ, Sherbondy M. Cirrhosis and chronic liver failure: part II. Complications and treatment. Am Fam Physician. 2006;74(5):767–76.
80. Use CfMPfH. Note for guidance on the evaluation of the pharmacokinetics of medicinal products in patients with impaired renal function. 2004. CHMP/EWP/225/02. European Medicines Agency, London, United Kingdom; 2013.
81. Periáñez Párraga L, Bosch P, Martínez-López I, Delgado Sánchez O, Martínez Sotelo J, Calleja HM. Evaluation of pharmaceutical intervention in patients with hepatic insufficiency in a hospital setting. Gastroenterol Hepatol Open Access. 2018;9(6):241–7.
82. Mahmud N, Gadsden MM, Goldberg DS. Is the pediatric end-stage liver disease score truly a detriment to pediatric liver allocation? JAMA Pediatr. 2018;172(11):1013–5.
83. Kamath PS, Kim WR. Is the change in MELD score a better indicator of mortality than baseline MELD score? Liver Transplant. 2003;9(1):19–21.
84. Dhiman RK, Saraswat VA, Rajekar H, Reddy C, Chawla YK. A guide to the management of tuberculosis in patients with chronic liver disease. J Clin Exp Hepatol. 2012;2(3):260–70.
85. Cho H-J, Koh W-J, Ryu Y-J, Ki C-S, Nam M-H, Kim J-W, et al. Genetic polymorphisms of NAT2 and CYP2E1 associated with antituberculosis drug-induced hepatotoxicity in Korean patients with pulmonary tuberculosis. Tuberculosis. 2007;87(6):551–6.

23 Clinical Applications of Pharmacogenetics in Improving Drug Safety

Katja S. Just and Julia C. Stingl

Abstract

Pharmacogenetics (PGx) impacts the individual risk for adverse drug reactions (ADRs). In particular, non-dose-related type B ADRs such as hypersensitivity reactions can be connected to pharmacogenetic variants mainly of the human leukocyte antigens (HLA) system. In addition, an increased risk for dose-dependent type A ADRs can be expected with pharmacogenetic variants altering drug metabolism activity of enzymes. Treatment recommendations exist to guide the use of PGx for the prevention of ADRs. However, challenges for the successful implementation of PGx for optimizing drug safety exist, including interethnic differences, the extrapolation of a phenotype from a genotype in multimedicated patients, and the needed infrastructure. Hence, the application of PGx is a promising approach for improvement of drug safety, but there are some limitations that need to be considered.

Keywords

Adverse drug reaction · Pharmacogenetics · Cytochrome P450 · Human leukocyte antigens (HLA) · Drug metabolism · Hypersensitivity reaction

K. S. Just · J. C. Stingl (✉)
Institute of Clinical Pharmacology, University Hospital RWTH Aachen, Aachen, Germany
e-mail: jstingl@ukaachen.de

Learning Objectives

- To understand the potential influence of pharmacogenetics on development of adverse drug reactions
- To know the current resources for improving drug safety by the use of pharmacogenetics
- To have an impression of relevant limitations and hurdles in the application of pharmacogenetics for improving drug safety

Key Points

- Hereditary variability and pharmacogenetics can impact adverse drug reaction occurrence
- Respecting certain pharmacogenetic variants may help to improve drug safety
- Mechanisms for development and management may be different based on the type of adverse drug reactions
- Some challenges and hurdles need to be overcome for successful application of pharmacogenetics in improving drug safety

J. Jose et al. (eds.), *Principles and Practice of Pharmacovigilance and Drug Safety*,
https://doi.org/10.1007/978-3-031-51089-2_23

1 Introduction

Pharmacogenetics (PGx) is the study of the inherited variability affecting individuals' responses to drug treatment [1]. PGx is an important component of personalized medicine, improving the efficacy as well as the safety of drug treatment [2]. Inherited variations in our genome affect structures that are important for drug efficacy and safety, and alter functionality. This involves pharmacokinetic and pharmacodynamic responses, as well as the immune system. Application of PGx in clinical practice could be useful for predicting, preventing, and managing adverse drug reactions (ADRs), thereby ensuring safer use of medications. The present chapter covers the mechanisms behind the role of PGx in development of different types of ADRs and their management, challenges in clinical applications of PGx in medication safety, and the needed infrastructure.

2 Role of Pharmacogenetics in Different Types of Adverse Drug Reactions

Different PGx mechanisms may be assumed for different types of ADRs. While type A, dose-dependent ADRs could be connected to PGx variants affecting drug metabolism, type B, non-dose-dependent ADRs, such as hypersensitivity reactions, can be connected to PGx variants affecting the immune system; refer to Chap. 1. Even if not directly dose related in itself, type B reactions may also depend on PGx variants in drug metabolism affecting immunological pathways. A recent PGx implementation study has shown that the prevalence of serious ADRs can be reduced by 30% when testing PGx variants affecting both type A and type B ADRs [3].

PGx variants are often single-nucleotide polymorphisms (SNPs) but may also occur as insertions, multiplications, or deletions with impact on functionality.

2.1 Type A Adverse Drug Reactions

Approximately 80–90% of all ADRs are estimated to be dose-dependent type A ADRs [4]. Therefore, it is important to consider the factors that may alter individual dose exposure.

In principle, an erroneously administered dose that is too high, i.e., a medication error, can be responsible for a type A ADR. However, not all dose-modifying factors are always known in the medication process. Individual drug metabolism affects the steady state concentration (Css) dependent on dose and clearance. If clearance is unusually low, the dose needs to be decreased correspondingly in order to achieve the same Css (and vice versa).

A distinction can be made between phase I metabolism, oxidation, reduction, and hydrolysis, i.e., functionalization reactions, phase II metabolism, conjugation, i.e., mainly solubility reactions, and drug transport, sometimes referred to as phase III metabolism [1]. Since most of the phase I reactions and also some phase II reactions change the functionality of a drug, i.e., inactivate or activate a substance, they play a significant role in the individual exposure of the active moiety of a drug.

Enzymes of the cytochrome P450 (CYP) system catalyze the majority of all phase I reactions in drug metabolism [1]. Drug-metabolizing phase II enzymes catalyze conjugation reactions that often serve to improve solubility and therefore excretion capacity, but in some cases they also lead to changes in functionality. One example here is the activation of morphine to the even more potent μ receptor agonist metabolite morphine 6-glucuronide by the phase II UDP-glucuronosyltransferase (UGT) enzyme. Due to a higher overlap in substrate specificity of the phase II enzymes compared to the phase I enzymes, pharmacogenetic variants affecting drug-metabolizing phase II enzymes are in general clinically less relevant for individual dose exposure and drugs that commonly cause ADRs have been found to be metabolized predominantly by polymorphic phase I enzymes [5]. However, there are some cases where pharmacogenetic variants in phase II enzymes have been shown to affect drug safety, and in these cases, pharmacogenetic testing is also recommended (e.g., UGT1A1 in irinotecan treatment).

The clearance of a drug can vary up to ten-fold due to PGx variants of drug-metabolizing enzymes [6]. Functional CYP polymorphisms may consist of gene deletions or gene mutations leading to inactive gene products, or gene mutations, gene duplications, and gene multiplications leading to activity or function alteration of the expressed CYP enzyme [7]. Based on the genotype, four different phenotypes of CYP enzymes may be assumed roughly:

- Ultrarapid metabolizers (UM) are carriers of functional alleles leading to high enzyme activity. This may be caused by higher expression caused by variants in the upstream region or also by gene duplications or multiplications.
- Normal metabolizers (NM) are carriers of two functional alleles (wild-type).
- Intermediate metabolizers (IM) are carriers of one functional and one defective allele or two partially defective alleles.
- Poor metabolizers (PM) are characterized by the complete absence of enzyme activity due to two completely defective alleles or gene deletions.

Depending on the drug, the variant phenotypes can lead to an inadequate response to the drug as well as to ADRs due to the changed dose exposure [5]. ADRs may occur in both higher and lower metabolic activities depending on the drug. Drugs—when administered in standard recommended doses—that are inactivated by polymorphic CYP enzymes would cause ADRs in low activity phenotypes (e.g., IM, PM). In contrast, drugs that are activated by polymorphic CYP enzymes (e.g., prodrugs) would cause ADRs in high activity phenotypes (e.g., UM). Prodrugs that are activated by a polymorphic enzyme are problematic in both UMs (too much activation) and PMs (no activation).

2.2 Type B Adverse Drug Reactions

Concerning PGx, Type B ADRs may be related to variants affecting the immune system's response to a drug. This is often connected to variants in human leukocyte antigens (HLA). HLA genes encode cell-surface proteins that are important for the immune system's function in presenting peptides derived from pathogens to T cells.

The main concept how PGx variants can lead to type B ADR is that a HLA variant can affect the immune system's response to a drug and may lead to often severe hypersensitivity reactions. The clinical picture may involve a range of severe hypersensitivity reactions that are not dose-related, from cutaneous reactions such as Stevens–Johnson syndrome (SJS) and toxic epidermal necrolysis (TEN), to single-organ reactions such as drug-induced liver injury (DILI), and systemic responses such as myelosuppression.

3 Treatment Recommendations

In cases of robust evidence that a certain genotype can have impact on a drug's safety, clinical treatment recommendations exist. These recommendations are documented in the drug label or Summary of product characteristics (SmPC) (open access available at https://www.pharmgkb.org) [8]. The underlying mechanisms may be different for type A and type B ADRs, and thus, the treatment recommendations can differ. Certain examples for treatment recommendations for types of ADRs are briefly discussed below.

Recommendations or even obligatory testing information can be found in the SmPC. Hence, some drug labels recommend to use a drug in a certain genotype only, whereas sometimes a certain genotype can lead even to contraindication. The drug label information can differ from country to country (e.g., between a North American and a European country), but are more or less comparable.

In the following, some examples are given and discussed.

3.1 Recommendations to Prevent Type A Adverse Drug Reactions

Concerning potential type A ADRs, many drugs are known in which phase I metabolism can be altered leading to different drug exposures and outcomes. Thus, clinical application of PGx to prevent type A ADRs could be used in different fields of medicine including for example oncology or cardiology.

Clinically relevant polymorphisms impacting drug safety are known for the CYP enzymes CYP2D6, CYP2C9, and CYP2C19 [1]. Hence, these will be focused on here. However, also other drug-metabolizing enzymes can have PGx variability with different drug outcomes. Two of the most important when it comes to risk of critical ADRs are dihydropyrimidine dehydrogenase (DPYD), an enzyme involved in the degradation of fluoropyrimidines (5-FU and precursors), and the phase II enzyme thiopurine S-methyltransferase (TPMT) involved in the metabolism of, e.g., azathioprine and 6-mercaptopurine. These examples are not "important" in the sense that many commonly used drugs are metabolized by them, but they are very important for those patients treated with just these drugs. Pharmacogenetic testing is here mandatory and mentioned in the SmPC [9, 10].

The concept of treatment recommendations is in general, that a certain genotype can be extrapolated to a phenotype (e.g., PM, hence a reduced CYP activity phenotype). If there is evidence that an altered CYP enzyme activity can impact dose exposure and/or outcome, drug dose modifications or the use of an alternative drug can be recommended.

Dose recommendations have already been developed for some drugs that can guide clinical adjustment of pharmacotherapy based on genotypes [8]. As examples, the vitamin K antagonist warfarin metabolized by polymorphic CYP2C9 and the opioid codeine metabolized by polymorphic CYP2D6 can be used [11, 12]. The example of opioid codeine is described below and the one with warfarin is discussed in Sect. 6.1.

3.1.1 Example—Opioids

The analgesic efficacy of codeine results from its active metabolite morphine. The metabolism from codeine to morphine is catalyzed by CYP2D6. Thus, in carriers of higher CYP2D6 activity (e.g., UM), a higher amount of active morphine will be available potentially leading to dose-dependent type A ADRs. In contrast, PM would result in decreased morphine exposure and are therefore at risk for insufficient pain relief. Different treatment guidelines on the use of opioids in PGx variants carriers exist. For example, Royal Dutch Association for the Advancement of Pharmacy-Pharmacogenetics Working Group (DPWG) [13] and the Clinical Pharmacogenetics Implementation Consortium (CPIC) guidelines [14] both recommend to avoid codeine in CYP2D6 UM due to potential serious type A ADRs. Likewise, the use of an alternative analgesic is recommended in PM, due to the potential of insufficient pain relief [11].

Comparable recommendations are given for the opioid tramadol, which does not exert μ receptor agonist properties by itself, but that is likewise metabolized predominantly by CYP2D6 to its active metabolite O-desmethyltramadol, whereas recommendations for other opioids such as hydrocodone or oxycodone are not as clear [11]. Cases of severe ADRs with the use of opioids such as codeine have been reported in children. Thus, the use of codeine in children (below the age of 12) and in women during lactation is contraindicated in drug labels approved by, for example, the United States Food and Drug Administration (US FDA) or the European Medicine Agency (EMA). In addition, according to the same drug labels, the use of codeine in patients being CYP2D6 UM is contraindicated due to an increased risk of severe ADRs. However, it must be emphasized that a PGx test and characterization of CYP2D6 activity are not currently obligatory before the use of codeine.

3.2 Recommendations to Prevent Type B Adverse Drug Reactions

Concerning type B ADRs, many drugs are known that can provoke often severe hypersensitivity reactions in certain PGx variant carriers. In many cases, carriers of a specific PGx variant are at high risk for a hypersensitivity reaction. However, since the variants often are rare, this means that the negative predictive value (NPV) of a PGx variant is close to 100%. An NPV of 100% shows a perfect test accuracy, meaning that the likelihood that someone who is not carrier of a certain variant does not experience the hypersensitivity reaction gets almost 100%. In contrast, the positive predictive value (PPV) may at the same time be around 40% as an example. This means that someone could be carrier of a certain variant, but will not necessarily experience the hypersensitivity reaction. Meanwhile, an NPV of 100% can mean that with a negative test result a drug can be used safely without the risk for a certain hypersensitivity reaction. However, at the same time, the PPV of 40% describes that of 10 people carrying the variant, only 4 are expected to in fact experience the ADR, meaning that the majority of carriers of a PGx variant would not experience the type B ADR. As a consequence, concerning prevention of ADRs, the NPV is of high interest.

Clinically relevant PGx variants with high NPVs are known above all in HLA-B. On the HLA-B gene, cell-surface molecules are coded that are important for hypersensitivity reactions via activation of CD8+ cytotoxic T cells. Nonsynonymous substitutions can lead to an increased activation of the immune system and thereby to type B ADRs [15]. Thus, in PGx testing, the presence of a certain PGx variant known to provoke a type B ADR can be tested. A wide variety of drugs can be affected by PGx variants. We will discuss the antiretroviral drug abacavir under Sect. 6.2 and the antiepileptic drug carbamazepine as an example below [16, 17].

3.2.1 Example—Carbamazepine

Carbamazepine is an antiepileptic drug used in the treatment of epilepsy, trigeminal neuralgia, and bipolar disorders. Carbamazepine can lead to severe cutaneous hypersensitivity reactions such as SJS or TEN, but also drug reaction with eosinophilia and systemic symptoms (DRESS) and maculopapular exanthema (MPE). Testing for the HLA-B*15:02 variant has an NPV of >99% to experience SJS or TEN, while the PPV is around 2%. Several recommendations exist not to use carbamazepine in carriers of the HLA-B*15:02 variant. This mechanism is also true for oxcarbazepine that can lead to SJS or TEN in HLA-B*15:02 carriers.

In addition, a variant of the HLA-A gene, HLA-A*31:01 is associated with hypersensitivity reactions to carbamazepine. These hypersensitivity reactions can present in a wider range from SJS or TEN to DRESS or MPE.

In conclusion, CPIC or DPWG guidelines recommended not to use carbamazepine or oxcarbazepine in carriers of the HLA-B*15:02 variant. In patients being carriers of the HLA-A*31:01 variant (and negative for HLA-B*15:02), alternative agents to carbamazepine are recommended [17].

Interestingly, the drug label information given about carbamazepine's PGx risk for type B ADRs varies largely among drug administration agencies. For example, the US FDA states PGx screening for the HLA-B*15:02 variant and that carbamazepine shall not be used in carriers of this variant. This variant is highly prevalent in Han-Chinese population, exposing those at higher risk to carbamazepine-associated SJS or TEN [17].

In contrast, the EMA recommends to test individuals of Han Chinese and Thai origin whenever possible, for HLA-B*15:02 allele prior to treatment with carbamazepine. Testing for HLA-B*15:02 allele in other Asian populations at genetic risk may be considered.

4 Challenges in Clinical Application

Although the use of PGx for prevention of ADRs is a promising approach, there are several challenges in clinical application that would need to be considered. This may lay in the interplay of PGx and other factors influencing drug safety, the interethnic differences in prevalence of PGx variants, and the challenges in phenotype extrapolation.

Changes in drug metabolism affecting type A ADRs can occur together with pharmacokinetic changes in relation to age, drug–drug interactions (DDI), and other individual factors. As an example, a patient cotreated with a drug that is a strong inhibitor of an enzyme could phenotypically be a PM, although the genotype indicates that the subject is an NM. The extent to which these factors add up and the form in which they interact are still largely unclear.

4.1 Interethnic Differences

The prevalence of genotypes can vary greatly depending on ethnicity. For example, about 1–3% of CYP2D6 UMs would be expected in Northern Europe, about 10% in Spain and in many Latin American countries, and up to 30% in Ethiopia and the Arabian peninsula [7]. Hence, different probabilities of PGx variants affecting drug safety should be expected based on ethnicity. However, this may still be a mechanistic view that needs to be considered carefully in a globalizing world. PGx variants are also passed on following a theory of inheritance. Therefore, ethnically expected probabilities of occurrence may result. Nevertheless, it is not clearly predictable which probability of occurrence is to be expected in the case of interethnic inheritance. Thus, the probability of a child being CYP2D6 UM when parents are from African and European origin cannot be clearly predicted.

This can be important if different *alleles are present based on ancestry. For example, a reduced CYP2C9 activity requiring lower warfarin dosages is expected in carriers of the CYP2C9 *2 and *3 alleles (see Sect. 6.1). This was shown to work for accurate dosing recommendations in Caucasians. However, in people of African ancestry, the CYP2C9 alleles *5, *6, *8, and *11 are needed in addition for accurate dosing [12]. Likewise, as already discussed above, the prevalence of the HLA-B*15:02 variant varies largely depending on ethnic origin.

4.2 Extrapolation of Phenotype from Pharmacogenetic Testing

The unambiguous extrapolation of a phenotype based on a genotype is questionable. This is a relevant point for the prevention of type A ADRs. In some cases, genotype–phenotype discrepancies may occur. This means that patients will present with a phenotype that deviates from the one that would be predicted based on the genotype. This can hamper the successful implementation of PGx to prevent ADRs. These limitations may arise from phenoconversion due to DDIs (see Sect. 6.3) or disease interactions, or based on the genotyping methodology used [18–20].

To what extent the interpretation of PGx additionally changes, for example, with age is unclear and may depend on whether a drug is primarily metabolized by a polymorphic enzyme or whether other nonpolymorphic metabolic pathways exist [21]. The metabolism of some drugs seems to be dependent on age in particular, since decreases in total liver volume, blood flow, etc. associated with age affect drug metabolism—irrespective of genotype. One might suspect an additive effect of age and PGx polymorphisms. However, most PGx studies examine drug exposure in younger adults, and clear data on the relevance of PGx in older adults are lacking [22]. Thus, PGx variants even of the polymorphic CYP enzymes CYP2D6 and CYP2C9 explain only a small proportion of the observable interindividual pharmacokinetic differences [23].

The same may occur for reduced liver function as well. The liver is the main organ for drug metabolism. It seems like the liver's drug-metabolizing capacity is preserved for a long time. However, how the liver's function impacts drug metabolism and the interplay with PGx variants is largely unclear.

Some situations are known in which phenoconversion can occur, making the application of recommendations difficult or even impossible. This can happen in the context of DDI, preexisting conditions associated with inflammatory states or even in pregnancy [18]. In a study analyzing ADRs as a reason for admission to the hospital emergency department (ADRED study), for example, the majority of all patients took at least one CYP2D6 substrate (64.5%), and for more than half of these drugs (54.4%), CYP2D6 was the major pathway of degradation, thus predisposing to drug interactions if more CYP2D6 substrates or even inhibitors were taken. With regard to possible saturation effects of the CYP2D6 enzyme, especially in the central nervous system (CNS) [24], it seems likely that the phenotype predicted on the basis of the genotype is not applicable here or that phenoconversion can occur. This feature of phenoconversion in discussed in Sect. 6.3. However, in which situations an NM predicted on the basis of the genotype changes phenotypically into a PM is unclear and requires detailed analysis in order to be able to apply personalized medicine in particular in multimedicated and/or older people. Recommendations are currently being developed to deal with interacting substrates of the same enzyme and thus the potential for phenoconversion [25].

The above-mentioned limitations could be even more important for drug safety concerning certain body compartments. The majority of drug metabolism takes place in the liver. However, drugs can also be metabolized extrahepatically, for example, in the gastrointestinal tract or in the CNS [6, 26]. While in the liver a range of drug-metabolizing enzymes are highly expressed, there can be alternative routes for drug metabolism in the case of a reduced activity (e.g., CYP2D6 PM), whereas for example in the CNS, less drug-metabolizing enzymes are expressed [6]. For example, the polymorphic metabolized drug codeine (see above) is also metabolized in the brain [27]. This may lead to a higher vulnerability for type A reactions of the CNS in reduced activity PGx variant carriers.

4.3 Needed Infrastructure

The successful implementation of personalized medicine in clinical care is a relevant challenge for a personalized approach to drug safety. Some hurdles have been identified in the past. These include the demonstration of an efficient cost-benefit ratio for PGx testing, which could serve as a basis for reimbursement by health insurers, but also the harmonization of laboratory methods and methods of data analysis, interpretation, and embedding in clinical recommendations for action [28]. Another relevant hurdle is sufficient pre- and postgraduate education in personalized medicine training in the application and interpretation of test results.

PGx diagnostics are to date primarily used for research purposes by individual laboratories, and data storage usually takes place in the laboratory infrastructure, thus available for clinical use only to a limited extent [29]. Here, autonomous data management for the patient with decentralized retrievable data could be a possible alternative to improve access to genotyping data [30].

In addition, it should be kept in mind that PGx testing to date is usually carried out as an exclusion process. Hence, several alleles of interest get defined (e.g., CYP2C9 *2, *3, HLA-B*15:02, see above) and detected in PGx assays. A wild-type allele (e.g., CYP2C9 *1) or a negative result, respectively (e.g., HLA-B*15:02 negative), is diagnosed if no variant allele of interest could be detected. This is a sufficient process concerning the prevention of type B ADRs. Since some alleles have an NPV close to 100%, an exclusion of such variants increases the safety largely. However, in drug metabolism activity, the genotype can explain only a small amount of observed variability [31]. In addition to the above-mentioned uncertainties in aging or reduced liver function and phenocopying by, e.g., DDIs, some variants occur only rarely, but may still have an impact on functionality. Thus, a large number of variants would be needed to be included in PGx testing, making the process even more expensive and more difficult to interpret. For example, more than 100 variants are known for CYP2D6 that only explain 60% of observed variability in activity [32]. Hence, the prevention of type A ADRs by the use of PGx is promising, but still complex to implement. However, a recent multinational prospective trial showed a reduction in ADRs by 30% with using preemptive PGx testing for 50 variants in 12 genes including many drug-metabolizing enzymes [3].

5 Summary and Conclusions

PGx impact the individual risk for ADRs. In particular, non-dose-related type B ADRs such as hypersensitivity reactions can be connected to PGx variants mainly of the HLA system. In addition, an increased risk for dose-dependent type A ADRs can be expected with PGx variants altering drug metabolism activity of enzymes. Treatment recommendations exist to guide the use of PGx for the prevention of ADRs. However, challenges for the successful implementation of PGx for optimizing drug safety exist including interethnic differences in prevalence of pharmacogenetic variants, the extrapolation of a phenotype from a genotype in patients, and the needed infrastructure. Hence, the application of PGx is a promising approach for improvement of drug safety at least for some gene/drug combinations with some aspects that need to be considered.

6 Case Studies

6.1 Case Study 1: Type A ADR with Warfarin in the Context of a PGx Variant

A 72-year-old Japanese woman is diagnosed with a central retinal vein occlusion. Therefore, treatment with warfarin gets started and INR levels measured. On day three, the lab results show an INR of 5.8 (target INR 2.0–3.0). The dose of warfarin is decreased. The INR result 2 days later is 5.6. Despite the fact that the warfarin dose is again decreased, the patient experiences severe epistaxis that can only be stopped with the help of the ENT specialists.

The PGx test results in a CYP2C9 *3/*3 genotype which results in a PM phenotype.

1. *What could be the reason behind the bleeding event and the high INR?*

   The vitamin K antagonist warfarin is metabolized predominantly by polymorphic CYP2C9. Polymorphic means that at least one variant exists that alters functionality and is frequently seen in a population. In cases of reduced CYP2C9 activity (e.g., IM, PM), warfarin is metabolized to a lesser extent, and a patient taking warfarin will be exposed to higher concentrations of warfarin. Thus, bleeding events may occur more often with reduced activity phenotypes.

2. *What could in addition lead to a higher risk of bleeding events in a CYP2C9 PM?*

   Warfarin shows its effect through inhibition of the vitamin K epoxide reductase complex 1 (VKORC1), which again can have relevant PGx variants. PGx variants in VKORC1 can lead to longer clotting time and bleeding events. Thus, a person being CYP2C9 PM is at higher risk for warfarin-associated bleeding events than a CYP2C9 IM, and the risk is even higher, if a VKORC1 variant exists concomitantly. In conclusion, patients being carriers of these variants may need lower warfarin doses for the same efficacy and prevention of dose-dependent ADRs. For example, in certain CYP2C9 alleles, lowering the warfarin dose by 15–30% is recommended [12]. While dose reductions may be useful, there are no CYP2C9 polymorphisms known causing increased enzyme activity that would result in treatment failure [7].

3. *Are PGx variants in CYP2C9 and VKORC1 also important for other vitamin K antagonists?*

   While there is strong evidence for a differing outcome in carriers of certain PGx variants with the use of the vitamin K antagonist warfarin, this seems not to be true for other vitamin K antagonists such as phenprocoumon. For phenprocoumon, differences in drug response may exist based on PGx variants, but clinically do not impact that strongly the occurrence of dose-dependent type A ADRs. This can be explained, though CYP2C9 is likewise involved in the metabolism of phenprocoumon, it is not the predominant enzyme as, for example, CYP3A4 plays a bigger role in the metabolism of phenprocoumon compared to warfarin. Hence, the involvement of polymorphic enzymes, in drug metabolism differs from substance to substance. And what is true for one substance cannot be easily transferred to another substance even in the case of the same drug class. Conclusively, there are dosing guidelines from different working groups available that recommend a lower dosage of warfarin in the case of a reduced activity genotype. For phenprocoumon, there was a previous dosing guideline from the DPWG on PGx associated dosing [33]. In contrast, the CPIC did not publish a dosing guideline for phenprocoumon as phenprocoumon is usually not used in the United States. However, the DPWG dosing guideline was changed in 2018, resulting in no recommendation for phenprocoumon dosing in CYP2C9-altered activity genotypes [34].

Comparably, the FDA included dosing recommendations for the use of warfarin on the base of PGx genotypes. Though this information is provided, there is no requirement to use it. The EMA, while not giving any specific pharmacogenetic testing recommendations for warfarin, informed that the efficacy is affected primarily when the metabolism by CYP2C9 is altered. In addition, neither the FDA nor the EMA annotates PGx in the drug label of phenprocoumon.

6.2 Case Study 2: Type B ADR with Abacavir in the Context of a PGx Variant

A 32-year-old man from Caucasian ancestry is diagnosed to be positive for the human immunodeficiency virus (HIV). He is started on antiretroviral therapy including abacavir. Seven days after starting the drug, he experiences an extended maculopapular exanthema, malaise, and high fever. After experiencing severe episodes of vomiting, he presents to the emergency department.

An abacavir-associated hypersensitivity reaction is diagnosed. Abacavir is withdrawn and the patient receives treatment with antihistamines and corticosteroids. Under this treatment, the symptoms resolve within a few days.

A note in his medical record is made and the patient is instructed that he should not receive abacavir again.

1. *How can this hypersensitivity reaction be diagnosed as related to the use of abacavir? Should a rechallenge be undertaken?*

   Abacavir is a nucleoside reverse transcriptase inhibitor that is used in the treatment of HIV infection. Some people can present with a hypersensitivity reaction including fever, rash, gastrointestinal symptoms, fatigue, cough, and dyspnea. If a hypersensitivity reaction is diagnosed, treatment with abacavir should be stopped immediately. A rechallenge that could be done in the context of an ADR causality assessment should not be done here, as it can lead to anaphylaxis and even be fatal.
2. *If the patient is found to be positive for carrying a relevant PGx gene for abacavir-related hypersensitivity reaction, how would this affect his drug treatment?*

   The PGx variant HLA-B*57:01 has a very high NPV with >99%, whereas risk for hypersensitivity reaction in the overall population is around 3%. Even though the PPV of the HLA-B*57:01 variant is around 50%, working groups such as CPIC or DPWG recommend not to use abacavir in any carriers of the HLA-B*57:01 variant irrespective of being a homozygous or heterozygous carrier. This is recommended as hypersensitivity reaction can be very serious, in some cases, even a life-threatening condition that should be prevented as far as possible [16].

   In concordance, several drug administration agencies such as the FDA and EMA restrict the use of abacavir to patients that have been tested prior to the use of abacavir and are not carriers of the HLA-B*57:01 allele.

6.3 Case Study 3: Complex Drug-Drug and Drug-Gene Interactions in the Context of PGx Variants

A 45-year-old woman of Caucasian ancestry presents to the emergency department with paresthesia in fingers of both hands and legs since 2 weeks. She seems highly agitated and slightly confused. Her heart rate is 110 bpm at rest.

The woman had an episode of a major depression and was started on the antidepressant venlafaxine 2 months ago. The symptoms are interpreted in line with a serotonin syndrome, a dose-dependent type ADR, that can occur with the use of venlafaxine. The woman confirms that in the first weeks of treatment with venlafaxine, she did not have the described symptoms. However, she mentions that she needed high doses of venlafaxine for sufficient treatment of her depression.

Her PGx tests result in CYP2D6 2N*1/*1, CYP2C19 *1/*2, and CYP2C9 *1/*1. This gets interpreted in the following way: For CYP2D6, a gene duplication of a functional allele is found; hence, a UM phenotype is assumed. In the case of CYP2C19, one reduced function allele is found leading to an IM phenotype. For CYP2C9, no nonfunctional variants were found leading to the interpretation of an NM phenotype.

1. *How are these enzymes involved in the metabolism of the drug venlafaxine?*

   The drug venlafaxine gets predominantly metabolized by CYP2D6 to the active metabolite O-desmethyl-venlafaxine, with CYP2C19 being involved in N-demethylation. Thus, despite the CYP2C19 IM phenotype that can result in reduced N-demethylation of venlafaxine, the CYP2D6 UM phenotype leads to increased O-demethylation of venlafaxine. However, due to the antidepressant activity of the O-desmethyl-metabolite, the active moiety may be similar in all CYP2D6 metabolizer groups. The higher dosages as described by the patient at the start of treatment may have increased the total active drug moiety.
2. *Do the PGx variants explain the occurrence of the ADR, a serotonin syndrome?*

   As the occurrence of a serotonin syndrome cannot be explained, the woman is queried more carefully for any changes in new onset diseases, changed medication or changed habits in food and nicotine. The woman tells that due to muscle cramps in her legs, she started approximately 3 weeks ago a treatment with quinidine by herself. As quinidine is a strong CYP2D6 inhibitor, the phenotype might not be UM as predicted by the genotype, but rather IM or PM due to CYP2D6 inhibition. The most likely explanation might be that her comedication with quinidine resulted in a reduced CYP2D6 activity that increased her exposure with active venlafaxine and thus resulted in dose-dependent type A ADR.

References

1. Evans WE, Relling MV. Pharmacogenomics: translating functional genomics into rational therapeutics. Science. 1999;286:487–91. https://doi.org/10.1126/science.286.5439.487.
2. Hamburg MA, Collins FS. The path to personalized medicine. N Engl J Med. 2010;363:301–4.
3. Swen et al. Ubiquitous Pharmacogenomics Consortium. A 12-gene pharmacogenetic panel to prevent adverse drug reactions: an open-label, multicentre, controlled, cluster-randomised crossover implementation study. Lancet. 2023;401(10374):347–56. https://doi.org/10.1016/S0140-6736(22)01841-4. PMID: 36739136.
4. Edwards IR, Aronson JK. Adverse drug reactions: definitions, diagnosis, and management. Lancet. 2000;356:1255–9. https://doi.org/10.1016/S0140-6736(00)02799-9.
5. Phillips KA, Veenstra DL, Oren E, Lee JK, Sadee W. Potential role of pharmacogenomics in reducing adverse drug reactions: a systematic review. JAMA. 2001;286:2270–9. https://doi.org/10.1001/jama.286.18.2270.
6. Stingl JC, Brockmöller J, Viviani R. Genetic variability of drug-metabolizing enzymes: the dual impact on psychiatric therapy and regulation of brain function. Mol Psychiatry. 2013;18(3):273–87. https://doi.org/10.1038/mp.2012.42.
7. Ingelman-Sundberg M, Sim SC, Gomez A, Rodriguez-Antona C. Influence of cytochrome P450 polymorphisms on drug therapies: pharmacogenetic, pharmacoepigenetic and clinical aspects. Pharmacol Ther. 2007;116(3):496–526. https://doi.org/10.1016/j.pharmthera.2007.09.004.
8. Whirl-Carrillo M, McDonagh EM, Hebert JM, Gong L, Sangkuhl K, Thorn CF, et al. Pharmacogenomics knowledge for personalized medicine. Clin Pharmacol Ther. 2012;92(4):414–7. https://doi.org/10.1038/clpt.2012.96.
9. EMA. EMA recommendations on DPD testing prior to treatment with fluorouracil, capecitabine, tegafur and flucytosine; 2020. https://www.ema.europa.eu/en/documents/referral/fluorouracil-fluorouracil-related-substances-article-31-referral-ema-recommendations-dpd-testing_en.pdf. Accessed 21 April 2023.
10. EMA. Jayempi: EPAR—Product Information; 2022. https://www.ema.europa.eu/en/documents/product-

information/jayempi-epar-product-information_en.pdf. Accessed 21 April 2023.
11. Crews KR, Gaedigk A, Dunnenberger HM, Leeder JS, Klein TE, Caudle KE, et al. Clinical pharmacogenetics implementation consortium guidelines for cytochrome P450 2D6 genotype and codeine therapy: 2014 update. Clin Pharmacol Ther. 2014;95(4):376–82. https://doi.org/10.1038/clpt.2013.254.
12. Johnson JA, Caudle KE, Gong L, Whirl-Carrillo M, Stein CM, Scott SA, et al. Clinical pharmacogenetics implementation consortium (CPIC) guideline for pharmacogenetics-guided warfarin dosing: 2017 update. Clin Pharmacol Ther. 2017;102(3):397–404. https://doi.org/10.1002/cpt.668.
13. Royal Dutch Association for the Advancement of Pharmacy- Pharmacogenetics Working Group (DPWG). https://www.pharmgkb.org/page/dpwg
14. Clinical Pharmacogenetics Implementation Consortium (CPIC). https://cpicpgx.org.
15. Rive CM, Bourke J, Phillips EJ. Testing for drug hypersensitivity syndromes. Clin Biochem Rev. 2013;34(1):15–38.
16. Martin MA, Klein TE, Dong BJ, Pirmohamed M, Haas DW, Kroetz DL. Clinical pharmacogenetics implementation consortium. Clinical pharmacogenetics implementation consortium guidelines for HLA-B genotype and abacavir dosing. Clin Pharmacol Ther. 2012;91(4):734–8. https://doi.org/10.1038/clpt.2011.355.
17. Phillips EJ, Sukasem C, Whirl-Carrillo M, Müller DJ, Dunnenberger HM, Chantratita W, Goldspiel B, Chen YT, Carleton BC, George AL Jr, Mushiroda T, Klein T, Gammal RS, Pirmohamed M. Clinical pharmacogenetics implementation consortium guideline for HLA genotype and use of carbamazepine and oxcarbazepine: 2017 update. Clin Pharmacol Ther. 2018;103(4):574–81. https://doi.org/10.1002/cpt.1004.
18. Klomp SD, Manson ML, Guchelaar HJ, Swen JJ. Phenoconversion of cytochrome P450 metabolism: a systematic review. J Clin Med. 2020;9(9) https://doi.org/10.3390/jcm9092890.
19. Nebert DW, Zhang G, Vesell ES. From human genetics and genomics to pharmacogenetics and pharmacogenomics: past lessons, future directions. Drug Metab Rev. 2008;40(2):187–224. https://doi.org/10.1080/03602530801952864.
20. Shah RR, Smith RL. Addressing phenoconversion: the Achilles' heel of personalized medicine. Br J Clin Pharmacol. 2015;79(2):222–40. https://doi.org/10.1111/bcp.12441.
21. Just KS, Schneider KL, Schurig M, Stingl JC, Brockmöller J. Falls: the adverse drug reaction of the elderly and the impact of pharmacogenetics. Pharmacogenomics. 2017;18(13):1281–97. https://doi.org/10.2217/pgs-2017-0018.
22. Dücker CM, Brockmöller J. Genomic variation and pharmacokinetics in old age: a quantitative review of age- vs. genotype-related differences. Clin Pharmacol Ther. 2019;105(3):625–40. https://doi.org/10.1002/cpt.1057.
23. Matthaei J, Brockmöller J, Tzvetkov MV, Sehrt D, Sachse-Seeboth C, Hjelmborg JB, et al. Heritability of metoprolol and torsemide pharmacokinetics. Clin Pharmacol Ther. 2015;98(6):611–21. https://doi.org/10.1002/cpt.258.
24. Just KS, Dormann H, Freitag M, Schurig M, Böhme M, Steffens M, et al. CYP2D6 in the brain: potential impact on adverse drug reactions in the central nervous system-results from the ADRED study. Front Pharmacol. 2021;12:624104. https://doi.org/10.3389/fphar.2021.624104.
25. Cicali EJ, Elchynski AL, Cook KJ, Houder JT, Thomas CD, Smith DM, Elsey A, Johnson JA, Cavallari LH, Wiisanen K. How to integrate CYP2D6 phenoconversion into clinical pharmacogenetics: a tutorial. Clin Pharmacol Ther. 2021;110(3):677–87. https://doi.org/10.1002/cpt.2354.
26. Zhang Y, Benet LZ. The gut as a barrier to drug absorption: combined role of cytochrome P450 3A and P-glycoprotein. Clin Pharmacokinet. 2001;40(3):159–68. https://doi.org/10.2165/00003088-200140030-00002.
27. Milne et al. Drug Metab Rev. 1996;28(3):345–472. https://doi.org/10.3109/03602539608994011.
28. Shuldiner et al. Clin Pharmacol Ther. 2013;94(2):207–10. https://doi.org/10.1038/clpt.2013.59.
29. Just KS, Turner RM, Dolžan V, Cecchin E, Swen JJ, Gurwitz D, Stingl JC. Educating the next generation of pharmacogenomics experts: global educational needs and concepts. Clin Pharmacol Ther. 2019;106(2):313–6. https://doi.org/10.1002/cpt.1471.
30. Blagec K, Koopmann R, Crommentuijn-van Rhenen M, Holsappel I, van der Wouden CH, Konta L, et al. Implementing pharmacogenomics decision support across seven European countries: The Ubiquitous Pharmacogenomics (U-PGx) project. J Am Med Inform Assoc. 2018;25(7):893–8. https://doi.org/10.1093/jamia/ocy005.
31. Lauschke VM, Ingelman-Sundberg M. Precision medicine and rare genetic variants. Trends Pharmacol Sci. 2016;37(2):85–6. https://doi.org/10.1016/j.tips.2015.10.006.
32. Ingelman-Sundberg M, et al. Integrating rare genetic variants into pharmacogenetic drug response predictions. Hum Genomics. 2018;12(1):26. https://doi.org/10.1186/s40246-018-0157-3.
33. Swen et al. Clin Pharmacol Ther. 2011;89(5):662–73. https://doi.org/10.1038/clpt.2011.34.
34. PharmGKB Annotation of DPWG Guideline for phenprocoumon and CYP2C9 (n.d.). https://www.pharmgkb.org/chemical/PA450921/guidelineAnnotation/PA166105004. Accessed 21 Feb 2023.

Further Reading

PharmGKB(R): www.pharmgkb.org
Institute of Clinical Pharmacology, University Hospital RWTH Aachen, Germany: https://seeme-app.azurewebsites.net/users/sign_in?locale=en

Index

J. Jose et al. (eds.), *Principles and Practice of Pharmacovigilance and Drug Safety*,
https://doi.org/10.1007/978-3-031-51089-2

Q

MIX
Papier aus verantwortungsvollen Quellen
Paper from responsible sources
FSC® C105338

If you have any concerns about our products,
you can contact us on
ProductSafety@springernature.com

In case Publisher is established outside the EU,
the EU authorized representative is:
Springer Nature Customer Service Center GmbH
Europaplatz 3, 69115 Heidelberg, Germany

Printed by Libri Plureos GmbH
in Hamburg, Germany